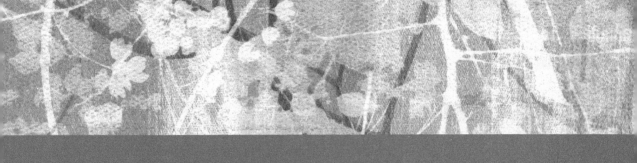

GERONTOLOGY

for the Health Care Professional

FOURTH EDITION

D1611482

Edited by

Regula H. Robnett, PhD, OTR/L, FAOTA
Professor, Department of Occupational Therapy
University of New England

Nancy Brossoie, PhD
Senior Research Scientist, Center for Gerontology
Virginia Tech

Walter C. Chop, MS, RRT
Professor Emeritus, Respiratory Therapy Department
Southern Maine Community College

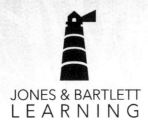

JONES & BARTLETT
LEARNING

World Headquarters
Jones & Bartlett Learning
5 Wall Street
Burlington, MA 01803
978-443-5000
info@jblearning.com
www.jblearning.com

Jones & Bartlett Learning books and products are available through most bookstores and online booksellers. To contact Jones & Bartlett Learning directly, call 800-832-0034, fax 978-443-8000, or visit our website, www.jblearning.com.

Substantial discounts on bulk quantities of Jones & Bartlett Learning publications are available to corporations, professional associations, and other qualified organizations. For details and specific discount information, contact the special sales department at Jones & Bartlett Learning via the above contact information or send an email to specialsales@jblearning.com.

15940-0

Production Credits

VP, Product Management: David D. Cella
Director of Product Management: Cathy L. Esperti
Product Assistant: Rachael Souza
Director of Production: Jenny L. Corriveau
VMO Manager: Sara Kelly
Vendor Manager: Juna Abrams
Director of Production: Julie Bolduc
Senior Production Editor, Navigate: Leah Corrigan
Director of Marketing: Andrea DeFronzo
Marketing Manager: Michael Sullivan
VP, Manufacturing and Inventory Control: Therese Connell

Composition: Exela Technologies
Project Management: Exela Technologies
Cover Design: Kristin E. Parker
Text Design: Kristin E. Parker
Director of Rights & Media: Joanna Gallant
Rights & Media Specialist: Robert Boder
Media Development Editor: Troy Liston
Cover Image (Title Page, Chapter Opener):
    © patpitchaya/Shutterstock
Printing and Binding: LSC Communications
Cover Printing: LSC Communications

Library of Congress Cataloging-in-Publication Data

Names: Robnett, Regula H., editor. | Chop, Walter C., editor. | Brossoie, Nancy, editor.
Title: Gerontology for the health care professional / [edited by] Regula H. Robnett, Walter Chop, and Nancy Brossoie.
Description: Fourth edition. | Burlington, MA : Jones & Bartlett Learning, [2020] | Includes bibliographical references and index.
Identifiers: LCCN 2018013913 | ISBN 9781284140569 (pbk. : alk. paper)
Subjects: | MESH: Geriatrics | Aged | Aging–physiology | Geriatric Assessment
Classification: LCC RA564.8 | NLM WT 100 | DDC 618.97–dc23 LC record available at https://lccn.loc.gov/2018013913

6048

Printed in the United States of America
23 22 21   10 9 8 7 6 5 4

Dedication

This edition is dedicated to:

The older adults who have shown us how to live productive, healthy, and happy lives and for reminding us that age is more than just a number.

Our authors for their tireless writing efforts and commitment in educating healthcare workers, from students to seasoned professionals.

Our families who sacrificed their needs and wants when our work on this edition had to come first.

We thank all of you.

—Regi, Nancy, and Walter

Brief Contents

Contents

Chapter 3   Aging in Place and the Continuum of Care 57

Ann O'Sullivan, OTR/L, LSW, FAOTA
Nancy Brossoie, PhD
Regula H. Robnett, PhD, OTR/L, FAOTA

Chapter 4   Loss, Grief, Death, and Dying 85

Regula H. Robnett, PhD, OTR/L, FAOTA
Nancy Brossoie, PhD

Chapter 5 Health Literacy and Clear Communication: Keys to Engaging Older Adults and Their Families. 109

Audrey Riffenburgh, PhD
Sue Stableford, MPH, MSB

Chapter 6 Policy Issues for Older Adults 129

Laney Bruner Canhoto, PhD, MSW, MPH

Chapter 7 The Physiology and Pathology of Aging 153

Kimberly Wilson, DNP, RN

Chapter 8 Cognitive and Psychological Changes Related to Aging . . . 189

Regula H. Robnett, PhD, OTR/L, FAOTA

Chapter 12 Perspectives on Oral Care in Healthy Aging and Prevention for the Older Adult 297

Marji Harmer-Beem, RDH, MS

Chapter 13 Sexuality and Aging 313

Nancy MacRae, MS, OTR/L, FAOTA

Chapter 14 Reframing Aging Issues to Ensure a Better Future . . . 345

Raven H. Weaver, PhD

Introduction

Thank you for choosing to open this textbook and read this page. *Gerontology for the Health Care Professional, Fourth Edition* is designed with you in mind. Our goal is to provide a textbook that is reader-friendly and includes information that easily translates to healthcare practices.

As you read each chapter, we encourage you to consider the interprofessional roles of each of the healthcare professions listed below. While this is not an exclusive list and, most of the time, only a small portion of all the possible professions will actually be involved in working with any given client, we encourage you to think about how each profession *could* be involved and when a consultation or referral would be in order. You may need to investigate some of the following professions to familiarize yourself with their roles and further research is certainly encouraged.

The most prominent healthcare professionals involved in gerontological care are:

- Alternative Medicine Practitioners
- Art Therapists
- Athletic Trainers
- Audiologists
- Cardiovascular Technologists
- Case Managers
- Counselors
- Dental Practitioners
- Dieticians/Nutritionists
- Emergency Medical Practitioners
- Gerontologists
- Horticulture Therapists
- Imaging Technologists
- Massage Therapists
- Medical Laboratory Practitioners
- Medical Records Health Information Specialists
- Music Therapists
- Neuropsychologists
- Nursing Practitioners
- Occupational Therapy Practitioners
- Orientation and Mobility Specialists (low vision)
- Orthotists
- Physical Therapy Practitioners
- Physician Assistants
- Physicians
- Polysomnographers
- Prosthetists
- Psychiatrists
- Psychologists
- Radiological Technologists
- Recreation Therapists
- Rehabilitation Teachers (low vision)
- Respiratory Therapists
- Social Workers
- Speech and Language Pathologists
- Visual Care Specialists

We are fortunate to be living in an information-rich age in which Internet resources are readily available as never before. Certainly not everything available online can be relied upon, and therefore we need to read what is out there in cyberspace with critical and questioning eyes. However, for individuals who want to learn, the floodgates have opened and the world of information is there for the learning.

▶ How This Text Is Organized

The *Fourth Edition* begins with chapters on the social, psychological, and biological aspects of aging, including:

- Demographics (Chapter 1)
- Social Relationships and Roles (Chapter 2)
- Community Living (Chapter 3)
- End of Life (Chapter 4)
- Communication (Chapter 5)
- Policy (Chapter 6)
- Physiology (Chapter 7)
- Cognition and Psychology (Chapter 8)

Later chapters explore issues that, although not exclusive to older people, are of primary importance to the older population. These issues include:

- Functional Performance (Chapter 9)
- Drugs (Chapter 10)
- Nutrition (Chapter 11)
- Oral Health (Chapter 12)
- Sexuality (Chapter 13)
- Future of Aging (Chapter 14)

▶ What Is New to the Fourth Edition

- NEW! Now in FULL color with a new and expanded art program!
- REVISED! Chapter 1 on demographics of aging offers more information about aging worldwide and the factors that contribute to a growing worldwide population.
- REVISED! Chapter 2 on social gerontology includes an expanded section on elder abuse.
- REVISED! Chapter 3 on community living has been expanded to include more information on aging in place and the continuum of care.
- NEW! New Chapter 4 on Loss, Grief, Death, and Dying.
- REVISED! Chapter 13 on sex and gender issues has been revised to reflect the lives of the LGBTQ community and other hidden populations.
- REVISED! Chapter 14 on the future of aging examines aging issues using community, family, and individual perspectives.
- NEW AND REVISED! Case Studies have been revised and additional ones added so there are two per chapter.
- UPDATED DATA! All information is updated to reflect current census data and statistics.

How to Use This Text

Gerontology for the Health Care Professional, Fourth Edition incorporates a number of engaging pedagogical features to aid in the student's understanding and retention of the material.

BEHAVIORAL OBJECTIVES

Upon completion of this chapter, the reader will be able to:

1. Differentiate between average life expectancy and maximum life span.
2. Compare and contrast the genetic and environmental theories of aging.
3. Explain the possible role of free radical formation in the aging process.
4. Identify common age-related changes related to the cardiovascular, respiratory, gastrointestinal, genitourinary, musculoskeletal, nervous, sensory, endocrine, immune, and integumentary systems.
5. Discuss health promotion for the aging process in relation to prevalent chronic diseases.

KEY TERMS

Atherosclerosis	Fecal incontinence	Osteoporosis
Average life expectancy	Free radical	Peptic ulcers
Cataract	Gastritis	Presbycusis
Chronic bronchitis	Hyposmia	Presbyopia
Chronic obstructive pulmonary	Hypothalamus	Sarcopenia
disease	Kyphosis	Senescence
Diabetes mellitus	Maximum life span	Urinary incontinence
Diaphragm	Metastasize	Xerostomia
Diverticulosis	Myocardial infarction	
Dysphagia	Osteoarthritis	

▶ Introduction

For hundreds of years, people have sought ways to live longer and slow down the aging process. Remedies have been promoted through abundant advertising and have included therapies such as special diets, vitamin supplements, cosmetic measures, and various other aids to help reduce the impact of aging. Even though researchers may study specific aspects of aging associated with their particular fields, a commonly held opinion is that the aging process is not linear, but multifaceted and influenced by individual biopsychosocial factors as well as external factors such as context, environment, and technology.

The **average life expectancy** (**TABLE 7-1**) in the United States has risen from about 47.3 years in 1900 to 78.8 years in 2015 (National Center for Health Statistics, 2017). This increase can largely be attributed to improvement in water supplies, sanitation, health technology, disease control, health promotion, and lower infant mortality rates (Forsberg & Fichtenberg, 2013). However, during the same period, there has been no change in the **maximum life span** (MLS), that is, the oldest age reached by an individual in a population, which is estimated to be about 120 years (Hayflick, 1997; Schneider, 1985). Although improvements in our standard of living have helped spare us from several causes of premature death, such as cholera, tuberculosis, and influenza, changes have done nothing to slow down the inherent aging process. In fact, any medical intervention that claims to slow down human aging must be shown to increase the MLS potential. But, to date, none have done so.

Behavioral Objectives at the beginning of each chapter help you focus on the most important concepts and can be used as a study tool to assess comprehension.

Each chapter lists the Key Terms that are highlighted throughout the text.

TABLE 7-1 Life Expectancy at Selected Ages, by Sex: United States 1900, 1950, 2014, and 2015

| | Life Expectancy at Exact Age (Years) | | | | | |
| | At Birth | | | At Age 65 | | |
Year	Both Sexes	Male	Female	Both Sexes	Male	Female
1900[1,2]	47.3	46.3	48.3			
1950[3]	68.2	65.6	71.1	13.9	12.8	15.0
2014[4]	78.9	76.5	81.3	19.4	18.0	20.6
2015[4]	78.8	76.3	81.2	19.4	18.0	20.6

[1] Death registration area only. The death registration area increased from 10 states and the District of Columbia (DC) in 1900 to the conterminous United States in 1933. See Appendix II, Registration area.
[2] Includes deaths of persons who were not residents of the 10 states and DC.
[3] Life expectancy estimates for 1950 are based on final Medicare data. Life expectancy estimates for 2014 and 2015 are based on preliminary Medicare data.
Data from National Center for Health Statistics. (2017). Health, United States, 2016: With chartbook on long-term trends in health. Hyattsville, MD: Centers for Disease Control and Prevention.

An unchanging MLS coupled with increasing life expectancy suggests two dimensions to the aging process. First, it supports the notion of distinguishing disease from aging. To illustrate, one of the most important chapters in the history of medicine has been the eradication of smallpox from the face of the earth through the use of vaccines. Although children who are immunized against smallpox have been spared a devastating infectious disease, they are not likely to age more slowly than nonimmunized children. Second, a MLS that has not likely changed in centuries points to the existence of a "biological clock" that predetermines humans' length of life. No such clock has been discovered, and it is perhaps an oversimplification of human physiology to suggest that one single mechanism in the body is responsible for aging. Nonetheless, it certainly appears that there are relatively fixed limits on how long the human body lasts.

A fixed life span, however, does not necessarily sentence adults to pain and suffering as they get older. Many of the physiologic changes associated with aging can be slowed to some extent with a healthy diet and consistent regimen of moderate exercise. Moreover, many of the chronic diseases prevalent in older adults are either preventable or modifiable with healthy lifestyle habits (**TABLE 7-2**). Reduction of dietary fat (especially saturated fats and cholesterol) lowers one's risk of coronary artery disease and stroke (i.e., occlusion or rupture of a cerebral artery) as well as breast and colon cancer (Spence, 2007; Tufts University, 2012). A program of increased physical activity increases one's resting and maximum cardiac output (the amount of blood pumped out of the heart per minute) while decreasing the chance of developing hypertension (American Heart Association, 2014). To the extent that exercise helps prevent obesity, it also

---

Oral Administration

Most drug absorption after oral administration occurs in the small intestine. Thus, the rate of gastric emptying needs to be considered. In the older patient, gut motility in general and gastric emptying in particular takes a longer amount of time (Cusack, 2004). However, research studies have resulted in mixed results as to the clinical relevance of these findings.

Generally, the slowed gastric emptying is reflected clinically in a time delay in attaining maximal drug concentrations in the blood without a change in maximal drug concentration. Studies on the absorption of drugs from the small intestine showed some changes in this parameter, but the changes uncovered were inconsistent and did not lend themselves to broad generalization. Thus, oral administration of drugs, in general, does not significantly affect the clinical response to drugs (Cusack, 2004; McLean & Le Couteur, 2004).

Transdermal Administration

Transdermal administration or medication administered through the skin, often through the use of a patch, is a convenient way to administer a steady amount of drug over a prolonged period (FIGURE 10-2). Examples of drugs administered though transdermal

FIGURE 10-2 Transdermal patches administer drugs (e.g., fentanyl and nicotine) over a prolonged period through the skin.
© Image Point Fr/Shutterstock

administration include estrogen (female hormone), fentanyl (an opioid painkiller), and scopolamine (treats motion sickness). Yet, as people age, they experience changes in how drugs are absorbed through the skin. The outer layer or epidermis thins with age and becomes dryer, allowing for a decreased absorption of drug through the skin. Thus, use of transdermal medications in older adults may lead to lower concentrations in the blood.

Drug Distribution

The next phase of pharmacokinetics is distribution. Drugs distribute throughout the body based on their **physicochemical properties**, that is, the relationship between the chemical structure of the drug and its interactions with the body. The most important of these properties is the **hydrophilicity** or **lipophilicity** of the drug—is it more attracted to water or to fat, respectively? As people age, lean body mass decreases, which leads to an increase in fat content in the body. With fat content increased, a fat-soluble drug will show a larger volume of distribution, which will lower its concentration and lower its therapeutic efficacy. The effect of aging on distribution is very much dependent upon the specific drug, so there is no consensus on the general effect of all fat-soluble drugs.

Drug Metabolism

Drug metabolism is an area where the complexities of pharmacokinetics in older people are most apparent. The liver is the major organ of drug metabolism, although the intestines, lungs, and kidneys also have important drug metabolizing enzymes. Fortunately, in the absence of disease, drug metabolizing enzymes are not significantly affected by aging (McLean & Le Couteur, 2004). Other changes, however, are more significant. One factor that relates directly to drug metabolism is blood flow through the

---

Tables and Figures throughout help with comprehension of key concepts and summarize important information for students.

Guidelines That Encourage Healthy Eating Patterns

1. **Follow a healthy eating pattern across the lifespan.** All food and beverage choices matter. Choose a healthy eating pattern at an appropriate calorie level to help achieve and maintain a healthy body weight, support nutrient adequacy, and reduce the risk of chronic disease.

   Follow a healthy eating pattern over time to help support a healthy body weight and reduce the risk of chronic disease.
   - A healthy eating pattern includes: fruits, vegetables, protein, dairy, grains, and oils.
   - A healthy eating pattern limits: saturated fats and trans fats, added sugars, and sodium.

2. **Focus on variety, nutrient density, and amount.** To meet nutrient needs within calorie limits, choose a variety of nutrient-dense foods across and within all food groups in recommended amounts.

   Choose a variety of nutrient-dense foods from each food group in recommended amounts. Examples include
   - Fruits: apples, grapes
   - Vegetables: lettuce, celery
   - Protein: chicken breast, unsalted walnuts
   - Dairy: fat-free milk
   - Grains: whole-grain bread
   - Oils: mayonnaise

3. **Limit calories from added sugars and saturated fats and reduce sodium intake.** Consume an eating pattern low in added sugars, saturated fats, and sodium. Cut back on foods and beverages higher in these components to amounts that fit within healthy eating patterns.

   Consume an eating pattern low in added sugars, saturated fats, and sodium. Examples include
   - Saturated fats: ice cream, burger
   - Added sugars: aerated drinks, muffin
   - Sodium: pizza, sandwich

4. **Shift to healthier food and beverage choices.** Choose nutrient-dense foods and beverages across and within all food groups in place of less healthy choices. Consider cultural and personal preferences to make these shifts easier to accomplish and maintain.

   Replace typical food and beverages choices with more nutrient-dense options. Be sure to consider personal preferences to maintain shifts over time. For example, replacing macaroni and cheese with vegetable salads.

5. **Support healthy eating patterns for all.** Everyone has a role in helping to create and support healthy eating patterns in multiple settings nationwide, from home to school to work to communities.

   Everyone has a role in helping to create and support healthy eating patterns in places where we learn, work, live, and play.

FIGURE 11-3 Dietary Guidelines for Americans 2015–2020.
Reproduced from U.S. Department of Health and Human Services, Office of Disease Prevention and Health Promotion. 2015-2020 Dietary Guidelines. www.health.gov/dietaryguidelines/2015/

Review material is included at the end of each chapter for classroom use, homework, or self-assessment: Case Studies, Learning Activities, and Review Questions.

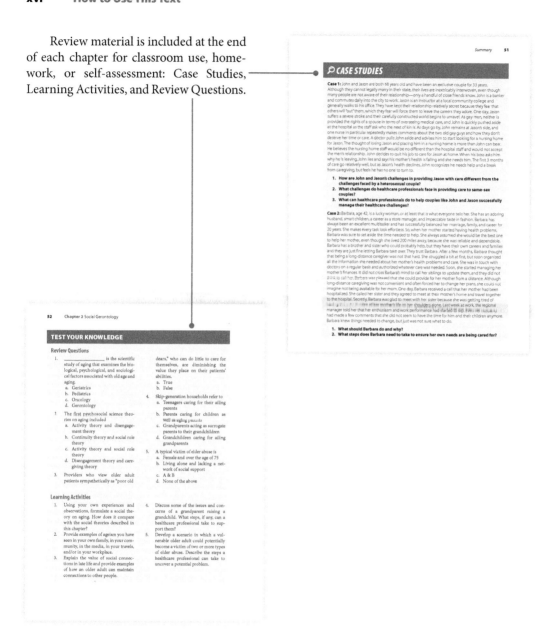

CASE STUDIES

Case 1: John and Jason are both 66 years old and have been an exclusive couple for 33 years. Although they cannot legally marry in their state, their lives are inextricably interwoven, even though many people are not aware of their relationship—only a handful of close friends know. John is a banker and commutes daily into the city to work. Jason is an instructor at a local community college and generally walks to his office. They have kept their relationship relatively secret because they fear that others will "out" them, which they fear will force them to leave the careers they adore. One day, Jason suffers a severe stroke and their carefully constructed world begins to unravel. As gay men, neither is provided the rights of a spouse in terms of overseeing medical care, and John is quickly pushed aside at the hospital as the staff ask who the next of kin is. As days go by, John remains at Jason's side, and one nurse in particular repeatedly makes comments about the two old gay guys and how they don't deserve her time or care. A doctor pulls John aside and advises him to start looking for a nursing home for Jason. The thought of losing Jason and placing him in a nursing home is more than John can bear. He believes the nursing home staff would be no different than the hospital staff and would not accept the men's relationship. John decides to quit his job to care for Jason at home. When his boss asks him why he is leaving, John lies and says his mother's health is failing and she needs him. The first 3 months of care go relatively well, but as Jason's health declines, John recognizes he needs help and a break from caregiving, but feels he has no one to turn to.

1. How are John and Jason's challenges in providing Jason with care different from the challenges faced by a heterosexual couple?
2. What challenges do healthcare professionals face in providing care to same-sex couples?
3. What can healthcare professionals do to help couples like John and Jason successfully manage their healthcare challenges?

Case 2: Barbara, age 42, is a lucky woman, or at least that is what everyone tells her. She has an adoring husband, smart children, a career as a store manager, and impeccable taste in fashion. Barbara has always been an excellent multitasker and has successfully balanced her marriage, family, and career for 20 years. She makes every task look effortless. So, when her mother started having health problems, Barbara was sure to set aside the time needed to help. She always assumed she would be the best one to help her mother, even though she lived 200 miles away, because she was reliable and dependable. Barbara has a brother and sister who could probably help, but they have their own careers and families and they are just fine letting Barbara take over. They trust Barbara. After a few months, Barbara thought that being a long-distance caregiver was not that hard. She struggled a bit at first, but soon organized all the information she needed about her mother's health problems and care. She was in touch with doctors on a regular basis and authorized whatever care was needed. Soon, she started managing her mother's finances. It did not cross Barbara's mind to call her siblings to update them, and they did not think to call her. Barbara was pleased that she could provide for her mother from a distance. Although long-distance caregiving was not convenient and often forced her to change her plans, she could not imagine not being available for her mom. One day, Barbara received a call that her mother had been hospitalized. She called her sister and they agreed to meet at their mother's home and travel together to the hospital. Secretly, Barbara was glad to meet with her sister because she was getting tired of [illegible] ... letting her mother's life on her shoulders alone. Last week at work, the regional manager told her that her enthusiasm and work performance had started to dip. Even her husband had made a few comments that she did not seem to have the time for him and their children anymore. Barbara knew things needed to change, but just was not sure what to do.

1. What should Barbara do and why?
2. What steps does Barbara need to take to ensure her own needs are being cared for?

TEST YOUR KNOWLEDGE

Review Questions

1. _____ is the scientific study of aging that examines the biological, psychological, and sociological factors associated with old age and aging.
   a. Geriatrics
   b. Pediatrics
   c. Oncology
   d. Gerontology

2. The first psychosocial science theories on aging included
   a. Activity theory and disengagement theory
   b. Continuity theory and social role theory
   c. Activity theory and social role theory
   d. Disengagement theory and caregiving theory

3. Providers who view older adult patients sympathetically as "poor old dears," who can do little to care for themselves, are diminishing the value they place on their patients' abilities.
   a. True
   b. False

4. Skip-generation households refer to
   a. Teenagers caring for their ailing parents
   b. Parents caring for children as well as aging parents
   c. Grandparents acting as surrogate parents to their grandchildren
   d. Grandchildren caring for ailing grandparents

5. A typical victim of elder abuse is
   a. Female and over the age of 75
   b. Living alone and lacking a network of social support
   c. A & B
   d. None of the above

Learning Activities

1. Using your own experiences and observations, formulate a social theory on aging. How does it compare with the social theories described in this chapter?
2. Provide examples of ageism you have seen in your own family, in your community, in the media, in your travels, and/or in your workplace.
3. Explain the value of social connections in late life and provide examples of how an older adult can maintain connections to other people.
4. Discuss some of the issues and concerns of a grandparent raising a grandchild. What steps, if any, can a healthcare professional take to support them?
5. Develop a scenario in which a vulnerable older adult could potentially become a victim of two or more types of elder abuse. Describe the steps a healthcare professional can take to uncover a potential problem.

▶ Instructor Resources

Qualified instructors will receive a full suite of instructor resources, including:

- More than 250 slides in PowerPoint format
- A test bank with chapter-by-chapter questions along with midterm and final tests
- Case studies along with potential answers
- An Instructor's Manual containing a summary, key terms and definitions, teaching tips, and a list of material and online resources

About the Authors

Regula H. Robnett, PhD, OTR/L, FAOTA
Professor
Department of Occupational Therapy
University of New England
Portland, Maine

Regi Robnett has 27 years of experience as an occupational therapist and over 30 years of experience working with older people in various capacities. She has worked at the University of New England for 22 years. Regi holds a PhD in Gerontology from the University of Massachusetts, Boston. She teaches courses in the biopsychosocial dimensions of older adults, communication, culture, and group process as well as research (often incorporating older adults and their concerns) and mental health. Regi enjoys doing community work to benefit older adults, often with her students.

Nancy Brossoie, PhD
Senior Research Scientist
Center for Gerontology
Virginia Tech
Blacksburg, Virginia

Nancy Brossoie is a senior research faculty member in behavioral and social science. Her primary research interests include aging in place, age-friendly communities, substance misuse in late life, and building community capacity to meet the needs of vulnerable populations. Nancy's expertise is informed by 17 years supervising home and community-based service delivery, evaluating programs and services at the state and community levels, and developing strategic plan initiatives for hospital systems, long-term care organizations, and mental health agencies.

Walter C. Chop, MS, RRT
Professor Emeritus
Respiratory Therapy Department
Southern Maine Community College
Portland, Maine

Walter Chop served as chair and professor in the Respiratory Therapy Department, Southern Maine Community College, for over 29 years. During his tenure at the college, he has also served as chair of Allied Health Sciences for 22 years. He has written numerous articles on both gerontology and respiratory care. For the past 10 years, he has been a member of the American Association for Respiratory Care Gerontology Committee.

Acknowledgments

It takes many individuals to create the final product that becomes a textbook. We thank everyone who has contributed to the process that has made the *Fourth Edition* of *Gerontology for the Health Care Professional* possible. Specifically,

- All the contributing authors whose hard work and dedication created the substance of this text: Jessica Bolduc, Ann O'Sullivan, Sue Stableford, Marji Harmer-Beem, Kathryn Thompson, Nancy MacRae, Laney Bruner Canhoto, Audrey Riffenburgh, Kimberly Wilson, David Mokler, and Raven Weaver.
- All the good people at Jones & Bartlett Learning, especially Cathy Esperti, Rachael Souza, Juna Abrams, Robert Boder, Troy Liston, and Sameer Jena.
- Our loving families, whose ongoing support and encouragement kept us going.

If we inadvertently left anyone out, we ask for your forgiveness.

Contributors

Jessica J. Bolduc, DrOT, MS, OTR/L
Staff Occupational Therapist, Mercy Hospital
Adjunct Faculty, University of New England
Portland, Maine

Laney Bruner Canhoto, PhD, MSW, MPH
Assistant Professor
Family Medicine and Community Health
University of Massachusetts Medical School
Worcester, Massachusetts

Marji Harmer-Beem, RDH, MS
Associate Professor
Dental Hygiene Program
University of New England
Portland, Maine

Nancy MacRae, MS, OTR/L, FAOTA
Associate Professor
Occupational Therapy Department
University of New England
Portland, Maine

David J. Mokler, PhD
Professor of Pharmacology and Chair
Department of Biomedical Sciences
College of Osteopathic Medicine
University of New England
Biddeford, Maine

Ann O'Sullivan, OTR/L, LSW, FAOTA
Trainer and Consultant
Scarborough, Maine

Audrey Riffenburgh, PhD
President, Plain Language Works, LLC
Founding Member, Clear Language Group
Albuquerque, New Mexico

Sue Stableford, MPH, MSB
Consultant and Trainer
Health Literacy, Plain Language, & Clear
    Health Communication

Kathryn H. Thompson, PhD, RD
Professor
University of New England College of
    Osteopathic Medicine
Biddeford, Maine

Kimberly Wilson, DNP, RN
Program Director of Accelerated Bachelor
    of Science in Nursing (ABSN)
Assistant Professor
Jefferson College of Health Sciences
Roanoke, Virginia

Raven H. Weaver, PhD
Assistant Professor
Washington State University
Pullman, Washington

Reviewers

Keciana Enaohwo, MS, MA, CHW-I
Houston Community College
Houston, Texas

Laura M. Horn, MEd, RD, LD
Professor
Cincinnati State Technical and
    Community College
Cincinnati, Ohio

Karen L. Madsen, FNP-BC
Assistant Professor
Missouri Southern State University
Joplin, Missouri

Susan C. Maloney, PhD, CRNP, FNP-BC
Assistant Professor
Edinboro University
Edinboro, Pennsylvania

Audrey McCrary-Quarles, PhD
Associate Professor
South Carolina State University
Orangeburg, South Carolina

Cindy Meyer, MEd, MSCPM, OTR/L, OTA/Retired
OTA Program Director
South Arkansas Community College
El Dorado, Arkansas

Margaret H. Teaford, PhD
Associate Professor Emeritia
Ohio State University
Columbus, Ohio

Linda J. Tsoumas, PT, MS, EdD
Professor of Physical Therapy
MCPHS University
Worcester, Massachusetts

Ann Marie Zvorsky, MSN, RN, CNE
Medical-Surgical Nursing Instructor
The Joseph F. McCloskey School of Nursing
    at Schuylkill Health
Pottsville, Pennsylvania

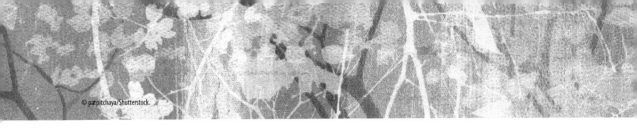
© patpitchaya/Shutterstock.

CHAPTER 1

Age Matters: Profiles of an Aging Society

Nancy Brossoie, PhD
Regula H. Robnett, PhD, OTR/L, FAOTA
Walter C. Chop, MS, RRT

CHAPTER OUTLINE

BEHAVIORAL OBJECTIVES

Upon completion of this chapter, the reader will be able to:

1. Explain terms used to describe and classify age.
2. Describe how populations are aging around the world.
3. Explain the difference between the terms lifespan and longevity.
4. Describe three key factors that influence population aging.
5. Describe the general characteristics of the U.S. population of adults age 65 years and older.
6. Describe the most common chronic health conditions among older adults.
7. Explain the types of services provided by formal and informal caregivers.
8. Identify the most common causes of death among older adults.
9. Discuss the impacts the U.S. baby boom generation is having on U.S. society.
10. Explain how marital status, income level, sex, and race can affect quality of life.

KEY TERMS

Activities of daily living
Baby boom generation
Biopsychosocial
Centenarian
Chronological age
Formal caregivers
Functional age
Gerontology

Incidence
Informal caregivers
Instrumental activities
    of daily living
Life expectancy
Lifespan
Longevity
Old

Old-old
Prevalence
Quality of life
Snowbirds
Successful aging
Super-centenarian
Total fertility rate
Young-old

▶ Introduction

We all start to age from the moment we are born. Aging is a lifespan process that influences every aspect of our lives. Yet, many people do not think about growing older or the issues that accompany growing older until they see their parents' health decline or experience health challenges of their own. The field of **gerontology** is the study of aging and age-related issues and the biological, sociological, and psychological (**biopsychosocial**) factors that influence aging and old age. As a heath care professional, you will need to have a basic grasp of aging and age-related issues, which this text attempts to provide.

The first step to learning about issues that influence and affect old age is to consider what the term "old age" implies. Old age is a subjective concept that can change over time and depends on cultural and social considerations. What we thought of as old in the 19th century is considered middle age now. What we considered old when we were 15, will vary greatly from when we are 40 or even 75!

Researchers define age in ways that help them study age in their fields of interest. Public health and health policy leaders rely on defining old age by **chronological age** (i.e., the length of time a person is alive) to inform policy and programs. Countries, including the United States use ages 60, 62, or 65 as benchmark ages or age eligibility thresholds for policies that affect older adults. Health scientists find **functional age** (i.e., the level at which a person can perform) is more useful than chronological age in determining an individual's health status. Social scientists often group older adults into age groups (e.g., ages 50–64, 65–74, 75–84, and 85+) that reflect similar life experiences and obligations, historical memories, and health problems within each group. Similarly, some researchers may apply terms to age groupings such as **young-old** (i.e., 50–64), **old** (i.e., 65–84), and **old-old** or oldest of old (ages 85 and older) to describe the stage of members in very late life. Within the old-old age group are two well-studied sub-groups—**centenarians** (i.e., persons at least 100 years old) and **super-centenarians** (i.e., persons at least 110 years old). How and why centenarians have been able to reach old age continues to be of great interest to scientists.

Whatever classification for age you choose to use in your work is a matter of preference, as long as you realize the limitations and variations implied by the term. A salient point to note and what is stressed throughout this text, is that there is a great amount of variability among older adults. Older adults are a heterogeneous group.

Some individuals retain a sound mind and body into late life, while other persons do not. Some people remain financially secure, while other individuals fall into poverty. While the aging process is not a one-size fits all experience, the fundamental processes are shared by all.

▶ Global Aging

Age, Sex, and Distribution

The world population is growing larger and getting older every year. The United Nations Department of Economic and Social Affairs (2017) reported that by mid-2017, the world population exceeded 7.5 billion people, an increase of 1 billion people since 2002. There are slightly more males than females (i.e., 102 males per 100 females) worldwide and they are distributed relatively equally across age groups as illustrated in **FIGURE 1-1**. As a group,

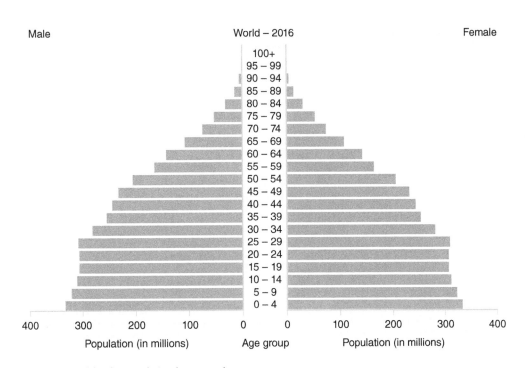

FIGURE 1-1 Worldwide population by sex and age group.

females tend to live longer than males, explaining less decline in group size later in life. The median age (i.e., the age in which half of the population is above and below) of the entire world population is 30 years, which is also illustrated by the width of the age group bars in Figure 1-1.

Worldwide population growth is expected to remain steady as the population increases by approximately 83 million people each year. **TABLE 1-1** includes estimates for total population growth in 2030, 2050, and 2100 as well as population data by world region.

Conversations about world population can be more effective if the world is discussed by geographic regions, such as Africa, Asia, Europe, Latin America and the Caribbean, Northern America, and Oceania. Even though the governments and policies of countries within a single region may differ, their geographic location unites them by shared and common resources, climate, lifestyles, and cultures.

As shown in **TABLE 1-2**, 60% of the world population lives in Asia (4.5 billion). China and India are the most populated countries in the entire world and account for 90% of Asia's population. Within Asia, adults age 25–59 represent nearly half (48%) of the region's population (see Table 1-2). The second largest populated world region is Africa and it contains 17% of the world population (1.25 billion). Africa's population is relatively young with 40% of the population age 0–14 years. Only 5% of Africa's population is age 60+ years. Conversely, Europe (the third largest populated region) is the "oldest" region with 25% of its population representing adults age 60+ years and 16% of its population age 0–14 years. The population in Latin America and the Caribbean (646 million) is slightly less than Europe (742 million people), but one quarter of its population (25%) are 0–14 years old and it is home to half as many older adults (12%). Northern America, which includes the United States, ranks 5th in population size among regions and includes 361 million people. Only 22% of the North America population is 60+ years old. The least populated

TABLE 1-1 Population of World and Population by Region, 2017

Region	Population (in millions)			
	2017	2030	2050	2100
World	7,550	8,551	9,772	11,184
Africa	1,256	1,704	2,528	4,468
Asia	4,504	4,947	5,257	4,780
Europe	742	739	716	653
Latin America & the Caribbean	646	718	780	712
Northern America	361	395	435	499
Oceania	41	48	57	72

Data from United Nations, Department of Economic and Social Affairs. (2017). *World Population Prospects: The 2017 Revision, Key Findings and Advance Tables.* Working Paper No. ESA/P/WP/248.

TABLE 1-2 World Population and Population by Age Groups and Region, 2017

Region	Total Population (in millions)	Population by Age Group (%)			
		0–14	15–24	25–59	60+
World	7,550	26	16	46	13
Africa	1,256	41	19	35	5
Asia	4,504	24	16	48	12
Europe	742	16	11	49	25
Latin America & the Caribbean	646	25	17	46	12
Northern America	361	19	13	46	22
Oceania	41	23	15	45	17

Data from United Nations, Department of Economic and Social Affairs. (2017). *World Population Prospects: The 2017 Revision, Key Findings and Advance Tables.* Working Paper No. ESA/P/WP/248.

region is Oceania, which is home to 41 million people; 17% of whom are age 60+ years.

The population differences by region illustrate the fact that population size alone does not predict the age composition of a population. Instead, demographers look to three key and interrelated factors: fertility rate, longevity, and migration.

Fertility Rates

The number of older adults in the world today is directly connected to the **total fertility rate** (TFR; i.e., the average number of live births a child-bearing women would have in her lifetime) at the time they were born. In the 1950s, the TFR in the regions of Africa, Asia, Latin American and the Caribbean was approximately five live births per woman, a veritable population explosion when compared to Europe's TFR, which was less than three lives births per woman during the same years. Consequently, countries

that experienced a high TFR in the mid-20th century are now faced with a growing economically inactive (i.e., retired or not working) older population that needs to be supported. Countries that experienced a low TFR at the same time, now tout a smaller aging population and are likely to be in a better position to provide members with economic and physical support.

War can dramatically impact TFR. During wartime, live births decrease because men and women are sent away from home to fight. However, post-war economies often generate socioeconomic growth that supports marriages, births, and an increased TFR. After World War II, the TFR skyrocketed in the United States and the large number of babies born between 1946 and 1964 have been subsequently referred to as members of the **baby boom generation**. Like the United States, South Korea also had a baby boom that is now entering old age. However, the years of birth for Korea's baby boomers (1955–1963) began with the end of the Korean War and not World War II (Howe, Jackson, & Nakashima, 2007).

By tracking fertility rates in a region, policy makers and service providers can better predict the needs of a population and prepare for change. When countries experience sudden changes in fertility rates, it dramatically affects the population balance. For example, South Korea is the fastest growing aging society. It doubled its aging population from 7% (1999) to 14% (2017) in just 18 years and it continues to rise at a rapid rate (Klassen, 2010). Perhaps more troublesome is that the TFR in South Korea is the lowest in the world at 1.25; meaning that the population is barely able to replace people who die (referred to as the fertility replacement rate). Declining birth rates are expected to dramatically impact the size and productivity of the South Korean labor force and the national economy. Simply put, when older adults stop working, there will be few workers to replace them. One fear is if South Korean industry leaders are faced with a decreasing labor pool, they may seek laborers and manufacturing deals in neighboring countries, further reducing the nation's productivity. Moreover, the South Korean government faces challenges in meeting increased healthcare costs and the need to develop a system of services and supports to address the needs of the growing older population.

In 2017, the country with the oldest population was Japan. One-third (33%) of its residents were age 60+. Japan was closely followed by Italy, (29%), Germany (28%), and Portugal (28%). Each of these countries also represents developed societies (i.e., high socioeconomic development) that boast high gross domestic products (GDP; i.e., the value of everything produced in a country) per capita (i.e., per person). By maintaining a high GDP, a country is better positioned to access, maintain, and provide resources, economic trade, and opportunities, which contribute to population health and **longevity** (i.e., the length of time lived).

Still, GDP ranking is not enough to predict if a county has a large aging population.

In 2017, the top five developed countries with the highest GDP per capita included the small governments of Qatar, Luxembourg, Macao, Singapore, and Brunei. The total populations of these countries were significantly different: 2.2 million, 590 thousand, 650 thousand, 5.6 million, and 423 thousand residents, respectively. Moreover, the percentage of the population aged 60+ in each country also varied considerably, ranging from 3% to 20%. Thus, wealth is also not a predictor for identifying if a country has a large population of older adults, even if that wealth can help provide services and products that promote longevity.

Longevity

Maintaining a healthy population across the **lifespan** (i.e., the period from birth to death) is directly influenced by access to health care (including pre-natal care), public sanitation, a well-balanced diet, education, and safe and secure communities. **Life expectancy** (i.e., the length of time a person is expected to live) is further influenced by the historical time in which a person lives, environment factors such as air and water quality, and any social and behavioral factors that affects the population such as smoking, obesity, homicide, and war.

Worldwide, life expectancy at birth is currently 70.8 years, an increase from 67.2 years since 2000. The greatest increases across world regions have occurred in Africa, which showed an increase of 6.6 years in the same period, after increasing less than 2 years in the prior decade. Despite the rapid increase, life expectancy in Africa is now just 60.2 years. The highest life expectancy is in Northern America (79.2 years) followed by Oceania (77.9 years), Europe (77.2 years), Latin America and the Caribbean (74.6 years) and Asia (71.8 years). When comparing population size with life expectancy, it become clear that population size alone does not translate to higher life expectancy. Clearly, other factors are at play.

Population Health

Obesity is becoming an epidemic health concern throughout the world with proportional increases in weight across all age groups and educational levels (Samper-Ternent & Al Snih, 2012). According to the World Health Organization (2017), the prevalence of obesity has tripled worldwide from 1975 to 2016, and is responsible for the deaths of at least 2.8 million people annually. The U.S. population leads the world in obesity for both men and women (**FIGURE 1-2**). By 2015, residents 50–74 years old had significantly poorer health with multiple health conditions compared to their British and European counterparts including hypertension, heart disease, diabetes, cancer, lung disease, and mobility impairments (National Institute on Aging, National Institutes of Health, & World Health Organization [2011]).

Since the 1980s, HIV/AIDS has been a worldwide health concern that is often overlooked in association with older adults. Human immunodeficiency virus (HIV) is a virus, which once acquired can be treated, but cannot be eradicated from the body. If left untreated, HIV can develop into acquired immunodeficiency syndrome (AIDS). Antiviral therapies (ART) have improved dramatically in effectiveness and can now control HIV so that it does not develop into AIDS. Persons affected can live long, relatively healthy lives with the virus largely under control (Centers for Disease Control and Prevention, 2017). About half of persons infected are already older than age 50 (Mills, Bärnighausen, & Negin, 2012). Undeveloped countries have not fared as well, especially sub-Sahara African countries where the prevalence of HIV among persons age 50+ is expected to exceed 10% by 2025. Moreover, persons over age 50 with HIV and receiving ART, still have a 30% higher risk of dying within 4 years compared to younger patients.

To combat population health problems, Mills et al. (2012) suggest that the world needs more geriatric clinicians. They are few in number in the United States and absent in many regions of the world. Training needs to include better geriatric training, improved rehabilitation services, and prevention outreach services to improve older peoples' ability to avoid disease and cope living with their health problems.

Migration

In addition to fertility rates and life expectancy, population size is influenced by migration patterns. In peaceful times, immigrants enter a country to gain education, engage in business, or to live with family members who have already relocated. Most countries have processes and procedures in place to regulate this form of immigration. Some immigrants stay for short periods of time, while others seek and obtain citizenship. A challenge for any society is when residents of a war-torn country or a country undergoing political unrest, want to leave and make their home in a neighboring country, as has been the case with Syrian refugees. As of 2015, an estimated 4.2 million people have fled the civil conflict in Syria and 2.2 million have settled in Turkey (Tumen, 2016). More often than not, immigrants are young adults with young families or with the intention of sending for them after getting settled. The persons left behind are people least able to support themselves and their communities such as women and children, older adults, poor people, and persons with disabilities.

The effect of mass migration on the departure and arrival countries can be staggering. Mass migration of a population places a strain on local and national economies, social services, housing, education, public health, and sanitation. In countries receiving large numbers of immigrants, the economy is unlikely to have job openings for all the new arrivals, resulting in increased enrollments in the public welfare system. In the country left behind, the future is also not bright for the persons who remained. The workers who used to support the economy and pay taxes to support community infrastructure (e.g., roads, hospitals, schools, and health care) are no

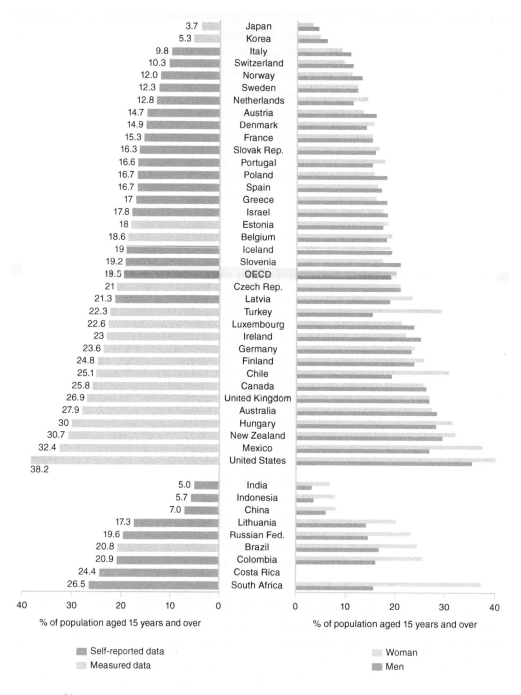

FIGURE 1-2 Obesity rates by country, 2015 or nearest year.

Data from OECD. (2017). Obesity update 2017. OECD Health Statistics. Retrieved from www.oecd.org/els/health-systems/Obesity-Update-2017.pdf.

longer contributing. The transactions of goods and services may stop. Older adults, who once depended on a state pension, may suddenly have no income. Without a large infusion of capital and manpower, many communities left behind after war and conflict simply fall apart and the population becomes impoverished and left with little hope for a better future.

Recognizing the influences on population size and health is needed to understand what it takes for people to age successfully. Gerontologists use population information as a guide to explore what it takes to provide a quality of life at the individual, societal, national, and global levels. A brief discussion about successful aging and quality of life is at the end of this chapter.

▶ Aging in the United States

Age and Age Groups

The U.S. Census Bureau estimated that the national population in 2016 was slightly more than 323 million people (Federal Interagency Forum on Aging-Related Statistics, 2016). The median age in the United States was 37.9 years, seven years higher than the world population median age. Among the 50 states, Maine had the oldest population with a median age of 44.5 years, while Utah had the youngest populations with a median age of 30.7 years (Statista, 2017). The average life expectancy in the United States for both sexes in 2016 was 78.8 years.

In 2016, adults age 65 and older made up 15.2% of the population, an increase of 0.3% from the previous year. As aforementioned, members of the baby boom generation were born from 1946 to 1964 and include approximately 76 million people. The individuals born in 1946 started turning age 65 in 2011. Since then, approximately 10,000 adults turn age 65 each day until 2029. Therefore, it is important to any analysis of the older population to include members born in all years of the baby boom generation, even if they have yet to reach age 65, as the sheer number of adults reaching old age will impact social policy and services.

In 2016, the percentage of adults by age breakdown was as follows:

- Age 45–54 (13.3%)
- Age 55–64 (12.8%)
- Age 65–74 (8.9%)
- Age 75–84 (4.4%)
- Age 85+ (1.9%)

Geographic Distribution

Older adults live in communities all across the United States. Some individuals live in the same towns where they were born and raised, and other individuals relocate several times during their lives, even in late life. Not surprisingly, where the older population resides in the United States is heavily influenced by the economy, health, and weather.

The outmigration of young adults due to poor job and economic prospects has left some regions with increased numbers of older adults. When industries fold and are not replaced with new industries drawing on the same labor force, individuals tend to seek work in other regions thus, leaving the non-active workforce behind. The density of older populations in post-industrial areas, such as Appalachia and the Midwest shown in **FIGURE 1-3**, help emphasize the effect of outmigration.

Older adults who migrate to new regions in the country, generally do so after retiring from the workforce. The pull of a new community is generally tied to several factors: a lower cost of living than the pre-retirement community, warmer and drier climate, and proximity to friends and family. As can be seen in Figure 1-3, the warmer climes of Florida, Arizona, and southern Utah draw older persons and thus, have dense older populations. Florida has long been known for its older demographic. Eighty percent of Florida counties (i.e., 53 of 67) have an above average proportion of older adults. In Sumter County more than half of its residents are reportedly age 65+. In 2010, the southern

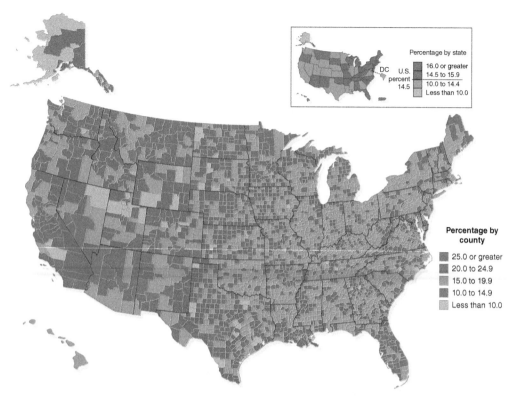

FIGURE 1-3 Percentage of population age 65+ by county and state in the United States in 2014.

Data from U.S. Census Bureau, Annual Estimates of the Resident Population for Selected Age Groups by Sex for the United States, States, Counties, and Puerto Rico Commonwealth and Municipios: April 1, 2010, to July 1, 2014 (PEPAGESEX).

regions of the U.S., had the largest number of individuals over age 65 whereas the northeast had the largest proportion of persons over age 65 (Statista, 2017).

However, not all persons relocate permanently to warmer states. The term **snowbirds** refers to older adults who move south for the winter to avoid the cold weather at home and all the heating bills and snow removal that accompany living in the cold. Many snowbirds make the trek south for a few years before settling down permanently in the south, while other snowbirds only want it to be an annual winter trip.

Sex

In contrast to the world population composition, in 2016, there were more females than males in the total U.S. population (i.e., 100 females per 96.9 males, or 50.8% females to 49.2% males). The gap widened between the sexes by age 65 with even fewer males (44.1%) than females (55.9%). Historically, this difference has been attributed to better health and health care among females, although with the rise in obesity, heart disease, and tobacco use in females, the gap has narrowed.

Race

The racial diversity of the older population in the United States is less diverse than that of the entire population and the younger population. Older adults are predominately White (78%) and non-Hispanic (92%). Only 9% of older adults are Black and 4% are Asian. This can be explained in part by the fact that the immigration rates of non-White and Hispanic populations into the

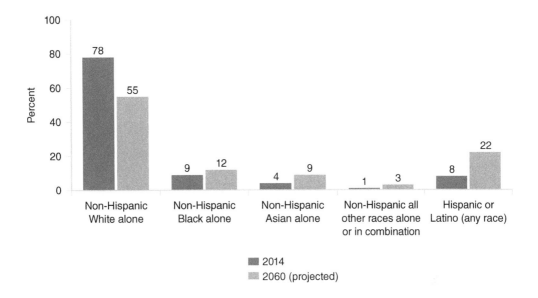

FIGURE 1-4 Older U.S. population by race and Hispanic origin.

Federal Interagency Forum on Aging-Related Statistics. (2016). *Older Americans 2016: Key Indicators of Well-Being.* Federal Interagency Forum on Aging-Related Statistics. Washington, DC: U.S. Government Printing Office.

United States were much lower when today's older adults were young, and today's older immigrants of color are not numerous enough to influence the national data. It is also important to remember that interracial marriages were illegal at the time many of today's older adults were getting married, so they were unlikely to marry outside of their race. The racial profile of older adults in 2014 is illustrated in **FIGURE 1-4**.

Marital Status

An important influence on quality of life and well-being are social relationships, including marriage. Because there are more women than men and women tend to live longer than men, it stands to reason that a higher percentage of older men are married than older women. In 2015, among adults age 65–74 years, about 74% of men were married although only 58% of women of the same age were married. The increased rate of married men continues across age groups (**FIGURE 1-5**). Not surprisingly, more women than men were widowed. Seventy-three percent of women age 85+ years

were widowed compared to 34% of men of the same age. What remains relatively consistent across age groups and sex are the rates of never married adults (3–6%) and divorced adults (6–17%). At the time of this writing, there is no reliable national relationship data on same sex marriages or partnerships among older adults.

Living Arrangements

One's living arrangement can also have a significant impact on health, quality of life and well-being. In 2015, 70% of men lived with a spouse yet, only 45% of women lived with a spouse. Expectedly, women were more apt to live alone (36%) than were men (20%). However, the trend for living alone has begun to decline after a fivefold increase (6–29%) from 1900 to 1990 (Stepler, 2016). Older persons of color are more apt to live alone than older White adults. Specifically, 46% of older Black women lived alone, and older Black men live alone three times more often than older Asian men. However, older men of color were more apt to live with relatives than their White

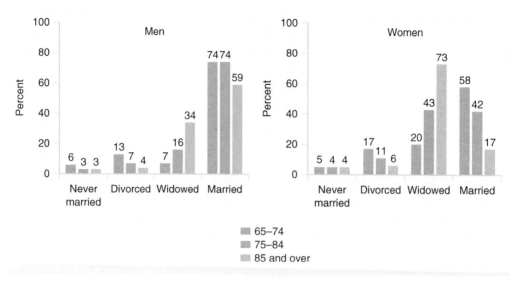

FIGURE 1-5 Marital status of older adults in the United States by sex and age group, 2015.

Federal Interagency Forum on Aging-Related Statistics. (2016). *Older Americans 2016: Key Indicators of Well-Being.* Federal Interagency Forum on Aging-Related Statistics. Washington, DC: U.S. Government Printing Office.

counterparts. Approximately 14% of Black and Hispanic men of color lived with a relative other than a spouse compared to only 4% of While men doing the same. Older people living alone are three times as likely to live in poverty and less likely to view their economic status as "living comfortably" (Stepler, 2016).

▶ Economic Status

Poverty

The economic status of older Americans is more varied than any other age group. Poverty among older adults was such a serious problem by the mid-20th century that in 1964 it was integrated into President Lyndon B. Johnson's War on Poverty legislation. This led to federal implementation of the Older Americans Act in 1965 in an effort to lift older citizens out of poverty. In 1966, 29% of people age 65+ years lived below the federal poverty threshold and 18% of children were deemed impoverished. By 2014, the rate for older adults in poverty dropped to 10–12% (depending on the

measure used), although the rate for children has hovered around 20% (**FIGURE 1-6**).

Poverty in late life is experienced differently by gender, age, and race. Not only are older women likely to live alone, they are more apt to live alone in poverty (12%). Moreover, as time passes, the chances of an older adult becoming impoverished increases. In 2014, the overall poverty rate for adults age 65+ years was 9%, compared to 12% of adults ages 75 and older experiencing poverty.

Persons of color experience greater rates of poverty than White men (5%) and women (10%). In 2014, older Black men, Hispanic men, and Asian men experienced poverty rates of 17%, 16%, and 13%, respectively. Yet, older women of color still experience the highest rates of poverty in late life. Older Black women (21%) and Hispanic women (20%) are four times as likely to be in poverty as older White men and twice as likely as older White women. Older Asian women (16%) experience poverty at nearly the same rate as Asian men yet, their rate is still triple the rate of older White men. Lifting older adults out of poverty is connected to the provision

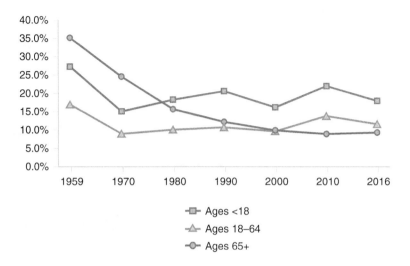

FIGURE 1-6 Poverty rates in United States over time.

Semega, J. L., Fontenot, K. R., & Kollar, M. A. (2017). *Income and poverty in the United States: 2016.* Report Number: P60-259. Washington, DC: U.S. Government Printing Office.

of need-based supplementary programs and services, discussed further in Chapter 6.

Income

Personal and household incomes of older adults are as diverse as they are among younger people. Due to many economic factors, the median income of older adults has risen in the past 40 years. In 1974 median income was reportedly $22,921 (in 2014 dollars) and by 2014, it reached $36,895. As **FIGURE 1-7** illustrates, the distribution of wealth among older adults is diverse. Using the federal poverty level as an income baseline, low income adults are identified as receiving income 100–199% above the poverty level, middle income adults receive 200–399% above the poverty level, and high income older adults receive income at least 400% above the poverty level.

Sources of Income

Variation in income size is reflective of the sources of income (e.g., personal savings, investments, retirement pensions, and Social Security). In 2014, nearly half (49%) of all households (including 86% of all older adults) received Social Security (i.e., an entitlement program that workers pay into and draw from upon leaving the workforce; see Chapter 6). By age 80, 90% of older adults receive Social Security. Less than half (41%) of older adults received income from a private retirement pension or annuity, and only 18% received income from a public pension fund. Selling or cashing in personal assets also provides a source of income and more than two thirds (67%) of older adults receive income from their assets. Conversely, 13% of older adults had little to no assets to draw upon and received public assistance (i.e., cash and non-cash) to supplement their income.

FIGURE 1-8 displays a chart comparing the sources of income by dividing the older population into quintiles (i.e., five graduated income categories with equal numbers of adults in each). The visual helps demystify the sources older adults rely upon for their incomes. Clearly, individuals with lower incomes rely more on Social Security than persons in the higher income groups.

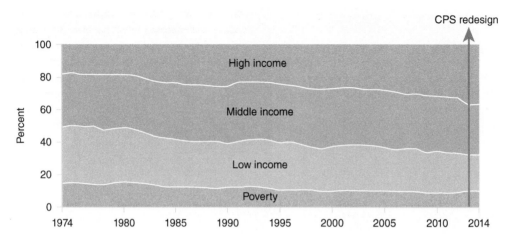

FIGURE 1-7 Income distribution in the United States among older adults, 1974–2014.

Federal Interagency Forum on Aging-Related Statistics. (2016). *Older Americans 2016: Key Indicators of Well-Being.* Federal Interagency Forum on Aging-Related Statistics. Washington, DC: U.S. Government Printing Office.

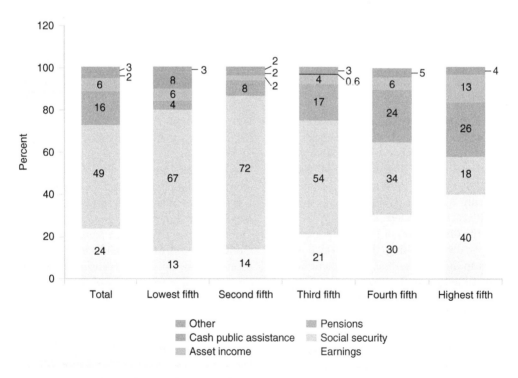

FIGURE 1-8 Percentile distribution of per capita family income for persons age 65+, by income quintile and source of income, 2014.

Federal Interagency Forum on Aging-Related Statistics. (2016). *Older Americans 2016: Key Indicators of Well-Being.* Federal Interagency Forum on Aging-Related Statistics. Washington, DC: U.S. Government Printing Office.

▶ Work and Retirement Status

Not all older adults leave the labor force once they reach age 65 or retire. Continued employment in some form can provide additional income, opportunities for socialization, and feelings of self-worth and contribution, which all contribute to improving quality of life and well-being. Approximately 29% of older adults have no retirement savings or pension plan (United States Government Accountability Office, 2015), which forces many people to continue to be active in the workforce. As illustrated in FIGURE 1-9, rate of participation of older adults in the workforce is expected to rise, whatever the reason.

Although finances are a leading factor for returning to or remaining in the labor force, other reasons cited for continuing to work included: boredom or extra time to engage, sought out by employer to train or mentor younger workers, and personal enjoyment and fulfillment (Tamburo, 2017). Additional information on work and retirement is presented in Chapter 2.

▶ Health Status

The health of older Americans is frequently discussed in terms of the **incidence** (i.e., the number of new cases reported) and **prevalence** (i.e., the total number of cases reported) of chronic health conditions and communicable diseases, functional limitations, vaccination rates, and self-reported health status.

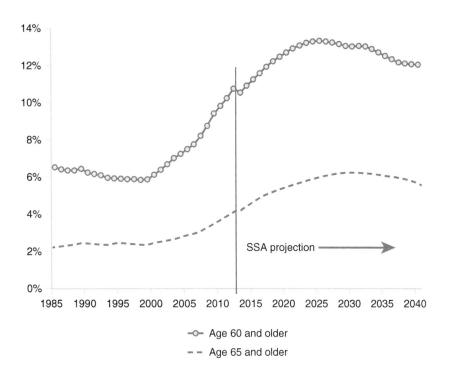

FIGURE 1-9 Percentage of older employed population age 60+.

Data from Burtless, G. (2013). *The impact of population aging and delayed retirement on workforce productivity.* (CRR WP 2-13-11). Chestnut Hill, MA: Center for Retirement Research.

Chronic Health Conditions

Chronic health conditions, such as heart disease, stroke, cancer, diabetes, and arthritis, are among the most costly health conditions to treat. Moreover, they are preventable if an individual commits to change the behaviors that lead to the condition. Multiple chronic health conditions are experienced by the majority of older adults; co-morbid conditions (i.e., multiple conditions at the same time) directly contribute to frailty and disability (**FIGURE 1-10**).

In 2014, the most frequently occurring health conditions for non-institutionalized older adults were uncontrolled hypertension (55.9%), diagnosed arthritis (49%), heart disease (29.4%), cancer of any type (23.4%), diabetes (20.8%), asthma (10.6%), and stroke (7.9%). Differences in prevalence rates between men and women were small. However, prevalence rates by race and ethnicity varied greatly for some conditions. White men and women led other races and ethnicities in the prevalence for heart disease (30.7%) and cancers (26%). However, Black men and women experienced hypertension (70.6%), stroke (10.6%), and diabetes (31.1%) more than other groups. Older adults of Hispanic origin (regardless of race) also had diabetes (32.3%) more often than other non-Hispanic racial and ethnic groups.

Functional Limitations

Functional limitations can be debilitating and thus, impact quality of life and well-being. In 2014, 22.6% of older adults reported a functional limitation that disabled them even if they used corrective devices (e.g., hearing aids, eyeglasses). More precisely, prevalence rates in functional limitations that created a disability (for both sexes and all races) included mobility (17.1%), hearing (4.2 %), vision (3.3%), self-care (3.0%), cognition (2.7%), and communication (1.2%).

Racial and ethnic differences emerged across some types of functional limitations. Specifically, non-Hispanic Black men and women were more likely to experience a disability in mobility (20.6%) compared to Hispanic older adults (16.9%) and non-Hispanic White older adults (13.3%). Additionally, Hispanic (4.6%) and non-Hispanic Black (4.0%) older adults were more than twice as likely

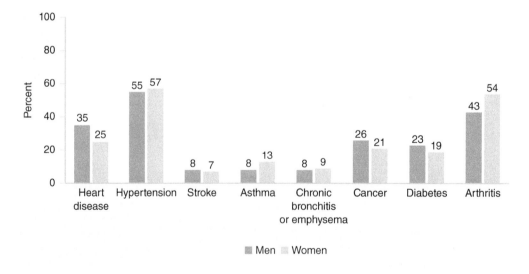

FIGURE 1-10 Percentage of people age 65+ who reported selected chronic conditions, by sex, 2013–2014.

Federal Interagency Forum on Aging-Related Statistics. (2016). *Older Americans 2016: Key Indicators of Well-Being.* Federal Interagency Forum on Aging-Related Statistics. Washington, DC: U.S. Government Printing Office.

as non-Hispanic White (1.7%) older adults to have a disability with cognition. An overview of the functional limitations older adults can face at the individual level is presented in Chapter 9.

Vaccinations

Vaccinations against influenza and pneumococcal disease are critical to maintaining health in late life. A compromised or weakened immune system has trouble combating disease and if infected, can lead to death. One preventive measure undertaken frequently by local healthcare systems, public health departments, and pharmacies is to offer free vaccination clinics each autumn as a strategy to get older adults inoculated. In 2014, 70.1% of older adults reported being vaccinated against influenza and 61.3% were vaccinated against pneumococcal disease. Historically, Black men and women have been far less likely to receive an influenza inoculation than White men and women. In 2014, only 57.4% of Blacks and 60.5% of Hispanics (of any race) received an influenza shot compared to 72% of non-Hispanic White older adults. The disparity suggests continued and alternative education and outreach efforts need to target persons of color.

Self-Rated Health

Despite the high prevalence of chronic health conditions and diseases in the second half of life, many older adults do not perceive that their health is bad or problematic. In 2014, 77.5% of older adults rated their health status as either good or excellent. Even 68.1% of persons age 85+ rated their health status as good or excellent. The reason older adults frequently rate their health higher than the people around them might rate it is because they tend to compare their ability to function against the functional abilities they see in other people of their own age. As a result, everyone knows someone who is worse off, so they themselves must be doing well!

▶ Caregivers

For many older adults, there comes a time when they need help with their **activities of daily living** (ADL; i.e., bathing, dressing, eating, toileting, and mobility) and **instrumental activities of daily living** (IADLS; housework, preparing meals, using a telephone, managing money, or shopping). Family caregivers frequently fulfill that role as an act of filial responsibility (or family obligation). Family caregivers are referred to as **informal caregivers** because they provide services without compensation.

Both care recipients and caregivers tend to be female (65% and 75%, respectively). Daughters (including biological daughters, step-daughters, and daughters by marriage) account for 19% of informal caregivers, followed by other relatives (22.3%), and spouses (21.2%). While the average age of the caregiver is 49.2 years, 35% of caregivers are age 65 or older. The average caregiver provides over 24 hours of care per week, and nearly one-fourth (24%) of caregivers provide care for more than 5 years. Fifteen percent of all caregivers provide care for at least 10 years.

Informal caregivers for persons with dementia (including Alzheimer's disease) provide on average, nine hours of service per day of care. Caregiving tasks include assistance with ADLs, IADLs, advocating for services and supports, and decision making on behalf of the care recipient (Family Caregiving Alliance, 2016). The challenges and stresses related to taking the responsibility for caring for a person with dementia are well documented as highly stressful and can negatively impact the health and well-being of the caregiver. In response, caregiver support groups and workshops are available to help caregivers cope successfully and maintain their own health.

If caregivers simply stopped performing caregiving tasks, the resultant demand for services and supports would overload the healthcare system in the United States. In 2013, the value of unpaid caregiving services was estimated to be $470 billion! That estimate is more than was reimbursed in the same year for Medicaid and home and community-based services combined (Family Caregiving Alliance, 2016). More information about the types of home and community-based services available in the United States is provided in Chapter 5.

Long-Term Care Services

In 2014, approximately 9 million people (including older adults and young persons with extensive physical impairments and disabilities) were provided long-term care services through multiple service venues that included adult day service centers, home health agencies, hospice centers, nursing homes, assisted living facilities, and residential care communities that offered services and supports needed to function in daily life. Since 1966, when federal service programs (e.g., Medicare and Medicaid) were introduced, the number of older adults accessing services and supports has more than tripled from 2.5 million to 9 million. The workers employed by organizations offering such services are referred to as **formal caregivers** because unlike family caregivers, they are paid to deliver care.

Among the 9 million care recipients, approximately 1.2 million adults age 65 and older lived in nursing homes (Administration on Aging, 2015). Although this number includes only 1% of persons ages 65–74 years, it increases to 10% of persons age 85+. Overall annual resident rates usually include 5% or less of the general older population. Eligibility for nursing home admission is determined by an assessment of personal health needs, functional limitations, limitations with ADLs and IADLs, and available resources and supports in the community. Adults age 85 and older represent the fastest-growing segment of the population needing nursing home care and 25% are eligible for placement. Understandably, adults of that age are typically in declining health, have growing unmet needs, and dwindling resources. However, the number of nursing home beds is increasing at half the rate needed to meet the demands of this expanding age group and the need is expected to increase as baby boomers reach late life.

Older adults who become long-term residents of nursing homes will, on average, spend all their savings and assets within one year (Tamburo, 2017). In 2017, the average estimated costs for nursing home care was $235 per day ($85,775 per year) for a shared room, with the lowest costs for care in the south and mid-west ($165 per day; $60,225 per year) and the highest costs in the northeast ($350 per day; $127,750 per year; American Elder Care Research Organization, 2017). Once personal funds are depleted, a resident may become eligible for public assistance such as Medicaid, which helps pay for some care. In 2013, 62.9% of all nursing home residents were paying for their care using Medicaid.

Considering the sharp increased demand ahead for home and community-based care and institutionalized care, the question on the minds of all policymakers and service leaders is, "Where will the funds come from to continue funding long-term care services and supports?"

▶ Death

Older adults generally experience health co-morbidities as they age and each health challenge affects another in some way. However, discussions about national mortality statistics necessitate that deaths are attributed to the primary cause of death listed on the death certificate and not to multiple health diagnoses. This can pose challenges in analyzing causes of death when an individual has been diagnosed with a primary health problem (e.g., Alzheimer's disease or cancer) but dies from another (e.g., heart failure). In response, international rules of reporting deaths have been implemented to provide a system that will provide the most accurate profile of mortality as possible, while recognizing caveats in reporting.

Causes

The negative health impacts of chronic health conditions include death. In 2014, the six leading causes of death for persons age 65 and older included conditions and diseases that can be controlled to some extent through healthy behaviors. As shown in **TABLE 1-3**, heart disease was the leading cause of death in 2014, followed by cancer, chronic lower respiratory disease, stroke, Alzheimer's disease, diabetes, unintentional injuries, and influenza and pneumonia.

When compared to rates in 2000, death rates in 2014 declined by about 20% for all causes except Alzheimer's disease and unintentional injury, which both rose. Rates for Alzheimer's disease increased in part due to improved diagnosis and reporting. Historically, a diagnosis of Alzheimer's disease was confirmed only upon autopsy of the brain after death. Therefore, the inclusion of Alzheimer's disease on death certificates, from which this data was collected, was likely more limited in 2000 than today.

Mortality from heart disease and cancer does not differ a great deal by sex, race, and ethnicity, although, differences do exist for some other causes of death. Specifically, diabetes is the fourth highest cause of death for non-Hispanic Black older adults (212 per 100,000) and Hispanic (all races) older adults (155 per 100,000) yet, is the seventh highest cause of death for non-Hispanic White older adults (106 per 100,000). Women had higher rates of death from Alzheimer's disease (222 per 100,000) than men (161,000 per 100,000), although, men experienced higher rates of death from unintentional injuries (131 per 100,000) than women (36 per 100,000).

Knowledge about causes of death helps us better understand life. Information about mortality can be used to develop interventions to delay or prevent health challenges, especially

TABLE 1-3 Leading Causes of Death Among U.S. Adults Aged 65 or Older in 2000 and 2014

Cause of Death	2000 Rates of Deaths (per 100,000)	2014 Rates of Deaths (per 100,000)
Heart disease	1,707	1,062
Cancer	1,124	915
Chronic lower respiratory diseases	305	277
Stroke	426	247
Alzheimer's disease	141	200
Diabetes	150	119
Unintentional injury	89	105
Influenza and pneumonia	169	97

Data from Federal Interagency Forum on Aging-Related Statistics. (2016). *Older Americans 2016: Key Indicators of Well-Being.* Federal Interagency Forum on Aging-Related Statistics. Washington, DC: U.S. Government Printing Office.

if we can connect them to client behaviors and habits. Our ability to "connect the dots" between the biopsychosocial influences in our clients' lives, will help us support them to age successfully and enjoy a quality of life.

▶ Aging Successfully

Successful Aging

The concept of **successful aging** was first introduced over 50 years ago in response to negative social beliefs about age and growing older. In 1987, Rowe and Kahn took a biopsychosocial approach to develop their model for successful aging (Rowe & Kahn, 1997). The model included three key factors representing each domain. Rowe and Kahn proposed that individuals aged successfully if they:

■ Lived free of disease and disability
■ Retained high cognitive and physical abilities
■ Maintained meaningful interactional social relationships

Each of the three domains interfaced with the other two. At first blush, the model seems ideal as it represents the best of a bio-psycho-social approach. However, critics argue that the model dismisses and diminishes people who do not live free of disease and disability, have low cognitive and physical abilities, or cannot maintain social relationships. Are we to conclude that they cannot and will not age successfully? Moreover, by what standards should society judge a person's ability to age successfully? Researchers continue to modify the model to address the criticisms and adapt the model to include other factors including spirituality. The overall concept is valid, yet for many researchers the focus of successful aging should focus more on quality of life.

Quality of Life in Old Age

Quality of life (QOL) is another subjective construct that is difficult to measure. Yet, researchers are in general agreement that it is influenced by the topics presented in this text, including but not limited to personal characteristics, living arrangement, physical and mental health status and health issues, social relationships, sexuality, and outlook on life. Because there is a lot of variance in rating quality of life, it is easy to understand how everyone can have a different sense of what it means.

The idea of living a quality life in old age is often dismissed by people who view it as a time of decline and suffering. Advertising campaigns, television, and social media tend to focus on "suffering" in old age (e.g., dementia, depression, cancer, arthritis, stroke), while ignoring evidence that people can live well and happily even with health problems. A recent study of centenarians found that a significant proportion of the oldest-old (over age 80) have lived with chronic health conditions (associated with the condition of "suffering") for decades. However, the majority of older adults do not "suffer" through life but rather learn to live well in spite of pain or bodily restrictions (Terry, Sebastiani, Andersen, & Perls, 2008). The word "suffer" should be used less frequently and only in regards to individuals who truly cannot enjoy life due to irascible pain or anguish. The vast majority of older adults do not fit into this mold.

Quality of life and what it means to individuals has been studied in different cultures around the world (Molzahn, Kalfoss, Makaroff, & Skevington, 2010). Findings indicated that older adults in developed countries often cited general health and attributes of physical health such as sleep quality, energy, and being free of pain as essential to having a good QOL. In contrast, older adults in less developed countries cited energy, happiness, and home environment as positive contributors to their QOL. Results from a study in the United States on QOL (Pew Research Center, 2013) showed that QOL cannot be tidily defined by older adults. **FIGURE 1-11** includes some of the indicators found to be important to U.S. older adults in achieving a good QOL.

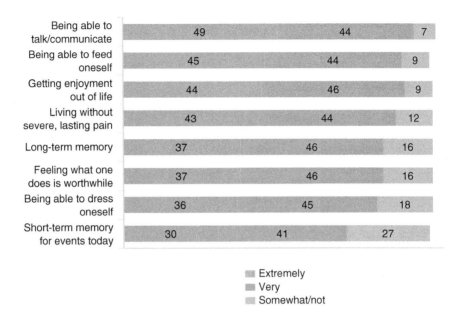

	Extremely	Very	Somewhat/not
Being able to talk/communicate	49	44	7
Being able to feed oneself	45	44	9
Getting enjoyment out of life	44	46	9
Living without severe, lasting pain	43	44	12
Long-term memory	37	46	16
Feeling what one does is worthwhile	37	46	16
Being able to dress oneself	36	45	18
Short-term memory for events today	30	41	27

FIGURE 1-11 Quality of life indicators in old age. Percent of U.S. adults who say each of these is important for a good life in old age.

Data from Pew Research Center. (2013). *Views on end-of-life medical treatments.* Retrieved from: http://www.pewforum.org/2013/11/21/chapter-6-aging-and-quality-of-life/.

Specifically, being able to communicate with others, living without severe pain, and getting enjoyment out of life was identified more important; but, higher in importance to older women than older men.

Life Satisfaction

Life experiences and hardships can challenge an individual yet, offer opportunities to strengthen insight, wisdom, and faith, which can actually promote satisfaction with life. When conceptualized in that way, it is easy to understand why people who experience difficulties, continue to find their lives satisfying and fulfilling. This contrast—a high level of satisfaction with life despite ongoing experiences with loss— is aptly referred to as "the paradox of aging" (Carstensen, Mikels, & Mather, 2006, p. 346).

Being satisfied with one's life also contributes to QOL. Ardelt (1997) explored life satisfaction in old age in terms of wisdom

(i.e., an integration of cognitive, reflective and affective elements including an awareness and acceptance of human limitations), which allows an individual to view life with humor, compassion, and detachment. The approach addressed some of the same issues brought forth by critics of Rowe and Kahn's model of successful aging (1997). That is, persons experiencing poor life conditions can still have high levels of life satisfaction. Ardelt's findings ultimately confirmed that participants' level of wisdom explained much of the variability in life satisfaction among older adults.

Well-being

Well-being is another subjective indicator often associated with quality of life. Steptoe, Deaton, and Stone (2015) theorized that well-being included three domains: evaluative well-being (i.e., life satisfaction), hedonic well-being (i.e., happiness, sadness, stress level, pain, anger), and eudemonic well-being (i.e., sense of purpose and life meaning). In examining how these influence QOL in older adults, they found that in English-speaking countries, life satisfaction levels tended to follow a U-shaped curve, with persons age 45–54 years having the lowest level and younger and older adults enjoying higher levels. Researchers generally agree that low levels of perceived well-being correlate with increased numbers of life stressors (e.g., child-rearing, work, family caregiving), which generally occur during mid-life. Older adults who transition into late life with few life stressors generally report positive levels of well-being.

▶ Summary

The world population is growing and aging, creating new opportunities for healthcare professionals to support people in the second half of life. The large and growing proportion of older adults, offers many opportunities for older individuals and the communities in which they live. Population data confirms that age is only a number and does not directly translate to declining health, poor quality of life, and dissatisfaction with life. Rather, older adults are a heterogeneous group with many members experiencing good health, engaging in productive activities, and maintaining their social connections. Not only do older adults have more time to pursue leisure and enjoyable productive activities, they have the time and inclination to help others as caregivers. Many older adults are also remaining in the workforce, some because they feel financially unable to retire, and others because they genuinely enjoy or appreciate the work. A key factor in allowing older adults to remain vibrant and active is good health, which can be promoted through physical, social, and cognitive engagement. The more healthcare professionals can support positive health gains and supportive environments, the greater the potential is for older adults to live happier, more fulfilling lives.

🔎 CASE STUDIES

Case 1: Joram is a 67-year-old man living in a nation torn apart by civil war. Initially, his community wasn't directly affected, and although many people were on edge, their lives remained relatively normal. He worked as a cook in a small local restaurant during the week, and on the weekends he spent time with his 32-year-old daughter, Aya, her husband, and their young children. Before long, war spread to their part of the country and life became more dangerous. Concerned for the well-being of their children, Aya and her husband decided to flee the country. They wanted Joram to join them, but he felt that he would only slow them down, and didn't want to leave the village he had called home all his life. Aya's family managed to escape to a neighboring nation, along with thousands of other refugees fleeing the war. Within months, the population of Joram's village went from several thousand people to just a few hundred, as the war continued to rage on.

1. **How will the loss of so many residents likely impact Joram's village?**
2. **What challenges will the neighboring nation to which Aya and her family fled likely experience as migrants continue to flow in?**

Case 2: Sharon and Karen are twin 65-year-old sisters who were born and raised in Connecticut. Sharon has chronic obstructive pulmonary disease (COPD) as a result of a decades-long smoking habit, and she is married to Paul. Together, Sharon and Paul have a 35-year-old unmarried son who lives in California. Karen and her husband, Joe, work full-time and have three children with whom they are close—a 36-year-old married daughter with 8-year-old twin girls, a 32-year-old divorced son with a 2-year-old daughter, and a single 28-year-old daughter who has gone back to college and lives with them, along with her 4-year-old son. A few months ago, Sharon and Paul retired and moved to Florida. They talked to Karen and Joe about moving south with them, but they decided not to. Today, Sharon and Paul are enjoying their new life in Florida, and are making the most of the warm weather and new friendships they have developed. The move has been beneficial for Sharon's health, even though she is still limited in what she can physically do. Karen and Joe are happy that they decided not to retire yet, and enjoy filling their days with productive activity alongside coworkers who are also friends. Although they miss one another, Karen and Sharon are both happy with the decisions they made.

1. **Explain why you think Sharon decided to move south to Florida.**
2. **What are some reasons Karen decided to stay in Connecticut?**
3. **Do you think Karen and Sharon are aging successfully? Why or why not?**

TEST YOUR KNOWLEDGE

Review Questions

1. The term _____ refers to the length of time a person is alive whereas _____ refers to the level at which a person can perform.
   a. Life expectancy, life span
   b. Chronological age, functional age
   c. Functional age, life expectancy
   d. Life span, chronological age

2. By tracking fertility rates in a region, policy makers and service providers can better predict the needs of a population and prepare for change.
   a. True
   b. False

3. In 2016, adults age 65 and older made up approximately _____ of the U.S. population.
   a. 5%
   b. 15%
   c. 30%
   d. 52%

4. Implementation of the Older Americans Act in 1965 was part of an effort to provide older citizens with free health care and incomes for the remainder of their lives.
   a. True
   b. False

5. The term _____ caregivers applies to workers who are paid to provide care and _____ caregivers refers to people who provide care without compensation.
   a. Informal, formal
   b. Volunteer, respite
   c. Formal, informal
   d. Respite, informal

Learning Activities

1. How is the world population and the population of older adults expected to change in the coming years, and what three factors do demographers look to when predicting the age composition of a population?

2. How does a country's total fertility rate (TFR) change during wartime, and why? How does it change again when wartime ends, and why?
3. Obesity is becoming an epidemic health concern. Why is this particularly important when considering the population of older adults?
4. Imagine that you are the caregiver for an older person with dementia. What types of tasks would you be responsible for in this role?
5. Think about what aging successfully means to you, and what you will need to do in order to become an older adult that has aged successfully. Develop a list of five personal goals or indicators that you can revisit as an older adult to determine if you have aged successfully.

References

Administration on Aging. (2015). *A profile of older Americans*. Administration on Aging, Administration for Community Living, U.S. Department of Health and Human Services. Retrieved from https://www.acl.gov /sites/default/files/Aging%20and%20Disability%20 in%20America/2015-Profile.pdf

American Elder Care Research Organization. (2017). How to Pay for Nursing Home Care / Convalescent Care. Retrieved from https://www.payingforseniorcare.com /longtermcare/paying-for-nursing-homes.html#cost -table

Ardelt, M. (1997). Wisdom and life satisfaction in old age. *Journals of Gerontology Series B: Psychological Sciences and Social Sciences, 52B*, P15–P27. doi:10.1093/geronb /52B.1.P15

Burtless, G. (2013). *The impact of population aging and delayed retirement on workforce productivity*. (CRR WP#2013-11). Chestnut Hill, MA: Center for Retirement Research.

Carstensen, L. L., Mikels, J. A. & Mather, M. (2006). Aging and the intersection of cognition, motivation, and emotion. In J. E. Birren & K.W. Schaie (Eds.), *Handbook of the psychology of aging* (pp. 343–362). Burlington, MA: Elsevier.

Centers for Disease Control and Prevention. (2017). HIV Basics. Division of HIV/AIDS Prevention, National Center for HIV/AIDS, Viral Hepatitis, STD, and TB Prevention, Centers for Disease Control and Prevention. Retrieved from https://www.cdc.gov/hiv /basics/index.html

Central Intelligence Agency. (2016). World Fact Book. Retrieved from https://www.cia.gov/library /publications/the-world-factbook/geos/xx.html

Family Caregiving Alliance. (2016). *Caregiver statistics: Demographics*. Retrieved from https://www.caregiver .org/caregiver-statistics-demographics

Federal Interagency Forum on Aging-Related Statistics. (2016). *Older Americans 2016: Key indicators of well-being*. Federal Interagency Forum on Aging-Related Statistics. Washington, DC: U.S. Government Printing Office. Retrieved from https://agingstats .gov/docs/LatestReport/Older-Americans-2016-Key -Indicators-of-WellBeing.pdf

Howe, N., Jackson, R., Nakashima, K. (2007). The aging of Korea: Demographics and retirement policy in the land of the morning calm. Global Aging Initiative (p. 52). Washington, DC: Center for Strategic and International Studies, Global Aging Initiative.

Klassen, T. (2010). South Korea: Ageing tiger. *Global Brief*. Retrieved from http://globalbrief.ca/blog/2010/01/12 /south-korea-ageing-tiger/

Molzahn, A. E., Kalfoss, M., Makaroff, K. S., & Skevington, S. M. (2010). Comparing the importance of different aspects of quality of life to older adults across diverse cultures. *Age and Ageing, 40*, 192–199. doi:10.1093/ ageing/afq156

Mills, E. J., Bärnighausen, T., & Negin, J. (2012). HIV and aging—preparing for the challenges ahead. *The New England Journal of Medicine, 366*, 1270–1273. doi:10.1056/NEJMp1113643

National Institute on Aging, National Institutes of Health, World Health Organization. (2011). *Global health and aging*. (NIH Publication no. 11-7737). Washington, DC: U.S. Government Printing Office. Retrieved from http:// www.who.int/ageing/publications/global_health.pdf

OECD. (2017). *Obesity update 2017*. OECD Health Statistics. Retrieved from https://www.oecd.org/els /health-systems/Obesity-Update-2017.pdf

Pew Research Center. (2013). *Views on end-of-life medical treatments*. Retrieved from http://www.pewforum .org/2013/11/21/chapter-6-aging-and-quality-of-life/

Rowe, J. W., & Kahn, R. L. (1997). Successful aging. *The Gerontologist, 37*(4), 433–440. doi:10.1093/geront/37.4.433

Samper-Ternent, R., & Al Snih, S. (2012). Obesity in older adults: Epidemiology and implications for disability and disease. *Reviews in Clinical Gerontology, 22*(1), 10–34. doi:10.1017/S0959259811000190

Semega, J. L., Fontenot, K. R., & Kollar, M. A. (2017). *Income and poverty in the United States: 2016.* Report Number: P60-259. Washington, DC: U.S. Government Printing Office. Retrieved from https://www.census.gov/library/publications/2017/demo/p60-259.html

Statista. (2017). Median age of the U.S. population 2016, by state. Retrieved from https://www.statista.com/statistics/208048/median-age-of-population-in-the-usa-by-state/

Stepler, R. (2016). *Smaller share of women ages 65 and older are living alone: More are living with spouse or children.* Washington, DC: Pew Research Centers. Retrieved from http://www.pewsocialtrends.org/2016/02/18/smaller-share-of-women-ages-65-and-older-are-living-alone/

Steptoe, A., Deaton, A., & Stone, A. A. (2015). Subjective wellbeing, health, and ageing. *The Lancet, 385*(9968), 640–648. doi:10.1016/S0140-6736(13)61489-0

Tamburo, J. (2017). Issues, impacts, and implications of an aging workforce. American Society on Aging. Retrieved from http://www.asaging.org/blog/issues-impacts-and-implications-aging-workforce

Terry, D. F., Sebastiani, P., Andersen, S. L., & Perls, T. T. (2008). Disentangling the roles of disability and morbidity in survival to exceptional old age. *Archives of Internal Medicine, 168*(3), 277–283. doi:10.1001/archinternmed.2007.75

Tumen, S. (2016). The economic impact of Syrian refugees on host countries: Quasi-experimental evidence from Turkey. *American Economic Review, 106*(5), 456–460. doi:10.1257/aer.p20161065

United Nations, Department of Economic and Social Affairs. (2017). *World Population Prospects: The 2017 Revision, Key Findings and Advance Tables.* Working Paper No. ESA/P/WP/248.

United States Government Accountability Office. (2015). Retirement security: Most households approaching retirement have low savings. (GAO-15-419). Washington, DC: U.S. Government Printing Office. Retrieved from https://www.gao.gov/assets/680/670153.pdf

World Health Organization. (2017). Obesity and overweight. Fact Sheet. Retrieved from http://www.who.int/mediacentre/factsheets/fs311/en/

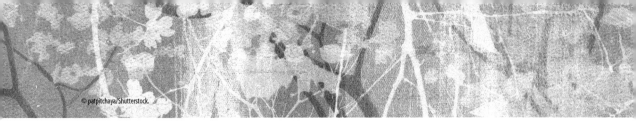
© patpitchaya/Shutterstock.

CHAPTER 2
Social Gerontology

Nancy Brossoie, PhD
Walter C. Chop, MS, RRT

CHAPTER OUTLINE

BEHAVIORAL OBJECTIVES

Upon completion of this chapter, the reader will be able to:

1. Define gerontology and how it differs from geriatrics.
2. Define ageism and explain why it is harmful to the health and well-being of older adults.
3. Identify and describe some of the social roles adults might hold in later life.
4. Describe the importance and focus of social relationships in late life.
5. Define elder abuse and describe the general characteristics of victims and abusers.
6. Define mandated reporter and describe the signs of potential abuse.
7. Explain why some older adults choose to work in late life.

KEY TERMS

AARP	Elder abuse	Older Americans Act (OAA)
Activity theory	Fictive kin	Polyvictimization
Adult Protective Services	Geriatrics	Sandwich generation
Ageism	Gerontology	Skip-generation household
Biopsychosocial	Grandfamilies	Self-neglect
Caregiver	Infantilizing	Senior Service America (SSA)
Continuity theory	Long-distance caregiver	Social roles
Convoy of support	Long-term care ombudsmen	Social Security
Discrimination	Mandatory reporters	Stereotypes
Disengagement theory	Older adults	Trusted individual

▶ Gerontology

The aging process begins the moment we are born. As we age, our bodies and minds grow, develop, and mature. During childhood, the course of our development is influenced by many factors, including our personal characteristics, our family background, how we are raised, where we grow up, and who raises us. Similarly, our development through adulthood continues to be influenced by our health, attitude, and behaviors and our interactions with family, friends, and the environment around us. Therefore, it is shortsighted to limit discussions about aging to matters of physical health and decline. Aging is a complex process influenced not only by health, but also by many other personal and social factors.

Gerontology is the scientific study of aging that examines the biological, psychological, and sociological (**biopsychosocial**) factors associated with old age and aging. The factors that affect how we age are broad in scope and diverse: biological factors include genetic background and physical health; psychological influences include level of cognition, mental health status, and general well-being; and sociological factors range from personal relationships to the cultures, policies, and infrastructure that organize society.

Although sometimes confused with the term gerontology, **geriatrics** is a medical term for the study, diagnosis, and treatment of diseases and health problems specific to **older adults**. Geriatricians (medical doctors who specialize in geriatrics) increasingly recognize the importance of social and psychological influences when treating patients. In this chapter, key issues in gerontology are presented to facilitate your understanding about the lifestyles of older adults and how these may influence health status.

In the field of social sciences, the term older adults is used to describe people age 65 years and older and is the preferred term when speaking about older individuals. The term patient is medically oriented and can refer to a person of any age. The term elderly has the social connotation of being white haired and frail. Because many people age 65 and older do not have gray hair and live vibrant healthy lifestyles, the term older adult has a more positive connotation, and therefore is preferred and used in this chapter.

▶ Historical Perspectives on Aging

Throughout history, older adults have been generally valued for the experience, insight, and wisdom they can share with others. Leadership is frequently bestowed upon older adults because of a social belief that wisdom and experience are acquired over time. However, conferring respect and responsibilities to older adults has not been consistent, and tends to occur more in preindustrial or agrarian societies where families are intergenerational and family members are dependent on one another for survival and support. For example, in 2004, hours before a tsunami in the Indian Ocean reached the shore, villagers from small fishing communities followed the leadership of their village elders and fled to safety. The suggestions of the elders were followed because the elders held the respect of the others and possessed the ability to interpret environmental cues that signaled impending danger, cues that were passed down to them from village elders long ago (Associated Press, 2004).

The image of the "wise old person" may be hard for those of us in the West to conceive, but in Eastern and indigenous cultures this is commonplace. West African teacher and author Malidoma Somé relayed the following description: "An elder is a repository for wisdom of the ancestors, the culture and the tribe. He or she is familiar with the various protocols for maintaining relationships with the other world and is keeper of the various 'recipes' that sustain the soul and spirit of the community. When elders are absent there is chaos and instability. The young are in charge but don't know where they are going" (Goodman, 2010, p. 415). Perhaps, we in the West can listen and learn from our elders as these other cultures do.

In industrial societies, older adults are generally less valued than they are in agrarian societies. During the 20th century, as industrialization in the United States expanded, family members became less dependent on each other for support, frequently leaving older adults to manage for themselves, which resulted in many older people living in poverty. In 1964, President Johnson launched the War on Poverty, which fought for institutionalizing civil rights, opportunities, and social services for all poor Americans to help lift them out of poverty. From that initiative, the **Older Americans Act (OAA)** of 1965 was passed into legislation. It specifically included language to address the needs and rights of older adults. The OAA is expected to be reauthorized indefinitely as one piece of legislation that represents the U.S. commitment to promoting the rights and welfare of older adults.

▶ Theories About Aging

Theories are used to guide research and help us make sense of the world around us. By using theory, we can better understand why individual behaviors or actions occur. In the early 1960s, when gerontology was a new field of research, the first psychosocial science theory on aging called **disengagement theory** was proposed by Cumming and Henry (1961). Guided by their observations of older adults in society, they proposed that older adults recognize that their health and abilities decline over time and their time as industrious citizens is limited before they die. In response, older adults intentionally remove themselves from their **social roles** and responsibilities to allow younger and healthier adults to take their place as productive members in society. At the time it was developed, the theory aligned well with social norms and social expectations of older adults. Society pressured adults to retire from the workplace at a preset age (e.g., mandatory retirement ages) and to relinquish their social responsibilities to younger people. However, the utility of disengagement theory was limited, because it did not it account for differences among individuals and did not accommodate the fact that if social norms were not enforced individuals would be less likely to disengage from life as the theory postulates.

In response to disengagement theory and to develop a better framework for examining old age, Havighurst (1961) attempted to explain aging through the use of **activity theory**. He posited that older adults are happier and healthier when they remain engaged in daily life and social interactions. He also suggested that as opportunities to be active change, older adults simply replace them with new ones to maintain their health and well-being. Although widely accepted as a positive view of aging, critics of activity theory suggest that it discriminates against individuals who do not have the resources to remain engaged or the interest in maintaining an active lifestyle.

The third major psychosocial theory used in gerontology is **continuity theory**. Originally proposed by Maddox (1965), it was further developed by Atchley (1989), who theorized that people remain consistent in how they live their life, manage their relationships, and exhibit their personalities even though they experience changes in their physical, mental, and social status. Continuity theory

can be used to help us understand the process by which older adults make decisions throughout adulthood. However, critics of continuity theory suggest it is based upon a healthy, wealthy, and male-oriented social model, and as such does not adequately account for the implicit social constraints placed on women, the chronically ill, or the role of social welfare programs in the lives of impoverished and needy older adults.

Social and behavioral scientists continue to build upon the three core theories to gain a better understanding of aging. Using a biopsychosocial approach, they combine the theoretical frameworks from the fields of psychology, sociology, and biology. They may also examine an issue utilizing a nuanced perspective (e.g., life course, feminist) or lens (e.g., LGBT, immigrant), which can open a window into the experiences and needs of the unique and often hidden populations not identified in other research. Our understanding of social science theories has grown exponentially in the last 50 years and is expected to continue at a fast pace as our aging population grows.

▶ Ageism

How we treat older adults is influenced by many social factors, including our own personal assumptions, expectations, and fears about growing older (Butler, 1969, 2008; Richeson & Shelton, 2006). Fears about aging are often based on our lack of understanding about the aging process. Unfortunately, many people believe that old age means being burdened with or suffering from physical disabilities, poor health, the inability to think clearly and quickly, and possessing a negative outlook on life. These inaccurate assumptions are examples of **ageism**, that is, the systematic labeling and **discrimination** against people who are old.

Ageism is based on **stereotypes**, myths about aging, and language that conjure up negative images of older adults. Ageism is to old age as racism is to skin color and sexism is to gender. Ageist thinking is detrimental to society and can result in limited opportunities (e.g., employment and workplace discrimination) and reduced access to resources (e.g., healthcare discrimination) for older adults. In its worst form, ageism leads to **elder abuse**, mistreatment, and neglect (Butler, 2008).

Ageist Stereotypes

Ageist comments place older adults into set roles or categories called stereotypes. For example, older adults are sometimes characterized as senile, grumpy, set in their ways and mannerisms, and slow to accept new ideas and learn new skills (**FIGURE 2-1**). Similarly, older adults also may be portrayed as eccentric or overly happy about life, perceiving it as rosy and carefree. When young family members witness ageist stereotyping in their own families and communities, they are likely to engage in ageist practices and thoughts themselves, as it can lead them to believe that older adults are different and perhaps unworthy of respect and kindness. Similarly, older adults who are subjected to ageist stereotyping often begin to accept the stereotypes as true, which consequently compromises their health, well-being, and longevity (Levy, Slade, Kunkel, & Kasl, 2002).

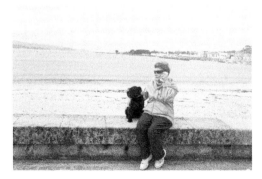

FIGURE 2-1 Most older adults are active, productive, and enjoy their lives.
© Tetxu/Shutterstock

Ageist attitudes permeate all facets of society, especially when money is involved. Negative connotations about older adults being "greedy geezers" first surfaced in the March 1988 issue of the magazine *The New Republic*. In that issue, older adults were described as wealthy with financial and social advantages, yet eager to siphon public money (e.g., **Social Security**) that should be dedicated to poor and needy children (Tagliareni & Waters, 1995). However, it must be realized that older adults paid into Social Security their entire working lifetime, and thus expect and are owed remuneration. Over the last 50 years, there has been a gradual improvement in attitudes toward older adults in the United States, thanks to greater public education and awareness, the OAA, and increased media attention. This, however, has done little to reverse deep undercurrents that run below the surface of ageism, as some people continue to view older adults as drains on public resources.

Myths About Aging

Older adults are not a homogeneous group. Even though collectively they may represent the same ideals and have shared the same historical experiences, they do not all look, think, or act alike. Older adults are as unique as members in any other group of people. Therefore, making blanket assumptions and generalizations about older adults simply perpetuates myths. The following statements are examples of myths that promote ageism. Although the statements may be accurate for some individuals, they are not true for older adults as a cohesive group (Butler, 2008; Richeson & Shelton, 2006; Palmore, 1990):

Myth 1: Older adults are either very rich or very poor.

Myth 2: Older adults are senile (have defective memory or are disoriented or demented).

Myth 3: Older adults are neither interested in nor have the capacity for sexual relations.

Myth 4: Older adults are miserable and unhappy with the state of their lives.

Myth 5: Older adults are very religious.

Myth 6: Older adults are unable to adapt to change.

Myth 7: Older adults are unable to learn new things.

Myth 8: Older adults generally want to live in nursing homes.

Myth 9: Older adults urinate on their clothing.

Myth 10: Older adults tend to be pretty much alike.

Ageist Language

Ageist language is insensitive to older adults, because it is used without much thought or understanding of how ageist terms hurt and degrade the individual. Some ageist terms include:

Geezer	Biddy
Hag	Fossil
Q-tip	Blue hair/Q tip
Boroi (Japanese slang for old and worn)	Old buck/codger
Old duffer	Old battleax
Dirty old man	Little (or dirty)
Old coot	old lady

Ageist phrases used in conversation also disparage older adults:

Over the hill	Set in their ways
Old school	One foot in the grave
Out to pasture	Ol' man _____
Older than dirt	(fill in name)
Gone senile	

Ageist Attitudes of Healthcare Professionals

Unfortunately, healthcare professionals are not immune to promoting ageist attitudes when treating their older patients (Alliance for Aging Research, 2003; Simkins, 2007). Providers who view older adult patients sympathetically as "poor old dears," who can do little to care for themselves, are actually placing little value on their patients' abilities. Calling an older patient "honey" or "dear" may be socially acceptable in some cultures, but generally carries a negative connotation. **Infantilizing** older adults by talking to them as if they were children with limited understanding, immature, or weak actually encourages dependency, because it devalues personal autonomy and individuality and does not promote person-centered care.

Other ageist terms used by medical professionals in describing patients in conversation or in medical charts include (Anti-Ageism Task Force, 2006):

"The wheelchair (or the stroke, hip fracture, etc.) in room number. . . ."

MFP (measure for pine box)

VAC (vultures are circling)

Bed blocker

GOMER (get out of my emergency room)

TMB (too many birthdays)

Research has shown that healthcare professionals are significantly more negative in their attitudes toward older patients than they are toward younger patients (Simkins, 2007). Although not appropriate, their negative attitudes can be attributed to several reasons:

- A need to justify why the medical needs of their older patient were not addressed or met.
- Feelings of frustration about not being able to manage the demands of the job.
- Feelings of helplessness due to not being able to save or cure patients' medical problems.
- Increased awareness or reminder of one's own life and mortality.

Awareness is the first step in overcoming an ageist attitude. To avoid making ageist comments and remarks as a healthcare professional, it is important to recognize and explore your personal feelings and attitudes about growing older. Stopping the spread of ageism is everyone's responsibility and starts at home.

Media Stereotyping of Older Adults

The media regularly perpetuate the stereotypes of older adults through inaccurate and sometimes demeaning portrayals of older adults in print, advertising, and entertainment. This is puzzling considering that older adults have the ability to purchase the products supporting the media, and thus should be able to facilitate changing attitudes in the industry. Yet, limited efforts have been made to alter how older adults are depicted. Perhaps, as more members of the baby boom generation reach old age, positive changes will emerge.

The entertainment industry plays a major role in perpetuating stereotypes. More often than not, older adults are portrayed as comical, stubborn, eccentric, and foolish. They are also often depicted as narrow-minded, sickly, poor, sexually dissatisfied, and slow to respond (Hilt & Lipshultz, 2016). Movie scripts tend to feature older adult characters only when they are reclusive (*Finding Forrester*), offer some extraordinary skill (*Space Cowboys*), dying (*The Notebook*), or facing their own mortality (*The Bucket List*). It is uncommon to watch older adult characters on the big screen portraying everyday people (*Return to Me*) in a manner that does not romanticize their lives (*Cocoon*), portray them as behaving comically (*Grumpy Old Men*), or proliferate the expectation that most people will get dementia (*Nebraska, Iris, On Golden Pond*).

Television show scripting is no different. Although we do see older adults on special programming, it is unusual to see a realistic portrayal of an older person on a television show (Hilt & Lipshultz, 2016). Again, this network programming decision is puzzling, considering that television shows are targeted for specific demographic audiences who are apt to buy the sponsors' products. Older adults watch television more than any other age group and generally have the discretionary income to buy the products advertised during commercials (Hilt & Lipshultz, 2016).

Yet, limited efforts have been made to accurately depict the lives of older adults on television, with the exception of selected actors such as Jane Fonda, Lily Tomlin, Judi Dench, Betty White, Maggie Smith, and a few noteworthy others.

Print and television advertisements also tend to portray older adults at their worst—when they have some kind of physical ailment or have the desire to look and feel younger. We see older actors in commercials for laxatives, skin moisturizers, gas elimination medications, analgesics, and hair coloring products, just to name a few. This would not be as detrimental to the image of the older adult if we also saw older adults in other types of commercials advertising general use products.

▶ Social Roles in the Second Half of Life

Social roles are useful in identifying, defining, and validating each member of a society. A social role not only defines a position, but also supports social norms and expectations that dictate behaviors and attitudes within social groups such as families, workplaces, and communities. Some social roles remain with us throughout our lives (e.g., friend, cousin, daughter), whereas other roles change or transform as new levels of accomplishment or development are reached. For example, a person may transition from being a student to a teacher or from a worker to a retiree. In late life, social roles are more apt to remain constant (e.g., neighbor, club member, and community resident); however, the level of participation in those roles may fluctuate as changes in health, finances, and mobility occur. Nonetheless, older adults continue to participate in many of their social roles, even when faced with diminished capacities and capabilities (Ferraro, 2001). Three new roles often taken on in the second half of life include retiree, grandparent, and **caregiver**.

Retiree

For many retirees, adjusting to changes in social role and status that accompany leaving the workforce can be difficult. When they were employed, they were granted a status that provided them with respect and support from their colleagues, friends, and acquaintances. However, transitioning from a position of daily recognition and involvement to one with limited recognition and possible isolation from other individuals can be psychologically difficult (Wang, 2007). Although no single solution exists for making the social adjustment into retirement, it can be made easier with planning and preparation. Retirement planning advisors strongly suggest that in addition to financial planning, older workers plan their retirement routines, hobbies, habits, and social interactions, so that they can remain engaged and socially connected, which will enhance their quality of life. Additional information about retirement planning is provided in this chapter under the heading Employment and Civic Engagement.

Grandparent

Grandparenting is a social role that many adults look forward to once their children leave home and establish their own lives. Because people are living longer, it is not uncommon for older adults to take on the role of great-grandparent or even great-great-grandparent. The U.S. Census Bureau estimated that approximately one in four adults in the United States were grandparents in 2010 (MetLife Mature Market Institute, 2011).

Grandparents generally welcome interactions with their grandchildren as a chance to relive their early years without balancing the stresses and responsibilities of caring for their own children the first time around. Grandparenting also offers them the possibility for sharing their wisdom and lived experiences with their grandchildren. A new grandchild can also be like a booster shot for some older couples, reawakening early days of marriage and the enthusiasm of early parenting (Berkman & Breslow, 1983).

Not surprisingly, the role of a grandparent is as varied as any other social role. Grandparents share multiple roles and responsibilities within families, and as such can be described as one of five distinct types (Neugarten & Weinstein, 1964):

- Distance figures (live far away and visit infrequently)
- Fun seekers (provide and engage in exciting opportunities)
- Surrogate parents (take on a parenting role)
- Formal (as patriarch or matriarch of the family)
- Reservoirs of family wisdom (sources of knowledge and expertise)

Yet, the role of a grandparent is not static. The role of a grandparent today needs to be responsive to the needs of the extended family. In the United States, one of the most important roles of a grandparent is that of a caregiver (**FIGURE 2-2**). Grandparents can support grandchildren in the broadest sense by providing child care, paying educational costs, and sometimes providing the deposit for large expenses such as a new house. The toy industry, especially, likes grandparents because they purchase approximately

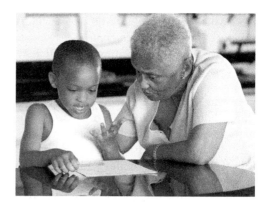

FIGURE 2-2 Grandparents often take on a surrogate parent role.

© Rolf Bruderer/Blend Images/Getty Image

25% of all toys, 40% of all children's books, and 20% of all children's video games (Howe, 2016).

Surrogate Parent

Increasingly, more grandparents are assuming a primary parental role in raising their grandchildren. In 2015, the U.S. Census estimated that 2.6 million grandparents had full responsibility for providing for their grandchildren's basic needs. Among them, one million children did not have a parent actively involved in their lives (U.S. Census Bureau, 2017a). These **grandfamilies** or **skip-generation households** are largely formed due to substance misuse (e.g., opioid addiction and alcohol dependence) and incarceration of parents (i.e., the grandparents' adult children).

The role of becoming a surrogate parent in late life can be demanding because it requires engaging in all aspects of a child's life, including associating with teachers and other parents who are much younger. This new social role can be quite fulfilling and simultaneously challenging—especially when undertaken with a fixed retirement income, managing personal health problems, balancing personal needs with parenting demands, and having to cope with the social stigma attached to the adult child's inability to parent. More and more communities are establishing community support programs for grandparents in an effort to provide a way to connect grandfamilies, help grandparents learn how to navigate social service systems, and provide needed counseling and legal resources.

Caregiver

Becoming a caregiver for a spouse, family member, or friend is another social role most people do not think about until they find themselves faced with providing care. An estimated 14.3% of all U.S. adults are a caregiver to person age 50+ (National Alliance for Caregiving & AARP Public Policy Institute, 2015). Caregiving responsibilities can emerge slowly or start suddenly after an illness or accident. Sometimes, the need for assistance is so imperceptible that neither the caregiver nor the care recipient recognizes the full extent of decline over time. For example, providing care to a spouse can be a lengthy and subtle process with the tasks gradually increasing in intensity before transitioning into a full time job and before other family members are even aware of the need.

When that time comes, adult children are apt to intervene, even though they are ill-prepared to take on the caregiving role. Although each family is different, researchers have found a common pattern in family caregiving within the United States. Generally, older adults depend on the oldest daughter (or daughter-in-law) to provide assistance with activities of daily living and rely on the eldest son for support with financial and estate matters (Suitor, Pillemer, Keeton, & Robison, 1996). This does not mean that other family members will not be asked to help or will not offer to help. It simply means that, culturally, older adults expect specific assistance from these offspring.

In many families, adult children are unaware of the daily routines, habits, and needs of their parents until a health crisis arises and additional support in the home is needed. Like their children, most older adults want to live independently and do not want to live with other family members (Bursack, n.d.). They also do not want to share their financial information or include their children in their decision-making processes. Older adults want to retain control over their lives. So, it comes as no surprise that many older adults resist accepting the role of care recipient. They are unwilling to relinquish their roles and responsibilities to other people, even when they know they could use help. Out of pride, some older adults remain adamant about not accepting support until they reach a point where they cannot function without it.

When additional support or care is needed, approximately 83% of support received comes from family members (National Alliance for Caregiving, 2005). One study estimated that 24% of caregivers of older adults lived with the person they were caring for, 42% lived within 20 minutes away, and 15% lived more than 1 hour away—referred to as **long-distance caregivers**. Nearly 7 million Americans are long-distance caregivers for an older relative (MetLife & National Alliance for Caregiving, 2008).

As family caregiving evolves and continues over time, it can demand more of the adult child caregivers' time, leaving less time for family care involving their own children. This can be especially challenging for caregivers simultaneously providing care to two or more generations. Adults found in this position are often referred to as the **sandwich generation**, because they are caught between two caregiving roles—caring for a child and caring for a parent (or even a grandparent).

Social Roles in Context

Most Western societies, including the United States and Western Europe, stress individualism (i.e., the needs of the individual are addressed before the needs of the group). Other cultures such as those found in Asia and the Pacific Islands are collectivist societies; that is, members place the needs of the family or collective group (which may be an intergenerational family) before the needs of the individual. Differences between individual and collective perspectives naturally inform how groups perceive older adults and place responsibility for providing care and support. Understanding how groups differ can assist in the planning and provision of effective healthcare services, no matter where the care is provided.

In an individualistic society, older adults are generally free to remain living independently and managing life as they see fit as long as they can afford it and they are not placing themselves or others in immediate danger. In a collectivist society, the resources of the older adults are pooled with other family resources. The activities of daily life are shared rather than lived separately. As a result, living expenses are reduced because the older adult lives with other family members. For example, in India, when a parent joins a young household, he or she is welcomed as a member of the household. Even though the household may not have planned to include the older adult, family members willingly make accommodations for the aging family member (Pinto & Sahur, 2001). In a Filipino household, the youngest daughter is expected to care for the older adult at home until she marries, and then moves the older adult with her to her husband's home (Torres, 2002).

The social role of the older adult within the household also varies by social expectations. Ethnic groups that revere elders as authority figures enable the older adults to reside in positions of power within the family and community. Other ethnic groups take an almost opposite view and see older adults in terms of added responsibility, if not burden, to family and society.

In the Vietnamese culture, a grandparent shares household authority with the father of the household. His or her place in the family is highly regarded (Hunt, 2002). In contrast, in the old Athabascan Indian culture in Alaska, older adults were seen as burdens—a drain on food and resources in the harsh and demanding climate. Older adults were expected to contribute as much as possible until the day when the chief of the tribe would leave them to die in the wilderness in an effort to preserve resources for the healthy and strong members of the tribe (Wallis, 1993).

Family life and respect for the knowledge and wisdom of elders are central to Asian culture. This has, however, decreased somewhat in the Asian American population with modernization and assimilation into American society. However, Asian cultures remain strongly collectivistic and believe family life is central to their existence (Brightman & Subedi, 2007; Kim-Rupnow, 2001).

Even though collectivism may appear to be an effective approach to managing family and social resources, sometimes it has not been perceived as beneficial to people with disabilities, including dementia. They are often viewed as an embarrassment to the family because they are not strong enough to contribute their fair share of family responsibilities. As a result, they are frequently disowned, abandoned, and left to beg on the streets to get their needs met, further increasing the collectivist society's disdain for them. Because individuals with special needs (i.e., physical, cognitive, and/or behavioral) generally do not have strong support from within the collectivist society to lead a productive and successful life, they are challenged to determine their own life course (Jezewski & Sotnik, 2001).

In the United States and in other individualistic societies, the strong belief in individualism has produced legislation that has protected the rights of people with long-term disabilities (e.g., the Americans with Disabilities Act) and has provided accommodations for people with physical and mental health needs in communities and the workplace. Coupled with legislation through the OAA, significant strides have continued to be made to ensure that older adults are legally protected to lead full and productive lives.

A great deal of research has been conducted in the United States on family dynamics and the roles and responsibilities of family members. The United States has become a mobile and independent society in which intergenerational households and the strong reliance on family as a source of sole support are no longer the norm. Yet, among some racial groups such as African Americans, families still tend to maintain extensive kin networks to provide help, especially to young family members and neighbors. Community-based institutions such as the church are also viewed as very important sources of physical and emotional support. Similarly, Hispanic Americans, who make up 17.8% of the U.S. population (U.S. Census Bureau, 2017b) maintain close family relationships that promote family solidarity. They have more contact with their children than their non-Hispanic counterparts (Garcia, 2001). As the number of older adults surpassing age 65 increases, additional studies will need to be conducted to examine how different ethnic groups are coping and meeting the needs of their aging parents.

▶ Social Relationships

Personal Relationships

Maintaining social relationships contribute to better physical health and provide emotional and psychological benefits, including better sense of belonging, increased self-worth, and feelings of security—all of which contribute to improved psychological well-being (Qualls, 2014). The importance of retaining personal relationships does not diminish as one ages. Older adults desire and engage in social relationships like younger adults, although their relationships are likely to reduce in number and type. Opportunities to socialize are also likely to lessen when personal health declines or mobility becomes more difficult.

Research on personal relationships has also shown that as we age and our health declines, we intentionally distance ourselves from some of our relationships, retaining only the ones from which we can benefit and know we can maintain (Berkman & Breslow, 1983). We do this because we recognize that relationships should be reciprocal. If we no longer have the ability, energy, or resources to exchange support, we let go of those relationships. The people we choose to retain in our social circle in late life tend to be people from whom we draw strength and value the most, like family members. Kahn and Antonucci (1980) aptly described the evolution of personal social network as a **convoy of support**, moving with the individual through life challenges and transitions. Relationships maintained in late life can serve a variety of purposes and take place within a variety of contexts. The following sections provide additional insights into some of the different types of relationships older adults enjoy and how they maintain them.

Computers and Social Media

Computers play a large role in keeping older adults connected to family and friends, reconnecting old friends, and developing new relationships. Accessing the Internet is gaining popularity as friends encourage friends to "get connected." A 2017 study by the Pew Research Center (2017a) indicated that 67% of adults age 65+ used the Internet, and among them 75% went online daily. Fifty-one percent of all older Internet users had Internet service in their home. All older Internet users tended to be more educated with higher incomes than nonusers. Similarly, owning a tablet or eReader (e.g., Nook, Kindle) was associated with advanced education and high income. In 2015, 25% of older adult users also reported playing online video games, an activity largely pursued by younger adults.

Like their younger counterparts, older adults are increasingly keeping in touch through email and social media rather than relying on letters and telephone calls, as their parents did. Computers have enabled older adults to remain in touch and stay current with activities in the lives of children, grandchildren, and friends who have moved away (**FIGURE 2-3**). In 2017, 34% of older adults reported using Facebook or Twitter, a 7% increase over the past 4 years (Pew Research Center, 2017a). Similarly, chat

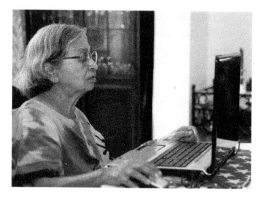

FIGURE 2-3 Email is an easy way for interested older adults to maintain communication with family and friends.
© Paul Maguire/Shutterstock

rooms and online dating services have also increased and enabled older adults to establish new relationships for companionship and love (Malta, 2007).

For older adults who have never used a computer, learning to operate one may be initially challenging. Among adults age 65+ who reported getting a new digital device, 73% reported needing someone else to set it up for them (Pew Research Center, 2017a). However, many community centers and libraries provide periodic classes on how to send email, surf the web, access social media sites, play games, and use word processing programs.

The Aging Couple

Like other adult couples, some older adults have been married or in a committed relationship for decades, whereas others have more recently become a couple later in life (**FIGURE 2-4**). Older men who find themselves single generally have no problem finding female companionship because, statistically, women continue to outlive men. The 2010 United States Census Bureau confirmed that assumption by reporting that by age 85 there were 100 women for every 54 men (U.S. Census Bureau, 2011).

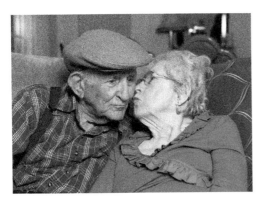

FIGURE 2-4 Expressions of love and affection.

© Fotoluminate LLC/Shutterstock

Couple relationships that have endured into old age have probably experienced and overcome many challenges and crises along the way. Health problems aside, one of the earliest challenges faced in later life occurs during transition into retirement. For some couples, it is a time of deep soul searching, redefining social roles as individuals, and wondering what the future of the couple relationship will be like (Silverstone & Hyman, 1992).

If a couple can successfully weather the challenges associated with retirement, their feelings for each other can actually become enriched and strengthened. However, problems can arise when each person struggles with the change at different times. For example, if one person is ready to retire while the other one is not or one wants to sell the family home and move to a warmer climate and the other does not, problems in the relationship often arise. Subsequently, some couples spend considerable time reflecting on the value, purpose, and usefulness of their relationship during this stage of life. For many, this is just another one of life's challenges that they will share and work through together. Others, however, will see it as a reason and opportunity to dissolve their relationship.

Many other couples choose not to grow old together. Maybe they have stayed together for the sake of the children or perhaps they became absorbed in work or other activities over the years to avoid having to deal with underlying relationship issues. These couples may share their lives but might not be emotionally engaged. They may be genuinely fond of each other but view their relationship as more of a business partnership than a marriage. Similar to a marriage of convenience, each partner "does his or her own thing." Sometimes, one or both partners engage in extramarital affairs (even into late life), which can bring about the final unraveling of the marriage.

The Pew Research Center (2017b) reports that, in 2016, 61% of adults ages 50+ were married and the rate of divorce has been steadily rising. In 1990, only 5% of older adults were divorced, yet by 2015 more than 10% were divorced. Research has shown that divorce rates are higher among second, third, or subsequent marriages, which are reflected in this data. However, it is important to note that divorce cannot be only attributed to persons with multiple marriages. Among the couples divorced in 2015, 34% had been in a first marriage lasting at least 30 years and 10% had a marriage lasting at least 40 years. Cohabitation with a sexual partner is also on the rise among older adults and corresponds to the divorce rate. Older adults ages 50+ represent 23% of all cohabiting adults—a rate increase of 75% since 2007. Unlike their younger counterparts, older cohabitants have a history of marriage and are often older. Thirteen percent of older adult cohabiters are aged 70+.

Although some relationships worsen or dissolve with age, others actually get better and experience a renewal or rebirth. Communication often improves and affection and intimacy can become recharged. Late life can be the most satisfying years of a marriage for the couple who finds contentment in their relationship and has come to accept one another for who they are (Silverstone & Hyman, 1992).

In many ways, late-life relationships among same-sex couples are no different than for opposite-sex couples. Aside from sexual orientation, the main difference is public visibility. For many lesbian (i.e., a woman is sexually attracted to women), gay (i.e., a man is sexually attracted to men), and bisexual (i.e., an individual has a sexual attraction to both men and women) elders born more than 65 years ago, a lifetime of social marginalization, persecution, and denial of civil rights because of sexual orientation has forced them to keep their partnerships secret. Even though many lesbian, gay, bisexual, and transgendered (LGBT) couples have built lives that contradict negative social identities, many remain reluctant to reach out to the greater community for support services in late life (Meisner & Hynie, 2009; National Resource Center on LGBT Aging, 2013). The challenge for healthcare professionals in offering services to members of the LGBT community is gaining access and providing care that respects their personal choice and right to self-determine care, just like those afforded members of the heterosexual community.

Aging Parent and Adult Child

Relationships between aging parents and adult children also tend to be as varied as spousal relationships. Within most families, there is a fair degree of positive involvement between generations. Many parents continue to provide emotional, physical, and financial support to their adult children and grandchildren to help them manage their lives. Ideally, support would be provided with good intentions with "no strings attached." However, an underlying reason for helping out younger family members may include a hope or unspoken agreement that help will be reciprocated in later years when needed (Silverstone & Hyman, 1992).

Unfortunately, strained relations can develop between a parent and child in adulthood. Verbal finger pointing—unfair fighting with "you never" or "you always" statements—can upset relationships, as can favoritism toward some family members over others. Sometimes, parental disapproval of a lifestyle or friends generates family disharmony. Feelings of disappointment coupled with shame may lead older parents to preserve their own public image instead of their sons' or daughters' needs and feelings. However, if affection and communication remain open between a parent and adult child, their psychological well-being will benefit and their relationship will grow stronger (Silverstone & Hyman, 1992).

One relatively recent challenge faced by many older adults has been the increased prevalence of substance misuse (i.e., dependence on alcohol and drugs) and incarceration rates among their adult children. Subsequently, many older adults are forced to deal with the addictive behaviors of their adult child (or grandchild), a task many are ill-prepared to undertake. Studies indicate that the problems of adult children are a significant cause of depression in older adults—the greater the child's problem, the greater the parent's depression. Older adults continue to want the best for their children, no matter what their age, and are often emotionally affected by the challenges and failures their offspring encounter (Dunham, 1995).

Never Married or Childless in Late Life

Approximately, 4% of the population in the United States age 65 and older has never married (Tamborinia, 2007). Also notable is the increase of women in the United States who have never borne a child (nearly 20%)—a rate that has nearly doubled since the 1970s (Tamborinia, 2007).

The reasons for remaining single and for not bearing children are numerous and personal. Still, social roles and expectations of older adults are often centered on being coupled and having families. This narrow perspective leads some people to wonder how never married and childless people receive support later in life and from whom.

Although some people may assume that never married and childless couples have been deprived of the emotional support of family in late life, research suggests otherwise. Happiness, life satisfaction, loneliness, and self-esteem appear to be unrelated to contact with adult children during late life (Connidis & McMullin, 1993). Many never married and childless couples have adjusted by adapting their social network to include relationships generally thought to be held by partners and children. These **fictive kin** are treated as family and linked by close emotional bonds (Jordan-Marsh & Harden, 2005). Sometimes, a niece or a nephew takes on the social role of a child or a sibling takes on some of the traditional roles of a spouse. Despite the social pressure to marry and bear children, individuals who do not conform to social pressure are not emotionally unstable in later life (**FIGURE 2-5**). Never marrying or remaining childless is not something to be pitied or viewed as a curiosity. It is simply another way of life.

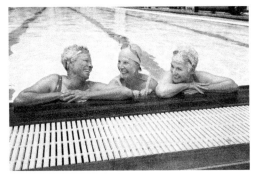

FIGURE 2-5 Friendships are sources of emotional and motivational support.
© Jupiter Images/DigitalVision/Getty Images

Friendships

Friendships established early in life often continue into old age, especially if they begin during midlife. Unlike relationships with family members who are connected by blood ties and replete with social roles and expectations, friendships exist because the individuals involved share similar interests and want to maintain the relationship. Like younger adults, older adults tend to establish friendships with people similar to themselves: same gender, similar social and economic status, and from the same town or community. However, as friendships deteriorate as a result of increased distance, poor health, or death, new ones are formed if the older adult has the access and opportunity to build a new connection. The ability to form new relationships is essential because an important outcome of friendship is enhanced psychological well-being. Research indicates that friendships have an even stronger influence on well-being than do familial relationships, although the precise relationship remains unclear (Adams, Leibbrandt, & Moon, 2011).

Studies have also shown that women have more friends than men do, because they view and engage in friendships differently (Antonucci, 2001). Women perceive friendships to be sources of ongoing emotional and physical support and prefer to surround themselves with friends who can help them address the daily challenges they face. When a friendship ends, it is replaced with a new one. Thus, women are intentional about managing their friendships so that they maintain the desired complement of friends to help them process the events in their life. Men, however, prefer to rely on their spouse, partner, or close family members for help and emotional support rather than friends. Males' friendships are based on specific activities such as a sport or a project rather than sharing feelings and processing a particular situation or event. As a result, men tend to require fewer friends than women do.

Like young adults, older adults nurture their friendships and feel a sense of loss when a friendship dissolves or becomes inactive. Poor health, new living arrangements, and loss in mobility frequently change the course of friendships and make sustaining them that much more difficult. As Kahn and Antonucci (1980) proposed in their "convoy of support" when maintaining relationships becomes too difficult to manage, older adults will break off some relationships because they recognize they cannot reciprocate support. Instead, they choose to place their energy and resources into their most valued relationships—those with their closest family and friends.

▶ Elder Abuse

Elder abuse is an insidious and often hidden problem, which is expected to increase as baby boomers reach old age. Elder abuse is a form of family or domestic violence, which can be defined as "intentional or neglectful acts by a caregiver or **trusted individual** that lead to, or may lead to, harm of a vulnerable elder" (Centers for Disease Control and Prevention, 2016). For some victims, their abuse is a continuation of abuse or violence that began years earlier, and for other victims, their abuse started in late life after they became more dependent on someone else for help, support, and care (Rennison, 2001).

Accurate statistics on the prevalence of elder abuse are hard to find because incidents are rarely reported, and when they are, how they are recorded varies by the reporting agency. In 2016, the CDC convened a panel of experts to come up with definitions to streamline the process. The first challenge they faced was determining who qualifies as an elder. Most organizations, like the American Medical Association (AMA), do not specify the age of an elder, whereas the OAA which funds aging services defines an

elder as a person age 60 or older. The second challenge was identifying how abuse is categorized. The AMA categorizes and reports abuse by physical or mental injury, sexual abuse, and withholding of necessary food, clothing, and medical care. The National Center on Elder Abuse (NCEA) advocates for more precise categorization that includes physical abuse, psychological abuse, sexual abuse, exploitation, neglect, abandonment, and **self-neglect** (**TABLE 2-1**). Regardless of the typology of abuse utilized, research indicates that each type of abuse does not necessarily occur in isolation. Rather, abuse may expand to include multiple forms of abuse known as **polyvictimization** (Ramsey-Klawsnik, 2017; Roberto, 2017).

In light of the data analysis challenges, a research team in New York triangulated data collected by agencies and programs responsible for serving victims with information collected by citizens age 60+. The team estimated that approximately 7% of the older population has experienced some form of abuse in the previous year; an estimate slightly lower than other research has indicated (Acierno et al., 2010). For every case reported in New York, approximately 24 cases went unreported. The rates of abuse vary by type of abuse, with the most frequent type of abuse reported being financial (Lifespan of Greater Rochester, Inc., Weill Cornell Medical Center of Cornell University, & New York City Department for the Aging, 2011).

Victims of Abuse

Like individual victims of domestic violence, victims of elder abuse are unique but share common characteristics. Many victims are isolated from their social networks and communities. Their isolation may be of their own choosing or may occur because their abusers have systematically isolated them to maintain more power and control over them. Many victims experience physical and mental health

TABLE 2-1 NCEA Definitions of the Seven Types of Elder Abuse[a]

Type	Definition
Physical	Use of force to threaten or physically injure a vulnerable elder.
Psychological	Verbal attacks, threats, rejection, isolation, or belittling acts that cause or could cause mental anguish, pain, or distress to an elder.
Sexual	Sexual contact that is forced, tricked, threatened, or otherwise coerced upon another person, including anyone who is unable to grant consent.
Exploitation	Theft, fraud, misuse or neglect of authority, and use of "undue influence" as a lever to gain control over an older person's money or property.
Neglect	Failure or refusal by a caregiver to provide for a vulnerable elder's safety, physical, or emotional needs.
Abandonment	Desertion of a frail or vulnerable elder by anyone with a duty of care.
Self-neglect	Inability to understand the consequences of one's own actions or inaction, which leads to, or may lead to, harm or endangerment.

[a]National Center on Elder Abuse (n.d.).

problems, some of which are exacerbated by ongoing abuse.

A typical victim of elder abuse is female, age 75+, lives alone, has physical or cognitive impairments, lacks a network of social support, and is reliant on other people for care and support. A victim's hesitancy to challenge or confront a perpetrator or report abuse to persons in a position to stop the abuse can be difficult for someone outside the relationship to understand. However, the victim's need for care and reliance on the perpetrator for support is so great that they tend to not report problems out of fear that they will be without services and support if they speak up. Moreover, they do not want other people to know they are in their current situation, they do not want to get the perpetrator in trouble (especially if the abuser is a close relative or friend), or they fear how the perpetrator might treat them after being reported. For many victims, the inconvenience

of being abused outweighs the perceived consequences of reporting; so they remain silent (Lafferty, 2009).

Self-Neglect Among Older Adults

A very challenging type of elder abuse to address and eliminate is self-neglect. The behaviors exhibited by individuals who self-neglect (e.g., not bathing, wearing clothes inappropriate for the weather, poor nutrition) challenge the social norms and values shared by the general population. Self-neglecting behaviors left unchecked can permeate all facets of life, including personal care, home environment, and personal relationships. Interventions that strive to reduce problems or alleviate conditions related to self-neglect are difficult to initiate and sustain because participants decide not to participate. When supporting individuals who self-neglect, it is imperative to honor their personal autonomy and legal right to live as they choose, if they are competent to make this decision, no matter how difficult or frustrating it may appear to you.

Perpetrators of Abuse

There is limited information available about perpetrators of elder abuse because victims are hesitant to identify them and file legal charges against them. In most cases, the relationship between a victim and a perpetrator has been established long before the abuse begins. Perpetrators present themselves to the elder and the elder's family as a good caring person or a supportive resource. Even if they did not initially plan to abuse their victim, perpetrators become savvy in manipulating how they present themselves, making it hard for individuals outside the victim/perpetrator relationship to recognize problems.

Although general public opinion is that most perpetrators are male offspring, available evidence suggests not all perpetrators are alike (Roberto, 2017). Among family members who provided care and perpetrated abuse, many typically relied on the elder for housing, financial support, and emotional support (Jackson & Hafemeister, 2012). Substance misuse (alcohol and drugs) is another characteristic among perpetrators (Jackson & Hafemeister, 2012). But, as found in cases of domestic violence, substance misuse may contribute to lowered inhibitions and poor decision-making but does not cause the abuse inflicted. The complex interdependent relationship between family perpetrators and their victims can be even more difficult to understand when the victim is cognitively impaired (Wiglesworth et al., 2010). Such abuse can be easily hidden or explained as the victim is unlikely to be believed if abuse is reported.

Perpetrators of financial abuse tend to be professionals (e.g., attorneys, financial planners, and conservators) entrusted with fiduciary care (MetLife Mature Market Institute, 2009). Legal guardians are also often involved with misappropriating assets and money through schemes that benefit themselves at the expense of the elders (United States Government Accountability Office, 2010). Healthcare providers can also be perpetrators of abuse. Reports of physical abuse, including use of physical restraint in feeding and toileting, hitting, beating, kicking, and sexual abuse, have been reported. Teaster and Roberto (2004) further found that having a diagnosis of Alzheimer's disease predicted physical abuse of an elder by staff. Moreover, residents perpetuated sexual abuse on other residents over 90% of the time. The forms of sexual abuse initiated included unwelcomed sexual interest in the body, sexualized kissing, fondling, and unwelcomed discussion of sexual activity (Teaster & Roberto, 2004).

Signs of Abuse

Because elder abuse can be a hidden problem that is easily overlooked or explained by health-related problems, the NCEA developed a list of signs of abuse to promote awareness among families and healthcare providers (**TABLE 2-2**).

Mandated Reporting

There is no federal law against elder abuse; however, all states have some form of law or laws against acts of elder abuse. These laws also provide for the reporting of suspected elder abuse. Depending on the state law, healthcare professionals, including doctors, nurses, rehabilitation therapists, and social workers, may be **mandatory reporters**. Therefore, it is vital that healthcare professionals continually assess for signs of abuse and report when they suspect a problem.

Some organizations have a protocol for reporting suspected abuse of children

TABLE 2-2 NCEA Signs of Abuse[a]

Type of Abuse	Signs of Abuse
Physical & Sexual	▪ Inadequately explained fractures, bruises, welts, cuts, sores, or burns. ▪ Unexplained sexually transmitted diseases.
Psychological	▪ Unexplained or uncharacteristic changes in behavior such as withdrawal from normal activities, unexplained changes in alertness, etc. ▪ Caregiver isolates elder (does not let anyone into the home or speak to the elder). ▪ Caregiver is verbally aggressive or demeaning, controlling, overly concerned about spending money, or uncaring.
Exploitation	▪ Lack of amenities a victim could afford. ▪ Vulnerable elder/adult "voluntarily" giving uncharacteristically excessive financial reimbursement/gifts for needed care and companionship. ▪ Caregiver has control of elder's money but is failing to provide for the elder's needs. ▪ Vulnerable elder/adult has signed property transfers (power of attorney, new will, etc.) but is unable to comprehend the transaction or what it means.
Neglect	▪ Lack of basic hygiene, adequate food, or clean and appropriate clothing. ▪ Lack of medical aids (glasses, walker, teeth, hearing aid, medications). ▪ Person with dementia is left unsupervised. ▪ Person confined to bed is left without care. ▪ Home cluttered, filthy, in disrepair, or having fire and safety hazards. ▪ Home without adequate facilities (stove, refrigerator, heat, cooling, plumbing, electricity, and parking). ▪ Untreated pressure "bed" sores (pressure ulcers).

[a]National Center on Elder Abuse (n.d.).

and elders, and healthcare professionals are encouraged to utilize the system at their workplace. Ultimately, the state and local **Adult Protective Service** (APS) agencies are the frontline responders investigating reports of abuse. Reports to law enforcement will eventually be connected to APS in most states, so either contact should be appropriate. APS missions vary state to state, but generally focus on protecting the rights of vulnerable adults and adults with disabilities. **Long-term care ombudsmen** (LTCO) are advocates for residents in long-term care facilities and are responsible for care provided within a

geographic region. The LTCO can directly receive reports of suspected abuse or work with APS to resolve elder abuse problems within a facility. For more information about the roles and responsibilities of a LTCO, visit ltcombudsman.org/about/about-ombudsman.

Reporting typically involves giving the name and contact information of the person suspected of being abused as well as specific details related to the suspected abuse. Reporting may also include the reporter giving his or her own contact information. Some states allow for anonymous reporting, in which the states protect the confidentiality of reporters.

▶ Employment and Civic Engagement

The U.S. Bureau of Labor Statistics projects that from 2014 to 2024, the fastest growing segments of the labor force will include workers age 65–74 and age 75+ (Toossi & Torpey, 2017). Although the number of older workers will be fewer than the number of younger workers, their participation rate (i.e., people working or actively seeking work) will exceed that of the entire labor force. The rationale for continuing to work is multifold. People are living longer and want to continue to work because they enjoy it, they want something interesting to do, they want to stay physically and mentally active, and they want to financially support themselves (AARP, 2014). Older workers who remain in the workforce generally occupy management and professional positions, followed by sales and office work, service work, production, and manual labor (Toossi & Torpey, 2017). Not surprisingly, jobs that place wear and tear on the body are less likely to appeal to an aging worker.

Older workers want to remain in the labor force (AARP, 2014). If not for financial gain, they want to engage in productive pursuits that provide meaning and validation to their lives. When asked about the ideal job, workers age 45–74 indicated that their ideal jobs were personally meaningful to them. Specifically, the ideal job would provide the opportunity to use personal skills and talents (92%), include a friendly work environment (92%), offer the chance to do something worthwhile (88%), offer respect from coworkers (82%), and respect from the boss (81%). The ability to work from home (36%), ethnic and racial diversity (40%), opportunity to work part-time (43%), and the opportunity to phase into retirement (53%) were ranked lowest in terms of requirements for an ideal job (AARP, 2014). Clearly, the benefits older workers look for in their work are personal and provide validation for the knowledge and skills they bring into the workplace.

Among workers age 65+, 40% work part-time (Toossi & Torpey, 2017). Ever more employers are now viewing older workers as an untapped resource to share experience and expertise with younger workers. The method of utilizing the skills and leadership of older workers is through "bridge employment," which typically occurs as the older worker transitions from full-time work to part-time work and then into full retirement. Many businesses and professions, now facing skills shortages, are beginning to view the retention of older workers as making good business sense. A retiring person who has been with an organization a long time possesses valuable institutional memory (i.e., understanding of the processes and decisions made in the past), which needs to be passed on to new personnel. Preserving organizational history is prompting some employers to seriously consider allowing loyal older workers to continue on a part-time basis, at least as they transition into retirement (Ng & Law, 2014).

Workplace Discrimination

The U.S. Age Discrimination in Employment Act (1967) prohibits employment discrimination against people age 40+. Yet, despite its existence, at least 60% of workers (age 45+) report being discriminated against in the workplace because of their age (AARP, 2014). Extensive research has been conducted on social attitudes toward older workers. Many employers and employees inaccurately perceive older workers to be rigid, inflexible, incapable of learning new skills, unproductive, and overpaid. It should, therefore, come as no surprise that the most common type of economic discrimination against older adults has been work related (AARP, 2014; Palmore, 1990). Research indicates that 80% of adults believe that most employers discriminate against older workers in hiring or on the job, and 61% of employers admit to doing so (AARP, 2014; U.S. Senate Special Committee on Aging, 1991). Discrimination against older workers ignores several overall advantages to hiring them, including low absentee rates, less turnover, low accident rates, less alcohol- and drug addiction-related issues, increased job satisfaction, and company loyalty (Palmore, 1990). Additionally, the experiences, knowledge, and insight older workers bring to the workplace are invaluable and cannot be easily replaced by a younger person with a limited work history who is working for lower wages.

Some employers believe that older workers are unable to keep pace with change and learn new technologies (AARP, 2014). For example, they may think that computers and computer software are far too difficult for older adults to learn to operate proficiently. Based on this assumption, employers are less likely to consider hiring older workers. However, evidence exists that older adults can and do learn new technological skills, including computer technology. According to adult learning theory, the learning strategies and styles of older adults may be different from younger adults, but they have the ability to learn and can become quite accomplished when given the opportunity to learn and study in a way that works for them (Knowles, 1984).

Work discrimination against older adults is most obvious when companies attempt to reduce costs by asking older workers to take early retirement, even seducing them into it by offering a tempting retirement package. The offer may initially appear to be a good financial move but may shortchange the worker of retirement income if not invested and managed wisely.

Retirement

Before the industrial revolution, retirement as a phase of life did not exist. Individuals worked until they became either disabled or too frail or infirm to do otherwise. They generally died shortly afterward. If they did live a long life, they were usually supported by family or by some charitable organization such as the local church. It was only in 1889 that Chancellor Bismarck of Germany established retirement for individuals reaching age 65. He chose the age of 65 as the beginning of retirement by adding 20 years to the then normal life expectancy of 45 years. Other European countries soon followed with similar retirement systems. In 1935, the United States was the first country to establish a nationalized pension system for people age 65 and older (Dewitt, 2010). Since then, other countries have followed suit, and today most offer a national pension to adults age 65 and older. Variations in the age of eligibility range about 5 years, with most notable differences between males and females. Some cultures stipulate that women cannot occupy the same positions as men or are required to step down from such positions at a younger age than a man, thus explaining differences in retirement.

Until 1967, retirement was compulsory for workers in the United States who reached age 65, regardless of their health status or abilities. Here again, we see another myth of aging that implies there is a general loss of ability that begins around age 65 or even earlier. However, in typically aging adults, there exists no sudden or general loss of ability at age 65 or at any other age (Palmore, 1990). Any losses that may occur among those aging typically generally do so gradually over many years. Even some disorders considered inevitable as we age (such as visual and hearing impairments) are now reversible or at least amenable to correction. Because of better health status, today's retirees can potentially spend 20 or more years in retirement (AARP, 2014). Many older adults continue working in the same or some new capacity, even after reaching retirement age. In sum, retirement is a stage of life that for some people begins with a change in employment status.

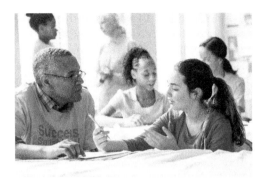

FIGURE 2-6 Many older adults continue to share their skills and expertise with the community after they retire.

© Kidstock/Blend Images/Getty Image

Preparing for retirement is not a task that should be taken lightly or without preparation (**FIGURE 2-6**). Retirement requires planning, planning, and more planning. And despite what the television commercials may say, it is not all about finances. Important considerations in the retirement decision-making process include:

- Financial and social resources
- Spouse's/partner's retirement plans
- Desire to continue working (e.g., part-time, full time, or on a flexible schedule)
- Need or desire to remain active in one's current profession
- Interest in starting a new career (reinventing one's self)
- Desire to volunteer and potential volunteer opportunities
- Desire to remain living in the same community (or to move)

Prior to retirement, some older adults begin developing hobbies or spare time occupations to engage in during retirement. Many daydream about being able to putter around their home and spend considerable time in their gardens, although good ideas, hobbies, and household activities are generally not intensive enough to fill the hours in a day (Allison, 1996). As many older adults with a few years of retirement behind them

frequently offer, you cannot just retire; you have to retire to something. Some older adults are determined to challenge themselves in pursuit of some activity that few, regardless of age, would choose to follow. Mary Harper, a 79-year-old great-grandmother, is one person who rose to such a challenge. Ms. Harper became the oldest person to sail across the Atlantic single-handedly. Although she broke a rib in severe weather, she later said, "The whole trip was worth it just to see the waves." In answer to why she did it alone, she explained that "it was something I wanted to do … but didn't want to be responsible for a crew" (Bennett, 1994). Another older adult who has refused to settle down to "quiet old age" is former U.S. President George H. W. Bush, who completed a skydive jump on his 80th, 85th, and 90th birthdays (Dooley, 2014). Some individuals continue to engage in lifelong passions. Such is the case for long-distance swimmer Diana Nyad. At age 64, she became the first person to complete the 110 mile ocean swim from Florida to Cuba (Associated Press, 2013). David Morrison of Milgrove, Ontario, Canada, had earlier in life performed folk music in local coffeehouses with friends Judy Lanza and the now famous actor Eugene Levy. A year prior to retirement, Morrison bought a new guitar and took up singing lessons. Three weeks after retiring as vice president of executive development for TD Bank, Morrison was on the verge of becoming a public performer again (Clements, 1993).

Advocacy Groups

Advocating for the rights and needs of older adults at the local, state, and national levels can be a daunting task. However, as increasing numbers of individuals reach the age of 65, the voices of advocates are becoming louder and stronger. This should come as no surprise because older baby boomers fought for the rights of disempowered groups in the 1960s and 1970s. Their involvement in civil rights, gay rights, and the feminist movement was generation shaping.

Three advocacy groups that help represent the needs of older adults are profiled in this section. The most recognizable organization that has demonstrated considerable success in representing the needs of adults age 50 and older is **AARP**, a nonprofit, nonpartisan organization. It was founded in 1958 as the American Association for Retired Persons with the agenda of addressing the social needs of retirees. Today, known as AARP (2017), it has expanded its scope of interests to include all aspects of life. In 2017, it boasted a membership of nearly 38 million people. The mission of AARP is simple: "To enhance the quality of life for all of us as we age." AARP advocates for social change through information, advocacy, and service as it represents adults of all ethnicities and cultures within the United States. All its publications (magazine, bulletins, and website) are instilled with the attitude that age is merely a number and life is what you make of it. Together with the AARP Foundation, research on topics of current interest, including prescription drug costs, grandparents raising grandchildren, and civic participation, is funded to generate information that can be used to promote positive social change.

The Gray Panthers was founded in 1970 by Maggie Kuhn and six other women who came together to discuss and address the issue of forced retirement at age 65. However, the first issue taken on by the fledgling organization was not age discrimination but rather opposition to the war in Vietnam. This was because the Gray Panthers did not want to be perceived as an organization that was only dedicated to fighting ageism. The Panthers believed philosophically that "gray power" should be on the cutting edge of social change by working with other organizations to "work for social and economic justice and peace for all people" (Gray Panthers Twin Cities, 2017). In 2015, the Gray Panthers reorganized and became the National Council of Gray Panthers Networks—a coalition of informal groups armed with national intergenerational support and organizational values that continue to honor maturity, unify generations, and actively engage in democracy to "create a humane society that puts the needs of people over profits, responsibility over power, and democracy over institutions" (Gray Panthers Twin Cities, 2017).

A third organization founded to address workplace and retirement issues is **Senior Service America (SSA)**, once known as the National Council of Senior Citizens, founded by the American Federation of Labor and Congress of Industrial Organizations (AFL-CIO) in 1961. Today, the organization's fundamental purpose is broader than the scope of retirement because the group advocates for political and legislative issues that affect older adults. Legislative issues that received the organization's attention in past years have included the OAA, Medicare, Medicaid, and employment training opportunities. Today, the SSA updates members through newsletters that report on how Congress is addressing the needs of older adults. The SSA and its partner organizations also provide employment and training opportunities to more than 10,000 adults nationwide (Senior Service America, 2017).

▶ Summary

The aging process begins the moment we are born and continues as our bodies and minds grow, develop, change, and mature. Gerontology is the scientific study of aging that examines the biological, psychological, and sociological (biopsychosocial) factors associated with old age and aging. The foundation for social science research in gerontology includes three theories about aging: disengagement theory, activity theory, and continuity theory. While none of the theories can explain social aging completely, each one helps inform our historical perspectives.

Ageism, a systematic stereotyping of and discrimination against people who are old, fosters the notion that older adults are not useful or valued. Ageism is fueled by numerous myths regarding aging and older adults as well as by language that conjures negative images of old persons. Ageism limits opportunities (employment and workplace discrimination) and access to health care and in its worst form can lead to elder abuse, mistreatment, and neglect.

Research has shown that healthcare professionals are significantly more negative in their attitudes toward older patients than they are toward younger patients. To avoid, even inadvertently, making ageist comments and remarks, it is important to recognize and explore your own feelings and attitudes as a healthcare professional. Stopping the spread of ageism is everyone's responsibility, and starts at the individual level.

The media regularly perpetuate the stereotypes of older adults through inaccurate and sometimes demeaning portrayals of older adults in print, advertising, and entertainment. This is puzzling, considering that older adults have the ability to purchase the advertisers' products that sponsor these media activities. Nonetheless, limited efforts continue to be made to accurately depict the daily lives of older adults through the media.

Social roles continue to be important in later life. However, relationships are sometimes dissolved as a result of poor health, limited mobility, and the inability to reciprocate support. Relationships with close family and friends are maintained before others because they are the source of most support. Some couples find later life to be a time of closeness after weathering life's storms together, some choose to separate and go their own ways, and some remain single and seek support from fictive kin. Relationships between aging parents and adult children tend to be as varied and challenging as spousal relationships, yet families can generally be counted on to provide support. Maintaining friendships continue to promote psychological well-being well into old age. Grandparenting has been, and remains, a rewarding and fulfilling experience in later life.

Attitudes toward work and retirement vary greatly as do the lifestyles of older adults. Many older adults choose to continue to work after retirement age because it not only provides a source of income, but also allows them to engage in productive pursuits that provide meaning and validation to their lives. For other individuals, retirement heralds the chance to pursue a special interest or hobby they never had time to do while working. Some people see it as an opportunity to travel or return to school to pursue a second career, whereas others view it with a bit of disappointment, especially if they previously held an influential position. For most individuals, however, retirement is a time of relaxation to be spent with spouse, children, grandchildren, and/or friends.

Several organizations advocate for the rights and needs of older adults at the local, state, and national levels: AARP, National Council of Gray Panthers Networks, and SSA. All three organizations were founded more than 40 years ago with the mission of bringing about social changes for older adults.

Understanding the social factors that affect older adults is essential when providing care. By developing an appreciation for the diverse backgrounds of older adults, we can better tailor interventions and meet clients' or patients' needs. Moreover, appreciation for social gerontology can only enhance how we interact with our own family members and think about our personal needs as we age.

🔍 *CASE STUDIES*

Case 1: John and Jason are both 68 years old and have been an exclusive couple for 33 years. Although they cannot legally marry in their state, their lives are inextricably interwoven, even though many people are not aware of their relationship—only a handful of close friends know. John is a banker and commutes daily into the city to work. Jason is an instructor at a local community college and generally walks to his office. They have kept their relationship relatively secret because they fear that others will "out" them, which they fear will force them to leave the careers they adore. One day, Jason suffers a severe stroke and their carefully constructed world begins to unravel. As gay men, neither is provided the rights of a spouse in terms of overseeing medical care, and John is quickly pushed aside at the hospital as the staff ask who the next of kin is. As days go by, John remains at Jason's side, and one nurse in particular repeatedly makes comments about the two old gay guys and how they don't deserve her time or care. A doctor pulls John aside and advises him to start looking for a nursing home for Jason. The thought of losing Jason and placing him in a nursing home is more than John can bear. He believes the nursing home staff would be no different than the hospital staff and would not accept the men's relationship. John decides to quit his job to care for Jason at home. When his boss asks him why he is leaving, John lies and says his mother's health is failing and she needs him. The first 3 months of care go relatively well, but as Jason's health declines, John recognizes he needs help and a break from caregiving, but feels he has no one to turn to.

1. **How are John and Jason's challenges in providing Jason with care different from the challenges faced by a heterosexual couple?**
2. **What challenges do healthcare professionals face in providing care to same-sex couples?**
3. **What can healthcare professionals do to help couples like John and Jason successfully manage their healthcare challenges?**

Case 2: Barbara, age 42, is a lucky woman, or at least that is what everyone tells her. She has an adoring husband, smart children, a career as a store manager, and impeccable taste in fashion. Barbara has always been an excellent multitasker and has successfully balanced her marriage, family, and career for 20 years. She makes every task look effortless. So, when her mother started having health problems, Barbara was sure to set aside the time needed to help. She always assumed she would be the best one to help her mother, even though she lived 200 miles away, because she was reliable and dependable. Barbara has a brother and sister who could probably help, but they have their own careers and families and they are just fine letting Barbara take over. They trust Barbara. After a few months, Barbara thought that being a long-distance caregiver was not that hard. She struggled a bit at first, but soon organized all the information she needed about her mother's health problems and care. She was in touch with doctors on a regular basis and authorized whatever care was needed. Soon, she started managing her mother's finances. It did not cross Barbara's mind to call her siblings to update them, and they did not think to call her. Barbara was pleased that she could provide for her mother from a distance. Although long-distance caregiving was not convenient and often forced her to change her plans, she could not imagine not being available for her mom. One day, Barbara received a call that her mother had been hospitalized. She called her sister and they agreed to meet at their mother's home and travel together to the hospital. Secretly, Barbara was glad to meet with her sister because she was getting tired of having the extra burden of her mother's life on her shoulders alone. Last week at work, the regional manager told her that her enthusiasm and work performance had started to slip. Even her husband had made a few comments that she did not seem to have the time for him and their children anymore. Barbara knew things needed to change, but just was not sure what to do.

1. **What should Barbara do and why?**
2. **What steps does Barbara need to take to ensure her own needs are being cared for?**

TEST YOUR KNOWLEDGE

Review Questions

1. _____ is the scientific study of aging that examines the biological, psychological, and sociological factors associated with old age and aging.
   a. Geriatrics
   b. Pediatrics
   c. Oncology
   d. Gerontology

2. The first psychosocial science theories on aging included
   a. Activity theory and disengagement theory
   b. Continuity theory and social role theory
   c. Activity theory and social role theory
   d. Disengagement theory and caregiving theory

3. Providers who view older adult patients sympathetically as "poor old dears," who can do little to care for themselves, are diminishing the value they place on their patients' abilities.
   a. True
   b. False

4. Skip-generation households refer to
   a. Teenagers caring for their ailing parents
   b. Parents caring for children as well as aging parents
   c. Grandparents acting as surrogate parents to their grandchildren
   d. Grandchildren caring for ailing grandparents

5. A typical victim of elder abuse is
   a. Female and over the age of 75
   b. Living alone and lacking a network of social support
   c. A & B
   d. None of the above

Learning Activities

1. Using your own experiences and observations, formulate a social theory on aging. How does it compare with the social theories described in this chapter?

2. Provide examples of ageism you have seen in your own family, in your community, in the media, in your travels, and/or in your workplace.

3. Explain the value of social connections in late life and provide examples of how an older adult can maintain connections to other people.

4. Discuss some of the issues and concerns of a grandparent raising a grandchild. What steps, if any, can a healthcare professional take to support them?

5. Develop a scenario in which a vulnerable older adult could potentially become a victim of two or more types of elder abuse. Describe the steps a healthcare professional can take to uncover a potential problem.

References

AARP. (2014). *Staying ahead of the curve 2013: The AARP work and career study*. Washington, DC: AARP. Retrieved from https://www.aarp.org/content/dam/aarp/research/surveys_statistics/general/2014/Staying-Ahead-of-the-Curve-2013-The-Work-and-Career-Study-AARP-res-gen.pdf

AARP. (2017). Home Page. Retrieved from http://www.aarp.org

Acierno, R., Hernandez, M. A., Armstadter, A. B., Resnick, H. S., Steve, K., Muzzy, W., & Kilpatrick, D. G. (2010). Prevalence and correlates of emotional, physical, sexual, and financial abuse and potential neglect in the United States: The National Elder Mistreatment Study. *American Journal of Public Health, 100*(2), 292–297. doi:10.2105/AJPH.2009.163089

Adams, K. B., Leibbrandt, S., & Moon, H. (2011). A critical review of the literature on social and leisure activity and wellbeing in later life. *Ageing & Society, 31*, 683–712. doi:10.1017/s0144686x10001091

Age Discrimination in Employment Act, 29 U.S.C. § 621 (1967).

Alliance for Aging Research. (2003). *Ageism: How Healthcare Fails the Elderly*. New York, NY: Alliance for Aging Research.

Allison, R. (1996). Easy steps to tone up retirement. *Advertising Age, 67*(45), 32.

Anti-Ageism Task Force. (2006). What is ageism? In *Ageism in America*. New York, NY: International Longevity Center. Retrieved from http://aging.columbia.edu/sites/default/files/Ageism_in_America.pdf

Antonucci, T. C. (2001). Social relations: An examination of social networks, social support, and sense of control. In J. E. Birren & K. W. Schaie (Eds.), *Handbook of the Psychology of Aging*. San Diego, CA: Academic Press.

Associated Press. (December 31, 2004). Elders' knowledge of the oceans spares Thai "sea gypsies" from tsunami disaster. Retrieved from http://www.freerepublic.com/focus/f-news/1311910/posts

Associated Press. (September 4, 2013). Diana Nyad finishes historic swim. Retrieved from http://www.espn.com/espnw/news-commentary/article/9626550/diana-nyad-becomes-first-person-complete-cuba-florida-swim-shark-cage

Atchley, R. C. (1989). A continuity theory of normal aging. *The Gerontologist, 29*(2), 183–190. doi:10.1093/geront/29.2.183

Bennett, D. (1994). Great grandmother goes solo. *Cruising World, 19*(12), 8–9.

Berkman, L., & Breslow, L. (1983). *Health and Ways of Living: The Alameda County Study*. New York, NY: Oxford University Press.

Brightman, J., & Subedi, L. A. (2007). *AAPI Culture Brief: Hawai'i*. Vol. 2(7). Honolulu: National Technical Assistance Center.

Bursack, C. B. (n.d.). *Do Parents Really Want to Live with Their Adult Children?* Retrieved from https://www.agingcare.com/articles/parents-living-with-adult-children-152285.htm

Butler, R. M. (1969). Ageism: Another form of bigotry. *The Gerontologist, 9*, 243–246.

Butler, R. M. (2008). *The longevity revolution*. New York, NY: Public Affairs.

Centers for Disease Control and Prevention. (2016). *Elder abuse surveillance: Uniform definitions and recommended core data elements*. Atlanta, GA: Centers for Disease Control and Prevention. Retrieved from https://www.cdc.gov/violenceprevention/pdf/ea_book_revised_2016.pdf

Clements, M. (December 12, 1993). What we say about aging. *Parade Magazine*, 4–5.

Connidis, I. A., & McMullin, J. A. (1993). To have or not to have: Parent status and the subjective well-being of older men and women. *The Gerontologist, 33*, 630–636.

Cumming, E., & Henry, W. E. (1961). *Growing old: The process of disengagement*. New York, NY: Basic Books.

Dewitt, L. (2010). The development of social security in America. *Social Security Bulletin, 70*(3). Retrieved from https://www.ssa.gov/policy/docs/ssb/v70n3/v70n3p1.html

Dooley, E. (June 12, 2014). George H. W. Bush marks 90th birthday by skydiving. Retrieved from http://abcnews.go.com/Politics/george-bush-marks-90th-birthday-skydiving/story?id=24103264

Dunham, C. C. (1995). A link between generations: Intergenerational relations and depression in aging parents. *Journal of Family Issues, 16*, 450–465.

Ferraro, K. F. (2001). Aging and role transitions. In R. H. Binstock & L. K. George (Eds.), *Handbook of Aging and the Social Sciences* (5th ed.). San Diego, CA: Academic Press.

Garcia, E. C. (2001). Parenting in Mexican American families. In N. B. Webb (Ed.), *Culturally Diverse Parent–Child and Family Relationships: A Guide for Social Workers and Other Practitioners*. New York, NY: Columbia University Press.

Goodman, L. (2010). Between two worlds: Malidoma Somé on rites of passage. *Sun Magazine*, p. 415.

Gray Panthers Twin Cities. (2017). Home Page. Retrieved from http://graypantherstwincities.org/

Havighurst, R. J. (1961). Successful aging. *The Gerontologist, 1*, 8–13. doi:10.1093/geront/1.1.8

Hilt, M. L., & Lipshultz, J. L. (2016). *Mass Media, An Aging Population, and the Baby Boomers*. New York, NY: Rutledge.

Howe, N. (May 17, 2016). *Brands now market to the extended family.* Retrieved from https://www.forbes.com/sites/neilhowe/2016/05/17/brands-now-market-to-the-extended-family/#435f0443c4df

Hunt, P. C. (2002). *An Introduction to Vietnamese Culture for Rehabilitation Service Providers in the U.S.* Buffalo, NY: Center for International Rehabilitation Research Information and Exchange.

Jackson, S. L., & Hafemeister, T. L. (2012). Pure financial exploitation vs. hybrid financial exploitation co-occurring with physical abuse and/or neglect of elderly persons. *Psychology of Violence, 2,* 285–296. doi:10.1037/a0027273

Jezewski, M. A., & Sotnik, P. (2001). Culture brokering: Providing culturally competent services to foreign born persons. Buffalo, NY: Center for International Rehabilitation Research Information and Exchange.

Jordan-Marsh, M., & Harden, J. T. (2005). Fictive kin: Friends as family supporting older adults as they age. *Journal of Gerontological Nursing, 31*(2), 24–31.

Kahn, R., & Antonucci, T. (1980). Convoys over the life course: Attachment, roles, and social support. In P. Baltes & O. G. Brim (Eds.), *Life-Span Development and Behavior.* New York, NY: Academic Press.

Kim-Rupnow, W. S. (2001). *An introduction to Korean culture for rehabilitation service providers.* Buffalo, NY: Center for International Rehabilitation Research Information and Exchange.

Knowles, M. (1984). *Andragogy in Action.* San Francisco, CA: Jossey-Bass.

Lafferty, A. (2009). Public perceptions of elder abuse: A literature review. National Centre for the Protection of Older People, 1–38. Retrieved from http://www.ncpop.ie/Year%201%20Reports/Microsoft%20Word%20-%20Review%202Public%20Perceptions%20of%20elder%20abuse_AL181109_Final_ILc21_01_10.pdf

Levy, B. R., Slade, M. B., Kunkel, S. R., & Kasl, S. V. (2002). Longevity increased by positive self-perceptions of aging. *Journal of Personality and Social Psychology, 83*(2), 261–270. doi:10.1037//0022-3514.83.2.261

Lifespan of Greater Rochester, Inc., Weill Cornell Medical Center of Cornell University, & New York City Department for the Aging. (2011). *Under the Radar: New York State Elder Abuse Prevalence Study.* Retrieved from http://ocfs.ny.gov/main/reports/Under%20the%20Radar%2005%2012%2011%20final%20report.pdf

Maddox, G. L. (1965). Fact and artifact: Evidence bearing on disengagement theory from the Duke Geriatrics Project. *Human Development, 8,* 117–130. doi:10.1159/000270296

Malta, S. (2007). Love actually! Older adults and their romantic internet relationships. *Australian Journal of Emerging Technologies and Society, 5*(2), 84–102.

Meisner, B. A., & Hynie, M. (2009). Ageism with heterosexism: Self-perceptions, identity, and psychological health in older gay and lesbian adults. *Gay and Lesbian Issues and Psychology Review, 5,* 51–58.

MetLife and National Alliance for Caregiving. (2008). *Since You Care: Long Distance Caregiving.* Retrieved from http://www.metlife.com/assets/cao/mmi/publications/sinceyou-care-guides/mmi-long-distance-caregiving.pdf

MetLife Mature Market Institute. (2009). Broken trust: Elders, family, and finances. Retrieved from https://www.metlife.com/assets/cao/mmi/publications/studies/mmi-study-broken-trust-elders-family-finances.pdf

MetLife Mature Market Institute. (2011). New insights for a new generation of grandparents. Retrieved from https://www.metlife.com/assets/cao/mmi/publications/studies/2011/mmi-american-grandparents.pdf

National Alliance for Caregiving. (2005). *Caregiving in the U.S.* Retrieved from http://assets.aarp.org/rgcenter/il/us_caregiving_1.pdf

National Alliance for Caregiving & AARP Public Policy Institute. (2015). *Caregiving in the U.S.* Retrieved from https://www.aarp.org/content/dam/aarp/ppi/2015/caregiving-in-the-united-states-2015-report-revised.pdf

National Center on Elder Abuse. (n.d.). *Frequently asked questions: Types of abuse.* Retrieved from https://ncea.acl.gov/faq/abusetypes.html

Neugarten, B. L., & Weinstein, K. K. (1964). The changing American grandparent. *Journal of Marriage and the Family, 26,* 199–204.

Ng, E. S., & Law, A. (2014). Keeping up! Older workers' adaptation in the workplace after age 55. *Canadian Journal on Aging, 33,* 1–14. doi:10.1017/S0714980813000639

Palmore, E. B. (1990). *Ageism: Negative and positive.* New York, NY: Springer.

Pew Research Center. (2017a). Tech Adoption Climbs Among Older Adults. Retrieved from http://assets.pewresearch.org/wp-content/uploads/sites/14/2017/05/16170850/PI_2017.05.17_Older-Americans-Tech_FINAL.pdf

Pew Research Center. (2017b). *Marriage and divorce.* Retrieved from http://www.pewresearch.org/topics/marriage-and-divorce/page/2/

Pinto, P. E., & Sahur, N. (2001). *Working with people with disabilities: An Indian perspective.* Buffalo, NY: Center for International Rehabilitation Research Information and Exchange.

Qualls, S. H. (2014). Yes, health and social relationships are inextricably linked. *Generations, 38,* 6–7.

Ramsey-Klawsnik, H. (2017). Older adults affected by polyvictimization: A review of early research. *Journal of Elder Abuse & Neglect, 29*(5), 299–312. doi:10.1080/08946566.2017.1388019

Rennison, C. M. (2001). *Intimate partner violence and age of victim, 1993–99* (NCJ 187635). Washington, DC: U.S. Department of Justice, Office of Justice Programs, Bureau of Justice Statistics. Retrieved from https://www.bjs.gov/content/pub/pdf/ipva99.pdf

Richeson, J. A., & Shelton, J. N. (2006). A Social Psychological Perspective on the Stigmatization of Older

Adults. In L. L. Carstensen & C. R. Hartel (Eds.), *When I'm 64*. Washington, DC: National Academies Press. Retrieved from https://www.ncbi.nlm.nih .gov/books/NBK83758/

Roberto, K. A. (2017). Perpetrators of late life polyvictimization. *Journal of Elder Abuse & Neglect, 29*(5), 313–326. doi:10.1080/08946566.2017.1374223

Senior Service America. (2017). Home Page. Retrieved from http://www.seniorserviceamerica.org

Silverstone, B., & Hyman, H. (1992). *Growing Older Together*. New York, NY: Pantheon Books.

Simkins, C. L. (2007). Ageism's influence on health care delivery and nursing practice. *Journal of Student Nursing, 1*, 24–28.

Suitor, J. J., Pillemer, K., Keeton, S., & Robison, J. (1996). Aged parents and aging children: Determinants of relationship quality. In R. Blieszner & V. H. Bedford (Eds.), *Aging and the Family*. Westport, CT: Praeger.

Tagliareni, E., & Waters, V. (1995). The aging experience. In M. A. Anderson & J. V. Braun (Eds.), *Caring for the Elderly Client* (pp. 2–15). Philadelphia, PA: F. A. Davis.

Tamborinia, C. (2007). The never-married in old age: Projections and concerns for the future. *Social Security Bulletin, 67*, 25–40.

Teaster, P. B., & Roberto, K. A. (2004). Chapter 7 sexual abuse of older women living in nursing homes. *Journal of Gerontological Social Work, 40*(4), 105–119. doi:10.1300/ J083v40n04_08

Toossi, M., & Torpay, E. (2017). *Older workers: Labor force trends and career options*. Washington, DC: U.S. Bureau of Labor Statistics. Retrieved from https://www.bls.gov /careeroutlook/2017/article/print/older-workers.htm

Torres, S. (2002). *Understanding persons of Philippine origin: A primer for rehabilitation service providers*. Buffalo, NY: Center for International Rehabilitation Research Information and Exchange.

U.S. Census Bureau. (2011). Age and Sex Composition: 2010. Retrieved from http://www.census.gov/prod /cen2010/briefs/c2010br-03.pdf

U.S. Census Bureau. (2017a). Facts for Features: Grandparent's Day 2017. Retrieved from https://www .census.gov/content/dam/Census/newsroom/facts -for-features/2017/cb17-ff14.pdf

U.S. Census Bureau. (2017b). The Hispanic Heritage Month: 2017. Retrieved from https://www.census .gov/content/dam/Census/newsroom/facts-for -features/2017/cb17-ff17.pdf

United States Government Accountability Office. (2010). *Guardianships: Cases of financial exploitation, neglect, and abuse of seniors* (GAO-10-1046). Retrieved from http://www.gao.gov/assets/320/310741.pdf

U.S. Senate Special Committee on Aging, American Association of Retired Persons, Federal Council on the Aging, and U.S. Administration on Aging. (1991). *Aging America, Trends and Projections*. Washington, DC: U.S. Department of Health and Human Services.

Wallis, V. (1993). *Two Old Women: An Alaska Legend of Betrayal, Courage and Survival*. Seattle, WA: Epicenter Press.

Wiglesworth, A., Mosqueda, L., Mulnard, R., Liao, S., Gibbs, L., & Fitzgerald, W. (2010). Screening for abuse and neglect of people with dementia. *Journal of the American Geriatric Society, 58*(3), 493–500. doi:10.1111 /j.1532-5415.2010.02737.x

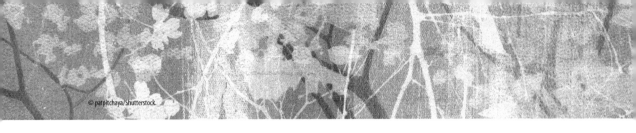
© patpitchaya/Shutterstock.

CHAPTER 3

Aging in Place and the Continuum of Care

Ann O'Sullivan, OTR/L, LSW, FAOTA
Nancy Brossoie, PhD
Regula H. Robnett, PhD, OTR/L, FAOTA

CHAPTER OUTLINE

BEHAVIORAL OBJECTIVES

Upon completion of this chapter, the reader will be able to:

1. Define aging in place and describe the benefits of aging in place.
2. Discuss the connection between housing, health care, and least restrictive environment.
3. Compare and contrast housing options along the continuum of care.
4. Discuss the role of person-centered care along the continuum of care.
5. Describe how technology has impacted health care, especially for older adults.
6. Discuss ways that health care professionals can support aging in place and productive aging with their clients.

KEY TERMS

Accessibility	Gerotechnology	Physiatrists
Activities of daily living	Home health	Productive aging
Adult day services	Instrumental activities of daily	Program of All-Inclusive Care
Aging in place	living	for the Elderly
Assisted living facility	Least restrictive environment	Rehabilitation
Assistive technology	Long-term care insurance	Reverse mortgage
Chore services	Meal services	Shared housing
Cohousing	Medicaid	Telehealth
Competency	Naturally occurring retirement	Telephone reassurance
Continuing care retirement	community	Transportation
community	Nonmedical home care services	Universal design
Eden Alternative	Person-centered care	Village model

▶ Introduction

Sentiments such as "There is no place like home" and "Home sweet home" can elicit pleasant memories and emotions when reflecting on homes and communities we claim as our own—attachments that can persist despite not living in those same places. Our home (be it a specific house or location) provides us with a sense of place that can connect us to a community greater than ourselves. But, most importantly, home is also the place that facilitates independence and the quality of life we embrace, especially when it includes modifications and supports that promote our health and well-being (Rowles & Ravdal, 2002).

The connection between home (however we personally define it) and health is well established and significant (Ball, 2004). Research across the life span has shown that living in safe and familiar surroundings with personal ties to the community contributes positively to good health, well-being, and quality of life. The healing and supportive power of home and community is strong!

With increased recognition of the connection between health and home, efforts over the last 30 years have become more intentional and widespread in providing services to people in the community where they live. In more recent years, the term **aging in place** personifies this approach and is considered the best option for managing the health care needs of the growing population of older adults.

▶ Aging in Place

Aging in place is typically defined as the ability to remain in one's own home or community as one ages (Centers for Disease Control and Prevention, n.d.). By aging in place, the benefits of remaining connected to home (house or location) can support the acute care needs and the compression of morbidity (i.e., reduction of the period of illness before death; Fries, Bruce, & Chakravarty, 2011), thereby shortening the length of time in institutional care and extending time spent living at home and in the community.

Critics of the aging in place concept have argued that not all older adults should stay in their homes as doing so would be detrimental to their health. For example, individuals who live in squalor, have cognitive impairments, self-neglect, or suffer abuse by household members would be sentenced to ongoing discomfort if they remained in their current situation. Proponents would agree and reiterate that the meaning of aging in place is not limited to the current residence or situation. For a person perceived as at-risk for staying in their home, remaining in the community in a new supportive living environment would be more beneficial, because communities hold the same cultural and social norms and behaviors that the individual embraced. Even within a long-term care setting, an older adult can remain engaged in the local community's culture and connections through staff and visitor interactions, and on-site activities. Thus, older adults who choose not to remain living in their current residence, can still age in place and do it quite successfully.

The notion of aging in place aligns well with how many older adults are already thinking about their futures. An AARP survey in 2014 (Harrell, Lynott, Guzmann, & Lampkin, 2014) revealed that among adults age 65+, 87% of respondents reported they intend to remain in their current homes for as long as possible. However, among persons age 50–64, only 71% were willing to remain in their communities. Reasons for the decrease were largely attributed to low-income respondents representing people of color living in metropolitan areas. Still, the intentions expressed by both groups support the general concept of aging in place.

The decision to age in place also supports an older adult's ability to remain as independent or autonomous as possible. The World Health Organization (2015) has identified autonomy as key priority for quality of life in aging, impacting dignity, integrity, freedom, and independence. Making choices about how one lives and controls how his/her basic needs are met is integral to achieving life satisfaction, well-being, and quality of life.

Independence

Like people in all age groups, older adults value their independence (MacDonald, Remus, & Laing, 1994). Nevertheless, how they define it can sometimes vary. In a study examining the link between housing and health, the study findings suggested that some people viewed independence as meaning they lived comfortably without needing regular assistance from anyone else, or that they lived in their own home and maintained the ability to make their own decisions. Yet, some participants shared a modified view by suggesting that maintaining independence could include accepting some help from families and friends but without becoming a burden.

One responsibility of health care practitioners is to facilitate the independence of persons under their care. With providers respecting their independence and freedom of choice, clients can regain mastery over their lives (Minkler, 1992). Therefore, it is imperative that practitioners ask clients what independence means to them, and then honor their goals toward reaching independence while supporting their efforts in working toward treatment goals.

When an individual requires assistance to complete their **activities of daily living** (ADLs; e.g., bathing, toileting, dressing, eating, walking) and **instrumental activities of daily living** (IADLs; e.g., housekeeping, budget management, using a telephone), a key therapeutic goal is to provide those supports in the **least restrictive environment** possible. That is, individuals should be provided the opportunity to live in an environment that provides them with the opportunities to function as normally as possible and be as independent as possible (a tenet of the continuum of care discussed later in this chapter).

Productive Aging

The ability to remain independent, active, and as high functioning as possible are core values associated with aging in place and **productive aging**—a term that refers to making valued contributions to one's life by engaging in enjoyable, meaningful, and useful activities (Kerschner & Pegues, 1998). Remaining productive through active engagement, physical activity, and pursuit of cognitive challenges is also associated with longevity (Terracciano et al., 2008). That is, people who live productive lives tend to live to the oldest ages. Although the scope and type of activities one can and might engage in as one ages may differ from those experienced earlier in life, engaging in them continues to benefit the body, mind, and spirit, and promote healthy and successful aging.

Competency

Promoting independence and productive aging is not always easy for the health care practitioner. The issue of **competency** can arise when supporting some older clients. In the course of providing support, health care professionals may question a client's behaviors and choices and their ability to comprehend the consequences of their actions, especially when those actions can place them or others at risk. Practitioners find themselves questioning a client's cognitive ability or competency to make decisions and may seek advice from other providers on how to proceed. Yet, competency is not for them to decide alone. Competency is a legal determination and only the court can determine if an individual is incompetent to make their own decision. Thus, until incompetency has been declared and a guardian appointed to oversee their care and services, practitioners are bound to respect their clients' choices and work with them to provide services and supports that align with their preferences, even if these conflict with the practitioner's choices.

Person-Centered Care

Respecting client wishes is a cornerstone of client-centered or **person-centered care**. The notion of providing care that meets the therapeutic needs of the individual rather than engaging in prescriptive care originated in the 1940s with psychologist Carl Rogers (Kirschenbaum, 2009). Clinicians used Roger's work to develop practical methods for working with clients with psychological, emotional, and social adjustment problems. Use of the person-centered approach gained widespread attention, and by 1980 advocates for people with intellectual and developmental disabilities started promoting its use nationwide as the foundation for person-centered planning in service delivery (Kirschenbaum & Jourdan, 2005). Today, many intake assessments administered to clients prior to entry into services and programs utilize a biopsychosocial approach to better understand an individual's needs, which is the first step to offering person-centered care services in the least restrictive environment.

Technology-Based Services

Person-centered care includes not only personal services, but also **assistive technology** (AT; i.e., assistive, adaptive, and rehabilitative devices that help users complete ADLs, IADLs). AT includes any product that is used to increase, maintain, or improve the functional capabilities of individuals needing specialized help. Examples of AT range from low tech (e.g., a dressing stick, sock aid, or spork [spoon /fork combination]) to high tech (e.g., smart home technology to regulate temperature, lighting, and security; medication dispensers; and monitors). AT can also be portable (e.g., hearing aids, smart phones, communication boards) or built into the environment (e.g., raised toilet, adjustable height sink, levered doorknobs). The type of AT utilized depends on the needs of the individual. As functional levels change, the AT used should also adapt to meet new needs so that the individual can remain as high functioning as possible. (Assistive Technology Industry Association, n.d.).

Gerotechnology is a term used to describe a professional field that focuses on technology specifically designed to support older adults. Developers in Asia, Europe, and the United States have taken the lead in using technologies to provide products that promote the health and welfare of older people. For example, a compact freezer/oven combination unit that can hold up to a month's worth of frozen meals was developed in Finland. All the user has to do is remove the meal from the freezer, place it in the oven, and push one button to cook the "home-cooked" meal. In Asia, where the older population is rapidly growing in size, researchers are seeking ways to utilize gerotechnology to meet the needs of large numbers of people with as little human assistance as possible. Specifically, researchers are currently developing vending machines that can dispense prepackaged hot and cold single container meals. In Japan, scientists have designed rooms with robots that take care of the people living in the room by monitoring their vital signs and even anticipating basic needs such as thirst or hunger (Dethflefs & Martin, 2006; Saunders, 2012).

Similarly, in the United States, the MED-Cottage is now being produced (N2Care, n.d.). MEDCottage is a modular home intended to be temporarily placed on a caregiver's property to house an individual needing oversight or assistance. The state-of-the-art monitoring equipment installed in the MEDCottage permits basic health functions to be monitored and tracked, affording privacy and independence to the resident. Not only does this portable unit provide medical support, it also helps the resident age in place and stay connected to family, friends, and community.

Technology is playing an ever larger role in health care, from wrist monitors that monitor vital signs 24/7 to avatars (i.e., virtual humans) that can guide older clients through the exercises taught to them by their physical therapist (Halloran, 2018). Other creative technological solutions currently under refinement for use outside the home and in the provision of services include virtual care coordinators, wellness communication platforms, and autonomous vehicles.

However, the products produced by gerotechnology may not be the panacea envisioned. There is little doubt that older adults can benefit from technology, but the products cannot replace the social interactions that emerge during direct contact with care providers. Heavy reliance on products can potentially be isolating. For example, an automated stuffed animal used for cuddling and social interaction cannot quite compare to engaging in human touch and conversation, even though it might superficially help improve mood. Also, individuals may perceive being watched or listened to continuously by electronic devices as intrusive and violating their personal space, interfering with their independence and ability to have a choice in how they live. Therefore, the judicious use of technological advances to make life easier and healthier is warranted. Continuous feedback can ensure its use is appropriate and acceptable to the client.

Universal Design

Clearly, AT can make life easier for many individuals and their families. Yet, for people of all ages, what is needed most are changes in how products and environments are designed.

Universal design addresses those needs. Universal design is "the design and composition of an environment so that it can be accessed, understood and used to the greatest extent possible by all people regardless of their age, size, ability or disability" (Centre for Excellence in Universal Design, 2014a). Simply put, universal design is good design. Products and environments that represent universal design are guided by seven principles (Centre for Excellence in Universal Design, 2014b):

1. Equitable use
2. Flexibility in use
3. Simple and intuitive use
4. Perceptible information
5. Tolerance for error
6. Low physical effort
7. Size and space for approach and use

An example of a product in everyday use in which universal design principles are utilized is the lever door handle. Compared to a traditional round door knob, a level door handle requires less manual dexterity and is easier to operate by individuals with arthritis or upper extremity weaknesses. Moreover, lever door handles are easier to use when carrying groceries or small children, or wearing gloves or mittens.

Buildings that incorporate universal design principles that enable people of all abilities to navigate without special accommodation can include features such as access ramps, one-story construction or single-level living areas, antiglare and nonslip floor finishes, easy-to-reach electrical switches and outlets, levered faucet handles and door knobs, and automated smart home technology (i.e., wireless and sensor controlled heating, cooling, lighting, security).

In the home, entryways are frequently modified using universal design features (**FIGURE 3-1**). Built environments that incorporate universal design facilitate engagement in daily life, which in turn promotes independence, personal well-being, and quality of life.

Even though universal design features promote **accessibility** (i.e., the ability to

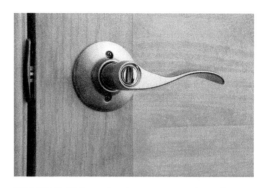

FIGURE 3-1 Objects that incorporate universal design principles enable people of all abilities to use them without special accommodation.
© James Brey/iStock/Getty Images Plus

navigate through an environment), the two terms are not interchangeable. The existence of accessible buildings and environments for everyone in the United States can be credited to the passage of the Americans with Disabilities Act (ADA) in 1990. Not only did the ADA guarantee that persons with disabilities have the same opportunities at work, school, and in the community as everyone else, but it also became the legal foundation for standards and guidelines in the built environment to accommodate the needs of people with physical and sensory challenges. For example, ADA guidelines and standards include requirements for the width of door frames and hallways to accommodate wheelchairs, no-rise thresholds, structural requirements of access ramps, and auditory and visual cues added to alarm systems, to name a few. State and local building requirements can differ from ADA standards only if they result in more stringent standards. A copy of the 2010 "ADA Standards for Accessible Design" can be found at www.ada.gov /2010ADAstandards_index.htm.

Continuum of Care

One way to think about and support older adults and their physical, emotional, and social needs is through a continuum of care service delivery model. The model provides a way to connect

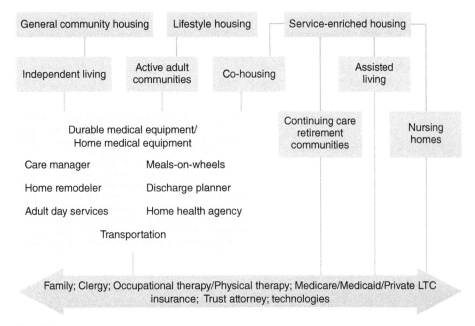

FIGURE 3-2 The continuum of care.

types of housing (i.e., general community housing, lifestyle housing, and service-enriched housing) with healthcare services in a way that supports aging in place in the least restrictive environments possible (**FIGURE 3-2**). Individuals may advance through the model by changing their living environments when healthcare needs become more intensive. Components of the continuum of care are presented next in this chapter by following the model moving from the least restrictive (independent living) to most restrictive (nursing home).

Independent Living

Understandably, the most desired living situation is an independent living arrangement in the community. Ideally, the option to live independently should exist for as long as possible. Types of housing that promote independent living include the same options available to adults at any age (e.g., apartment, townhouse, single-family dwelling, etc.).

There is one age-restricted independent living option that caters specifically to older adults—retirement communities. Retirement communities can range from publicly accessible housing developments to gated communities with keyed access. Housing options in a retirement community can be diverse and may include single-family homes, mobile homes, or space for parking motorhomes. Regardless of housing type, acceptance into a retirement community is generally based on age (e.g., age 55 and older) or retirement status. Many retirement communities charge a monthly homeowner's association fee to cover costs for community landscaping and upkeep, community center activities, and property management costs.

The first and possibly the most famous retirement community in the United States was Sun City, Arizona, developed by Del Webb (Recreation Centers of Sun City, Inc., 2016). The first model homes in Sun City opened in 1960 and 2000 homes sold in the first year. In the years that followed, more Del Webb retirement communities opened across the U.S. sunbelt, where many retirement communities are located today. Sun Cities were unique because they offered more than independent living to residents, they offered an active leisure lifestyle.

Active Adult Communities

Sun City, Arizona, is also a model of an active adult community. It was intentionally designed to provide all the amenities a person age 55+ could use without leaving the community. The original development included recreational facilities, stores, and a post office, which expanded to include churches, medical care, and a long-term care facility. The notion of retiring to an active adult community in a warm sunny climate continues to appeal to many people. However, active adult communities like Sun City require that residents have the financial resources to purchase their homes and pay fees, which is out of reach for the majority of older adults.

Not all active adult communities are intentionally designed like Sun City. Some emerge out of an existing community or neighborhood as residents' age in place or older residents move into available housing units. Three other examples of active adult communities are described in this section: naturally occurring retirement communities, Village model, and subsidized senior housing.

Naturally Occurring Retirement Community

A **naturally occurring retirement community** (NORC) is a demographic term used to describe a neighborhood, multiunit dwelling (e.g., apartment building), or group of buildings (e.g., apartment complex) in which the majority of residents are older adults. NORCs are not designed to be retirement communities, they just evolve into areas in which the majority of residents are older adults. NORCs tend to be located

in densely populated areas and the majority of NORC residents have called the area home for many years (United Hospital Fund, 2015).

The evolution of a community into a NORC community occurs over time. As residents age, they first look to each other to get their needs met. As needs increase, these small group efforts unite to form a NORC program to better serve the needs of all residents. NORC representatives often work with the local housing and transportation authorities and health and social service providers to gain better resident access to local services and supports. Some services may be provided for a fee, which the member pays when accessed. NORCs may also receive public and private funds to sustain programming and support current and future residents' ability to age in place. **TABLE 3-1** is an example of the range of services and supports provided by one of the 54 NORCs in operation in the State of New York (New York Department for the Aging, 2017). The descriptions of some of these services are provided in subsequent sections in this chapter.

In St. Louis, the Jewish Federation partnered with Washington University to study the needs of older adults in a local NORC. The team recognized the need for wellness programming, social activities, resident councils, and information exchanges. Moreover, a transportation program was also launched to help residents with their grocery shopping. However, when the residents shared that they really wanted transportation to attend cultural events instead (because they were already getting help with groceries), the transportation program was revamped to offer popular day trips. As this example illustrates, NORCs are designed to be receptive to resident needs by bringing services and supports rather than requiring that they move to be closer to the services they need (Opp, n.d.).

Village Model

The **Village model** originated in Beacon Hill, Massachusetts, in 1999, and has since expanded to over 270 communities in the

TABLE 3-1 Services Provided by a NORC in New York City

Senior Center: EDUCATIONAL ALLIANCE COOP VILLAGE NORC		
Address & Phone Number	**Hours**	**Services Offered**
465 GRAND STREET NEW YORK, NY 10002 (212) 358-8489	▪ MONDAY 9:00–5:00 ▪ TUESDAY 9:00–5:00 ▪ WEDNESDAY 9:00–5:00 ▪ THURSDAY 9:00–5:00 ▪ FRIDAY 9:00–5:00	▪ NORC CASE ASSISTANCE ▪ NORC EDUCATION/RECREATION ▪ NORC FRIENDLY VISITING ▪ NORC HEALTH ASSISTANCE ▪ NORC HEALTHCARE MGT ▪ NORC NE HEALTH PROMO ▪ NORC TELEPHONE REASSURE ▪ NORC TRANSPORTATION ▪ NORC-SSP CASE MANAGEMENT
How to Get There		
For information on how to get to this Senior Center, visit the Maps page on MTAs website or call MTAs Transit and Travel Info Line at (718) 330-1234.		

Data from New York Department for the Aging. (2017). NORC services. Retrieved from https://a125-egovt.nyc.gov/egovt/services/service _detail.cfm?contract__cont_dfta_id=N3101

United States, Australia, and New Zealand (Village to Village Network, n.d.). The Village model is a resident-governed community service and support model. Members live in their own homes but work with other Village members to coordinate needed nonmedical services and care they might need (e.g., transportation, chore service). As a member's needs increase, the Village works with them to identify resources and connect with services and supports in the community.

Like other congregate housing options, engagement with other members in the Village can help reduce social isolation, promote relationships and interdependence among members, and reduce overall healthcare costs. Moreover, they are similar to NORCs, in that they help older adults obtain needed health and social services in order to increase their ability to age in place. Yet, unlike NORCs, Villages are formed and governed by members

and funded by annual membership dues rather than fee-for-service programs or grants.

Homes of members enrolled in Villages can be located in small or large geographic areas. Regardless of location, members commit to collaborating with one another through volunteering, establishing group service contracts with providers, advocating for the needs of older adults, and organizing educational and social events (Greenfield, Scharlach, Graham, Davitt, & Lehning, 2012).

Challenges with sustainability at Villages are shared by other cohousing models. Funding sources are decreasing and members are struggling to maintain services and supports on their limited incomes. Recruiting residents that represent a diverse population is also difficult. In cohousing, residents are generally recruited by word of mouth, which results in a membership that is not racially and economically diverse. The same exclusivity also limits the recruitment of young members who are needed to sustain the community (Lehning, Davitt, Scharlach, & Greenfield, 2014).

Subsidized Senior Housing

Subsidized housing programs are funded through the U.S. Housing and Urban Development (HUD) and implemented at the state and local levels. In 1959, HUD created a housing program (Section 202) specifically for housing older adults. Since then, funds have been allocated to provide monies to build multiunit senior housing structures and to supplement the monthly rents paid by residents (HUD, n.d). In 2016, older adults constituted at least one-third of all subsidized housing in the United States.

Unfortunately, need has surpassed the number of available units, in part because funding for construction of new housing complexes has not been available since 2011 (Cisneros & Martinez, 2016). Senior housing sites are age-restricted apartments accepting residents age 62 and older (or lower, depending on the funding source). Apartments are usually one bedroom with a kitchen and a bath. Accessibility features include grab bars, access ramps, and nonskid flooring. Tenants must meet income eligibility requirements that are at or below 50% of the area median income. In 2015, the typical occupant in senior housing was 79 years old and had an annual income of $10,018 per year ($834 per month; Joint Center for Housing Studies, 2017). Rent is calculated by various methods, but does not exceed more than 30% of monthly adjusted income (HUD, 2002). This is the same housing cost standard (i.e., all housing costs should not exceed 30% of the adjusted monthly income) applied to applicants seeking mortgages to buy a home.

Critics of subsidized government housing are quick to point out that eligible older adults are being placed on waiting lists for more than a year before being offered a unit, which may or may not be in their preferred area (National Low Income Housing Coalition, 2016).

Additionally, the quality of the housing available is below acceptable standards. Units are not being maintained, updated, or replaced (Cisneros & Martinez, 2016). For persons who are able to access subsidized housing, it can offer an affordable, safe, and secure environment. But individuals who are not able to secure affordable housing that supports their service needs, are at extreme risk of becoming homeless (discussed further in this chapter).

Congregate Living Arrangements

Congregate living arrangements may resemble any other apartment or house, offering private bathrooms and kitchen facilities, and with features to support independent functioning (e.g., grab bars, access ramps, nonslip floors). They usually offer group dining, housekeeping, and socialization opportunities and provide at least a minimum level of assistance in accessing personal assistance or health services from an outside agency. By entering into a congregate living arrangement, an individual is in a good position to receive needed supports from the housing operator while remaining as independent as possible. More specific examples of congregate living arrangements include cohousing and shared housing.

Cohousing

Cohousing is a type of collaborative housing in which residents actively participate in the design and operation of their own neighborhoods (The Cohousing Association of the United States, 2017a). Whereas NORCs develop where people are already living, cohousing communities are intentional communities with private homes and common facilities and operate using consensus governing, shared responsibilities, and mutual assistance.

Early cohousing communities were not designed expressly for older adults. The idea that a child would benefit from being raised by a community shaped the development of the first cohousing community in

Copenhagen, Denmark, in 1972. Over the years, Denmark has improved upon cohousing community designs and boasts that 1% of the population live in cohousing communities (Lietaert, 2007).

In 2017, there were more than 150 cohousing communities in the United States (The Cohousing Association of the United States, 2017b). According to a 2012 survey of community leaders (Margolis, 2015), a typical cohousing community population includes people who are White, female, and not married. Over 80% of residents are age 40 or older and 40% are age 60 and older. Approximately, 47% of residents have incomes of $50,000–$99,000 per year, suggesting a middle income appeal. More than one-third (37%) of residents report holding atheist or agnostic religious views compared to 29% of the general population. Most residents have earned college degrees and share a strong connection to nature and spirituality. Activities in the communities are consensus driven and include stewardship of the earth, promotion of renewable energy, and shared empathy for the challenges faced by people around the world.

Communities operate from value statements that guide their development. For example, in New Mexico, Sand River Cohousing describes itself with the following value statements (Sand River Cohousing, n.d.):

- We respect the diversity of paths to personal growth. Deepening our connections to the natural world and others in the place that we live is a significant part of conscious aging.
- We live in a respectful, egalitarian community which uses a modified consensus process to guide our decision making. We are creating a peaceful, aesthetically pleasing environment that nurtures a sense of community and individual contentment.
- We value one another and the expression of mutual caring. We cherish and

celebrate our diverse origins, joys, talents, beliefs, and life experiences.
- We affirm a sustainable future by conserving resources and living ever more lightly on the Earth.
- We offer service to the larger community both as individuals and as representatives of Sand River.

At ElderSpirit Community in Virginia, the cohousing community was developed specifically for persons age 55 and older. The community includes privately owned homes and apartments for renters, who must qualify as low-to-moderate income households. ElderSpirits mission statement recognizes the importance of spirituality in late life. To that end, "Members believe that spiritual growth is the primary work of those in the later stages of life. Agreeing that freedom of religion is fundamental, we encourage one another in the search for meaning and commitment to the spiritual path of our choice. Through face-to-face relationships, we offer and receive support, express our needs and convictions, listen carefully to each other, and strive to act responsibly, considering our good, the good of the other, and the good of the community" (ElderSpirit, 2017).

A challenge faced by ElderSpirit and other long-standing cohousing communities is that the influx of younger residents to replace older residents is not occurring as quickly as first envisioned. Residents are living longer and healthier. Although that is desirable, the mutual support each resident is able to provide the community lessens with age. As a result, the scope and intensity of support the community can provide can decline if young and healthy residents are not integrated into it. Because residents are generally recruited by word of mouth, the membership may not be racially and economically diverse. The same exclusivity also limits the recruitment of young members who are needed to sustain the community (Lehning, Davitt, Scharlach, & Greenfield, 2014).

Shared Homes

Unlike cohousing, **shared housing** is less formal and may take place in any home in the community. In this arrangement, people might share expenses or exchange services for rent. For example, a homeowner needing help might have someone complete the housework and yard chores in exchange for free lodging. An adult might opt to share a home to reduce expenses (e.g., rent, utilities), to share chores, and for companionship. Shared housing arrangements can also be intergenerational. A grandmother could move in with an adult child and contribute to the household expenses or live in exchange for day care or any other arrangement made with the family.

▶ Community-Based Services and Supports

Home and Community-Based Services

In an effort to support independence and choice and reduce admission into long-term care facilities (presented in subsequent sections in this chapter), community providers offer a variety of services and supports in the home, which are called home and community-based services (HCBS) and are one aspect of the larger system of long-term care services and supports (LTCSS).

LTCSS include an array of services and supports for people who need assistance to function in everyday life. An estimated 70% of persons over the age of 65 will need long-term care services at some point in their lives (Genworth Financial, 2013). Care services selected can include personal care, rehabilitation, social services, AT, health care, home modifications, care coordination, assisted transportation, and more. Services may be needed on a regular or intermittent basis over a period of days,

months, or years. Moreover, they may be delivered in individual homes, in assisted living or supportive housing, in adult day centers, or in nursing facilities or other institutional settings.

The need for long-term care is usually measured by assessing limitations in an individual's capacity to perform or manage ADLs and IADLs. Although it is easy to assume that most older people need a lot of assistance, over 88% of individuals age 75 and older do not need any assistance with ADLs and over 80% have no functional limitations requiring assistance with IADLs (Adams, Kirzinger, & Martinez, 2012)!

Nursing homes and old age homes used to be places where old and frail adults were often sent to live when they started needing help. Today, no more than 5% of persons age 65+ live in institutional settings. More specifically, only 1% of people between ages 65 and 74 and 11% of adults over age 85 live in institutions (Administration on Aging, 2016). Most people who need LTCSS, therefore, live at home or in community settings, not in institutions.

The vast majority of adults (78%) in the United States receiving care receive it at home from family caregivers. An additional 14% of care recipients receive a combination of family care (i.e., informal care) and paid help (i.e., formal care); only 8% rely on formal care alone (Thompson, 2004). Still, family caregivers are expected to continue to provide the greatest proportion of long-term care services in the future (Family Caregiver Alliance, n.d.).

Home Health Services

When family members are unable to provide necessary and skilled medical care, **home health** services are typically accessed. Skilled care refers to services requiring a high level of skill, which can only be provided by credentialed professionals, to ensure safe and effective care. In 2014, there were 16,400 Medicare- or Medicaid-certified home care and hospice providers in the United States. Collectively, they offered an estimated 6.3 million patients nursing care, therapeutic services (e.g., occupational, physical, and respiratory therapies, and speech-language pathology services), home health aide services (i.e., basic health and personal care), case management, and therapeutic counseling (i.e., psychological, nutritional) (Harris-Kojetin et al., 2016). Home health care services are included in a treatment plan only when they are deemed medically necessary. Moreover, only an authorized heath care provider can order them. By offering skilled care at home, health care costs are dramatically less than costs accrued during care in a skilled care facility. Home health care spending in 2015 reached $88.8 billion and the Medicare and Medicaid programs (Centers for Medicare and Medicaid Services, 2016) paid for over 80% of care provided.

Program of All-Inclusive Care for the Elderly

One innovative community-based long-term care program that is a reimbursed by Medicare (since 1997) is the **Program of All-Inclusive Care for the Elderly** (PACE). The PACE model was first piloted in San Francisco, California, in 1973, offering services to people age 55 and older needing a level of care normally provided in a nursing home (Tanaz & Anderson, 2009). PACE originated out of public interest to reduce LTCSS expenditures. The PACE model offered care using an alternative setting and approach. PACE developers recognized that older adults wanted to age in place and could benefit from accessing services and supports in their immediate neighborhood. After all, better access should lead to better utilization, better health, and lowered long-term costs.

In 2017, there were 123 PACE programs operating 233 PACE centers across 31 states. These PACE programs collectively served over 40,000 participants (National PACE Association, 2017a). Each program is required to provide all healthcare services "on site" at a capitated (or fixed) rate. That is, the reimbursement for providing care is the same for each participant regardless of their diagnoses or therapeutic needs. This behooves PACE programs to keep on top of the health care needs of each participant on a daily basis.

PACE programs include a comprehensive set of medical and supportive services, including meals, counseling, respite, medication management, transportation to and from the site, and an adult day program. Participant outcomes from attending PACE program have been positive. Participants gained improved health status and quality of life, lower mortality rates, increased choice in how time is spent, and greater confidence in dealing with daily challenges (National PACE Association, 2017b).

Aging Network Services

As highlighted in Chapters 6 and 14, the Older American's Act (OAA) continues to carve out federal funds for nonmedical services to support older adults. State and local area agencies on aging and tribal and native organizations are responsible for setting eligibility requirements and implementing services and supports within their service catchment areas. Programs offered reflect local needs, and as such may vary from region to region. Services provided may include nonmedical services such as case management, homemaker/companion services, personal care, adult day services (ADS), transportation, and meal services.

Nonmedical home care services offer assistance such as daily care, housekeeping, meal preparation, medication reminders, transportation, and companionship. Individuals providing such services may not need to hold special accreditation to perform their duties (some states regulate service delivery more than others do). Often, the regulations in place are connected to the provider. Specifically, formal (agency) providers are regulated, whereas informal (privately hired) providers are not regulated.

Consumers of nonmedical services are frequently offered the option of hiring and managing the employment of persons providing them with services (referred to as consumer-directed care). Workers might be placed with care recipients through the agency that employed them, they could be independent contractors managing their own work, or they may be hired directly by the care recipient, who in turn manages their employment. Many families directly employ workers to provide care and pay for their services when insurance does not reimburse (referred to as out-of-pocket care costs).

Adult day services (ADS) offer programs of activities, health monitoring, socialization, and assistance with ADLs for individuals requiring daily supervision and oversight. Attendance allows individuals to continue to live in their homes and receive needed care in a supportive, professionally staffed, community-based setting. ADS also benefit family caregivers by providing time away from caregiving to engage in work or receive needed time off (i.e., respite) from caregiving. ADS programs can also offer caregivers educational programs and support groups (MetLife Mature Market Institute, 2010b).

In 2010, 55% of ADS fees were paid through public funding such as Medicaid Home and Community-Based Waiver Programs, Veteran's Administration, and state and local funding. Twenty-six percent were paid privately and the remaining payers split among grants, donations, internal funding, and private insurance (MetLife Mature Market Institute, 2010b).

The use of ADS programs can decrease caregiver stress, so that caregivers can better function in their workplaces and enjoy time with their families. Because of ADS, the caregivers studied were better able to deal with problem behaviors, had an improved ability

to be adaptable, and showed decreased signs of stress, anger, and depression. They also reported a decreased sense of subjective burden (Dabelko-Schoeny & King, 2010).

More specifically, Zarit and colleagues (2011) found that caregivers' stress decreased significantly on days that the care recipient (who lived with them) was in an ADS program compared to days not in the ADS program. ADS participation also contributed to less disturbing "dementia" behavior and better sleep patterns among attendees. Ultimately, effective ADS programs could help to delay institutionalization for those at risk by providing caregivers needed support so that they could extend the time they are able to undertake this vital role.

In addition to the services already described, HCBS also includes single use and long-term use services such as **transportation**, **meal services**, and **chore services**. In some regions, transportation services are supplemented by volunteer transportation services designed specifically to transport individuals to medical appointments or pharmacy visits. Meal service options include the well-known Meals on Wheels program, in which delivery volunteers are trained to assess recipient health status during their visits and report changes in health status to the agency for follow up. Congregate meal sites are also operated in local gathering spots to offer socialization and activities in addition to a meal. **Telephone reassurance** programs are designed to support the needs of people who have limited socialization opportunities or do not have family nearby to check on them. Typically, a volunteer telephones the participant each day at a specified time. During the call, they talk about the recipient's health, any unmet needs, and plans to go into the community that day. Again, if a volunteer suspects problems, they report back to a designated person for follow up. The value of each of these services not only lies in its direct purpose (to transport, feed, and support), but the opportunities for socialization that can lead to decreased isolation and improved well-being.

▶ Service-Enriched Communities

Although reasons for staying in one's familiar home may be compelling, for some older adults, the decision to move may be the necessary or preferred option. People relocate for various reasons, including health challenges, limited finances, social isolation, distance from family or friends, wanting fewer home management responsibilities, experiencing a loss of functional ability, and/or seeking a more moderate climate. Although there are many living options for older adults, not all options are available to persons who need them. This section highlights several possibilities for people who are still independent yet may need some assistance on a day-to-day basis.

Continuing Care Retirement Community

Continuing care retirement community (CCRC) campuses are specifically designed to provide a spectrum of lifetime care to residents in the community. Ideally, residents enter the CCRC in the independent living setting and move to more supportive housing within the community if medical and/or personal care services are needed. To join a CCRC, residents typically pay an initial fee and a monthly administrative fee. In return, they are provided access to housing and services that meet their personal needs. Housing within the CCRC may include freestanding houses, townhomes, or apartments. Depending on the community, housing is purchased by the individual or rented. Services available may include medical or nonmedical. Some services may be automatically integrated into specific housing options. Although CCRCs can have a not-for-profit entity in its structure, the cost for entering CCRCs is out of the financial reach for most older adults. Some CCRCs offer some low-income housing opportunities, but those organizations are limited.

Assisted Living Facility

Assisted living facility (ALF) is a broad term used to describe several types of congregate living arrangements, including adult group homes, board and care homes, personal care homes, and assisted living facilities. In some states, the terms are interchangeable. Regardless of the name, ALFs provide people who could potentially live independently if offered support with ADLs (e.g., hygiene) and IADLs (e.g., medication administration). Whether ALFs offer nursing services or help with medication administration varies by state.

In most cases, residents pay monthly rent and additional fees for the services they receive. Medicare does not pay for housing and services provided in assisted living communities. Medicaid does not typically pay for room and board in these settings either, but depending on the state may cover other costs for eligible individuals. Some long-term care insurance policies may cover residential care as may some Veterans' benefits.

Most ALF apartments are "homelike," with residents encouraged to bring their own furniture and belongings. Community or shared spaces such as dining rooms, libraries, and activity rooms are provided to promote social interactions. Although the initial move into an ALF may be unsettling and discomforting, residents can trust that as health issues arise they will receive the care needed to remain in their new home for as long as possible.

In 2014, there were approximately 30,200 assisted living residences in the United States, housing more than 1 million people (Harris-Kojetin et al., 2016). Facility sizes vary greatly as do fees charged and services provided. Residences typically provide 24/7 supervision, up to three meals per day in a group dining room, personal care, social activities, housekeeping, help with medications, and arrangements for transportation.

Some ALFs specialize in serving people with specific health conditions such as dementia to ensure both their safety and their engagement in meaningful activities. Individuals considering a move to an ALF should clarify with each site how the staff will be able to meet their care needs, and at what point another move would be needed to find the best fit for anticipated future changes. The average cost for assisted living in the United States in 2017 was $3,750 per month, with the lowest cost in Georgia ($2,800) and significantly higher prices in parts of the northeast. The highest rate was in Delaware ($6,015; Genworth Financial, 2017).

Nursing Facilities

Many individuals with disabilities that interfere with their self-care skills are eligible to receive care within a nursing facility because of their physical or cognitive impairments. The decision to move into a facility is generally no longer a choice, but rather it is largely predicated on the need for medical care and assistance that is greater than what is available in the home by family or HCBS providers. In the continuum of care, long-term nursing home care is viewed as the most restrictive home environment.

Nursing facilities provide around-the-clock care with the services of registered nurses, licensed practical nurses, and nursing aides. A complement of physicians and therapists is typically associated with a facility, but may not be on site every day. As the need for reducing LTCSS costs has increased, the emphasis on nursing care has been changing. Services in nursing homes are shifting away from long-term care toward rehabilitation therapies. Residents are often admitted for periods of up to 90 days to receive rehabilitation services that improve their functioning to the point that they are able to transfer into a less restrictive environment (including their home) to convalesce.

Oversight of nursing home care is performed by federal and state entities. Regulations may vary state to state, although organizations that receive Medicare and Medicaid reimbursement must comply with federal regulations and standards. CMS periodically audits and surveys facilities that participate in the Medicare program to ensure that they comply with all state and federal requirements. Facilities that fail to comply can be shut down or lose their ability to be reimbursed for services provided. Agencies and facilities opting for additional accreditation, such as those provided by The Joint Commission (TJC) or the Community Health Accreditation Program (CHAP), are subject to additional requirements related to the care provided.

In spite of the need for long-term care facilities and the oversight provided, there still seems to be widespread fear and hatred of nursing homes due to the negative experiences many families have had in the past (Harmon & Harmon, n.d.). In an effort to quell consumer anxiety and to be more transparent about the quality of care provided, CMS provides survey ratings of CMS-regulated nursing homes through the Nursing Home Compare website (www.medicare.gov/NursingHome Compare/search.aspx). Users can compare nursing homes based on ratings of health inspections, staffing, adherence to residents' rights, and pharmaceutical services.

Rehabilitation

The process of helping someone regain the highest possible level of functioning after an injury or illness is called **rehabilitation** (informally referred to as "rehab"). Rehabilitation specialists, including **physiatrists** (i.e., physicians specializing in rehabilitation), nurses, and therapy practitioners in the fields of occupational therapy, physical therapy and speech-language pathology, work with clients in the home, community, residential facility settings, nursing homes, and hospitals. Rehabilitation services are provided at different levels of intensity, depending on the client's needs. In an acute rehabilitation setting such as a rehabilitation hospital or nursing home, a resident generally receives three or more hours of skilled therapy each day. Through medical management and therapy, individuals are expected to make significant gains in a reasonable and expected period of time (Medicare Rights Center, 2017). Therapists, rehabilitation nurses, and physiatrists are experts in judging whether this is likely to occur given various factors and the person's current condition. For example, after a stroke or cerebrovascular accident (CVA), an individual can often make good progress in regaining strength, balance, and motor control to do desired tasks. If excellent and quick gains are made, the person may return home directly from the rehabilitation unit. However, if gains are slow or insignificant, an individual may need alternative placement (e.g., assisted living or a nursing facility) prior to or instead of going home. Alternatively, if the individual's level of endurance cannot withstand the intensity of acute level rehabilitation, he or she may receive lower intensity therapy services in a skilled nursing facility. Detailed information about SNF rehabilitation services can be found at www.medicare.gov/coverage/skilled-nursing-facility-care.html.

Rehabilitation includes exercise, education, and training/retraining in ADLs, IADLs, mobility, communication, and other functional tasks as needed. By participating in rehabilitation services, many people have been able to return to their former level of independence and their former living situations. This is accomplished by restoration of function and/or using compensatory measures and environmental adaptations to make up for lost skills.

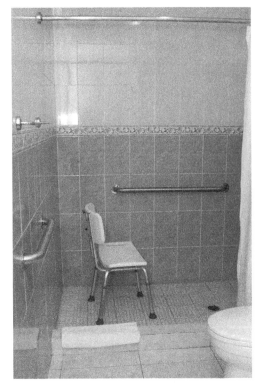

FIGURE 3-3 An accessible walk-in shower.
© Abalcazar/E+/Getty Image

▶ Person-Centered Approaches to Institutional Care

In the United States, there is a cultural shift in the values and principles on which institutional care is assessed and based. The health care system is leaning toward offering person-centered care, but continues to struggle with being prescriptive. However, there are some examples of successful person-centered approaches in the United States and abroad, which can serve as models for change.

In Europe, long-term care facilities seem to have more private rooms with private bathrooms and standard walk-in showers (FIGURE 3-3); and access to outdoors and walking paths (FIGURE 3-4). Some facilities even have cafés that are open and inviting to the public. When you walk into these facilities, the smell of baked goods is pleasing. Local community members looking for light fare at a reasonable cost or as a convenient place to meet friends may frequent the cafés, which also helps residents maintain their connections to the community.

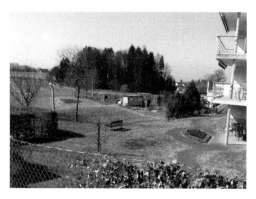

FIGURE 3-4 Access to outdoor spaces contributes to better health and well-being.

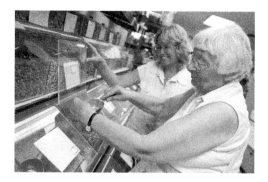

FIGURE 3-5 Persons with dementia can benefit from receiving help completing daily chores such as shopping.

© Imagegami/iStockphoto/Getty

Hogeweyk

A creative and imaginative approach to caring for elders, specifically persons with Alzheimer's disease, is offered in Hogeweyk. This village-styled nursing home was established near Amsterdam in 2009. Hogeweyk was developed on the site of a former nursing facility and its campus was transformed into a typical European village. Residents live in one of 23 units with other residents who share similar lifestyles. Each of the units or suites is decorated in a specific style (e.g., country, traditional, cosmopolitan) that conforms to the resident's taste. These units are chosen by the residents based on their lifestyle preferences so that they can continue to live in the way to which they are accustomed. Each unit houses six or seven residents and has a caretaker that assists with home management, outings, and shopping for food at the village store.

The residents in Hogeweyk are provided access to the entire campus in an effort to provide them with a sense of "normalcy." They can shop for food with their suite mates, stroll the grounds, socialize, and even get a haircut (Weller, 2017). Yet, all their activities and access occurs within a locked compound from which they cannot leave. Their activities are real, yet the backdrop of their daily life is not. All the staff working at Hogeweyk are trained in caring for persons with Alzheimer's disease

using a person-centered approach. They provide residents the opportunity to engage in activities because it helps promote a sense of normalcy and usefulness, which promotes improved personal well-being (**FIGURE 3-5**).

While proponents of Hogeweyk view the model as truly inventive and creative, critics call it a scary version of the *Truman Show*, because its operations are based on deceiving residents (Charter, 2012). Readers are encouraged to form their own opinion about Hogeweyk and what they would want should they need care in the future. A 2013 interview by Sanjay Gupta with the director of Hogeweyk is available at www.youtube.com/watch?v =LwiOBlyWpko

Eden Alternative

The **Eden Alternative** was developed by Bill Thomas in the 1990s after he became the medical director of a nursing care facility in upstate New York. Dismayed by the "institutionalized absence of life" (Gawanda, 2014, p. 115), he sought innovative ideas to improve the lives of the residents and to combat the "three plagues of nursing home existence: boredom, loneliness, and helplessness" (Gawanda, 2014, p. 116). Thomas fought (with the health department and the home's administrative staff) to bring in live plants and animals, including dogs, cats, rabbits, hens, and parakeets. Following the influx of pets, amazing events started happening. People who had been nonambulatory started walking so they could "walk the dog," people named and adopted the parakeets, and perhaps most important, the number of prescriptions required per resident decreased by 50%, while mortality also decreased 15%. Thomas contended that people need a reason to live, and in this case, the menagerie of animals offered that purpose, which was the opportunity to take care of another living being (Gawanda, 2014, p. 125).

The Eden Alternative model embraces 10 principles (Eden Alternative, 2016):

1. The three plagues of loneliness, helplessness, and boredom account for the bulk of suffering among our Elders.
2. An Elder-centered community commits to creating a Human Habitat where life revolves around close and continuing contact with people of all ages and abilities, as well as plants and animals. It is these relationships that provide the young and old alike with a pathway to a life worth living.
3. Loving companionship is the antidote to loneliness. Elders deserve easy access to human and animal companionship.
4. An Elder-centered community creates opportunity to give as well as receive care. This is the antidote to helplessness.
5. An Elder-centered community imbues daily life with variety and spontaneity by creating an environment in which unexpected and unpredictable interactions and happenings can take place. This is the antidote to boredom.
6. Meaningless activity corrodes the human spirit. The opportunity to do things that we find meaningful is essential to human health.
7. Medical treatment should be the servant of genuine human caring, never its master.
8. An Elder-centered community honors its Elders by de-emphasizing top-down, bureaucratic authority, seeking instead to place the maximum possible decision-making authority into the hands of the Elders or into the hands of those closest to them.
9. Creating an Elder-centered community is a never-ending process. Human growth must never be separated from human life.
10. Wise leadership is the lifeblood of any struggle against the three plagues. For it, there can be no substitute.

Development of the Eden principles helped lay the groundwork for inspiring other nursing facilities to transform their own culture into a person-centered culture that promotes health, well-being, and quality of life. Bill Thomas continues to advocate for facility administrators to replace their "top-down" prescriptive focus on care with a "bottom-up" strategy that emerges from resident need, so that the quality of nursing home care will improve. Facilities interested in adopting the Eden Alternative approach can participate in a training available through Eden Alternative.

Throughout the world, the push is on for the proliferation of more inventive person-centered care models to meet the needs of the growing size of the older population. By not segregating older adults from the rest of society and by viewing their needs as a continuum of care, new and innovative alternatives are more likely to emerge. Providing quality long-term care will ensure a better quality of life for persons needing such care (OECD, 2014).

▶ Special Topics and Issues

Telehealth

Ongoing technological developments in health care are enabling an array of new services to be provided away from the medical center. **Telehealth** is a way to visit with and monitor patients outside the medical setting, using ordinary telecommunications and physiological assessment devices such as stethoscopes, pulse oximeters, and blood glucose meters. These devices are altered to transmit information via phone lines.

Telehealth is a cost-saving measure for providers and patients because it eliminates costs associated with travel to remote locations. Technologically advanced service extenders such as telehealth may be harkening the dawn of a new age of home health care, especially in rural areas. When combined with in-home care as needed, telehealth interventions may actually help to prevent hospital readmissions (Dinesen et al., 2012).

As the use of telehealth spreads, the potential for more uses in providing services and supports will emerge. Current efforts are studying telehealth as a method of communication to conduct community support groups, provide continuing education opportunities to providers, and to train caregivers in how to provide basic nursing skills. Clearly, telehealth has the potential to connect individuals and communities that are otherwise isolated from one another.

Paying for LTCSS

As highlighted in chapters 6 and 14, nearly half of all reimbursements for LTCSS are paid through Medicare. However, **Medicaid**, a need-based program managed by state governments, can cover more HCBS service costs than Medicare. Currently, Medicaid pays for

49% of long-term care costs (Congressional Budget Office, 2013).

As life expectancy continues to rise, the need for ongoing long-term care will increase. Some people are purchasing **long-term care insurance** as a way to pay for services they may need in the future while protecting their financial assets. In 2014, an estimated 8.1 million policies were in place (American Association for Long-Term Care Insurance, 2014). Depending on the individual policy purchased, long-term care insurance may cover personal care and homemaking assistance at home, ADS, assisted living, nursing facility care, or other services. Because LTC insurance is relatively new, there is limited long-term data available to suggest that it is a sound investment for the future. However, it is becoming increasingly available as part of insurance package options in the workplace.

Homelessness

Homelessness rates of older adults are on the rise. Although the aged homeless population is much smaller in number than younger age groups, its growing size is raising concerns because more older adults will be living on low fixed incomes in the future and lack the ability to obtain affordable housing—a direct pathway toward homelessness (Sermons & Henry, 2010). When income and housing needs are compounded by chronic health problems, including mental health problems and addiction, long-term homelessness can result. As illustrated in **FIGURE 3-6**, the homeless population of persons age 65 and older is expected to increase 33% by 2020 (from 44,172 in 2010 to 58,772 in 2020) and will continue to rise through 2050 (Sermons & Henry, 2010).

For health care practitioners, the way to help combat homelessness is to remain attentive to each client's biopsychosocial needs. Observe their environment and become aware of their daily routines for potential unmet needs. Use the service referral mechanism in

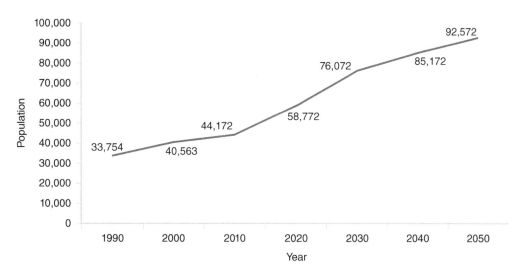

FIGURE 3-6 The rising population of older adults who are homeless.

National Health Care for the Homeless Council. (September 2013). Aging and Housing Instability: Homelessness among Older and Elderly Adults. In Focus: A Quarterly Research Review of the National HCH Council, 2:1. [Author: Sarah Knopf-Amelung, Research Associate] Nashville, TN: Available at: www.nhchc.org.

place in your agency to help connect clients with services that will reduce their risk for homelessness.

Home Modifications

In light of the fact that most people want to remain in their own homes for as long as possible, changes will likely need to be made in the home to keep the older residents safe and comfortable. Many times, older homeowners do not think about modifying their homes until they experience debilitating health problems that reduce their ability to be mobile and function independently in their homes. For these individuals, a physician should refer them to an occupational therapist or a physical therapist for a comprehensive home evaluation. The therapist will evaluate their home and how they function in it to identify areas that could be modified or strategies that they can implement to stay safe and remain as independent as possible.

When modifications to the home are required or just desired, it is up to the home-owner to secure a contractor to make the changes. The National Association of Home Builders (NAHB) offers professional training and Certified Aging in Place Specialist (CAPS) certification to builders and contractors who can provide the expertise needed to modify homes as directed by therapists and home-owners (Age in Place Network, n.d.).

Some modifications will involve extensive remodeling such as building a bathroom on the first floor or creating no-step thresholds to increase accessibility. Entry steps may need to be replaced by a ramp to allow for wheelchair access. Doorways may need to be widened to accommodate a wheelchair or chair lifts may need to be added to existing stairways. Kitchens may need to be remodeled to allow easy access under the counters and ease of retrieving items (**FIGURE 3-7**).

Even though universal design features promote accessibility within an environment, the process of adapting a home to fit changing physical needs may be so substantial that moving to a different home or building a new home is more cost-effective. However, existing

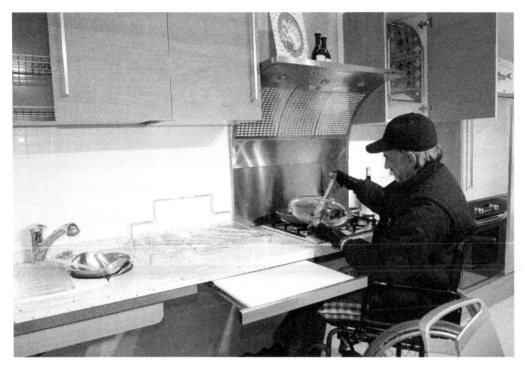

FIGURE 3-7 Accessibility features can make kitchen tasks possible for persons with physical limitations.
© paolo siccardi/age fotostock

homes may not be any more amenable to change than the current home. Older homes with typical multi- or split-level layouts do not generally have single-level living areas. Moreover, they are likely to have narrow doorways and inaccessible spaces for persons with limited mobility or using a wheelchair. Newly built homes may have more accessible features than older homes, but still may not offer the modifications needed unless the home is built with the modifications in mind. This, of course, may come at additional cost to the homeowner and is out of financial reach for the majority of older adults.

Some home modifications are less drastic and require little modification to the home. These changes may be perceived as more acceptable and affordable to homeowners:

- Adding raised toilet seats and grab bars in the bathroom

- Stabilizing or eliminating scatter and area rugs
- Improving lighting levels
- Using shower seats or bath transfer benches
- Eliminating clutter, tripping hazards (such as cords in pathways), and excess furniture
- Ensuring that smoke and carbon monoxide detectors are available and working
- Resetting the water heater to a lower temperature (not exceeding 120°F)
- Removing door thresholds
- Moving commonly used items into easily reached spaces

Not all older homeowners need to make all these changes to remain safe, although these accommodations are unlikely to cause harm to anyone who uses them (**FIGURE 3-8**).

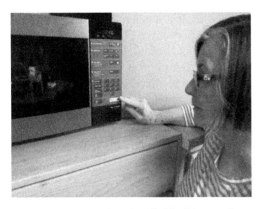

FIGURE 3-8 Marge, who is legally blind, has made simple adaptations to her microwave so she can continue to use it.

Courtesy of Marge's family

In addition to making home modifications, the individual needing the changes can learn compensatory strategies from a therapist to remain safe in the home. An occupational therapist or a physical therapist can help the individual learn to do the following:

- Transfer in and out of the tub or shower safely
- Use a walker or cane to compensate for decreased balance or strength
- Use safe techniques when using kitchen appliances
- Use alternative techniques for completing the daily tasks
- Use joint protection and energy conservation techniques
- Compensate for changes in eyesight, memory, and hearing

Reverse Mortgages

A home equity conversion mortgage or **reverse mortgage** is one financial planning option that makes it possible for many older people to afford to stay in their own homes. Through this federally insured program, borrowers use their home as collateral, and the

bank sets up either an annuity or a line of credit to be drawn from as needed until the home is sold or the loan repaid. This allows homeowners with inadequate monthly income, but substantial home equity, to remain in their own homes. When the homeowner sells the home or dies, the bank recovers its investment from the proceeds of the sale (National Council on Aging, n.d.).

Overall, reverse mortgage programs sound ideal for aging in place. However, critics of reverse mortgage programs suggest there are program caveats that can cause problems for some homeowners. Program users can face bankruptcy if they cannot pay monthly fees, overdraw on the equity of their home, or outlive the equity available. In some cases, the value of the house decreases and upon sale, the bank demands payment for the balance of the initial appraisal from which the equity was drawn. Regulations on lenders have tightened, thus reducing some of the problems, but they still exist.

According to the National Reverse Mortgage Lenders Association, reverse mortgages were first offered in 1990 when approximately 150 loans were secured. The number of reverse mortgage loans peaked in 2009 with 114,692 loans. In fiscal year 2016, fewer than 49,000 loans were offered (National Reverse Mortgage Lenders Association, n.d.). Still, use of reverse mortgages appears to be of interest to older adults.

▶ Summary

Home provides the foundation for maintaining health, well-being, and quality of life for older adults. A home "fulfills many needs: it is a place of shelter and security, inspires a sense of belonging and mastery, and allows the person to be him- or herself, reinforcing (by the presence of significant personal items) their life and identity" (Minkler, 1992). People of all ages deserve the opportunity to live in homes that not only provide safe shelter, but also offer environments to engage in desired occupations. For older adults, finding places that ensure supported and enjoyable living is sometimes challenging but not impossible. Whether home is a house, an ALF, or one of the many other housing options described in this chapter, it should provide the resident with a sense of being in the right place—the pleasing feeling of being home, not just existing. Regardless of type, homes need to be safe, affordable, and accessible to provide the least restrictive environment possible. If a resident feels safe and secure, they are able to focus on their health and social needs. Enjoyable surroundings provide opportunities to participate in personally meaningful activities, which can help promote a healthy, productive, and fulfilling aging experience.

🔍 CASE STUDIES

Case 1: Carmella, a 72-year-old widow with no children, lives alone. She is on a fixed income, but she owns her home, which is located in a rapidly growing neighborhood. Carmella has been relatively healthy for most of her life, but now her vision is failing, she was diagnosed with osteoporosis last year, and she does not have the strength and stamina that she once did. With her husband gone and most of her friends having moved away, she has few opportunities for socialization. Her biggest fear is that someday she might fall and break her hip and no one will find her. Carmella does not really want to leave her home, but she knows that it is time for something to change.

1. **If Carmella decided to move out of her home, which housing option would you recommend for her and why?**
2. **Do you think Carmella is a good candidate for a reverse mortgage? Why or why not?**
3. **If Carmella decides to stay in her home, what services might be most beneficial to her and why?**

Case 2: After he retired, Martin rented a room in a house with three roommates, one of whom owned the house. He and another roommate shared expenses in lieu of paying rent, while the third roommate lived there for free in exchange for performing home maintenance, running errands, and helping out with any other necessary tasks. Seven years ago, the homeowner died and Martin decided to move into an ALF. He has made many friends over the last few years and rarely had any significant health problems in that time. A few months ago, he suffered a stroke that did not affect his mental capacity, but caused mild paralysis and some difficulty speaking. Martin can still perform most ADLs and IADLs with minimal assistance, although it takes a bit longer than it used to. During a recent visit from his son and daughter-in-law, he overheard them in the hall discussing the possibility of moving him into a nursing home. Martin does not feel that he belongs in a nursing home and is frightened that his son might be able to force him to move into one.

1. **What type of housing did Martin live in before moving to the assisted living facility, and how do you know?**
2. **Based on Martin's current situation, do you think he needs to be moved to a nursing facility? Why or why not?**
3. **Martin is afraid that his son will force him to move into a nursing home. Is his son able to make this determination on his own? Why or why not?**

TEST YOUR KNOWLEDGE

Review Questions

1. The benefits of remaining connected to one's home can potentially shorten the length of time in institutional care and increase the time spent living at home and in the community.
   a. True
   b. False

2. A key therapeutic goal is to provide services and supports in the _____ as possible.
   a. Best medical environment
   b. Most family-like environment
   c. Least restrictive environment
   d. Least hospital-like environment

3. _____ includes not only personal services, but also assistive technology, which can help users complete activities of daily living and instrumental activities in daily living.
   a. Least restrictive environment
   b. Continuum of care
   c. Person-centered care
   d. Gerotechnology

4. The continuum of care service delivery model provides a way to connect _____ with _____ in a way that supports the least restrictive environments possible.
   a. Transportation, recreation
   b. Housing, healthcare
   c. Healthcare, transportation
   d. Recreation, housing

5. Long-term care services and supports (LTCSS) include an array of services and supports for people who need assistance to function in everyday life. Home and community-based services (HCBS) are one component of the LTCC system that supports personal independence and choice while increasing admissions into long-term care facilities.
   a. True
   b. False

Learning Activities

1. The seven principles of universal design are:
   a. Equitable use
   b. Flexibility in use
   c. Simple and intuitive use
   d. Perceptible information
   e. Tolerance for error
   f. Low physical effort
   g. Size and space for approach and use

   Discuss how these seven principles specifically support the needs of older adults. Provide specific examples.

2. Identify five things in your current home environment that you think you will need to change and will not need to change if you were an older person with mobility problems. Compare your answers with the group. What can you learn from the answers of others?

3. Research three different cohousing communities. In what ways are they similar and in what ways are they different. Identify steps each type of community could take to increase the diversity of its members and continue to be financially sustainable.

4. Research continuing care retirement communities (CCRCs). Identify the

advantages and disadvantages of living in a CCRC. What steps could a CCRC take to become more environmentally accessible to its residents?

5. Telehealth is an emerging technology. Identify a health issue that interests you. How can telehealth contribute to addressing the problem? Compare your answers with the group.

6. People can benefit a great deal from receiving person-centered care across the continuum of care. Initiate a group discussion on the positive and negative implications for embedding it in the health care and housing systems across the continuum of care. (HINT: financial, regulatory, public health).

References

Adams, P. F., Kirzinger, W. K., & Martinez, M .E. (2012). Summary health statistics for the US population: National Health Interview Survey, 2011. *Vital Health Statistics, 10*, 18. Retrieved from http://www.cdc.gov/nchs/data/series/sr_10/sr10_255.pdf

Administration on Aging (2016). *A profile of older Americans: 2016.* Washington, DC: U.S. Department of Health and Human Services. Retrieved from https://www.acl.gov/sites/default/files/Aging%20and%20Disability%20in%20America/2016-Profile.pdf

Age in Place Network. (n.d.). *Introduction to certified aging in place specialists (CAPS).* Retrieved from http://ageinplace.com/aging-in-place-professionals/certified-aging-in-place-specialists-caps/

American Association for Long-Term Care Insurance. (2014). Long-term care insurance facts-statistics. Retrieved from http://www.aaltci.org/long-term-care-insurance/learning-center/fast-facts.php

Assistive Technology Industry Association. (n.d.). What is AT? Retrieved from https://www.atia.org/at-resources/what-is-at/

Ball, M. S. (2004). *Aging in place: A toolkit for local government.* Community Housing Resource Center, Atlanta, GA: Atlanta Regional Commission.

Centers for Disease Control and Prevention. (n.d.). *Healthy Places Terminology.* Retrieved from https://www.cdc.gov/healthyplaces/terminology.htm

Centers for Medicare and Medicaid Services. (2016). *National health expenditures 2015 highlights.* Retrieved from https://www.cms.gov/Research-Statistics-Data-and-Systems/Statistics-Trends-and-Reports/NationalHealthExpendData/downloads/highlights.pdf

Centre for Excellence in Universal Design. (2014a). *What is universal design?* Retrieved from http://universaldesign.ie/What-is-Universal-Design/

Centre for Excellence in Universal Design. (2014b). *The 7 principles.* Retrieved from http://universaldesign.ie/What-is-Universal-Design/The-7-Principles/

Charter, D. (2012). *For the Alzheimer victims lost in time, a new village of care.* Retrieved from http://www.thetimes.co.uk/tto/news/world/europe/article3370109.ece.

Cisneros, H., & Martinez, M. (2016). Former HUD secretaries: America's elderly desperately need more affordable housing. *Housingwire.* Retrieved from https://www.housingwire.com/articles/print/37090-former-hud-secretaries-americas-elderly-desperately-need-more-affordable-housing

Congressional Budget Office. (2013). *Rising demand for long-term services and supports for elderly people.* Retrieved from https://www.cbo.gov/sites/default/files/113th-congress 2013-2014/reports/44363-ltc.pdf

Dabelko-Schoeny, H., & King, S. (2010). In their own words: Participants' perceptions of the impact of adult day services. *Journal of Gerontological Social Work, 53*(2), 176–192.

Dethflefs, N., & Martin, B. (2006). Japanese technology for aged care. *Science and Public Policy, 33*, 47–57. doi:10.3152/147154306781779163

Dinesen, B., Haesum, L. K., Soerensen, N., Nielsen, C., Grann, O., Hejlesen, Toft, E., & Ehlers, L. (2012). Using preventive home monitoring to reduce hospital admission rates and reduce costs: A case study of telehealth among chronic obstructive pulmonary disease patients. *Journal of Telemedicine and Telecare, 18*, 221–225. doi:10.1258/jtt.2012.110704

Eden Alternative. (2016). *Mission, vision, values, principles.* Retrieved from http://www.edenalt.org/about-the-eden-alternative/mission-vision-values/

ElderSpirit. (2017). Home page. Retrieved from http://elderspirit.org

Family Caregiver Alliance. (n.d.). *Caregiving.* Retrieved from https://www.caregiver.org/caregiving

Fries, J. F., Bruce, B., & Chakravarty, E. (2011). Compression of morbidity 1980–2011: A focused review of paradigms and progress. *Journal of Aging Research,* 10 pp. doi:10.4061/2011/261702

Gawanda, A. (2014). *Being mortal: Medicine and what matters in the end.* New York: Henry Holt and Company, LLC.

Genworth Financial. (2013). *Compare cost of care across the United States (2013).* Retrieved from https://www.genworth.com/corporate/about-genworth/industry-expertise/cost-of-care.html.

Genworth Financial. (2017). *Compare long-term care costs across the United States.* Retrieved from https://www.genworth.com/about-us/industry-expertise/cost-of-care.html

Greenfield, E., Scharlach, A., Graham, C., Davitt, J., & Lehning, A. (2012). *A national overview of villages: Results from a 2012 organizational survey.* New Brunswick, NJ: Rutgers School of Social Work.

Halloran, M. (2018). *Innovation in senior living: Michele Holleran examines nonprofit providers.* Leading Age. Retrieved from https://www.leadingage.org/resources/innovation-senior-living-michele-holleran-examines-nonprofit-providers

Harmon, L. C., & Harmon, K. M. (n.d.). *We don't like nursing homes.* Retrieved from http://www.alzheimersreadingroom.com/2010/03/we-dont-like-nursing-homes.html.

Harrell, R., Lynott, J., Guzmann, S., & Lampkin, C. (2014). *What is livable? Community preferences of older adults.* (20144-1) Washington, DC: AARP Public Policy Institute. Retrieved from https://www.giaging.org/documents/what-is-livable-report-AARP-ppi-liv-com.pdf

Harris-Kojetin, L., Sengupta, M., Park-Lee, E., Valverde, R., Caffrey, C., Rome, V., & Lendon, J. (2016). Long-term care providers and services users in the United States: Data from the National Study of Long-Term Care Providers, 2013–2014. *Vital & Health Statistics. Series 3, Analytical and Epidemiological Studies, 38,* pp. x–xii. Retrieved from https://www.cdc.gov/nchs/data/series/sr_03/sr03_038.pdf

Joint Center for Housing Studies. (2017). *America's rental housing.* Joint Center for Housing Studies. Cambridge, MA: Harvard University.

Kerschner, H., & Pegues, J. A. (1998). Productive aging: A quality of life agenda. *Journal of the American Dietetic Association, 98,* 1445–1448. doi:10.1016/S0002-8223(98)00327-7

Kirschenbaum, H. (2009). *The life and work of Carl Rogers.* Alexandria, VA: American Counseling Association.

Kirschenbaum, H., & Jourdan, A. (2005). The current status of Carl Rogers and the person-centered approach. *Psychotherapy: Theory, Research, Practice, Training, 42,* 37–51. doi:10.1037/0033-3204.42.1.37

Lehning, A., Davitt, J., Scharlach, A., & Greenfield, E. (2014). *Village sustainability and engaging a diverse membership: Key findings from a 2013 national survey.*

Baltimore, MD: University of Maryland School of Social Work.

Lietaert, M. (2007). *The growth of cohousing in Europe.* The Cohousing Association of the United States. Retrieved from http://www.cohousing.org/node/1537

MacDonald, M., Remus, G., & Laing, G. (1994). Research considerations: The link between housing and health in the elderly. *Journal of Gerontological Nursing, 20,* 5–9.

Margolis, D. (2015). *Demographics of cohousing survey data and national norms.* Retrieved from http://www.cohousing.org/2015/docs/research

Medicare Rights Center. (2017). *How do I qualify for care in a rehabilitation hospital?* Retrieved from https://www.medicareinteractive.org/get-answers/medicare-covered-services/hospital-services-inpatient-part-a/how-do-i-qualify-for-care-in-a-rehabilitation-hospital

MetLife Mature Market Institute. (2010a). *Aging in Place 2.0: Rethinking solutions to the home care challenge.* Retrieved from https://www.metlife.com/assets/cao/mmi/publications/studies/2010/mmi-aging-place-study.pdf

MetLife Mature Market Institute. (2010b). *The MetLife National Study of Adult Day Services: Providing support to individuals and their family caregivers.* Retrieved from https://www.metlife.com/assets/cao/mmi/publications/studies/2010/mmi-adult-day-services.pdf

Minkler, M. (1992). Community organizing among the elderly poor in the United States: A case study. *International Journal of Health Services, 22,* 303–316.

N2Care. (n.d.). *MEDCottage: The story.* Retrieved from http://www.medcottage.com/the-story-.html

National Council on Aging. (n.d.). *Reverse mortgages.* Retrieved from https://www.ncoa.org/economic-security/home-equity/reverse-mortgages/

National Low Income Housing Coalition. (2016). *Closed waiting lists and long waits await those seeking affordable housing, according to new NLIHC survey.* Retrieved from http://nlihc.org/press/releases/7202

National PACE Association. (2017a). *Find a PACE program in your neighborhood.* Retrieved from http://www.npaonline.org/pace-you/find-pace-program-your-neighborhood

National PACE Association. (2017b.). *PACE in the states.* Retrieved from http://www.npaonline.org/sites/default/files/March%202017%20-%20PACE%20in%20the%20States.pdf

National Reverse Mortgage Lenders Association. (n.d.). Retrieved from https://www.nrmlaonline.org/category/industry-news-reference/industry-statistics

New York Department for the Aging. (2017). *NORC services.* Retrieved from https://a125-egovt.nyc.gov/egovt/services/service_detail.cfm?contract__cont_dfta_id=N3101

OECD. (2014). *Long-term care.* Retrieved from http://www.oecd.org/els/health-systems/long-term-care.htm

Opp, A. (n.d.). *Productively aging: St. Louis's naturally occurring retirement community.* American Occupational Therapy Association. Retrieved from http://www.aota.org/news/centennial/40313/aging/40617.aspx

Recreation Centers of Sun City, Inc. (2016). *Sun city history.* Retrieved from http://suncityaz.org/discover/history/

Rowles, G. D., & Ravdal, H. (2002). Aging, place and meaning in the face of changing circumstances. In R. S. Weiss & S. A. Bass (Eds.), *Challenges of the third age: Meaning and purpose in later life* (pp. 81–114). New York, NY: Oxford University Press.

Sand River Cohousing. (n.d.). Home page. Retrieved from http://www.sandriver.org/

Saunders, P. (November 12, 2012). *Japan proposes robots to help elderly as population implodes.* LifeNews.com (Tokyo). Retrieved from http://www.lifenews.com/2012/11/12/japan-proposes-robots-to-help-elderly-as-population-implodes/

Sermons, M. W., & Henry, M. (2010). *Demographics of homelessness series: The rising elderly population.* Washington, DC: Homelessness Research Institute.

Tanaz, P., & Anderson, G. (2009). Program of All-Inclusive Care for the Elderly. *Health Policy Monitor.* Retrieved from http://old.npaonline.org/website/download.asp?id=3034&title=PACE_-_Health PolicyMonitor_-_2009

Terracciano, A., Löckenhoff, C. E., Zonderman, A. B., Ferrucci, L., & Costa, P. T. (2008). Personality predictors of longevity: Activity, emotional stability, and conscientiousness. *Psychosomatic Medicine, 70,* 621–627. doi:10.1097/PSY.0b013e31817b9371

The Cohousing Association of the United States. (2017a). Home page. Retrieved from http://www.cohousing.org/

The Cohousing Association of the United States. (2017b). The cohousing directory. Retrieved from http://www.cohousing.org/directory

Thompson, L. (2004). *Long-term care: Support for family caregivers.* Washington, DC: Long-Term Financing Project, Georgetown University Press.

United Hospital Fund. (2015). *NORC blueprint: A guide to community action.* Retrieved from http://www.norcblueprint.org/about/

U.S. Department of Housing and Urban Development. (2002). *Fact sheet: How your rent is determined for public housing and housing choice voucher programs.* Retrieved from https://www.hud.gov/sites/documents/DOC_11689.PDF

U.S. Department of Housing and Urban Development. (n.d.). *Section 202: Supportive housing for the elderly program.* Retrieved from https://www.hud.gov/program_offices/housing/mfh/progdesc/eld202

Village to Village Network. (n.d.) Home page. Retrieved from http://www.vtvnetwork.org

Weller, C. (2017). Inside the Dutch 'dementia village' that offers beer, bingo, and top-notch healthcare. *Business Insider.* Retrieved from http://www.businessinsider.com/inside-hogewey-dementia-village-2017-7/#hogeweyk-started-in-1993-as-your-typical-hospital-style-nursing-home-but-the-staff-soon-realized-there-was-a-better-more-humane-way-to-offer-care-1

World Health Organization. (2015). *World report on aging and health.* Geneva, Switzerland: World Health Organization. Retrieved from www.who.int/ageing/publications/world-report-2015/en/

Zarit, S. H., Kim, K., Femia, E. E., Almeida, D. M., Savla, J., & Molenaar, P. C. M. (2011). Effects of adult day care on daily stress of caregivers: A within-person approach. *Journals of Gerontology Series B: Psychological Sciences and Social Sciences, 66B,* 538–546. doi:10.1093/geronb/gbr030

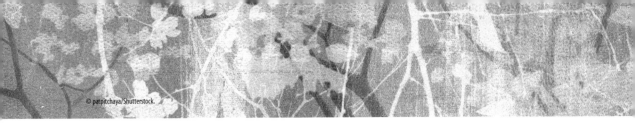
© patpitchaya/Shutterstock.

CHAPTER 4

Loss, Grief, Death, and Dying

Regula H. Robnett, PhD, OTR/L, FAOTA
Nancy Brossoie, PhD

CHAPTER OUTLINE

BEHAVIORAL OBJECTIVES

Upon completion of this chapter, the reader will be able to:

1. Define and explore the meaning of loss and ways to cope with loss.
2. Describe and discuss theories about the grieving process.
3. Explore definitions of death and the meaning of a good death.
4. Examine components of advanced directives.
5. Compare and contrast end-of-life care options.

KEY TERMS

Active euthanasia	Developmental loss	Organ and tissue
Advanced directive	Do not resuscitate (DNR)	donation
Attachment theory	Dual process model	Palliative care
Beehive theory	of grief	Passive euthanasia
Brain death	Euthanasia	Persistive vegetative
Burnout	Good death	state (PVS)
Cardiopulmonary resuscitation	Grief	Phase process model
(CPR)	Healthcare power of attorney	Physician-assisted suicide
Circumstantial loss	(HCPOA)	Premature death
Clinical death	Hospice care	Rituals
Compassion fatigue	Individual or personal	Stage process model
Complicated grief	autonomy	Suicide
Compression of morbidity	Living will	Talk therapy
Death	Loss	Task-based model
Death with Dignity Act (DWDA)	Natural death	Terminally ill

▶ Introduction

Losing a relationship with a loved one or cherished friend through **death**, illness, or accident can be emotionally painful at any age, even though most personal losses are experienced in late life. Still, a single **loss** can cause significant upheaval in the lives of the persons affected. In any 30-month period (2.5 years), approximately 70% of people aged 65+ experience a significant loss (e.g., death of a spouse or close friend; Williams, Sawyer Baker, Allman, & Roseman, 2007). In spite of its prevalence, few among us are experts at managing our own losses much less supporting other people who are grieving. We typically fumble through our exchanges with little understanding of the grieving process and how to respond. Moreover, few healthcare professionals (aside from individuals directly working with patients who are terminally ill) have a solid understanding of the death and dying process, which also influences the grieving process.

In this chapter, key concepts on loss, **grief**, death, and dying are presented to help healthcare professionals understand the losses a client may be experiencing as well as how to manage their own grief. The ability to effectively cope with loss connected to client care is paramount for a long productive career in health care. Feelings of distress should not be suppressed or tucked away prematurely. Expressing emotions through crying, laughter, sharing feelings, and even lamenting are natural and normal and necessary (Jackins, 1978). In our role as healthcare professionals (as well as family members and friends), it behooves us to increase our understanding and comfort level with managing grief, death, and the dying process.

▶ Loss and Grief

Loss

Losses are an inevitable part of life. The feelings associated with a loss can emerge after an incident (e.g., injury, accident, or death) or event (e.g., natural disaster or divorce). Loss can also originate from less visible causes, including changes in social role (e.g., widower, divorce, or retiree), responsibility (e.g., increased or decreased caregiving tasks), or personal expectation (e.g., shift in retirement plan). Clearly, losses can be anticipated or unanticipated and are often out of one's control. Regardless of source or timing, experiencing a loss is a universal feeling of grief that develops after being deprived of someone or something of value.

Despite the negative connotation in its definition, philosophers such as Friedrich Nietzsche have conceptualized loss as helping a person gain better perspective and understanding of life and eventually rediscovering joy. Nietzsche (1889) wrote: "What does not kill me, makes me stronger" (p. 8) and Kahlil Gibran (1923) penned: "The deeper that sorrow carves into your being the more joy you can contain" (p. 28). Many people who have contemplated their own losses believe that, while they did not choose to experience loss, good came of the situation through their own personal growth.

Researchers have also studied loss and its meaning, and have found it difficult to develop a generalizable theory about loss because it is so individualized. A loss for one person may not be experienced as a loss to another person. One type of loss (e.g., death) may hold more gravity than another loss (e.g., a minor accident). However, Wilson (2013) categorized loss into two categories: circumstantial and developmental. **Circumstantial losses** are typically unexpected incidents or events that negatively affect daily life (e.g., divorce, illness, and house fire). **Developmental losses** are anticipated events or milestones that occur as a function of personal growth and maturation. Developmental loss begins at birth in giving up the warmth and comfort of the womb. It continues into adulthood as developmental milestones are met (e.g., leaving the family home, retirement) as well as undergoing changes in physical health associated with old age (e.g., poor eyesight, loss of muscle mass, impaired memory recall).

Viktor Frankl (1905–1997), an Austrian neurologist and psychiatrist, has been considered an eminent scholar on the subject of loss. During the holocaust, he was a prisoner in the concentration camps. In an effort to preserve his own intellect and sanity, he decided to observe fellow prisoners and take note of how they defined loss and extracted meaning in their lives. In his book, *Man's Search for Meaning* (1946, 2006), he recalled his contemplative study and concluded that while humans often cannot control life events, they can control their response to these events. Frankl subsequently developed *logotherapy*, a therapeutic approach that is based on the belief that the ability to attach meaning to life is key to motivation and life preservation.

Through specific theories on loss and personal anecdotes, how individuals cope with loss (i.e., emotionally deal with an experience involving loss) has generated a great deal of interest as it is integral to many therapeutic interventions. A great deal of research and study has been focused on coping with loss directly associated with the death of a loved one. Death holds different meanings for individuals, families, and cultures. Everyone affected may appropriately utilize different coping strategies to manage their grief.

Coping with the loss of a loved one can be incredibly difficult and take time to overcome. Even though logic and social norms may dictate how to respond to death, people still can be overcome with feelings of confusion, sadness, anxiety, and depression when affected by death. Over time, feelings of sadness generally disappear. However, grief (i.e., mental suffering or anguish) can be particularly difficult to overcome and may require professional intervention to improve personal coping skills and functioning.

Grief

Grief can be defined as "keen mental suffering or distress over affliction or loss; sharp sorrow; painful regret" (Random House, 2017). Moreover, grief is personal, intimate, and intense and affects an individual emotionally, socially, mentally, and spiritually. It is not uncommon for people to interchange the terms grief/grieve and mourn/mourning. Yet, the terms have different meanings. Grieving refers to the state of internal suffering, whereas mourning is an outward expression of that distress (**FIGURE 4-1**). For example, social conventions often dictate that a woman wear black clothing after the death of her spouse or that a family hold a wake that includes excessive drinking and stories and tributes to the deceased. Like most mourning rituals, both of the previous activities were developed to help people manage their grief. The effects of grief can take a physical and emotional toll on an individual. However, people who receive emotional and social support from their family, friends, and community are better positioned to resolve their acute feelings of loss.

Everyone expresses their grief differently, as it is a highly individualized experience. Typical reactions include a range of feelings such as sadness, guilt, confusion,

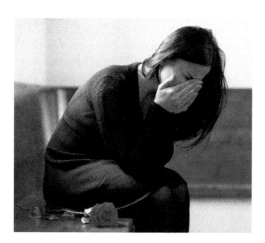

FIGURE 4-1 Mourning, unlike grief, is an outward expression of distress.
© Syda Productions/Shutterstock

loneliness, disbelief, denial, anger, happiness, fear, acceptance, shock, hatred, anxiety, emptiness, relief, and helplessness. The grieving process takes time as individuals learn to live with and manage their loss (Attig, 1996; Worden, 2009).

▶ Theories on Managing Grief

Theories behind how grief is managed have systematically emerged over the last 100 years. Sigmund Freud (1856–1939), founder of modern psychoanalysis, introduced the idea of grief management as early as 1917 (Freud, 1917). Freud, a firm believer in the benefits of **talk therapy** between patient and therapist, proposed that individuals should confront their grief by identifying and talking about issues that make it difficult for them to accept their losses. Patients were encouraged not to dwell on the deaths of their loved ones but to "move on" with their lives, so that their "broken" hearts and spirits could heal and their health would not be compromised. By engaging in grief therapy, Freud proposed that a patient could learn to cut ties to the deceased, readjust to life without the deceased, and form new relationships.

Freud's approach was simple, direct, and perhaps even elegant. However, it may not suffice. In fact, Freud reportedly did not "move on" from his own daughter's death and continued to mourn her for more than 30 years (Hall, 2011). Still, his influence on grief work cannot be underestimated, even though his approach was prescriptive and managed grief in a linear manner. As practitioners gained experience working with Freud's model, they reported that the underlying elements in it were sound but insufficient in resolving grief, which was found to be more complex and dynamic (Hall, 2011).

Attachment Theory

John Bowlby (1977), father of **attachment theory**, found that Freud's work aligned well with his theory on attachment. According to attachment theory, personal attachments to nurturing figures (e.g., mother or father) are initially focused on meeting basic needs such as safety and security, with the level and nature of the attachment changing over time. Bowlby maintained that we mourn persons with whom we have the closest attachments. However, even close relationships are complex and can have a degree of ambivalence, both of which impact the grieving process. Freud first brought up the ambivalent relationship as a component of relating to the deceased. Utilizing Bowlby's theory, Bradley and Cafferty (2001) found that older widowed adults whose relationships with their now deceased spouses had included high levels of quarreling and tension, tended to display more depression, guilt, self-reproach, and "disordered mourning" after the spouse's death. Conversely, spouses who had maintained healthy relationships were more likely to display signs of "uncomplicated grief", which included signs of sadness and pleasant memories, but rarely feelings of guilt.

Stage Process Model

Elisabeth Kübler Ross (1926–2004) was a Swiss American psychiatrist and thanatologist (an expert in the study of dying), who is best known for her **stage process model** for managing grief. In her book *On Death & Dying* (1969) she outlined five stages of grief, which corresponded with the stages she saw people go through after receiving medical confirmation that they were dying. She concluded that the emotional and psychological stages dying people experience help them come to terms with their own impending death.

Kübler Ross (2005) proposed five progressive stages of grief:

1. *Denial*: Refusing to accept the situation by relying on a defense mechanism of thoughts such as "this can't be true," even when one knows intellectually that the loss is real.
2. *Anger*: Directing frustration and anger toward oneself, other people, God, and/or the deceased. The grieving person may believe the situation is not fair and question "why me?"
3. *Bargaining*: Trying to negotiate with their God or higher power. They may promise to behave better (e.g., live a healthier lifestyle) if allowed to live.
4. *Depression*: Experiencing feelings of sadness, regret, loss, and/or anticipatory grief. Symptoms may result in a diagnosis of clinical depression.
5. *Acceptance*: Intentionally detaching from the problem and feeling like "it's going to be okay." Although not happy about the situation, people in the acceptance stage move on with life. Growth may occur (Kübler Ross, 2005).

General acceptance of the stage model was swift because it aligned well with stages practitioners were seeing in their patients and it appealed to their desire to provide them with closure. However, guiding patients through stages of grief remained difficult because grief was not experienced as a linear process and the timing of stages was not the same for everyone. Multiple studies have since focused on the model's effectiveness in managing grief, and findings are inconclusive. Grief is not linear, and therapeutic interventions need to account for its complexities as well as differences by gender, culture, and type of loss.

Still, Kübler Ross's model remains a useful guide for basic grief work (**FIGURE 4-2**). Since its

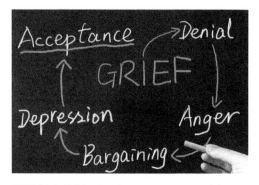

FIGURE 4-2 Kübler Ross's stage process model of grief.
© Raywoo/Shutterstock

development, theorists have used it to launch phase models of grief work, which posit that everyone's journey with grief is different and their unique responses will guide their transitions between stages or phases, as they work to resolve their grief.

Phase Process Model

There are several **phase process models** of grief that support grief work and enhance patient self-efficacy. Two influential models are the **Dual Process Model of Grief** (Stroebe & Schut, 1999) and the **Task-Based model** (Worden, 2009). In the Dual Process Model, resolving grief is dynamic and oscillates between two orientations. That is, the grief work process shifts between coping with loss (e.g., via therapy, avoidance, denial) and reorienting to daily life (e.g., adjusting to new routines and changes in lifestyle). When adopting this model approach, avoidance and denial, two responses often viewed as negative, are embraced as potentially helpful, especially when an individual needs to focus on another issue precipitated by the loss, such as adjusting to changes in daily routine.

Similarly, Worden's Task-Based Model (2009) accommodates an individual's need to work through tasks or phases to work through grief. He identifies the four tasks to be completed:

- Accept the reality of the loss.
- Work through the pain of grief.
- Adjust to an environment in which the deceased is missing.
- Find an enduring connection to the deceased while embarking on a new life.

The tasks do not need to be completed in any particular order and may be revisited for further exploration as time goes by. The practitioner's role is to be responsive to the individual's needs and help guide him or her through the tasks as the need presents.

Similar to other phase theorists, Edwin Shneidman (1918–2009), a clinical psychologist devoted to suicide prevention, purported that the grieving process has many interlaced emotional "themes" that can appear, disappear, and reappear again. One of the analogies he used to describe the grief process is the "**beehive theory**," which depicts the bereaved individual as going back and forth between acceptance and denial and bewilderment and pain. Thus, Shneidman also concluded that due to the amorphous nature of grief, it should not be viewed as a linear process (Shneidman, 1993). He also confirmed the inevitable: "Dying is the one thing—perhaps the only thing—in life that you don't have to do," he once wrote. "Stick around long enough and it will be done for you" (Dicke, 2009).

In this section, a few key theories were highlighted to demonstrate the types of theories guiding grief management. Researchers continue to test the theories, but have yet to come up with a single model that is effective with every person. Grief is a unique experience and how you process it may be different from your family members and friends. Grief can produce, heighten, or alter feelings, physical sensations, cognition, and behaviors. Lindemann (1944; as cited in Worden) provided descriptions of those personal responses to grief, presented in **TABLE 4-1** (Worden, 2009).

TABLE 4-1 Personal Aspects Related to the Grieving Process

Feelings	Physical Sensations	Cognitions	Behaviors
Sadness	Hollowness in the stomach	Disbelief	Sleep disturbances
Anger	Tightness in the chest and throat	Confusion	Appetite disturbances
Guilt and self-reproach	Oversensitivity to noise	Obsessive thoughts about or preoccupation with the deceased (e.g., ruminations)	Absentminded behavior
Anxiety	The feeling that nothing is real (depersonalization)	The sense of the deceased person's presence	Social withdrawal
Loneliness	Breathlessness	Hallucinations (both visual and auditory are common)	Dreams of the deceased
Fatigue (such as apathy or listlessness)	Weakness of the muscles		Avoidance of reminders of the deceased
Shock and feeling numb	Lack of energy		Searching or calling out
Yearning	Dry mouth		Crying and/or sighing
Emancipation (which may be an uncomfortable feeling)			Restlessness or hyperactivity
Relief (especially if the deceased had suffered)			Attachment to items or places that remind survivor of the deceased

Modified from Worden, 2009, pp. 18–30.

▶ Coping with Loss and Grief

Complicated Grief

With the support of a social network and an arsenal of coping strategies, it is possible to effectively process grief informally, that is, without the support of professionals. Most people do come through the acute bereavement period and reach what is known as "integrated grief," when they can successfully reengage in life and find contentment (Shear, Ghesquiere, & Glickman, 2013). However, when the grief process becomes too intense or complicated, or persists longer than a year, professional help may be needed in order to cope.

The therapeutic diagnosis of "persistent complex bereavement disorder" (American Psychiatric Association [APA], 2013), commonly known as **complicated grief**, applies to individuals who are unable to manage their grief and experience symptoms such as intense sorrow, yearning, and emotional pain during the majority of days for more than 12 months. Among individuals who develop complicated grief, adults age 61 and older experience it at twice the rate of younger adults (up to 70%), with women most affected (Kersting, Brahler, Glaesmer, & Wagner, 2011; Shear et al., 2013). Up to 20% of older bereaved individuals may experience complicated grief (Sung et al., 2011). Burton and colleagues (2012) found older adults experiencing complicated grief were unable to think optimistically, meet the needs of other persons, develop and reach personal goals, stay calm, or laugh (**FIGURE 4-3**). Moreover, additional studies also suggested complicated grief contributed to a lack of sense of control and self-worth (Shear et al., 2013). Persons afflicted also tend to deal with their grief using ineffective or dysfunctional methods such as preoccupation with death or inability to carry out daily occupations (APA, 2013). Latham and Prigerson (2004) reported a nearly sevenfold risk of "high suicidality" scores after approximately 6 months in a study

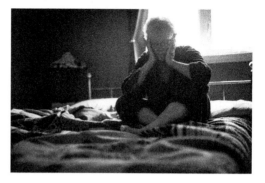

FIGURE 4-3 People who experience complicated grief may not be able to successfully complete their day-to-day activities.
© Lopolo/Shutterstock

of over 300 grieving older adults, with that risk factor rising even higher at the 11-month mark following the death. These researchers also cited increased risks in bereaved people for major depressive episodes, increased anxiety, decreased physical health, and increased substance misuse, even after accounting for potentially confounding variables such as posttraumatic stress syndrome (PTSD) and an initial major depression diagnosis.

Risk factors or red flags indicating a person may be at risk for experiencing complicated grief include witnessing a violent death (especially of a loved one), losing someone with whom they maintained a high level of dependence, experiencing high levels of anxiety, and exhibiting an insecure attachment style (Wilson, 2013, p. 37). Moreover, individuals who have low levels of social support, limited religious or spiritual support, low socioeconomic status, and physical disability or illness are at more risk for experiencing complicated grief than their counterparts (Alexander & Klein, 2012, pp. 94–95).

Dr. Therese Rando, a clinical psychologist and Clinical Director of The Institute for the Study and Treatment of Loss in Warwick, Rhode Island, has developed a theory on complicated mourning (i.e., the outward or culturally-based display of grief). She hypothesized that complicated mourning is more contextually based, individualized, and voluntary than "normal" grief. The three phases of active mourning include avoidance, confrontation, and accommodation. Within the three phases, six steps or "Rs" of mourning occur:

1. *Recognition* of the loss occurs during the initial avoidance phase. The person begins to acknowledge the loss and seeks to understand the death.
2. *Reaction* to the loss or separation, including feelings of pain and sadness. One expresses these feelings during the second confrontation phase.
3. *Recollection* and *re-experiencing* the past relationship with the deceased. Also during the confrontation phase, one reminisces about former experiences, including the feelings that occurred at the time.
4. *Relinquishing* also occurs in the confrontation phase. During this time, one begins to let go of the attachment to the deceased.
5. *Readjustment* occurs during the final accommodation phase. While one does not forget the past, new relationships, new ways of adapting, and a new identity may be established.
6. *Reinvesting* also happens in the final phase of mourning (accommodation). During this time, the mourner begins to put more energy into new ventures, including new life goals and new friendships (Rando, 1993).

▶ Supporting a Person Who Has Sustained a Loss

For many people, talking about their personal loss is difficult, especially when it involves the death of someone special to them. May Sarton, a well-known writer, chronicled her experiences before her own death, which her dear friend Susan Sherman later shared. Sarton and Sherman noted which response strategies seemed to help them during Sarton's dying process and which ones did not (*Signs of Love: Health and Aging*, 1997; see **TABLE 4-2**).

To move past any awkwardness in talking with a grieving individual, Marasco and Shuff (2010) suggested taking a deep breath and remembering that no matter what happens, the grieving person is in the more difficult and painful situation. They also advised keeping in mind that each person and each circumstance is different and that preplanned strategies may not always be effective. But, if you focus on being a good listener, the grieving person likely will guide your exchange. Many times it is more beneficial to simply be present rather than engaged in conversation.

Rituals

Rituals play an important role in society and are often utilized for coping with loss and grief, and to assist moving through the mourning process. Rituals can be personal, faith based, or social, and can be undertaken as an individual or as a group. Participating in a ritual can strengthen feelings of social connectedness and belonging, offer psychological support, and provide meaning to the loss. A ritual can include a traditional activity such as serving a birthday cake with candles at a birthday party honoring the deceased or it can be symbolic such as laying a token at a gravesite. Individualized or culturally-based rituals can directly support the healing process, help reduce anxiety, and promote regaining sense of control. Individuals involved in the process may find comfort by being among like-minded others (Norton & Gino, 2014). There can be a downside to rituals, however, when they become overly rigid (or overly ritualistic as found in persons with obsessive compulsive disorder; Norton & Gino, 2014). In the case of such unhealthy ritualistic behaviors, professional assistance may be warranted.

Some people engage in annual remembrance events to help retain connections with

TABLE 4-2 Helpful and Not Helpful Responses to a Person Who Has Experienced Loss

Helpful	Not Helpful
Offer specific support (What can I pick up at the store for you today?; I'm going to do your dishes)	Using euphemisms such as "He was old; it was for the best" or "She's in a better place"
Listen	Avoiding the topic of death or the person grieving
Ask what the person wants to talk about or share	Omitting the person from social events with friends
Use plain language	Touching, fondling, or petting that is not welcomed
Support the efforts of other people (friends, religions, and professionals)	Saying "it's OK, or you'll be OK" or sugarcoating the situation or infantilizing the grieving person
Heartfelt sharing and empathetic friendship	Making assumptions about what the person wants or needs
Be willing to say goodbye when it is time	Avoiding topics that cause discomfort
Use humor	Changing the subject when the grieving person wants to talk

Data from *Signs of love: On health and aging* (1997).

other individuals who have also experienced loss. For example, lighting a candle in a church or participating in a walkathon to support persons who have died or are battling cancer are common ways to honor a deceased person or group of persons. Engaging in a ritual or charity event can help an individual reflect on the past, focus on the present, and provide hope for the future.

Montross-Thomas and colleagues (2016) have found that rituals also play an important role in the self-care of healthcare professionals, especially among individuals who work with dying patients/clients. In a field that often demands long hours, limited professional support and organizational oversight, increased responsibilities on providers, and ever-changing caseloads, healthcare professionals are at high risk for experiencing **burnout** and **compassion fatigue**. These providers are often confronted with intense emotional situations, and it is uncommon for other people to consider the care needed by these caregivers who devote their lives to caring for others.

Burnout

Job burnout can occur in any profession. It is caused by excessive and prolonged stress caused by the work environment. Common signs include emotional exhaustion, feeling detached from patients and their care, and a lack of personal accomplishment. Providers who are experiencing burnout are at high risk for making mistakes in their work and often become cynical about their work (Gallagher, 2013; Koh et al., 2015).

Compassion Fatigue

Compassion fatigue can occur within helping professions and is sometimes referred to as secondary or vicarious trauma, a cousin of PTSD (Gallagher, 2013; Orpustan-Love, 2014). It is often associated with burnout, but has a different underlying cause. Compassion fatigue affects individuals (e.g., caregivers, healthcare professionals) affected by trauma experienced by someone else (e.g., patient/client). Signs of compassion fatigue include lack of self-care, low levels of compassion, and loss of boundaries with a patient/client (Koh et al., 2015; Orpustan-Love, 2014).

To combat burnout and compassion fatigue, studies have shown that self-care strategies such as maintaining physical health, engaging in an increased variety of clinical roles, pursuing hobbies, relying on meditation techniques, maintaining realistic expectations about work, limiting work to 40 hours a week, and engaging in rituals can reduce risk (Koh et al., 2015; Montross-Thomas, Scheiber, Meier, & Irwin, 2016; Orpustan-Love, 2014). Examples of rituals relied upon by end-of-life providers include attending the funeral of the deceased, offering condolences to the family/bereaved, writing in a journal, writing poetry, lighting a candle, saying a prayer, taking a walk, visiting the hospital chapel, or sitting quietly in the car after a death. The use of these important self-care and rituals can enhance one's ability to demonstrate compassion and find meaning and satisfaction with work (Koh et al., 2015; Montross-Thomas et al., 2016; Orpustan-Love, 2014).

▶ Death and Dying

Death

On the surface, death is a simple concept to understand—a dead person is simply no longer alive. Yet, determining when death actually occurs can be complicated. In the 1800s, there were great fears that individuals who were comatose would be presumed dead and erroneously buried. So, Victorian caskets included a shovel, a bell, or a periscope just in case the "dead" person woke up; at least that is what legends suggest. A scary thought, indeed. Since the mid-1900s, as life-sustaining technology (e.g., heart defibrillators, respirators, and organ transplants) and the use of **cardiopulmonary resuscitation** (CPR) have become mainstream in medical care, healthcare practitioners have significantly improved at recognizing death. However, defining the point of death remains contentious. In this chapter, we present the criteria followed in the United States while recognizing other countries may follow different rules.

Clinical death occurs when the heart stops circulating blood throughout the body and the lungs are unable to oxygenate the blood—two functions necessary to sustain human life. When those two functions cease, clinical or physical death has occurred. It is possible, however, to resuscitate (i.e., revive or bring back to life) an individual who is clinically dead by using CPR or a form of mechanical technology to restart the functioning of the heart and lungs. However, timing is extremely important when bringing a person back from clinical death, because a brain deprived of oxygen for too long will cease to function properly or not at all.

Brain death generally follows a devastating brain injury and occurs when three key processes occur: coma, apnea, and lack of brainstem reflexes. More specifically, brain death may be diagnosed when there is:

- No spontaneous movement in response to stimuli.
- No spontaneous respirations for at least 1 hour.
- Lack of responsiveness to painful stimuli.
- No eye movement, blinking, or pupil response.
- No postural activity, swallowing, yawning, or vocalizing.

- No motor reflexes.
- A flat electroencephalogram (EEG) for at least 10 minutes.
- No change in criteria in 24 hours.

When all these conditions occur, life support is considered futile except to preserve organs for donation to a living being (Goila & Pawar, 2009).

However, sometimes the brain does not completely cease to function when damaged. Brain activity in the cortex (where complex thinking processes occur) may cease but primal functions regulated in the brain stem (e.g., blinking, swallowing, and breathing) can remain strong. When this condition occurs, the individual is said to be in a **persistive vegetative state** (PVS) and there is no possible return to normal functioning. Modern technology is credited with the rise in prevalence of PVS, as healthcare providers strive to keep their patients alive through the use of technology that can regulate the heart and lungs. However, at what cost? Critics suggest there is no quality of life for persons in a PVS, their health-care costs tend to be high, and their ability to interact with family and friends is nonexistent, which increases the family's anxiety and stress.

The idea of prolonging life through medical intervention just because it is available does not appeal to most people. Understandably, most people prefer to live a long fulfilling life and die a **natural death** (i.e., dying at an old age at a time when the body stops functioning on its own) rather than live a long life dependent on machines or others for care. Some people might opt to use machines to keep themselves alive to avoid **premature death** (i.e., dying at a young age) due to accidents and unknown medical problems. In a perfect world, everyone would live to a very old age (100+, perhaps) and then naturally (and painlessly) pass away. But because that is unlikely to happen, the best one could hope and work towards is the **compression of morbidity** before death (i.e., the personal and systemic burden caused by illness is reduced to the shortest time possible; Fries, 2005).

Perspectives on Death

Regardless of personal feelings about death, it is important not to assume that anyone is, *or is not*, prepared to die. Even at very advanced ages, people may still possess enthusiasm for life, whereas even younger people may have accepted that death is near. A personal example illustrates: An older friend, aged 89, was just as vital and engaging as ever. She began to share that she was "ready to go" and enjoyed discussing what she thought she would find "on the other side." On a recent Friday night, she enjoyed a pedicure and dinner with her group of friends as she had done many times. The following Sunday, she sustained a massive stroke and died within a few days. Her best friend, on the other hand, is nearly 95 years old. She is also actively engaged in life and living independently in an apartment. She had her hip replaced at age 93 and says she hopes to attend her youngest granddaughter's wedding 6 months in the future. She is not "ready to go" but does realize that she could "exit" (her words) anytime. These two older women illustrate two distinct approaches to coming to terms with death and serve as a reminder for healthcare professionals to leave personal judgments and assumptions at the door, and to listen if a person wants to talk about death.

Conversations about death and dying, regardless of the underlying cause, are shaped by our own experiences and perspectives. In U.S. society, death tends to be talked about in hushed tones, relegated to a family matter (if addressed at all), and not publically examined. As a result, fear and anxiety about death can ensue. Fear of death typically peaks in young adulthood when the realities of the permanence of death and first-hand experiences with death often emerge. Not knowing or understanding what happens to the mind and body before, during, and after the dying process can create anxiety. Moreover, questions about whether or not people possess a soul or spirit and the possibility of an afterlife can generate more questions and angst.

▶ Seeking a Good Death

Perhaps because there are so many unknowns about the dying process and perhaps because society values personal choice, people are interested in controlling the circumstances surrounding their own death so that they can experience a **good death**. A good death means something different for everyone, but most of us would agree that we hope our deaths are pain-free and without distress and suffering for ourselves, our families, and our caregivers. We also want our end to be aligned with our own and our families' wishes and reasonably consistent with clinical, cultural, and ethical standards (Institute of Medicine, 2014).

Having choices and the ability to make an informed decision regardless of what other people may think is the best treatment or the morally correct treatment that is valued in U.S. society. People like to be in control of every aspect of their lives, including death. Having the ability to make a choice is a part of having **individual or personal autonomy**. On the surface, the freedom to choose one's course of treatment and course of death seems like an obvious right that every adult should expect to have throughout adulthood. But the right to die is a more complex matter that crosses legal, political, and social boundaries.

Suicide is simply the act of taking one's own life by using "self-directed injurious behavior with an intent to die as a result of that behavior" (National Institute of Mental Health, n.d.). Suicide is an illegal act in most states and viewed as morally reprehensible in most cultures. One might wonder, "So what difference does it make that it is illegal? The person is killing themselves!" In states where it is illegal, persons who attempt suicide face legal prosecution—in part, as a deterrent to future attempts. Many states view suicide as being on the continuum of assault and murder; which are also illegal.

In 2014, an estimated 1.1 million adults reported engaging in nonfatal suicide attempts (Lipari, Piscopo, Kroutil, & Miller,

2015), while 41,149 persons actually completed suicide (National Center for Injury Prevention and Control, 2015). Men continue to account for 77% of all suicides (National Center for Injury Prevention and Control, 2015), although suicide rates among women have been rising steadily since 1999 (Curtin, Warner, & Hedegaard, 2016). White males and females are also much more likely to commit suicide than other racial groups (Curtin et al., 2016). The suicide rates of young (25–44; 24.3 per 100,000) and middle aged (45–64; 29.7 per 100,000) men are high, but do not compare to the high rates of men aged 75+ (38.8 per 100,000; Curtin et al., 2016).

The reasons for the high rates of suicide among men aged 75+ can be linked to bereavement (Martikainen & Valkonen, 1996) and the growing stress in managing changing life roles and responsibilities such as caregiving for a spouse (something most men were never trained to do) and adjusting to a new social identity upon retirement and as friends and loved ones pass away. Like half of all men of all ages committing suicide, the majority of older men who completed suicide used a firearm (Curtin et al., 2016).

The rising rates of suicide in late life are especially concerning as the number of men reaching old age increases. Today's older men are unlikely to use therapeutic counseling services/mental health services or suicide hotlines to talk about the issues bothering them. Moreover, there are limited numbers of programs developed specifically for older adults to address suicide. Thus, future efforts need to focus on responding to this concerning problem (Young et al., 2012).

Unlike suicide, **euthanasia** is an act of killing another being and takes two forms—passive and active. **Passive euthanasia** involves "standing by" and not taking action to prevent an inevitable death by allowing "nature to take its course." Pneumonia was a condition historically referred to as an old man's friend. By letting pneumonia go untreated, the illness could shorten a life that otherwise would be filled with disease and debilitation. Passive euthanasia is illegal, unless strict medical and legal documentation is in place to support the lack of actions taken.

Conversely, **active euthanasia** involves taking direct action to shorten life. A veterinarian engages in active euthanasia when it "puts down" an animal by injecting it with drugs to stop its heart. Like suicide, active euthanasia with humans is illegal, with one exception. The U.S. legal system views the practice of lethal injection—in which a person is injected with a fatal solution of drugs that cause death—as an acceptable course of action in cases of capital punishment. In no other situation is active euthanasia or lethal injection considered legal.

Unlike euthanasia, **physician-assisted suicide** involves taking one's own life under the guidance of a physician. Physician-assisted suicide is currently legal in some countries in Western Europe (i.e., Netherlands, Belgium, Luxembourg, and Switzerland) and only in a few U.S. states (California, Colorado, Oregon, Vermont, Washington) plus the District of Columbia. U.S. residents have been known to travel to countries in Western Europe to end their lives when they are unable to do so in their own states. One poignant example is showcased in a 2010 episode of the PBS series *Frontline* titled *The Suicide Tourist*, which follows Craig Ewert as he travels to Switzerland to end his own life after being diagnosed with amyotrophic lateral sclerosis (ALS). For more information, visit: www.pbs.org/wgbh/pages /frontline/suicidetourist/.

For a long time, there has been an undercurrent of public interest in having the right to die where and when a person chooses. In 1980, the Hemlock Society began right to die advocacy by raising awareness and advocating for individual "choice, dignity, and control at the end of life" (Hemlock Society of San Diego, n.d.). Today, other organizations such as Compassion and Choices and the World Federation of Right to Die Societies continue the mission in advocating for the right to die without legal prosecution of the physician assisting the suicide.

In 1994, the people in the State of Oregon voted to enact the first **Death with Dignity Act** (DWDA) to allow physician-assisted suicide. After much public debate about the acts' merits, they re-voted and passed it into law in 1997. The Act provides **terminally ill** patients (i.e., diagnosed with a health condition from which there is no reasonable hope of recovery) a means in which to obtain a physician's order for medications to end their life. The process in Oregon and other U.S. states differ, but include strict guidelines with state (government) oversight in an effort to ensure participants are making informed decisions on how and when they want to die. After a person enters the program, they always have the option *not* to end their own life. Historically, more individuals utilize the Death with Dignity Act each year than actually end their life using it (Public Health Division, Center for Health Statistics, 2017). In 2016, 204 people obtained prescriptions; yet, only 133 people actually took them. Among those considering physician-assisted suicide, the underlying health problem was a malignant neoplasm (78.9% of participants). More than 88% were enrolled in hospice services and died at home. The top four end-of-life concerns shared by participants included losing autonomy (89.5%), being less able to engage in activities making life enjoyable (89.5%), loss of dignity (65.4%), and being a burden on family, friends/caregivers (48.9%).

Critics of Death with Dignity laws continue to express concerns that an individual registered in a program may be enrolled without adequate counseling about other available treatment options to prolong their life, or may self-administer a lethal dose of medication while not fully comprehending the outcome. Moreover, critics are concerned that individuals who are incapable of giving informed consent (e.g., people with cognitive impairments) are being lured into a program as a way to end their own life. However, advocates insist that the program enrollment process is stringent with strict guidelines that specify a timeline for decision-making, counseling, working with individual support networks, and obtaining the lethal medications. No program allows an individual to enroll and immediately consume a lethal dose of medications.

Advanced Directives

Planning for end-of-life care needs to begin before life-threatening illness, diseases, or accidents occur. Adults of all ages should have discussions with their family or significant others about their wishes and put together a set of legal documents called an **advanced directive**. By compiling a personalized advanced directive, you are making your end-of-life choices known, including who will speak for you in emergencies if you cannot speak for yourself.

Advanced directives often include multiple documents that outline preferred end-of-life care. Specifically, a **living will** instructs healthcare providers how an individual wants to be treated if they become seriously ill or are terminally ill or cannot communicate their wishes. Life-saving treatments extend beyond what typically might first come to mind, that is, CPR and automated external defibrillators (AEDs). Less obvious life-saving treatments may also include mechanical ventilation, blood transfusions, surgery, radiation, hydration, nutrition, and antibiotics. A living will is used to specify the problems or conditions for which you want life-saving treatments to be used and not to be used; your personal preference for pain relief; ethical, spiritual, or religious preferences related to your care; and any other specific instructions you want others to know. Clearly, there is a need for a thoughtful discussion about the benefits and risks of life-saving treatments and being able to articulate your personal preferences with healthcare providers and family members before you create a living will so that it represents your wishes. Living will templates can be found online or a lawyer can provide a template. Aging with Dignity is a not-for-profit organization that offers forms and guidance to people considering these important life and death decisions. The forms include personal, emotional, and spiritual questions such as who will make healthcare

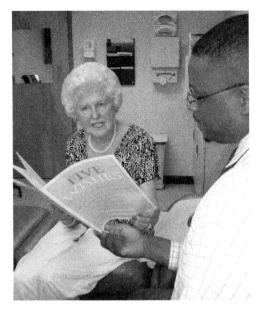

FIGURE 4-4 The not-for-profit organization, Aging with Dignity, provides the "Five Wishes" document which is accepted as an advanced directive in 42 states and the District of Columbia.

Courtesy of Aging with Dignity

decisions if the person becomes incapacitated, the potential type of medical and comfort care desired, and what the person wants loved ones to know. Most states accept the "Five Wishes" document (**FIGURE 4-4**) as legally binding if it is filled out correctly. (The document is available at agingwithdignity.org)

A **healthcare power of attorney** (HCPOA) is an individual appointed to speak on a person's behalf when he or she cannot speak or express their own wishes. An HCPOA is different from a power of attorney who is identified to complete a specific non-healthcare task on an individual's behalf (e.g., sell a vehicle) or a financial power of attorney who is responsible for an individual's finances when he or she is unable to manage them. It is important to include an HCPOA in an advanced directive, as only a HCPOA can make healthcare decisions about the treatment a person will or will not receive.

Another document sometimes included as part of an advanced directive is a

Do Not Resuscitate (DNR) order, also called a no code order. DNRs are usually signed when an individual has serious multiple chronic illnesses or is in the last stages of a disease or terminal illness. This legally binding order directs healthcare practitioners and emergency responders to withhold life-saving treatments such as CPR and advanced cardiac support in the event that the heart was to stop. Once a DNR is ordered, the individual may wear a special bracelet and a copy of the DNR should be retained in their living area and/or in their medical record so that all providers are aware of the order.

If a person is able to give informed consent and sign a DNR, no one else can revoke it. If a physician signs a DNR on their behalf, no one else can revoke it. If an individual has appointed someone as their HCPOA, that person may sign a DNR on the individual's behalf and no one else can revoke it (except for the individual). Having ongoing conversations with a HCPOA will help ensure that the HCPOA can effectively represent an individual's end-of-life wishes when the time comes. Social media frequently distributes images of people who tattoo the words "do not resuscitate" on their neck or chest as a way of ensuring their wishes not to be resuscitated are honored. Unfortunately, a DNR requires multiple signatures—the individual, a physician, and sometimes witnesses. A tattoo does not meet the criteria for use as a legal document (Smith & Lo, 2012).

Another document to include in an advanced directive includes direction for **organ and tissue donation**. According to the National Foundation for Transplants (n.d.), more than 121,000 people are waiting for organ or tissue transplants. Every 11 minutes, another name is added to the list, and every day 22 people die while waiting for a transplant. Unfortunately, only 45% of Americans have registered as organ and tissue donors. One person can make a difference by becoming a donor and potentially saving 8 lives and providing help to 50 additional people.

According to the U.S. Department of Health and Human Services, in 2016, more than 1 million tissue transplants and 82,000 corneal transplants were performed. Kidney transplants led organ transplants with 19,062, followed by 7,842 liver transplants, 3,191 heart transplants, 2,327 lung transplants, 798 kidney/pancreas transplants, 215 pancreas transplants, 147 intestine transplants, and 18 heart/lung transplants. More than 80% of organ donations come from deceased donors and less than 20% come from living donors (e.g., kidney donors).

Because there are not enough donors available to meet the current need, potential recipients are prioritized and placed on a waiting list. Their ranking is influenced by the potential success of the transplant and other factors including age, blood type, health of immune system, and prior donor status. Allocating in this way assures the best distribution of a limited number of organs. Unfortunately, organs are also allocated based on distance from the recipient. For example, a kidney can remain out of a body 24–36 hours before transplant, but a heart can only last 4–6 hours so is available only to persons nearby.

Many people are hesitant about becoming organ and tissue donors because they may have misconceptions about the process or believe it is not supported by their religion. In response, the National Foundation for Transplants (n.d.) offers the following facts:

- Almost anyone can be an organ donor, regardless of age or medical history.
- All major religions in the United States support organ donation.
- Donors can still have open casket funerals, and organ donation does not cost the donor's family any money.
- If a person is hospitalized, the medical staff provides the best possible care, regardless of organ donor status. Donation is only considered after a patient dies.
- Donors are needed for all races and ethnic groups. Transplant success rates increase when organs are matched between members of the same ethnic background.
- Signing the back of your license or a donor card is not enough. To officially register as an organ donor, visit www.donatelife.net and register as donor.

▶ End-of-Life Care Options

When medical treatments for a serious illness are no longer effective or when a terminal illness is diagnosed, discussions about a new plan of care generally include **palliative care** or comfort care. Palliative care involves treating symptoms to keep the individual comfortable rather than trying to cure the illness. Pain management is only one approach used in palliative care. Other strategies include antibiotics, nutrition, and other interventions that help the individual maintain the best quality of life possible. For example, a person in late stages of Alzheimer's disease may have an impacted tooth removed if it is causing pain and undue stress. Or an individual may receive oral inhalation treatments to make breathing easier, even though they are dying from lung disease. Palliative care attempts to keep an individual comfortable, not to cure an illness or disease.

Hospice

For individuals diagnosed with a terminal illness or injury, **hospice care** offers compassionate care that includes palliative care. The term hospice is derived from the Latin word "hospes," meaning both host and guest. As early as the 11th century, Roman Catholics in Europe set up hospices as retreats of hospitality for travelers and way stations for the weary, sick, and dying. Those hospices were commonplace through the middle ages (Cagle et al., 2014). More recently, physician Dame Cicely Saunders founded St. Christopher's Hospice for terminally ill patients in 1967 as the first modern hospice in London.

In the United States, legislation for hospice care was introduced in the 1970s but it did not pass into law until 1982, with a Medicare bill granting benefits nationally for Medicare recipients starting in 1986. Since that time, the number of hospice patients has steadily increased. An increasing number of people are dying while under hospice care, as it continues to be financially supported by Medicare and other insurance plans.

Hospice care can only be received after an individual has been certified by two physicians as having 6 months or less to live (National Hospice and Palliative Care Organization, 2017). Every 6 months, the recipient is either recertified to receive another 6 months of services or released if the illness has gone into remission and they do not require services. Recipients can be recertified to reenter the program and receive services at a later date.

In 2015, of the 1.38 million Medicare beneficiaries receiving hospice services, only 13% of hospice recipients received services for more than 6 months. The mean length of service was 69.5 days, but the median number of days of services received was 23 days. Among all Medicare hospice recipients in 2015, 88.3 % died in hospice care and 6.9% were discharged as they were no longer deemed terminally ill (National Hospice and Palliative Care Organization, 2017).

During the same year, hospice care was utilized predominately by individuals age 80+ (64.4%), Whites (86.8%), and females (58.7%; National Hospice and Palliative Care Organization, 2017). Among them, approximately 45% had at least four chronic health conditions (Kaiser Family Foundation, 2016), although the top three primary diagnoses included cancer (27.7%), cardiac and circulatory problems (19.3%), and dementia (16.5%). Persons with dementia received the most days of care: a mean of 105 days and a median of 56 days of care (National Hospice and Palliative Care Organization, 2017).

Of all persons enrolled in Medicare in 2014 who also died in the same year, 46% utilized hospice services, an increase from 21% in 2000 (Kaiser Family Foundation, 2016). The vast majority (97.8%) of hospice care is provided in the home, yet only 53% of the $15.9 billion costs paid by Medicare were for home-based care, indicating that the cost of care provided in nursing facilities and acute care settings is proportionately higher.

According to the National Hospice and Palliative Care Organization (2017), there are approximately 4,000 hospice agencies (62.8% with a for-profit tax status) throughout the United States. These agencies employ approximately 6,000 healthcare workers who work exclusively in this segment of health care (Green, 2015). Additionally, over one half million volunteers deliver hospice services to recipients and their families (National Hospice and Palliative Care Organization, 2017).

A hallmark of hospice care is that it utilizes an interdisciplinary team to offer support to the recipient and the family. The interprofessional approach helps support the recipient's quality of life by providing comfort and care in the recipient's preferred surroundings without pain and invasive medical treatment. In addition to basic nursing services providing palliative care, other types of services available are homemaker/companion services, pastoral care, social services support, recreational and rehabilitation therapy, nutrition/meal services, and social network support. The interdisciplinary approach embraces a biopsychosocial or holistic approach to maintain the well-being of recipients. **TABLE 4-3** illustrates the differences between approaches used in traditional medical care and hospice care.

Studies on the overall value of hospice services have found that recipients tended to be more mobile, less anxious, and less depressed. Family members and hospice staff were also perceived as more accessible (**FIGURE 4-5**; Rhodes, Mitchell, Miller, Connor, & Teno, 2008).

TABLE 4-3 Comparisons Between Traditional Medical Care and Hospice Care

Traditional Medical Care	Hospice Care
Fragmented	Holistic (multidisciplinary, interdisciplinary, or interprofessional teams)
Cure is goal	Cure is not the goal; palliative care is the goal
Death is seen as a failure	Ensure a good death
Focus on the physical	Biopsychosocial and spiritual
Physician directed	Client directed (family involved)
Pain meds feared as addictive	Client in control of pain meds
Hospital or institution	Home or hospice facility (client and family choice)
Symptoms treated in isolation	Symptom control
Death ends care	Bereavement care up to 1 year post

Data from Peat (1988) and Understanding Hospice (n.d.).

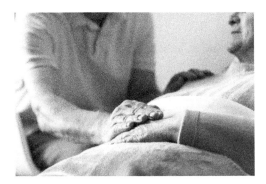

FIGURE 4-5 Hospice care settings make it easier for loved ones to visit than hospital settings.

© Photographee.eu/Shutterstock

Working with Dying Patients

Working with dying individuals is often referred to as a calling. It is not easy to watch individuals live to their final days and moments, yet some healthcare providers are more comfortable with the dying process. As a healthcare practitioner, it is important that you maintain your professional perspective and remember that the dying process is not about you. Your role is to support the dying person and their family. Key points to remember include the following:

- Offer words of kindness and support.
- Refrain from judging anyone or expressing discontent.
- Treat everyone with respect and dignity.
- Listen and watch.
- Reflect on the situation to learn more about yourself.

▶ Summary

This chapter has explored definitions and the historical perspectives of death, and touched on some cultural and personal perspectives of the dying and grieving processes. Certainly, over time, our concept of death has changed as we are able to enable living (in a technical sense) over a long period of time through technology.

An overview of some theories of grief and the grieving process included those of Freud, Kübler-Ross, Shneidman, Bowlby, Rando, and Worden. These theorists, including some thanantologists, provided differing perspectives on grief by explaining experiences of people who are dying or coping with a significant loss. There is no singular response to grief; each individual needs to cope with loss in their own way. Yet, understanding differing viewpoints can help inform professional practices and be useful as a springboard to managing personal responses to loss. Understanding differing perspectives on death and dying can help a healthcare professional gently educate a client who may be struggling in their own grieving process. The perspectives provided are not prescriptive, only educative. Sometimes it seems to help knowing that what one is experiencing is not abnormal, but rather just part of everyday life. Perhaps, one or two theories resonated with your own experience in the realm of loss.

As a society, we have become increasingly removed from death and the dying process with our increased reliance on technology. Instead of dying at home surrounded by family, more people die in institutions such as hospitals or hospice facilities. As a result, our perspectives on death and have evolved and our desire to control our own deaths have increased with the implementation of death with dignity laws, use of palliative care, and reliance of advanced directives to guide end-of-life care. Hospice services continue to be relied upon, but remain underused; perhaps because going into "hospice care" signals a resignation that hope for a cure no longer exists.

This chapter is not intended to make the reader a grief counselor, but it has been included to increase knowledge about loss, grief, death, and dying. Since older adults are more likely to experience loss than young adults, the likelihood that you will encounter someone in the throes of grieving is very likely. Our advice is simple—dare to extend empathy to a person who has sustained a loss; listen intently, be nonjudgmental, and simply and genuinely be present. You can make a difference.

🔍 CASE STUDIES

Case 1: Mary Jo lost her partner of 47 years about 6 months ago. She was Jim's primary caregiver over the course of his cancer treatment that lasted 2 years. For the last month of his life, Jim and Mary Jo were able to receive assistance from hospice services, for which Mary Jo was extremely grateful because this allowed her to keep Jim at home, which is where he wanted to spend his last days of life. Since Jim's death, Mary Jo has spent most of her time alone in the big house they shared. Friends have called wanting her to go out with them, but she always has an excuse (usually, she is too tired, has too much to do, or not feeling that well). Mary Jo and Jim had no children. Mary Jo has no known health problems and is retired from a career at the post office. She belongs to a church, but has not attended since the funeral. Her former hobbies included knitting, baking for friends and family (siblings and nieces and nephews), and shopping.

1. Discuss how the grieving process might be impacting Mary Jo's life. Have you any concerns?
2. Discuss how hospice may or may not be able to help Mary Jo at this time. How do you think hospice helped prior to Jim's death?
3. If you were asked to go and visit with Mary Jo as a healthcare professional, what would you expect and what are some of the ways you might be helpful to Mary Jo.

Case 2: Carter has been a grief counselor in a hospice program for about 10 years. When he first entered the profession, he felt a personal connection to each of his clients and was genuinely moved by their experiences. He put a great deal of effort into his work and felt a sense of accomplishment when his clients progressed to the point where they no longer needed him. In the last year or two, his enthusiasm for his work has started to dwindle. Rather than feeling energized by his work, Carter instead finds it emotionally exhausting, and he no longer looks forward to meeting with his clients. Although he intellectually understands what they are going through, he finds himself fighting the urge to tell his clients, "Stop complaining! Everybody goes through this sooner or later! It doesn't matter, life goes on!" Carter knows that what he is feeling is not appropriate, but is not sure what he should do.

1. Is Carter experiencing burnout or compassion fatigue? How can you tell and what caused it?
2. What can Carter do to improve his situation?

TEST YOUR KNOWLEDGE

Review Questions

1. The difference between circumstantial and developmental losses is that
    a. circumstantial losses are brief and transitory, while developmental losses are long term.
    b. circumstantial losses are expected, while developmental losses are random.
    c. circumstantial losses are unexpected, while developmental losses are generally anticipated.
    d. circumstantial losses generally have positive outcomes, while developmental losses are always negative.

2. Which of the following is true about Rando's stages of grief?
   a. The stages explain the exact step-by-step process of grief
   b. The stages are always followed in a specific order
   c. The stages are guidelines but each person responds differently
   d. The stages explain why people have grief that comes and goes

3. Clinical death occurs when
   a. there are no spontaneous movements (and motor reflexes are not evident).
   b. the lungs are no longer able to oxygenate the blood (and blood stops circulating).
   c. the person is not breathing on their own.
   d. the person does not respond to painful stimuli.

4. Physician assisted suicide is
   a. illegal in the United States.
   b. legal but only for the terminally ill.
   c. legal in parts of Europe.
   d. frowned upon by all the world's religions.

5. How do Hospice and traditional care compare?
   a. Hospice care and traditional care both end at death
   b. The patient is given control over pain medication in traditional care
   c. Hospice is curative
   d. Hospice focuses on symptom control

Learning Activities

1. If a person lost a limb in an automobile accident, would that be considered a circumstantial loss or a developmental loss, and why?
2. Select any two of the five progressive stages of grief and provide a specific example of each.
3. The six steps of mourning, in no particular order, are readjustment, reaction, recognition, recollection, reinvesting, and relinquishing. The three phases of active mourning include avoidance, confrontation, and accommodation. Identify which step(s) of mourning are associated with each phase of active mourning.
4. Describe what a good death means for you.
5. Do you agree with Death with Dignity laws? Why or why not?

References

Alexander, D., & Klein, S. (2012). Mental health, trauma, and bereavement. In P. Wimpenny & J. Costello (Eds.), *Grief, loss and bereavement: Evidence and practice for health and social care practitioners*. Chapter 6 (pp. 91–110). New York: Routledge.

American Psychiatric Association. (2013). *Diagnostic and statistical manual of mental disorders* (5th Ed.) (DSM-5). Washington, DC: Author.

Attig, T. (1996). *How we grieve: Relearning the world (understandings and perspectives)*. New York, NY: Oxford University Press.

Bradley, J. M., & Cafferty, T. P. (2001). Attachment among older adults: Current issues and directions for future research. *Attachment & Human Development, 3*(2), 200–221.

Burton, C. L., Yan, O. H., Pat-Horenczyk, R., Chan, I. S., Ho, S., & Bonanno, G. A. (2012). Coping flexibility and complicated grief: A comparison of American and Chinese samples. *Depression and Anxiety, 29*, 16–22.

Cagle, J., Tucci, A., Carrion, I., Van Dussen, D., Claassen, L., Plant, A., … Little, S. A. (2014). *Understanding hospice: Getting the answers*. Washington, DC: Hospice Foundation of America. Retrieved from https://hospicefoundation.org/hfa/media/Files/8-5x11_booklet_Hospice_Cagle_Sept1.pdf

Curtin, S. C., Warner, M., Hedegaard, H. (2016). *Increase in suicide in the United States, 1999–2014*. NCHS data brief, no 241. Hyattsville, MD: National Center for Health Statistics.

Dicke, W. (2009). *Edwin Shneidman, authority on suicide, dies at 91*. Retrieved from http://www.nytimes.com/2009/05/21/us/21shneidman.html

Frankl, V. (1946, 2006). *Man's search for meaning*. Boston, MA: Beacon Press.

Fries, J. F. (2005). The compression of morbidity. *The Milbank Quarterly, 83*(4), 801–823.

Freud, S. (1917). Mourning and melancholia. *The standard edition of the complete psychological works of Sigmund Freud, volume XIV (1914–1916): On the history of the psycho-analytic movement, papers on metapsychology and other works*. pp. 237–258.

Gallagher, R. (2013). Compassion fatigue. *Canadian Family Physician, 59*, 265–268.

Gibran, K. (1923). *The prophet*. New York, NY: Alfred A. Knopf.

Goila, A. K., & Pawar, M. (2009). The diagnosis of brain death. *Indian Journal of Critical Care Medicine, 13*, 7–11. doi:10.4103/0972-5229.53108

Green, K. (2015). *Careers in hospice care*. Career Outlook, U.S. Bureau of Labor Statistics. Washington, DC: U.S. Bureau of Labor Statistics.

Hall, C. (2011). Beyond Kubler-Ross: Recent developments in our understanding of grief and bereavement. *InPsych, 33*(6). Retrieved from https://www.psychology.org.au/publications/inpsych/2011/december/hall/

Hemlock Society of San Diego. (n.d.). *About Us*. Retrieved from http://www.hemlocksocietysandiego.org/

Institute of Medicine. (2014). *Dying in America: Improving quality and honoring individual preferences near end of life*. Washington, DC: The National Academy of Sciences.

Jackins, H. (1978). *The human side of human beings*. Seattle: Rational Island Publishers.

Kaiser Family Foundation (2016). *10 FAQs: Medicare's role in end-of-life care*. Retrieved from http://files.kff.org/attachment/10-FAQs-Medicares-Role-in-End-of-Life-Care

Kersting, A., Brahler, E., Glaesmer, H., & Wagner, B. (2011). Prevalence of complicated grief in a representative population-based sample. *Journal of Affective Disorders, 131*, 339–343. doi:10.1016/j.jad.2010.11.032

Koh, M. Y. H., Chong, P. H., Neo, P. S. H., Ong, Y. J., Yong, W. C., Ong, W. Y., Shen, M. J. L., & Hum, A. Y. M. (2015). Burnout, psychological morbidity and use of coping mechanisms among palliative care practitioners: A multi-centre cross-sectional study. *Palliative Medicine, 29*, 633–642. doi:10.1177/0269216315575850

Kübler Ross, E. (1969). *On death and dying*. New York, NY: The Macmillan Company.

Kübler Ross, E. (2005). *On grief and grieving: Finding the meaning of grief through the five stages of loss*. New York, NY: Simon & Schuster Ltd.

Latham, A. E., & Prigerson, H. G. (2004). Suicidality and bereavement: Complicated grief as psychiatric disorder presenting greatest risk for suicidality. *Suicide and Life-Threatening Behavior, 34*(4), 350–362.

Lipari, R., Piscopo, K., Kroutil, L. A., & Miller, G. K. (2015). *Suicidal thoughts and behavior among adults: Results from the 2014 National Survey on Drug Use and Health. NSDUH Data Review*. Rockville, MD: SAMHSA.

Marasco, R., & Shuff, B. (2010). *About grief: Insights, setbacks, grace notes, taboos*. Ivan R. Dee. Books.google.com

Martikainen, P., & Valkonen, T. (1996). Mortality after the death of a spouse: Rates and causes of death in a large Finnish cohort. *American Journal of Public Health, 86*(8), 1087–1093.

Montross-Thomas, L. P., Scheiber, C., Meier, E., & Irwin, S. A. (2016). Personally meaningful rituals: A way to increase compassion and decrease burnout among hospice staff and volunteers. *Journal of Palliative Medicine, 19*, 1043–1050. doi:10.1089/jpm.2015.0294

National Center for Injury Prevention and Control. (2015). *Suicide: Facts at a glance 2015*. Atlanta, GA: Centers for Disease Control and Prevention, Division of Violence Prevention.

National Foundation for Transplants. (n.d.). *Facts about organ donation*. Retrieved from http://www.transplants.org/facts-about-organ-donation

National Hospice and Palliative Care Organization. (2017). *NHPCO facts and figures: Hospice care in America*. Alexandria, VA: National Hospice and Palliative Care Organization.

National Institute of Mental Health. (n.d.). *Suicide*. Retrieved from https://www.nimh.nih.gov/health/statistics/suicide/index.shtml

Nietzsche, F. (1889). *Götzen-Dämmerung (Twilight of the Idols)*. Liepzig: Verlag von C. G. Neumann (translation [1990] London: Penguin Classics Revised ed. Language: English; ISBN-10: 0140445145; ISBN-13: 978)

Norton, M. I., & Gino, F. (2014). Rituals alleviate grieving for loved ones, lovers, and lotteries. *Journal of Experimental Psychology: General, 143*(1), 266.

Peat, M. (1988). *Current physical therapy.* Toronto: B.C. Decker, Inc.

Public Health Division, Center for Health Statistics. (2017). *Oregon Death with Dignity Act: Data summary 2016.* Portland, OR: Oregon Health Authority.

Orpustan-Love, D. (2014). The unintentional arm of compassion fatigue. *Academic Exchange Quarterly, 18.* Retrieved from http://rapidintellect.com/AEQweb/index.htm

Rando, T. (1993) *Treatment of complicated mourning.* Champaign, IL: Research Press.

Random House. (2017). *Random House dictionary.* New York, NY: Random House, Inc. Retrieved from www.dictionary.com

Rhodes, R. L., Mitchell, S. L., Miller, S. C., Connor, S. R., & Teno, J. M. (2008). Bereaved family members' evaluation of hospice care: What factors influence overall satisfaction with services? *Journal of Pain and Symptom Management, 36,* 365–371. doi:10.1016/j.jpainsymman.2007.12.004

Shear, M. K., Ghesquiere, A., & Glickman, K. (2013). Bereavement and complicated grief. *Current Psychiatry Reports, 15,* 1–7. doi:10.1007/s11920-013-0406-z

Shneidman, E. S. (1993). *Suicide as psychache: A clinical approach to self-destructive behavior.* Northvale, NJ/London: Jason Aronson, Inc.

Smith, A. K., & Lo, B. (2012). The problem with actually tattooing DNR across your chest. *Journal of General Internal Medicine, 27,* 1238–1239. doi: 10.1007/s11606-012-2134-1

Stroebe, M., & Shut, H. (1999). The dual process model of coping with bereavement: Rationale and description. *Death Studies, 23,* 197–224. doi:10.1080/074811899201046

Signs of love: On health and aging (1997). UNE Media Services/Maine Women Writers Collection, Biddeford, ME.

Sung, S. C., Dryman, M. T., Marks, E., Shear, M. K., Ghesquiere, A., Fava, M., & Simon, N. M. (2011). Complicated grief among individuals with major depression: Prevalence, comorbidity, and associated features. *Journal of Affective Disorders, 134*(1), 453–458.

U.S. Department of Health and Human Services. (n.d.). *Organ donation statistics.* Retrieved from https://www.organdonor.gov/statistics-stories/statistics.html

Williams, B. R., Sawyer Baker, P., Allman, R. M., & Roseman, J. M. (2007). Bereavement among African American and White older adults. *Journal of Aging & Health, 19,* 313–333.

Wilson, J. (2013). *Supporting people through loss and grief: An introduction for counsellors and other caring practitioners.* Retrieved from https://ebookcentral.proquest.com Publisher: Jessica Kingsley ISBN: 1-84905-376-6, 978-1-84905-376-1

Worden, J. W. (2009). *Grief counseling and grief therapy.* New York, NY: Springer Publishing.

Young, I. T., Iglewicz, A., Glorioso, D., Lanouette, N., Seay, K., Ilapakurti, M., & Zisook, S. (2012). Suicide bereavement and complicated grief. *Dialogues in Clinical Neuroscience, 14,* 177–186.

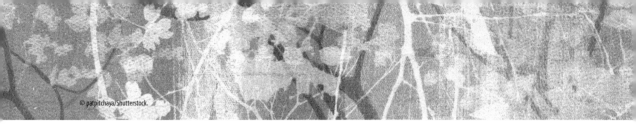

© patpitchaya/Shutterstock.

CHAPTER 5

Health Literacy and Clear Communication: Keys to Engaging Older Adults and Their Families

Audrey Riffenburgh, PhD
Sue Stableford, MPH, MSB

CHAPTER OUTLINE

BEHAVIORAL OBJECTIVES

Upon completion of this chapter, the reader will be able to:

1. Define the term *health literacy*.
2. Describe the health literacy skills of older adults according to their performance on the 2003 National Assessment of Adult Literacy (NAAL) as well as according to other research studies.
3. Describe the impact of older adults' limited health literacy skills on their health.
4. Describe the role of health system communication, processes, and demands.
5. List six plain language standards for verbal patient teaching.
6. Compare the reading level of health materials with the reading abilities of the majority of older adults and discuss the mismatch or gap between them.
7. List 5–10 plain language standards for written information.
8. List three health professional organizations and three federal agencies that publish standards or policies related to health literacy.
9. Discuss how you can address health literacy in your health career.

KEY TERMS

Health literacy
The Joint Commission
Limited literacy skills
Literacy

Numeracy
Plain language
Plain language guidelines
Reading levels

Sensory deficits
Shame-free environment
Teach back

▶ A Patient's Experience of Health Communication

Meet Cecilia. She is 78 years old and lives independently in the same town as her daughter and her grandchildren. She has arthritis, which makes it a little hard for her to get around. She takes precautions by wearing a medical alert device, although she has refused to get rid of her small area rugs. Early one morning, she trips on one and falls to the floor. She pushes her emergency medical button and this begins her journey into the unfamiliar land of health care.

During Cecilia's three days in the hospital, both she and her well-educated daughter, Rita, encounter many difficulties understanding and making decisions about care. Everything is unfamiliar—the care routines, the words used to explain things, the medicines prescribed. Time with doctors and nurses is short, with little time to ask questions or process the answers. Hospital surgeons repair Cecilia's broken hip, but now she faces additional challenges: managing pain and medications, learning exercises to regain strength and mobility, using unfamiliar assistive devices, choosing a rehab facility, and transitioning from hospital to rehab to home. Cecilia and Rita struggle to make sense of complex consent forms, written care and discharge instructions, and verbal information that fly by quickly.

▶ Understanding and Using Health Care: Why Older Adults Often Struggle

Health Literacy Challenges

As Cecilia and Rita face these unexpected and complex challenges, there are many factors at play. These factors are related to two general categories: (1) individuals' skills, knowledge, and capacities and (2) the demands and complexities of healthcare systems (Brach et al., 2012; Koh, Brach, Harris, & Parchman, 2013; Nielsen-Bohlman, Panzer, & Kindig, 2004; Centers for Disease Control and Prevention [CDC], 2009a). This interaction of factors greatly influences an individual's **health literacy**. A definition of individual health literacy is "the degree to which an individual has the capacity to obtain, communicate, process, and understand health information and services in order to make appropriate health decisions" (Patient Protection and Affordable Care Act, 2010).

Contemporary use of the term health literacy also includes the complexities and challenges presented by healthcare organizations. These organizations have a responsibility to ensure that patients and their families can understand and use information and services they need for their health. In recognition of this responsibility, a definition of health literacy for organizations has been developed. "Healthcare organizations that make it easier for people to navigate, understand, and use information and services to take care of their health" are called *health literate organizations* (Brach et al., 2012, p. 1).

Health literacy challenges everyone, albeit in varying circumstances and to varying degrees. The results of the most recent U.S. survey of adult literacy skills, which included health-related items, revealed that only 12% of adults scored in the *proficient* level for health literacy (Kutner, Greenberg, Jin, & Paulsen, 2006). In addition, 36% of U.S. adults scored at the *below basic* or *basic* levels. Significantly, older adults scored the lowest of all age groups—about 60% had *below basic* or *basic* health literacy skills (Kutner et al., 2006). Yet, as the age group using the most health care, they most likely need better skills to care for themselves effectively.

An example of one of the health literacy tasks labeled as *intermediate* was: "Determine what time a person can take a prescription medication, based on information on the prescription drug label that relates the timing of medication to eating" (Kutner et al., 2006, p. 6). Essentially, this means that a majority of older adults, due to their lack of an intermediate level of health literacy skills, cannot read, understand, and use this type of medication label (**FIGURE 5-1**). Yet, one needs to remember that this age group takes the most medications!

We now look at some of the challenges that cause older adults to struggle with understanding and using healthcare organizations and systems.

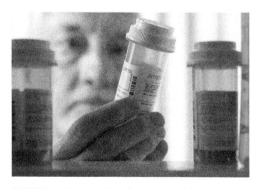

FIGURE 5-1 Many older adults are unable to read, understand, and use prescription drug labels.
© Burlingham/Shutterstock

Organizational Barriers

When patients and families enter a healthcare environment, there are a great many things they need to know or quickly learn to effectively understand and use the healthcare services. The organization's system demands and complexities create barriers to patients, families, and caregivers.

Healthcare organizations are under tremendous pressure in competitive markets with shifting regulations and financial stresses. This pressure often leads to the creation of systems and processes that can be challenging for patients and providers alike. For example, healthcare organizations may impose time pressures on providers and staff to move patients through the system very quickly.

In addition, providers and staff usually have little to no training in verbal communication skills. This despite many studies that indicate an increased risk of malpractice lawsuits due to ineffective communication and the ability to create and maintain a good relationship with patients (Olson & Windish, 2010; Posner, Severson, & Domino, 2015; Trudeau, 2016). Providers often communicate quickly, using unfamiliar medical vocabulary for unfamiliar concepts. In most systems, neither providers nor staff typically check for patients' comprehension (Karliner et al., 2012).

Patients and their families may also struggle to understand print and web-based information. Many healthcare systems pay scant attention to creating and providing print and web-based materials that are appropriate for the **literacy**, **numeracy**, and English language skills of much of the public.

Individual Factors

In addition to the challenges presented by organizations, individuals' skills and abilities come into play. Remember Cecilia's and Rita's situation? Consider that they are both likely to have limited knowledge of medical principles, the anatomy of the hip, and of new tasks they need to accomplish. Cecilia may have **sensory deficits** such as vision or hearing problems. Just as she needs to learn new tasks, she may also be experiencing cognitive decline from the stress of the situation, the effects of pain medication, and possibly depression. The emotional strain of the situation is likely to be significant for both of them, given the sudden new demands and changes in both their lives.

Like Cecilia and Rita, many older adults as well as their families and caregivers struggle with the same issues when thrust into the unfamiliar land of health care. They might struggle in a clinic, a pharmacy, a mental health setting, etc. They may feel rushed, afraid, and too intimidated to ask questions when they do not understand. Other challenges patients may face include mastering arcane health insurance systems; having the specialized vocabulary, knowledge, and skills to manage their own health; and using multiple information formats (such as booklets, charts, and tables) in multiple locations to accomplish multiple tasks.

Additional barriers to adequate health literacy can include diminished cognitive skills along with language and cultural differences. Many health-related tasks require adequate processing speed, attention span, memory, and reasoning capacity (Wolf et al., 2009), which some older adults may not possess, especially during the stress and confusion of being in a healthcare context. Recent research also highlights the negative impacts of impaired vision or hearing on cognitive abilities (Chen, Bhattacharya, & Pershing, 2017; Lin et al., 2013; Peelle, Troiani, Grossman, & Wingfield, 2011; Rogers & Langa, 2010).

Older adults may also experience barriers to using the Internet to obtain health information or using a patient portal in an electronic health record. In this electronic age, one might think that everyone knows how to use a computer, and that "print is dead," and that the Internet is the major source of health information. However, according to a Pew Internet survey on online use, about 9 in 10 U.S. adults use the Internet but only 4 in 10 people over the age of 65 do so (Internet/broadband fact sheet, 2016). Moreover, only half of U.S. adults over the age of 65 have Internet access at home.

Older people may also lack experience using technology and/or navigating the Internet (Taha, Sharit, & Czaja, 2014). Other studies show that web-based health information is usually at high **reading levels** (Friedman, Hoffman-Goetz, & Arocha, 2006; Walsh & Volsko, 2008) similar to printed materials. Therefore, even if older adults do access health information, this material may be too difficult to be helpful (**FIGURE 5-2**). Many U.S. adults struggle with limited literacy, numeracy skills, and/or limited English proficiency. We look at these factors and their impact on health literacy in more detail in this chapter.

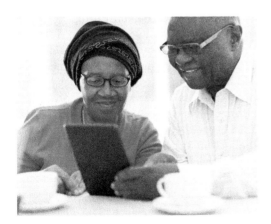

FIGURE 5-2 While some older adults may have access to web-based health information, they may find that it is at a level they cannot fully understand.

© Michael Jung/Shutterstock

▶ Literacy, Numeracy, and Health Literacy Challenges

For individuals, proficient *health literacy* depends on the building blocks of literacy and numeracy skills (Smith, Curtis, O'Conor, Federman, & Wolf, 2015). These building blocks support the development of knowledge, skills, and capacities needed for health literacy to emerge. These three concepts are related but distinct. This section addresses these three concepts and their interrelationship.

Literacy

The term *literacy* includes a constellation of skills, including reading (e.g., word recognition, fluency, drawing inferences from text), writing, speaking, and listening as well as other skills such as thinking analytically and making decisions. In the National Assessment of Adult Literacy (NAAL), 43% of all U.S. adults scored at the *below basic* or *basic* levels (Kutner, Greenberg, & Baer, 2005). (The other levels are *intermediate* and *proficient*.) However, almost 60% of adults aged 65 and older scored at the *below basic* or *basic* levels. Compared to all other age groups, adults aged 65 and older had the lowest average scores (Kutner et al., 2005).

Given the **limited literacy skills** of older adults, it is easy to see how they would struggle with understanding health information. Well over 800 studies have documented the mismatch between the literacy demands of most health and medical information and adult literacy skills (Rudd, 2010).

Numeracy

Limited numeracy skills are increasingly being recognized as an independent cause for concern, compromising patients' abilities to understand and act on health information (Smith et al., 2015). The term *numeracy* refers to a variety of skills, including basic computing, measuring and timing medicines, assessing risk, calculating percentages and statistics, interpreting food labels, and reading medical devices (Apter et al., 2008). In the NAAL survey mentioned earlier, more than 70% of U.S. adults aged 65 and over scored at *below basic* or *basic* numeracy levels (Kutner et al., 2006).

▶ Impacts of Literacy and Health Literacy Skills: Two Major Keys to Good Health

Research studies conducted over the past 20 years have highlighted the huge impact both literacy and health literacy skills can have on health and health outcomes (Al Sayah, Majumdar, Williams, Robertson, & Johnson, 2013; Batista, Lawrence, & Sousa, 2017; Peterson et al., 2011). Nearly 100 studies document a relationship between limited *literacy* skills and a variety of adverse health outcomes, including greater risk of hospitalization, lower medication adherence (Federman et al., 2014), and less knowledge of self-care guidelines for chronic conditions such as asthma and diabetes (Al Sayah et al., 2013; Berkman, Sheridan, Donahue, Halpern, & Crotty, 2011; Rudd, Anderson, Oppenheimer, & Nath, 2007).

In addition, inadequate *health literacy* is independently associated with greater risk of hospital admission (Mitchell, Sadikova, Jack, & Paasche-Orlow, 2012; Moser, Robinson, Biddle, & Pelter, 2015), higher likelihood of using emergency departments (Herndon, Chaney, & Carden, 2011), lower use of preventive health services such as flu and pneumonia shots (Fernandez, Larson, & Zikmund-Fisher,

2016), poorer physical and mental health (Wolf, 2005; Wu, Moser, DeWalt, Rayens, & Dracup, 2016), and higher all-cause mortality (Baker et al., 2007; Moser et al., 2015).

▶ The Impact of National Policies on Health Literacy Practice

From an *organizational* perspective, health literacy means attending to the communication demands placed on patients (and their families and caregivers) and how well or poorly an organization accommodates their communication needs. The responsibilities of medical offices, clinics, and systems are well articulated in a National Academy of Medicine (formerly the Institute of Medicine) report *Ten Attributes of Health Literate Health Care Organizations* (Brach et al., 2012). This report makes it clear that most organizations place health literacy demands on most adults that are significantly beyond their reading, numeracy, listening, and question-asking skills. Situational stress further compromises ability to absorb and process information.

Think of Cecilia and her daughter having to suddenly cope with a broken hip. They are thrust into trying to understand, decide, and consent to unfamiliar surgery, medications, and care. As an elder, Cecilia cannot process information as quickly as she used to, and has also arrived at the hospital without her glasses. Even her well-educated daughter is baffled by the consent forms and fast-paced verbal information shared in medical language.

These kinds of communication disconnect results in serious consequences for care systems as well for patients and their families. Major national groups responsible for accrediting hospitals and licensing physicians, establishing professional practice standards, and issuing policies are speaking out about the problem. Federal agencies have played a key role in raising awareness and promoting health literacy as well.

▶ Accrediting, Standard Setting, and Policy Organizations

The Joint Commission, which accredits hospitals around the country, points out in a report that communication failures are the underlying root cause of 65% of *sentinel events*—instances of serious patient harm. The Commission urges hospitals to make effective communications a priority to protect patient safety (The Joint Commission, 2007).

The Commission's 2010 *Roadmap for Hospitals* encourages the use of **plain language** at all points of patient care from admissions to discharge, to increase patient and family understanding (The Joint Commission, 2010). The Roadmap integrates health literacy with cultural competence, and reflects new accreditation requirements for hospitals to meet the oral and written communication needs of all patients, including those with speech, hearing, and other possible disorders that compromise their communication abilities.

The National Committee for Quality Assurance (NCQA) 2017: Recognition Standards for a Patient-Centered Medical Home include a new competency which states that the practice "Builds a health-literate organization … and act(s) to establish processes that address health literacy to improve patient outcomes" (*NCQA Patient-Centered Medical Home Standards and Guidelines*, 2017, p. 46)

The National Board of Medical Examiners now requires medical students to demonstrate communication competence on the U.S. Medical Licensing Examination. Students must pass this exam to earn their medical degree and enter a residency program. In encounters with simulated patients, examinees need to "demonstrate skills in providing information by use of terms the patient can understand… statements need to be clear and understandable and the words need to be those in common usage" (Federation of State Medical Boards of the United States and the National Board of Medical Examiners, 2017, p. 10).

The American Medical Association (AMA) played an early leading role in alerting physicians and other care providers about the health literacy problem and in supporting solutions. The AMA is one of a growing number of health profession organizations to publish policy statements, along with white papers alerting physicians about the dangers of "medspeak" and how to improve communications (Ad Hoc Committee on Health Literacy, Council for Scientific Affairs, 1999; American Medical Association, 2006; Killian & Coletti, 2017; Weiss, 2007) (**FIGURE 5-3**).

Allied health profession's organizations, including the American Dental Association, the American Occupational Therapy Association, and the American Physical Therapy Association, have urged consideration of health literacy in policy statements and by promoting resources for student

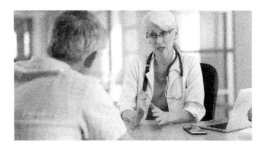

FIGURE 5-3 The American Medical Association (AMA) was instrumental in alerting healthcare providers about the health literacy problem and in providing ways to improve communication between providers and patients.

and practitioner learning (ADA Council on Access Prevention and Interprofessional Relations, 2009; American Physical Therapy Association, 2008; Braveman, Gupta, & Padilla, 2013).

The National Academy of Medicine, a highly esteemed nonprofit organization that serves as an independent advisor to government and the private sector, has long focused on health literacy. The Academy's Health Literacy Roundtable, established in 2006, is comprised of leaders from academia, industry, government, foundations, and patient/consumer representatives who meet biannually to address health literacy topics. Their informed discussions and evidence-based white papers have resulted in numerous publications linking health literacy and key healthcare issues such as health equity, patient safety, medication labeling, health insurance, and more. Publications are publicly available on their website (National Academy of Medicine, n.d.).

A 2017 report from the Academy, *Vital Directions for Health and Health Care*, links attention to health literacy with the changing expectations of health care to improve quality, achieve better outcomes, and reduce costs. It includes a recommendation to communicate with people in a way "appropriate to literacy" to "ensure that people, including patients and their families, are fully informed, engaged, and empowered as partners in health and health care choices..." (Dzau et al., 2017, p. 11).

▶ Federal Government Agencies

The federal government issued the Plain Writing Act in 2010, requiring all information from the government created for the public be written in plain language (Plain Writing Act. Public Law 111–247 111th Congress,

2010). This law has supported federal agencies and departments in creating additional policies, revamping written and electronic communications, and developing publicly accessible tools and training programs.

The Centers for Disease Control and Prevention (CDC) offers an extensive array of materials on a dedicated web section, including a highly regarded, skills-based training program (CDC, n.d.). The CDC also offers an assessment tool for written materials—the Clear Communication Index (CDC, 2016), which uses a numerical rating system to evaluate characteristics of printed matter. Low ratings of organizational materials can be a "wake-up call" to pay attention to health literacy and plain language.

The National Institutes of Health (NIH) promotes health literacy on their website: "Saves Lives. Saves Time. Saves Money." The NIH offers materials, resources, and training to support the statement (National Institutes of Health, n.d.).

The Agency for Healthcare Research and Quality (AHRQ) offers the Health Literacy Universal Precautions Toolkit (Brega et al., 2015) to help healthcare professionals and care systems learn how to systematically address and embed health literacy practices into clinical care.

The AHRQ also publishes the Consumer Assessment of Healthcare Providers and Systems (CAHPS) surveys, which ask patients to assess the quality of care they received after a hospital stay, physician-group visit, homecare services, hospice services, and more (Agency for Healthcare Research and Quality, 2014). Notably, many survey questions pertain to communication and the level of ease or difficulty encountered in understanding both oral and written information. Results from this survey affect hospital reimbursement rates.

The Department of Health and Human Services (HHS) promotes health literacy and plain language as part of updated Cultural and Linguistic Access Standards (CLAS)—a set of 15 action steps intended to advance health equity, improve quality of care, and help eliminate health care disparities. The Standards require "easy-to-understand print and multimedia materials and signage…" (U.S. Department of Health and Human Services, Office of Minority Health, 2012, p. 1).

The Office of Disease Prevention and Health Promotion within HHS promotes the National Action Plan to Improve Health Literacy. The plan outlines concrete action steps for all sectors of our society to address health literacy, including schools, workplaces, and healthcare systems (U.S. Department of Health and Human Services, Office of Disease Prevention and Health Promotion, 2010).

▶ The Business and Legal Case for Health Literacy

Beyond standards, legislation, policies, tools, and exhortations lies a business case for attending to this issue. The Centers for Medicare and Medicaid Services (CMS) use the standardized patient satisfaction data captured in CAHPS surveys to help determine merit-based incentive payments for physician groups (Centers for Medicare and Medicaid Services [CMS], 2017). As noted above, one of the major areas surveyed is how well providers communicate.

Similarly, Medicare hospital reimbursements for patients with traditional Medicare are based partly on "Value-Based Purchasing," a program that rewards hospitals not only for excellence in care practices and outcomes, but also for achieving high HCAHPS (Hospital Consumer Assessment of Healthcare Providers and Systems) scores. This hospital version asks patients with a recent hospital stay to rate their satisfaction with communication from nurses and doctors, as well as communication about their medications and discharge instructions (CMS, 2015).

One large business consulting firm has published research showing that hospitals with superior patient experience, as measured by HCAHPS scores, generate 50% higher financial return than hospitals with average scores (Stephan, 2016).

Finally, the business case includes "risk avoidance," the term lawyers use to advise clients about limiting liability and thus their costs. One major way healthcare providers and systems can avoid needless risk is to assure informed consent (**FIGURE 5-4**). This means that the written and verbal information is understandable to the patient or the patient's agent. Studies have shown that most written consents for surgeries and procedures require high levels of literacy skills, which most patients do not have (Institute of Medicine, 2015). Poor communication, including poor consent practices, is a major cause of malpractice claims (Posner et al., 2015; Spector, 2010; Trudeau, 2016). A Temple University toolkit summarizes research about consent forms, tells care providers and systems why they need to pay attention to this issue, and shows them how to do it (Fleisher et al., n.d.).

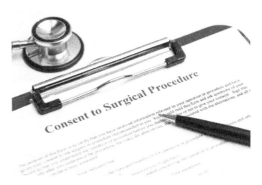

FIGURE 5-4 Using understandable consent forms is one way healthcare providers can limit their liability.

© Sherry Yates Young/Shutterstock

▶ Clear Health Communication: An Often Overlooked Necessity

Despite the research studies, standard setting, and policy advances, public health and health-care organizations often treat communication as an afterthought. Other issues command higher priority. Or perhaps providers and others assume that adults working in health disciplines know how to speak, teach, and write well enough to get their points across. Although clear communication is essential to good health outcomes, it does not happen automatically, as Cecilia's experience as well as research studies show.

A large and only partially answered question is how to best communicate, both verbally and in writing, so that patients, families, and their caregivers do understand critical health information. What works to motivate leaders of healthcare systems to systematically address communication challenges? What are the best solutions from both the patient and the system perspectives?

Researchers have some partial answers, although much remains to be learned. One major national research review, completed in 2004, noted that we still have more questions than answers (Dewalt, Berkman, Sheridan, Lohr, & Pignone, 2004). An update of that review, published in 2011, confirmed and somewhat expanded the original results (Berkman et al., 2011). The reviews *have* shown that using specific patient teaching techniques such as **"teach back"** and certain plain language writing techniques such as avoiding jargon increase the likelihood that adults will be able to understand and use health information (Davis et al., 1998; DeWalt et al., 2006; Schillinger et al., 2003; Wali, Hudani, Wali, Mercer, & Grindrod, 2016; Wolf et al., 2011).

The organizations that have drawn national attention to this problem—The Joint Commission, the American Medical Association, the federal government, and others—have proposed similar solutions. The Joint Commission report contains 35 specific recommendations for improving communication in hospitals and across the continuum of care. Major emphasis includes teaching and writing in plain language (The Joint Commission, 2007). Similarly, the AMA guide, *Help Patients Understand*, states: "...clinicians can best serve their patient populations by providing all patients with easy-to-understand information" (Weiss, 2007, p. 15). Also, the federal government devotes multiple websites to teaching employees and others how to communicate effectively in plain language (U.S. Department of Health and Human Services, Office of Disease Prevention and Health Promotion, n.d.).

▶ What Is Plain Language? How Will I Know It If I Hear It?

Multiple organizations promote effective verbal communication strategies. Two sources are the *Health Literacy Universal Precautions Toolkit* (Brega et al., 2015) and *Communicating with Older Adults* (Gerontological Society of America, 2012). The AMA guide (referenced earlier) reflects best practices included in these sources. Here are the six verbal communication tips that the AMA recommends that all physicians adopt to improve patient understanding (Weiss, 2007, p. 29). (The authors provide additional comments.)

1. *Slow down.* This is especially important to help older adults who may have hearing loss and who do not mentally process information as rapidly as when they were younger.

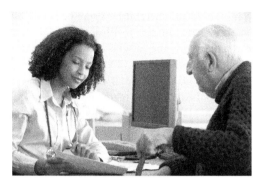

FIGURE 5-5 The AMA recommends six verbal communication tips for providers and their patients, including show or draw pictures.

© Monkey Business Images/Shutterstock

2. *Use plain, nonmedical language.* Another way to say this is to use everyday language or conversational language. Pretend you are talking with a relative or neighbor. Our usual spoken language is far simpler than formal communication.

3. *Show or draw pictures* (**FIGURE 5-5**). This is helpful in written materials as well. We know from research that pictures help older adults learn and remember information (Houts, Doak, Doak, & Loscalzo, 2006). Similarly, using models can increase patient understanding. For example, anatomical models can help patients understand how their bodies work. Food models can demonstrate healthy food choices and appropriate portion sizes.

4. *Limit the amount of information and repeat it.* This means prioritizing information to the three to five most important points. Most adults can remember only three things from a healthcare visit.

5. *Use the teach-back technique.* Sometimes, this is called the "show-me" or "demonstrate-back" or the "teach-to-goal" technique. This means,

have patients state in their own words what they are to do or demonstrate how they will perform a certain action such as use of a medical device. So, a provider might say something such as: "Ms. Smith, how will you explain what we've discussed to your family when you get home?" or "Ms. Smith, I want to make sure I've given clear directions. Would you tell me in your own words the key steps to take when you get home?" This gives the provider a chance to learn what the patient understands and to fill in or repeat missing information. The essential element of this technique is for the provider to take responsibility for being clear and not to "grill" the patient as if it were a test with shame attached for failure.

6. *Create a **shame-free environment**: Encourage questions.* Some providers say: "*What* questions do you have?" instead of the more common "*Do* you have any questions?" By asking "What questions do you have?" it is assumed that the adult does have some questions and now will feel more comfortable asking them.

Three additional tips also help older adults learn more effectively from healthcare visits:

1. *Frame the conversation first.* This means, tell the adult what you will be talking about before launching into the discussion. This helps prepare him or her to listen and hear information with understanding. So, you might say: "Ms. Smith, I'd like to start you on a new medicine. Let me explain what it is, how to take it, and how it should help." Then, go on with your teaching points.

2. *Encourage older adults to bring a friend or family member to the visit.* Another set of eyes and ears, or

someone to actually take notes, can help the patient remember what was discussed during the visit. However, the provider still needs to address the client, not the friend or family member. Often, older adult clients are ignored, especially when a younger person attends the visit with them.

3. *Give plain language written information that reminds the patient of what to do, how to do it, and why.* Most of us forget up to 50% of what we have heard as soon as we leave the exam room (Kessels, 2003). We all need reminders about actions and next steps. Many older adults also find it helpful to have written information to share with family members who have not been at the clinical visit but help care for them.

If some of these techniques had been used with Cecilia and her daughter, would they have been less confused and more able to partner with the team in making care decisions? If the healthcare providers had given easy-to-read discharge instructions and used the teach-back technique, would they have realized that Cecilia and Rita were struggling to understand many aspects of this traumatic situation? Perhaps, Rita could have learned how to better prepare for her mother's inevitable homecoming and the many adjustments to living space, medication management, and daily routines that would be needed. Cecilia's daughter faces huge caregiving tasks ahead.

▶ What Is Plain Language? How Will I Know it if I See it?

Cecilia did not bother trying to read the printed information handed to her. Even Rita, her well-educated daughter, had trouble

reading and understanding some of it due to unfamiliarity with the medical terms and jargon along with the fatigue and stress caused by the medical trauma. This outcome is not surprising, given the high reading demands of most health and medical information. Although plain language is not a total solution to a complex problem, it is a great starting point for creating more accessible print and web-based materials (Drake et al., 2017). Plain language principles also apply to designing information for other media such as DVDs and social media applications.

Many groups publish **plain language guidelines**, including federal agencies, healthcare organizations, insurance companies, private consulting firms, and the Plain Language Association International. Guidelines and checklists are easy to access online. Try using them when you are creating easier-to-read information (Lane, Blanco, Ford, & Mirenda, 2005; Plain Language Association International, 2017; CDC, 2009b).

Plain language guidelines accepted by multiple expert groups include:

- *Content*: Information is accurate, up-to-date, and limited. The focus is on behavior—what the reader needs to *do*. The average reader can use and remember no more than about five major points at one time. If a topic is complex, such as managing a parent's broken hip, break it up into smaller sections so that an adult can read small amounts at a time.

- *Structure/organization*: Structure and organize information from the user's perspective. This means putting the most important information first and creating small chunks with good headers or subtitles. Some adults read just the subtitles, so headings really need to convey key points. Health writers typically lead with explanations about anatomy or statistics about how many people have a certain problem. Plain language reverses this and begins with clear action messages. The background information comes later, if deemed to be important at all, because it is less critical. Do you think that initially Cecilia and her daughter could focus on the number of broken hips across the country and their surgical outcomes?

■ *Writing style*: Talk directly to the reader in a positive, friendly tone as much as appropriate and possible. As noted earlier, most adults best understand everyday language. These are typically short words (one or two syllables) common in spoken language. When medical terms are used such as the name of a condition, a pronunciation should be given and the term explained. Sentences should also be short, about 12–15 words on average. Use mostly active voice and explain general principles with concrete examples. For example, instead of writing about regular exercise, write about walking most days of the week for at least one-half hour. To engage your readers even further, use testimonials or short example stories of older adults who share the reader's concerns or who have solved a common problem.

■ *Appearance and appeal*: The first few seconds that an adult looks at a document (or a website) create a lasting impression. So, we need to make sure our print materials and websites are attractive, inviting, and look easy to read. This almost always means plenty of white space, not a page crammed full of print or a home page with too many visual distractions. The size of the print needs to be large enough for reading ease (usually about 13- or 14-point typeface for older adults), and the print/paper contrast should be sharp with dark print and light paper. Limit the use of fancy typefaces, underlining, and other visual tricks. Use appropriate images to humanize materials and show adults how to do recommended action steps.

One of the best-kept secrets about plain language is that it takes practice to write simply and clearly. One key to success is planning what you want to write (or say) before you sit in front of the computer and start writing. You must know both your audience and your purpose well. Ask yourself over and over: Who will use this? What do they need to know to take the action(s) I am recommending? How can I suggest this in a way that is appropriate and compelling to the intended audience?

Showing what you have written to prospective users before you make many copies of it is also important. Be brave and ask for feedback and ways to make your material more clear. You will be surprised at what your trial readers do not understand and the great ideas they will offer to improve your document.

▶ A Call to Action

Will using plain language and other clear health communication techniques ensure that older adults can read, understand, and use the information? Will it help to address our major national concerns with patient safety, quality, and costs of care? There is no *one* solution to the complex problem of communicating effectively with diverse patients and audiences. We do know from research that well-planned and simply written information, as well as the use of teach back, can make a big difference in the level of understanding.

But, simply knowing what to do is not the same thing as doing it, and many factors can interfere with adults taking actions beneficial to their health. Understanding, however, is almost always the first step, whether in getting preventive vaccines, managing a chronic condition, preparing for a medical test, or following discharge and medication instructions.

Healthcare providers have a challenge and an opportunity to enrich their practices and the lives of their clients or patients as well as their families. Healthcare professionals must take the lead in learning effective verbal and written communication techniques. Good health and health care are too complex, too important, and too costly for us to continue bumbling along with materials that are too hard to read and verbal teaching that patients cannot effectively remember and use. Online resources and training programs are listed in the references. You may also attend workshops to learn more.

Healthcare organizations and systems also have a role—building health literate organizations. This means allocating resources to develop policy, train providers and staff, develop or purchase plain language written materials, and evaluate ongoing efforts to shift cultural norms. This effort, wherever it takes place—in a hospital, pharmacy, primary care office, behavioral health or specialty clinic—supports patient or client engagement and a culture of safe, patient- or client-centered care.

Communication excellence is not only the right thing to do. It is essential to thrive in this new era of "pay for performance" and "bundled care." As payment models continue to shift to reimbursing for episodes and results of care and measuring them more accurately, effective communication will play an increasingly important role. Only if patients engage in their care as partners with their providers, and understand what to do and how to do it, will we be able to bend the cost curve. Only healthcare delivery systems and healthcare professionals that adapt will survive and thrive.

There are millions of "Cecilias"—millions of older adults and their families and caregivers managing health conditions who will benefit from the extra care we take with our communications. And the healthcare systems in which we serve will benefit as well.

$\mathcal{P}$ CASE STUDIES

Case 1: Arnold, a 62-year-old plumber, had been experiencing a series of symptoms, including increased thirst, frequent urination, and unusual weight loss. After some prodding from his wife, he went to see his family physician, Dr. Lopez. The doctor gave him a physical exam, ordered some blood work, and scheduled a follow-up appointment. On the return visit, Arnold sat down with the doctor to discuss his diagnosis. Dr. Lopez explained, "You have noninsulin-dependent diabetes or type 2 diabetes, which is a chronic condition that affects the way your body metabolizes glucose. Insulin is a pancreatic hormone that transforms dietary glucose into energy for your cells. If you had type 1 diabetes, it would mean that your pancreas produces little or no insulin. However, with type 2 diabetes, your pancreas produces sufficient amounts of insulin, but your cells are no longer utilizing it efficiently, which causes fluctuation in your blood glucose levels. To treat your condition, you'll need to start eating a healthy diet, start exercising regularly, and monitor your blood sugar. I'm writing you a prescription for Metformin and a glucose monitor." After finishing his explanation, Dr. Lopez asked Arnold if he had any questions. Slightly stunned, Arnold just shook his head and replied, "No." Dr. Lopez also told him that his practice has a diabetes fact sheet posted on their website and suggested that he look it up and read it. Arnold thanked him and left. He went to the pharmacy to have his prescription filled and also bought a bottle of glucosamine, a dietary supplement used by some people to treat joint pain. When his wife asked what the glucosamine was for, Arnold said, "I think I'm supposed to be taking it. The doctor mentioned it a few times."

1. **What are some reasons why Arnold likely did not understand what Dr. Lopez told him?**
2. **What could Dr. Lopez have done to better present the information in a way that Arnold would understand?**
3. **Was it a good idea for Dr. Lopez to refer Arnold to his practice's website for more information? Why or why not?**

Case 2: Dr. Falk and Dr. Keller operate a family medical practice. One afternoon, as they ate lunch in the break room, they discussed an article about health literacy that Dr. Falk was reading in a national news magazine. "There's been a growing trend toward healthcare organizations becoming health literate," Dr. Keller said. "The statistics are pretty surprising," Dr. Falk replied. "More than half of the people surveyed had only basic or below basic health literacy skills." "Do you think it's something we should look into at our practice?" Dr. Keller asked. "I think we should," Dr. Falk replied. While they were talking, Amanda, the office manager, and Jean, one of the nurses, came into the break room to get some coffee. They overheard what the doctors were discussing, and Amanda asked Jean, "What does health literacy mean?" Jean answered, "I think it refers to understanding your own health and knowing what you need to do to stay healthy."

1. **Is Jean's explanation of health literacy accurate? Why or why not?**
2. **Do you agree that Dr. Falk and Dr. Keller should address the issue of health literacy in their practice? Why or why not?**
3. **What are some resources that Dr. Falk and Dr. Keller can use to improve the level of health literacy at their practice?**

TEST YOUR KNOWLEDGE

Review Questions

1. Which statement most accurately describes the contemporary use of the term health literacy?
   a. An individual's literacy and numeracy skills used in a healthcare context
   b. The communication methods and approaches used in healthcare interactions and systems
   c. Confusion resulting from hard to understand medical terms
   d. Both a and b combined

2. Which statement about older adults' literacy skills is *true*?
   a. Those over 65 scored the highest on the 2003 National Assessment of Adult Literacy.
   b. Literacy skills tend to increase with age because of practice.
   c. Limited literacy skills are associated with greater health risks.
   d. Literacy skills are not related to hospital admission rates.

3. Which of these statements is *true*?
   a. Government agencies encourage attention to health literacy but lack support from health professions and health organizations.
   b. Various health professions and organizations encourage attention to health literacy but lack support from government agencies and payment systems.
   c. Neither government agencies nor health professions organizations play a role in communication between patients and providers.
   d. Both government agencies and health professions organizations encourage attention to health literacy and back it up with policies and standards.

4. Which of the following statements about written plain language is *true*?
   a. Plain language means simply using familiar words and does not include paying attention to any elements beyond words.
   b. Plain language dumbs down complex information and may not be 100% accurate.
   c. Plain language is conversational, meaning that it's simple and clear.
   d. Plain language insults patients because it can be so boring.

5. _____ have been shown to increase the likelihood that adults will use vital healthcare information.
   a. Detailed written materials
   b. TV shows
   c. Medically based instructions
   d. Teach back techniques

Learning Activities

1. View the American College of Physicians Foundation video *Health Literacy* (www.youtube.com/watch?v =ImnlptxIMXs&feature=related) and discuss it with your fellow students. This video is a great kick off to start building an understanding of how patients struggle in medical situations. However, it is important to remember that the video does not address the barriers organizations present for patients.

2. Download the handouts from the *Ask Me Three* program (www.npsf .org/?page=askme3). Discuss how the handouts might promote patient-provider interaction.

3. Interview one or more older adults and ask them about their communication with healthcare providers. What helps them understand how to care for themselves? What are the challenges? What are they not able to understand both in written information they are given and in the face-to-face communications with their providers?

4. Complete a health literacy audit of a local healthcare facility, preferably a hospital. Use the audit tool designed by Dr. Rima Rudd at Harvard School of Public Health, *Assessing the Health Literacy Environment* (www .hsph.harvard.edu/healthliteracy /environments/). Or, choose selected elements from the tool and create a mini audit tool that can be completed more easily. *The Health Literacy Universal Precautions Toolkit* is located on the same website. It includes audit tools, as well.

5. Use the checklists in one of the audit tools (noted earlier) to evaluate health and medical materials for plain language. Or, use the CDC tool, the Clear Communication Index (www.cdc.gov/ccindex/tool/index .html) or the AHRQ tool, the PEMAT (www.ahrq.gov/professionals /prevention-chronic-care/improve /self-mgmt/pemat/index.html). How well do the materials meet plain language guidelines?

6. Read and evaluate the executive summary from one or more of the reports issued by the Health Literacy Roundtable during the past 15 years (www.nap.edu/initiative/roundtable -on-health-literacy).

7. Look for research articles that link health literacy and your health occupation. A search in major databases will reveal articles published in most health fields, including nursing, physical and occupational therapy, social work, nutrition, pharmacy, dentistry, and medicine.

8. Complete the online training program offered by the CDC (www.cdc .gov/healthliteracy/, scroll down to the section on Training).

9. Try writing a one-page, easy-to-read information piece related to a specific issue in your field. If you have a clinical practicum and access to patients, ask some of them for suggestions of what to include and for feedback about your first draft. Practice using your piece for patient teaching along with the teach-back method.

10. Learn more about the Cultural and Linguistic Access Standards (CLAS) and the role of plain language (www.thinkculturalhealth.hhs.gov /assets/pdfs/EnhancedNational CLASStandards.pdf).

References

ADA Council on Access Prevention and Interprofessional Relations. (2009). *Health literacy in dentistry action plan: 2010–2015.* Retrieved from http://ada.org/sections /professionalResources/pdfs/topics_access_health _literacy_dentistry.pdf

Ad Hoc Committee on Health Literacy, Council for Scientific Affairs, A. M. A. (1999). Health literacy: Report of the Council on Scientific Affairs. *The Journal of the American Medical Association, 281*(6), 552–557. https://doi.org/10.1001/jama.281.6.552

Agency for Healthcare Research and Quality. (2014). *CAHPS: Assessing health care quality from the patient's perspective. Program brief.* Rockville, MD. Retrieved from https://www.ahrq.gov/sites/default/files/wysiwyg /cahps/about-cahps/cahps-program/14-p004_cahps.pdf

Al Sayah, F., Majumdar, S. R., Williams, B., Robertson, S., & Johnson, J. A. (2013). Health literacy and health outcomes in diabetes: A systematic review. *Journal of General Internal Medicine, 28*(3), 444–452. doi:10.1007 /s11606-012-2241-z

American Medical Association. (2006). *An ethical force program consensus report: Improving communication, improving care. American Medical Association.* Chicago, IL: AMA.

American Physical Therapy Association. (2008). Blueprint for teaching cultural competence in physical therapy education. *American Physical Therapy Association,* (June), 1–9. Retrieved from https://www.apta.org /Educators/Curriculum/APTA/CulturalCompetence/

Apter, A. J., Paasche-Orlow, M. K., Remillard, J. T., Bennett, I. M., Ben-Joseph, E. P., Batista, R. M., ... Rudd, R. E. (2008). Numeracy and communication with patients: They are counting on us. *Journal of General Internal Medicine, 23*(12), 2117–2124. doi:10.1007/s11606 -008-0803-x

Baker, D. W., Wolf, M. S., Feinglass, J., Thompson, J. A., Gazmararian, J. A., & Huang, J. (2007). Health literacy and mortality among elderly persons. *Archives of Internal Medicine, 167*(14), 1503–1509. doi:10.1001 /archinte.167.14.1503

Batista, M. J., Lawrence, H. P., & Sousa, M. D. L. R. (2017). Oral health literacy and oral health outcomes in an adult population in Brazil. *BMC Public Health, 18*(1), 60. doi:10.1186/s12889-017-4443-0

Berkman, N. D., Sheridan, S. L., Donahue, K. E., Halpern, D. J., & Crotty, K. (2011). Low health literacy and health outcomes: An updated review. *Annals of Internal Medicine, 155*(2), 97–107. doi:10.7326/0003-4819 -155-2-201107190-00005

Brach, C., Keller, D., Hernandez, L. M., Baur, C., Parker, R., Dreyer, B., & Schillinger, D. (2012). *Ten attributes of health literate health care organizations.* Washington,

DC: The National Academies Press. Retrieved from http://www.ahealthyunderstanding.org/Portals/0/Documents1/IOM_Ten_Attributes_HL_Paper.pdf

Braveman, B., Gupta, J., & Padilla, R. (2013). AOTA's societal statement on health disparities. *American Journal of Occupational Therapy, 67*(6(S)), S7–S8. doi:10.5014/ajot.2013.67S7

Brega, A., Barnard, J., Mabachi, N., Weiss, B., DeWalt, D., Brach, C., & West, D. (2015). *AHRQ health literacy universal precautions toolkit* (2nd ed.). Rockville, MD. Retrieved from www.ahrq.gov/professionals/quality-patient-safety/quality-resources/tools/literacy-toolkit/index.html

Centers for Disease Control and Prevention. (n.d.). Health literacy. Atlanta, GA. Retrieved September 1, 2017, from https://www.cdc.gov/healthcommunication/pdf/healthliteracy.pdf

Centers for Disease Control and Prevention. (2009a). *Improving health literacy for older adults: Expert panel report 2009.* Atlanta, GA. Retrieved from https://www.cdc.gov/healthliteracy/pdf/olderadults-508.pdf

Centers for Disease Control and Prevention. (2009b). *Simply put: A guide for creating easy-to-understand materials* (3rd ed.). Atlanta, GA. Retrieved from https://www.cdc.gov/healthliteracy/pdf/simply_put.pdf

Centers for Disease Control and Prevention. (2016). The CDC Clear Communication Index (CCI). Atlanta, GA. Retrieved from https://www.cdc.gov/ccindex/index.html

Centers for Medicare and Medicaid Services. (2015). *Hospital value-based purchasing.* Baltimore, MD. Retrieved from https://www.cms.gov/Outreach-and-Education/Medicare-Learning-Network-%0AMLN/MLNProducts/downloads/Hospital_VBPurchasing_Fact_Sheet_ICN907664.pdf%0A

Centers for Medicare and Medicaid Services. (2017). *2017 Consumer Assessment of Healthcare Providers and Systems (CAHPS) for the merit-based incentive payment system (MIPS) survey via CMS-approved survey vendor reporting.* Baltimore, MD. Retrieved from https://qpp.cms.gov/docs/QPP_CAHPS_for_MIPS_Fact_Sheet.pdf

Chen, S. P., Bhattacharya, J., & Pershing, S. (2017). Association of vision loss with cognition in older adults. *JAMA Ophthalmology, 135*(9), 963–970. doi:10.1001/jamaophthalmol.2017.2838

Davis, T. C., Berkel, H. J., Arnold, C. L., Nandy, I., Jackson, R. H., & Murphy, P. W. (1998). Intervention to increase mammography utilization in a public hospital. *Journal of General Internal Medicine, 13*(4), 230–233. doi:10.1046/j.1525-1497.1998.00072.x

Dewalt, D., Berkman, N. D., Sheridan, S., Lohr, K. N., & Pignone, M. P. (2004). Literacy and health outcomes: A systematic review of the literature. *Journal of General Internal Medicine, 19*(12), 1228–1239. doi:10.1111/j.1525-1497.2004.40153.x

DeWalt, D., Malone, R., Bryant, M., Kosnar, M., Corr, K., Rothman, R., … Pignone, M. (2006). A heart failure self-management program for patients of all literacy levels: A randomized, controlled trial. *BMC Health Services Research, 6,* 30. doi:10.1186/1472-6963-6-30

Drake, B. F., Brown, K. M., Gehlert, S., Wolf, L. E., Seo, J., Perkins, H., … Kaphingst, K. A. (2017). Development of plain language supplemental materials for the biobank informed consent process. *Journal of Cancer Education, 32*(4), 836–844. doi:10.1007/s13187-016-1029-y

Dzau, V. J., McClellan, M. B., McGinnis, J. M., Burke, S. P., Coye, M. J., Diaz, A., … Zerhouni, E. (2017). Vital directions for health and health care: Priorities from a National Academy of Medicine initiative. *National Academy of Medicine.* Retrieved from https://nam.edu/vital-directions-for-health-health-care-priorities-from-a-national-academy-of-medicine-initiative/

Federation of State Medical Boards of the United States and the National Board of Medical Examiners. (2017). *Step 2 clinical skills (CS): Content description and general information.* Philadelphia, PA. Retrieved from http://www.usmle.org/pdfs/step-2-cs/cs-info-manual.pdf

Federman, A. D., Wolf, M. S., Sofianou, A., Martynenko, M., O'Connor, R., Halm, E. A., … Wisnivesky, J. P. (2014). Self-management behaviors in older adults with asthma: Associations with health literacy. *Journal of the American Geriatrics Society, 62*(5), 872–879. doi:10.1111/jgs.12797

Fernandez, D. M., Larson, J. L., & Zikmund-Fisher, B. J. (2016). Associations between health literacy and preventive health behaviors among older adults: Findings from the health and retirement study. *BMC Public Health, 16*(1), 596. doi:10.1186/s12889-016-3267-7

Fleisher, L., Raivitch, S., Miller, S. M., Partida, Y., Martin-Boyan, A., Soltoff, C., & Courter, P. (n.d.). A practical guide to informed consent. Retrieved from http://www.templehealth.org/ICTOOLKIT/html/ictoolkitpage1.html. Accessed September 1, 2017.

Friedman, D. B., Hoffman-Goetz, L., & Arocha, J. F. (2006). Health literacy and the World Wide Web: Comparing the readability of leading incident cancers on the internet. *Medical Informatics and the Internet in Medicine, 31*(1), 67–87. doi:10.1080/14639230600628427

Gerontological Society of America. (2012). *Communicating with older adults: An evidence-based review of what really works.* Washington, DC: Gerontological Society of America. Retrieved from https://www.geron.org/publications/communicating-with-older-adults

Herndon, J. B., Chaney, M., & Carden, D. (2011). Health literacy and emergency department outcomes: A systematic review. *Annals of Emergency Medicine, 57*(4), 334–345. doi:10.1016/j.annemergmed.2010.08.035

Houts, P. S., Doak, C. C., Doak, L. G., & Loscalzo, M. J. (2006). The role of pictures in improving health communication: A review of research on attention, comprehension, recall, and adherence. *Patient*

Education and Counseling, 61(2), 173–190. doi:10.1016/j.pec.2005.05.004

Institute of Medicine. (2015). *Informed consent and health literacy: Workshop summary*. Washington, DC: National Academies Press.

Internet/broadband fact sheet. (2016). Retrieved September 19, 2017, from http://www.pewinternet.org/fact-sheet/internet-broadband/

Karliner, L. S., Auerbach, A., Nápoles, A., Schillinger, D., Nickleach, D., & Pérez-Stable, E. J. (2012). Language barriers and understanding of hospital discharge instructions. *Medical Care, 50*(4), 283–289. doi:10.1097/MLR.0b013e318249c949

Kessels, R. (2003). Patients' memory for medical information. *Journal of the Royal Society of Medicine, 96*(5), 219–222. doi:10.1258/jrsm.96.5.219

Killian, L., & Coletti, M. (2017). The role of universal health literacy precautions in minimizing "medspeak" and promoting shared decision making. *AMA Journal of Ethics, 19*(3), 296–303. doi:10.1001/journalofethics.2017.19.3.pfor1-1703

Koh, H. K., Brach, C., Harris, L. M., & Parchman, M. L. (2013). A proposed "health literate care model" would constitute a systems approach to improving patients' engagement in care. *Health Affairs (Project Hope), 32*(2), 357–367. doi:10.1377/hlthaff.2012.1205

Kutner, M., Greenberg, E., & Baer, J. (2005). *National Assessment of Adult Literacy (NAAL): A first look at the literacy of America's adults in the 21st century* (NCES 2006-470). U.S. Department of Education. Washington, DC: National Center for Education Statistics. Retrieved from http://nces.ed.gov/naal/pdf/2006470.pdf

Kutner, M., Greenberg, E., Jin, Y., & Paulsen, C. (2006). *The health literacy of America's adults: Results from the 2003 National Assessment of Adult Literacy* (NCES 2006-483). U.S. Department of Education. Washington, DC: National Center for Education Statistics. Retrieved from https://nces.ed.gov/pubs2006/2006483_1.pdf

Lane, P., Blanco, M., Ford, L., & Mirenda, H. S. (2005). *The health literacy style manual*. Reston, VA: Maximus. Retrieved from http://www.coveringkidsandfamilies.org/resources/docs/stylemanual.pdf

Lin, F. R., Yaffe, K., Xia, J., Xue, Q. L., Harris, T. B., Purchase-Helzner, E., … Simonsick, E. M. (2013). Hearing loss and cognitive decline in older adults. *JAMA Internal Medicine, 173*(4), 293–299. doi:10.1001/jamainternmed.2013.1868

Mitchell, S. E., Sadikova, E., Jack, B. W., & Paasche-Orlow, M. K. (2012). Health literacy and 30-day postdischarge hospital utilization. *Journal of Health Communication, 17*(Suppl. 3), 325–338. doi:10.1080/10810730.2012.715233

Moser, D. K., Robinson, S., Biddle, M. J., Pelter, M. M., Nesbitt, T. S., Southard, J., … Dracup, K. (2015). Health literacy predicts morbidity and mortality in rural patients with heart failure. *Journal of Cardiac Failure, 21*(8), 612–618. doi:10.1016/j.cardfail.2015.04.004

National Academy of Medicine. (n.d.). NAS Roundtable on Health Literacy publications page. Retrieved September 1, 2017, from http://nationalacademies.org/hmd/Reports.aspx?filters=inmeta:activity=Roundtable+on+Health+Literacy.

National Institutes of Health. (n.d.). Clear communication: Health literacy. Retrieved September 1, 2017, from https://www.nih.gov/institutes-nih/nih-office-director/office-communications-public-liaison/clear-communication/health-literacy

NCQA Patient-Centered Medical Home Standards and Guidelines. (2017). Washington, DC.

Nielsen-Bohlman, L., Panzer, A., & Kindig, D. (2004). *Health literacy: A prescription to end confusion*. Washington, DC: National Academies Press. Retrieved from http://www.nap.edu/catalog/10883/health-literacy-a-prescription-to-end-confusion

Olson, D. P., & Windish, D. M. (2010). Communication discrepancies between physicians and hospitalized patients. *Archives of Internal Medicine, 170*(15), 1302–1307. doi:10.1001/archinternmed.2010.239

Patient Protection and Affordable Care Act. (2010). U.S. Public Law 111 (148), 1.

Peelle, J. E., Troiani, V., Grossman, M., & Wingfield, A. (2011). Hearing loss in older adults affects neural systems supporting speech comprehension. *The Journal of Neuroscience : The Official Journal of the Society for Neuroscience, 31*(35), 12638–12643. doi:10.1523/JNEUROSCI.2559-11.2011

Peterson, P. N., Shetterly, S. M., Clarke, C. L., Bekelman, D. B., Chan, P. S., Allen, L. A., & Magid, D. J. (2011). Health literacy and outcomes among patients with heart failure. *Jama, 305*(16), 1695–1701.

Plain Language Association International. (2017). Plain Language Association International (PLAIN). Retrieved September 9, 2017, from http://plainlanguagenetwork.org/

Plain Writing Act. Public Law 111-247 111th Congress, Pub. L. No. 124 STAT. 2862 (2010). U.S. Congress. Retrieved from http://www.gpo.gov/fdsys/pkg/PLAW-111publ274/pdf/PLAW-111publ274.pdf

Posner, K., Severson, J., & Domino, K. (2015). The role of informed consent in patient complaints: Reducing hidden health system costs and improving patient engagement through shared decision making. *Journal of Healthcare Risk Management, 35*(2), 38–45. doi:10.1002/jhrm.21200

Rogers, M. A. M., & Langa, K. M. (2010). Untreated poor vision: A contributing factor to late-life dementia. *American Journal of Epidemiology, 171*(6), 728–735. doi:10.1093/aje/kwp453

Rudd, R. E. (2010). Improving Americans' health literacy. *New England Journal of Medicine, 363*(24), 2283–2285. doi:10.1056/NEJMp1008755

Rudd, R., Anderson, J. E., Oppenheimer, S., & Nath, C. (2007). Health literacy: An update of medical and public health literature. In J. P. Comings, B. Garner, &

C. Smith (Eds.), *Review of adult learning and literacy, Vol 7* (pp. 175–203). Mahwah, NJ: Lawrence Erlbaum Associates.

Schillinger, D., Piette, J., Grumbach, K., Wang, F., Wilson, C., Daher, C., … Bindman, A. B. (2003). Closing the loop: Physician communication with diabetic patients who have low health literacy. *Archives of Internal Medicine, 163*(1), 83–90. doi:10.1001/archinte.163.1.83

Smith, S. G., Curtis, L. M., O'Conor, R., Federman, A. D., & Wolf, M. S. (2015). ABCs or 123s? The independent contributions of literacy and numeracy skills on health task performance among older adults. *Patient Education and Counseling, 98*(8), 991–997. doi:10.1016/j.pec.2015.04.007

Spector, R. (2010). The plaintiff's attorneys share perspectives on patient communication. *Journal of Healthcare Risk Management, 29*(3), 29–33.

Stephan, J.-P. (2016). U.S. hospitals that provide superior patient experience generate 50 percent higher financial performance than average providers, Accenture finds. Retrieved from https://newsroom.accenture.com/news/us-hospitals-that-provide-superior-patient-experience-generate-50-percent-higher-financial-performance-than-average-providers-accenture-finds.htm. Accessed September 1, 2017.

Taha, J., Sharit, J., & Czaja, S. J. (2014). The impact of numeracy ability and technology skills on older adults' performance of health management tasks using a patient portal. *Journal of Applied Gerontology, 33*(4), 416–436. doi:10.1177/0733464812447283

The Joint Commission. (2007). *What did the doctor say?: Improving health literacy to protect patient safety. Joint Commission Public Policy Initiative.* Oakbrook Terrace, IL.

The Joint Commission. (2010). Advancing effective communication, cultural competence, and patient- and family-centered care: A roadmap for hospitals. Retrieved from http://www.jointcommission.org/assets/1/6/ARoadmapforHospitalsfinalversion727.pdf

Trudeau, C. R. (2016). Health literacy: The missing link to reducing risks and improving outcomes. *Hospitals and Health Systems Rx, 18*(3), 1–4.

U.S. Department of Health and Human Services, Office of Disease Prevention and Health Promotion. (n.d.). Health.gov, Health Literacy and Communication, Resources. Retrieved September 1, 2017, from https://health.gov/communication/resources.asp

U.S. Department of Health and Human Services, Office of Disease Prevention and Health Promotion. (2010). *National action plan to improve health literacy.* Washington, DC. Retrieved from https://health.gov/communication/hlactionplan/pdf/Health_Literacy_Action_Plan.pdf

U.S. Department of Health and Human Services, Office of Minority Health. (2012). *The national standards for culturally and linguistically appropriate services in health and health care.* Washington, DC. Retrieved from https://www.thinkculturalhealth.hhs.gov/clas/standards

Wali, H., Hudani, Z., Wali, S., Mercer, K., & Grindrod, K. (2016). A systematic review of interventions to improve medication information for low health literate populations. *Research in Social and Administrative Pharmacy, 12*(6), 830–864. doi:10.1016/j.sapharm.2015.12.001

Walsh, T. M., & Volsko, T. A. (2008). Readability assessment of internet-based consumer health information. *Respiratory Care, 53*(10), 1310–1315. Retrieved from http://www.ncbi.nlm.nih.gov/entrez/query.fcgi?cmd=Retrieve&db=PubMed&dopt=Citation&list_uids=18811992%5Cnhttp://rc.rcjournal.com/content/53/10/1310.full.pdf

Weiss, B. D. (2007). *Help patients understand. Manual for clinicians* (2nd ed.). Chicago, IL: American Medical Association Foundation. Retrieved from http://med.fsu.edu/userFiles/file/ahec_health_clinicians_manual.pdf

Wolf, M. S. (2005). Health literacy and functional health status among older adults. *Archives of Internal Medicine, 165*(17), 1946–1952. Retrieved from http://archpedi.jamanetwork.com/article.aspx?articleid=486704

Wolf, M. S., Davis, T. C., Curtis, L. M., Webb, A., Bailey, S. C., Shrank, W. H., … Wood, A. J. (2011). Effect of standardized, patient-centered label instructions to improve comprehension of prescription drug use. *Medical Care, 49*(1), 96–100. doi:10.1097/MLR.0b013e3181f38174

Wolf, M. S., Wilson, E. A. H., Rapp, D. N., Waite, K. R., Bocchini, M. V, Davis, T. C., & Rudd, R. E. (2009). Literacy and learning in health care. *Pediatrics, 124*(Suppl. 3), S275–S281. doi:10.1542/peds.2009-1162C

Wu, J.-R., Moser, D. K., DeWalt, D. A., Rayens, M. K., & Dracup, K. (2016). Health literacy mediates the relationship between age and health outcomes in patients with heart failure. *Circulation: Heart Failure, 9*(1), e002250. doi:10.1161/CIRCHEARTFAILURE.115.002250

CHAPTER 6

Policy Issues for Older Adults

Laney Bruner Canhoto, PhD, MSW, MPH

CHAPTER OUTLINE

BEHAVIORAL OBJECTIVES

Upon completion of this chapter, the reader will be able to:

1. List the eligibility criteria for Social Security, Medicare, and Medicaid.
2. Describe what is provided through Social Security.
3. Understand how Social Security, Medicare, and Medicaid are accessed.
4. Explain the differences among Social Security and Supplemental Security Income.
5. Describe what is covered under Medicare and Medicaid.
6. Compare and contrast Medicare and Medicaid.
7. Explain the programs available through the Aging Network and their structures.
8. Describe how the Americans with Disabilities Act impacts health care.
9. Explain how long-term services and supports are funded in the United States.

KEY TERMS

Aging Network	Long-term services and	Medigap
Americans with	supports	Older Americans Act
Disabilities Act	Medicaid	Social Security Act
Area agencies on aging	Medicaid waivers	State units on aging
Long-term care insurance	Medicare	Supplemental Security Income

▶ Introduction

Public policy issues affect everyone at all stages of life and in many different ways. Education policy requires certain behaviors of children and their parents. Transportation policy affects how people travel, whether on the interstate system that President Eisenhower began, on public transportation, or in environmentally friendly "green" vehicles. For older adults, specific policies have a real impact on their lives, including finances (Social Security) and health care (Medicare and Medicaid). Healthcare professionals need to know what these policies are, whom they cover, what services and benefits they provide, and how to access them to be able to fully help older clients and patients.

The specific policies covered in this chapter include income policies (Social Security and Supplemental Security Income, two distinct and separate policies) and healthcare policies (Medicare and Medicaid, also two distinct and separate policies). The specific federal policy for this population, the **Older Americans Act** (OAA), is discussed as an important foundation for services for older adults. A civil rights policy, the **Americans with Disabilities Act** (ADA), is also reviewed for its impact on older adults who may have a disability.

This chapter is organized into two main sections. In the first section, a high-level overview of the ever-evolving nature of policy and a historical perspective on elder policy is presented, with some emphasis on healthcare reform legislation under presidents Obama and Trump, to the extent possible in 2018 given the evolving situation. In the second section, "Policy Issues"—specific policies

related to older adults, organized by topic—are described, including an overview, a brief history, a description of eligibility criteria, an explanation of benefits, and instructions on how to access the policy or program.

▶ Policy Overview

The Ever-Evolving Nature of Policy

Just as science and medical care have evolved over the years, so too have public policies. The issues described in this chapter are current as of early 2018; however, they are ever-changing. Prime examples of this are the Patient Protection and Affordable Care Act (ACA) of 2010 (P.L. 111–148), President Obama's healthcare reform legislation and the current President Trump's efforts to repeal and replace certain features of the ACA. In 2018, this has remained a fluid and evolving situation. The policies discussed in this chapter are current at this time; however, it must be noted that as new healthcare legislation is passed, at least some of the provisions will affect older adults. Currently, the late 2017 repeal of the ACA's individual mandate no longer requires most individuals living in the United States to have health insurance through employer-based insurance, health insurance exchanges, or the optional expansion of state programs, including **Medicaid** (Henry J. Kaiser Family Foundation, 2013, 2018). Therefore, it appears that the current legislature is pushing to significantly reduce the strength of the ACA mandates, and limit some of the financial incentives for state to expand Medicaid, which may remain optional. For example, his executive order of October 2017 (Executive Order 13813) changed the way ACA is being implemented.

There are some specific provisions in ACA that affect older adults. These provisions include drug rebates and discounts for Medicare beneficiaries and the eventual closing of the Part D "doughnut hole" (a prescription drug coverage gap in Medicare), the creation of a center to provide funds to states to implement programs for individuals who are dually eligible for **Medicare** and Medicaid, and the expansion of home- and community-based services (HCBS) benefits for Medicaid populations. Under Medicare, older adults receive an annual wellness visit and additional preventive screenings like mammograms and colonoscopies with no deductibles or copayments. With the ACA, Medicare and Medicaid fraud and abuse protections were expanded. The ACA seeks to enhance quality of care for all individuals, including older adults, through the implementation and evaluation of better coordination strategies and programs (like the accountable care organizations and dually eligible [Medicare and Medicaid] initiatives; Medicare.gov, n.d.). These benefits for older adults remain, but potential reforms under President Trump may impact these and other benefits in the years to come.

As another example of the evolution of policy, if this chapter had been written right after the ACA was passed, one of the major benefits that would have been provided to the growing numbers of older adults was the Community Living Assistance Services and Supports (CLASS) provision. The CLASS Act was to be a national voluntary HCBS insurance program designed to provide a cash benefit, after an initial 5-year vesting period, to individuals who needed nonmedical services to remain in the community. The program was to be funded through payroll deductions. However, this provision was determined to be unsustainable through the proposed funding mechanism and was repealed (National Law Review, 2011). Additionally, if the Supreme

Court decision (which upheld much of the ACA) had struck down the entire law, this chapter might be focused less on Medicaid and more on private pay options for older adults.

Historical Perspectives on Elder Policy

Policies and programs for older adults in the United States are a relatively recent development. In the past, there were relatively few older adults and the community—typically families—took care of aging individuals. Older adults without family were often relegated to poorhouses, subsisting on meager charity based on poor laws (Gelfand, 2006).

With the passage of the **Social Security Act** in 1935, there was a dawning awareness of the need for policies and programs to assist individuals as they grew older (**FIGURE 6-1**).

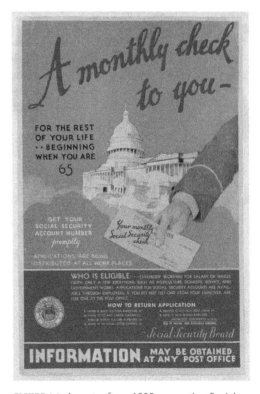

FIGURE 6-1 A poster from 1935 promoting Social Security benefits and detailing how to apply.
Library of Congress, Prints & Photographs Division, [LC-DIG-ppmsca-07216]

Much of the early policy focus for older adults was on finances and retirement, with amendments to Social Security expanding eligibility and eliminating limits in the 1950s and 1960s. Social Security has had a tremendous impact on the poverty rate of older adults, helping about 15 million older adults out of poverty in 2015 (Romig & Sherman, 2016).

During the 1960s, social service programs and funds, precursors to the current **Aging Network** of service providers, were also allocated for older adults. In 1961, the first White House Conference on Aging was held, followed by the establishment of the Commission on Aging in 1962. The Aging Network really took shape with the OAA of 1965, which created the Federal Administration on Aging (AoA) and **state units on aging** (Administration on Community Living, n.d.).

In fact, 1965 was an enormous year for both elder policy and healthcare policy affecting older adults. Medicare was established, creating federal healthcare insurance for older adults. Medicaid was also enacted, creating healthcare assistance programs at the state level for individuals with low income or resources (including older adults and people with disabilities).

In 1990, the ADA was enacted, calling for the integration of people with disabilities (including older adults) into employment, services, and health care. Following the "independent living" philosophy, disability advocates who fought for the ADA are now influencing how services are provided to older adults (Gibson, 2003). All these policies and programs exist today, though with amendments and specific changes dictated by current circumstances, politics, and demographics.

▶ Policy Issues

The policies discussed in this chapter are divided into several topic areas: Income, Health Care, Older Adults and Disabilities,

and **Long-Term Services and Supports.** Income policies relate to providing for some level of economic security and financial ability for individuals who are aging and may no longer be working or may have a disability. Healthcare policies provide a level of health care either through insurance or a safety net system. The policy area of Older Adults and Disabilities include policies that provide services, supports, or civil right protections for people who are aging or who have disabilities (or both). Finally the topic area of Long-Term Services and Supports is discussed, which includes elements and policy implications from all of the above topic areas.

Income Policies

Social Security

Social Security is the Old-Age, Survivors, and Disability Insurance (OASDI) program. It is funded through taxes on workers and employers. These taxes are paid into the Federal Old-Age and Survivors Insurance Trust Fund (better known as the Social Security Trust Fund). The current taxes pay for current benefits. Workers today are funding Social Security benefits for today's beneficiaries.

Much of the debate on Social Security revolves around whether Social Security will be able to pay out benefits to future generations of beneficiaries. This debate involves demographic and actuarial projections, which are uncertain. For example, life expectancy will play into the exact prediction of when the trust fund will be exhausted (i.e., when expenses exceed the total trust fund income). The number of individuals in the workforce will be another factor. Even as baby boomers are retiring in greater numbers, if the relative good health they enjoy compared to past generations induces some baby boomers to delay retirement, then these individuals will continue to pay into

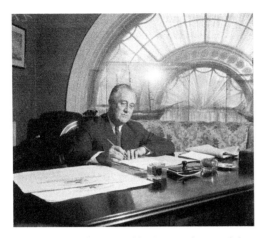

FIGURE 6-2 President Franklin Roosevelt signed the Social Security Act in 1935.

Library of Congress, Prints & Photographs Division, photograph by Harris & Ewing, [LG-DIG-hec-47244]

the trust fund rather than get "paid" from the trust fund.

History   (Social Security Administration, 2005) President Franklin Roosevelt signed the Social Security Act in 1935 (**FIGURE 6-2**); over the years, the act has been amended to evolve with the social, economic, and political tenor of the time. Social Security, at the federal level, was enacted to decrease the poverty rate among older adults, which was high during the Great Depression of the 1930s.

When it was enacted, Social Security covered all workers in commerce and industry (except for railroads). These categories excluded farm workers, domestic workers, and teachers, categories that were composed predominantly of women and minorities. The exclusions have been eliminated over time through amendments to the Social Security Act.

In addition, amendments in 1939 added spouses and children under the age of 18 years for dependent benefits, in cases where the worker was still alive, and survivor benefits, when a worker experienced a premature death. Amendments in 1950 created cost of living allowances (COLAs), which increased Social Security amounts (which until then had been a static amount) by a certain percent increase. Further amendments allowed for additional COLAs, until legislation in 1972 created automatic COLAs.

In the 1980s, there was a concern about the financing of Social Security. This concern led to the taxation of Social Security benefits and the slow increase in the retirement age from 65 to 67 in the 2000s. Other amendments have allowed older adults to remain in the workforce and still receive some Social Security benefits and, most recently, have excluded prisoners from receiving Social Security benefits.

Whom It Covers   (Social Security Administration, 2017b) Although this is a chapter on policy issues for older adults, Social Security is not just a policy solution for older adults or for retired workers. Non-elder beneficiaries of Social Security include workers with disabilities and dependents and survivors of workers who have participated in Social Security. Social Security covers workers who have earned enough credits through work. Typically, for people born in 1929 or later, they will need to have worked for at least 10 years to earn the 40 work credits needed to qualify for Social Security. Workers usually earn four credits for each year of work.

Individual workers can begin collecting Social Security benefits at age 62 (although workers with disabilities and dependents and survivors of workers may begin receiving Social Security benefits earlier). The benefit is greater for individual workers who wait until their full retirement age, which is based on their birth year. The benefit is reduced by 0.5% for each month Social Security benefits are begun before the worker reaches full retirement age. Almost 60% of new Social Security beneficiaries elect to start benefits before reaching full retirement age (Federal Interagency Forum on Aging-Related

TABLE 6-1 Full Retirement Age	
Year of Birth	**Full Retirement Age**
1943–1954	66
1955	66 and 2 months
1956	66 and 4 months
1957	66 and 6 months
1958	66 and 8 months
1959	66 and 10 months
1960 or later	67

Reproduced from Social Security Administration. *Understanding the Benefits* (SSA Publication No. 05-10024). Washington, DC: U.S. Government Printing Office, 2012: 9.

Statistics, 2016). See **TABLE 6-1** to determine the full retirement age.

Workers need not stop working completely to receive Social Security; however, depending on how old the worker is and how much he or she makes, the monthly Social Security benefit amount may be reduced until the worker reaches the full retirement age. Workers can also delay the start of Social Security benefits until age 70, which will increase their benefits by a certain percentage, depending on year of birth (8% for people born in 1943 or later; Social Security Administration, 2017a).

Social Security also covers spouses and, in certain cases, former spouses of workers. Spouses may collect Social Security benefits based on their husband's or wife's work history or on their own, depending on which amount is higher. Former spouses may collect if they were married to the worker for 10 or more years and have been divorced for at least 2 years (if the worker is not receiving benefits) and not remarried. Survivors of workers may collect Social Security benefits if they are 60 years or older or 50 years or older with a disability; children and parents of deceased workers may also collect benefits, under certain conditions.

Benefits (Federal Interagency Forum on Aging-Related Statistics, 2016) Social Security was originally developed as a floor or foundation for workers' retirement income and not meant to be the only source of income (**FIGURE 6-3**). Currently, however, statistics show that Social Security provides the largest part of older adults' income: in 2014, 49% of family income for individuals 65 or older was from Social Security, with earnings (24%), pensions (16%), and asset income (6%) rounding out the other main sources of income. For older adults with the lowest income, Social Security accounts for about 67% of their income. Benefits for Social Security depend on a worker's earnings, retirement age, working status, and relationship to the worker (in the case of spouses, dependents, and survivors).

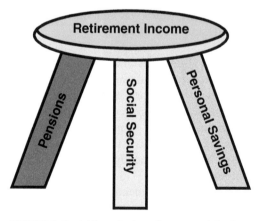

FIGURE 6-3 Social Security benefits were originally intended to be a small portion of retirement income, not the largest portion.

Given the role of pensions in older adults' income, a brief note on pensions is useful. Pension or retirement income typically comes in one of two forms: defined benefit or defined contribution programs. Initially, companies offered defined benefit programs. These pension programs were created such that individuals worked for a certain amount of time and then were guaranteed a specific amount (benefit) upon retirement as a lifetime annuity. Companies began moving away from those types of programs and now usually offer defined contribution programs like 401(k) accounts, where employees and employers set aside a specific amount into the program (defined contribution), which together with investment returns then determines the amount of the benefit upon retirement. As noted, regular income of any pension type provides less than one-fifth of the income for individuals 65 years or older (Federal Interagency Forum on Aging-Related Statistics, 2016). This, however, may not include income that is taken from other retirement accounts (like individual retirement accounts [IRAs]) because these amounts are often taken irregularly.

How to Access   (Social Security Administration, 2017b) Workers who are retiring should apply for Social Security benefits 3 months before they want to begin receiving benefits. Applications can be made online (www.socialsecurity.gov/applyforbenefits), on the telephone (1-800-772-1213, TTY 1-800-325-0778), or in person by making an appointment at the local Social Security office. Specific documentation is needed for the application process, and staff at the Social Security office can help to obtain the necessary documentation in the proper format.

Benefits are delivered electronically, either through direct deposit to a bank account or through a prepaid debit card program.

Supplemental Security Income

The Social Security Administration also operates the **Supplemental Security Income** (SSI) program (Social Security Administration, 2017c). The SSI program provides a monthly monetary payment for eligible individuals with little or no income and low resources. While the Social Security Administration operates SSI, Social Security and SSI are funded through different mechanisms. Whereas Social Security is funded through payroll taxes and eligibility is based on whether an individual or a member of his or her family paid into the system, SSI is financed through the U.S. Treasury's general funds.

Whom It Covers   Eligibility criteria include individuals who are 65 years or older, individuals who are legally blind, or individuals who are determined to be disabled. Many of these individuals may also receive Social Security benefits, as noted earlier, but an individual does not have to be receiving Social Security to receive SSI. Certain individuals are not allowed SSI benefits; these persons include fugitives from the law, individuals in prison or jail, individuals in publicly funded institutions, and individuals who only qualify for SSI because they transferred or gave away resources.

Benefits   The amount of the SSI benefit will be determined by an individual's income, resources, and living arrangement. For each of these categories, SSI has specific rules. SSI benefits also vary by who is paying for their room, board, and utilities. Often, individuals who receive SSI are eligible for Medicaid, although (as shown later in this chapter) each state has different eligibility requirements for Medicaid. Also, most states supplement SSI benefits with an additional monetary payment each month. Furthermore, states can choose to have the federal government administer the entire benefit amount of federal SSI plus state supplement, have the federal government administer the entire benefit amount for some categories of recipients but not others (dual administration states), or administer the state supplement on its own. This arrangement matters to individuals when they need to contact someone about their benefit.

How to Access   Applications can be made on the telephone (1-800-772-1213, TTY 1-800-325-0778) or in person by making an appointment at the local Social Security office. No online SSI applications are available. Benefits are paid electronically, through direct deposit, a debit card program, or an electronic transfer account.

Healthcare Policies

Medicare

Medicare is a social insurance program for older adults and certain other people. Social insurance is a government-sponsored program for which participation is generally mandatory for a defined population. A social insurance program's benefits and eligibility are defined by law and the program is funded through taxes from or on behalf of participants (Committee on Social Insurance of the American Academy of Actuaries, 1998). Medicare and Social Security are both examples of social insurance.

History   (Henry J. Kaiser Family Foundation, 2015) Medicare was created as the insurance program for older adults in 1965 when President Lyndon B. Johnson signed H.R. 6675 (PL 89-97). Much of the early years of Medicare, through the 1970s, saw the expansion of eligible groups and covered services. For example, the Social Security Amendments of 1972 expanded Medicare to allow coverage for individuals with end-stage renal disease. Also in 1972, covered services were expanded to include some chiropractic and rehabilitation therapy services.

In 1981, however, Congress became more concerned about slowing Medicare's growth and so put in place a variety of laws to limit Medicare spending. Laws were enacted that increased deductibles, instituted different payment methodologies for hospitals and physician services, and limited benefits such as home health and therapy services. For example, the Omnibus Budget Reconciliation Acts (OBRAs) of 1987, 1989, and 1993 modified payments to Medicare providers and changed physician billing. In 1988, the Medicare Catastrophic Coverage Act expanded coverage with a prescription drug benefit and caps on out-of-pocket expenses, and increased hospital and nursing facility benefits. However, by 1989, most of that act had been repealed. The Balanced Budget Act of 1997 continued the trend of implementing new payment methods for Medicare providers, including home health services and outpatient rehabilitation services. In 2003, with the Medicare Modernization Act, Medicare coverage was expanded to prescription drugs.

Current discussion revolves around the sustainability of Medicare and how it should be funded. Medicare is financed through payroll taxes kept in a trust fund, general revenues, premiums, and state payments (for certain benefits). Specifically, what people pay into the system is paying for the Medicare benefits of eligible individuals now. Debate centers on how long the Part A Hospital Insurance trust fund will remain solvent (insolvency will occur when the trust fund runs out of money to pay for Medicare benefits), with actuaries looking over a 70-year time horizon. The ACA enacted several provisions to slow Medicare spending and ensure the solvency of the trust fund while improving benefits and the quality of care for beneficiaries. At present, because of healthcare reforms, the trust fund is expected to remain solvent at 100% through 2029; after that date, the trust fund is predicted to remain between 81% and 88% solvent through 2091 (Van De Water, 2017).

Whom It Covers   (Henry J. Kaiser Family Foundation, 2015) Medicare covers people who are 65 years and older, certain people under 65 years with long-term disabilities, and adults with end-stage renal disease requiring dialysis or transplant. The inclusion of this specific disease category occurred in 1972 and was driven by Shep Glazer, who appeared before the House Ways and Means Committee while receiving dialysis. Since 2000, persons with the diagnosis of another specific disease, amyotrophic lateral sclerosis (ALS), are also allowed to enroll in Medicare upon diagnosis instead of waiting the 24 months as other adults with disabilities must do after a qualifying disability/disease.

Benefits   (U.S. Department of Health and Human Services, 2014) Medicare is composed of several different benefits or "parts," which provide specific help in covering certain healthcare services. Part A is also known as Hospital Insurance, and it covers inpatient hospital care, limited skilled nursing facility care (nursing homes), hospice, and home health care. Part B, also known as Medical Insurance, covers doctor/provider services, outpatient care, home health care, durable medical equipment, and some types of preventative services (Centers for Medicare and Medicaid Services, n.d.). Part C is Medicare Advantage plans, which include Part A and B services and are run by private insurance companies. Part D is the Medicare Prescription Drug Coverage, and is also run by private insurance companies (Henry J. Kaiser Family Foundation, 2017a).

Part A is financed through payroll taxes, paid by both employers and employees, and kept in the Hospital Insurance trust fund. The payroll tax was 1.45% for employees and employers (total 2.9%) for all but higher income taxpayers (Cubanski & Neuman, 2017). Part A covers a semiprivate hospital room (unless a private room is medically necessary), meals, nursing services, and other medically necessary supplies and services. Part A accounted for 29% of Medicare spending in 2016 (The Boards of Trustees, 2017). People with Medicare Part A are covered if there is an order from a doctor that the illness or injury requires inpatient hospital care, if the type of care can only be given in a hospital, if the hospital accepts Medicare, and if the hospital's utilization review process/entity approves of the hospital stay. Although Part A pays for the hospital stay, deductibles, coinsurance, and lifetime reserve days determine the amount that each Medicare hospital patient pays during a stay.

Part A also covers some skilled nursing facility care. Specifically, for up to 100 days, Medicare covers skilled nursing care, medications, supplies and equipment, medical social services, dietary counseling, physical therapy, occupational therapy, and speech-language pathology services—all as necessary to meet the patient's health/medical goals. To be covered, the Medicare recipient must have Part A with days left in the benefit period, a qualifying hospital stay, and a medical need for daily skilled care. A benefit period is how Medicare measures hospital and skilled nursing facility care. It begins on the first day a beneficiary received inpatient hospital or skilled nursing facility care and ends when the beneficiary has not had hospital or skilled nursing facility care for 60 days. There is no limit to the number of benefit periods. Similar to hospital stays, the person will be charged based on the number of days in a skilled facility.

Part A covers home health services, including intermittent skilled nursing care, physical and occupational therapy, and speech-language pathology services. There are certain limitations to coverage for these services. To be covered, skilled nursing services must be only intermittent. Therapy services must be reasonable in amount and frequency and specific, safe, and effective to treat the condition. In addition, the condition must be expected to improve with such treatment or else only a skilled therapist can safely create a maintenance program. Individuals receiving this benefit must have a doctor's order and the doctor must certify that the person is homebound (meaning they should not leave their house in their condition, they cannot leave home without help, and they cannot leave home without considerable and taxing effort). The benefit covers all costs for health-care services—individuals must pay 20% of any durable medical equipment.

Part B or Medical Insurance covers medically necessary services (such as doctor visits) and supplies and services to prevent illness. Unlike Part A, Part B is funded through a premium system and general revenues. Part B accounted for 28% of Medicare spending in 2016 (The Boards of Trustees, 2017).

Part B benefits include clinical research, ambulance services, durable medical equipment, mental health services, therapy services, and second opinions. Part B also provides an annual wellness visit, known as the "Welcome to Medicare" preventive visit, during the first 12 months of Part B coverage (under ACA provisions). Medicare beneficiaries who have had Part B coverage for longer than 12 months receive yearly wellness visits. Additionally, tobacco cessation counseling and screenings are covered under Medicare Part B. Some services are never covered by Medicare Part A or B, including routine dental and vision care, hearing aid fitting, long-term nonskilled (custodial) nursing care, dentures, and regular foot care.

Part C (Medicare Advantage) consists of plans from private insurance companies that cover Part A and Part B benefits for individuals enrolled in the plans. Monthly premiums vary by plan. Part C accounted for 29% of Medicare spending in 2017 (The Boards of Trustees, 2017), with over 19 million individuals enrolled in Medicare Advantage plans (Henry J. Kaiser Family Foundation, 2017b).

All Part C plans must cover emergency care as well as all the services covered by Part A and Part B or "original Medicare." The only exception is hospice, which is covered by basic Medicare even if there is a Part C/Medicare

Advantage plan in place. Part C plans do not have to cover any service that is not medically necessary; however, these plans may offer benefits that are not covered under original Medicare such as vision, hearing, or dental care.

Part D covers prescription drugs, and each private insurance plan has different lists of drugs that are covered. Similar to Part C/Medicare Advantage, Part D is funded through premiums that vary by plan. Part D accounted for 15% of Medicare spending in 2017 (The Boards of Trustees, 2017). For some Part D plans, the lists (or formularies) are organized into tiers, with different tiers costing a beneficiary a different amount. Older adults and their healthcare providers should determine the formulary as well as the rules and limits for their specific Part D coverage (such as prior authorization requirements, quantity limits, and step therapy, in which a lower cost drug must be trialed before a higher cost medication is approved).

Most Part D plans have a coverage gap called "the doughnut hole." This gap occurs when a beneficiary and his or her Part D plan have spent a certain amount of money on prescriptions. After that amount is reached, the beneficiary must pay for all prescriptions until a yearly limit on out-of-pocket costs is reached, and then the Part D plan again begins to help pay the prescription's cost. The ACA provides some relief for Medicare beneficiaries in the doughnut hole. First, the ACA closes the coverage gap by 2020. Second, if an individual reaches the coverage gap, there is a discount on covered brand name drugs (although the full amount is counted toward the yearly limit) until the limit is reached. Third, beneficiaries in the coverage gap receive a discount on generic prescriptions (Medicare.gov, n.d.).

Many older adults purchase additional coverage to supplement their original Medicare (Parts A and B). This coverage is known as **Medigap** insurance policy because it fills in certain gaps in the original Medicare (U.S. Department of Health and Human

Services, 2017). These gaps are costs that original Medicare does not pay, including coinsurances, deductibles, and copayments. Other gaps in the original Medicare such as services not covered (e.g., long-term nonskilled care, vision, etc.) are typically not covered with a Medigap policy. Medigap policies require premiums to be paid by the individual, which vary by plan. Medigap policies in the majority of states are standardized and identified by a letter, A–N, signifying exactly what the plan covers. (Exceptions to this standardization are in Massachusetts, Minnesota, and Wisconsin, which organize Medigap plans in a different way.)

For individuals with low incomes and little to no resources, states provide several programs to assist with paying for premiums. These programs include the Qualified Medicare Beneficiary (QMB) program, Specified Low-Income Medicare Beneficiary (SLMB) program, Qualifying Individual (QI) program, and Qualified Disabled and Working

Individuals (QDWI) program. Each program has certain income and resource limits and pays for certain types of premiums and/or deductibles. Any individual who qualifies for one of these programs also qualifies for Extra Help, a Medicare program designed to assist with Medicare prescription drug coverage.

How to Access (U.S. Department of Health and Human Services, 2014) For individuals already receiving Social Security, Social Security will contact them about 3 months before they turn 65 years to make decisions about their Medicare coverage (discussed later in this chapter). A person can receive Medicare at the age of 65 years, even if he or she delays the receipt of Social Security retirement benefits. To apply for Medicare for older adults, a person needs to be 64 years and 9 months old (**FIGURE 6-4**). Individuals who have been determined to be disabled and are receiving Social Security disability benefits are eligible for

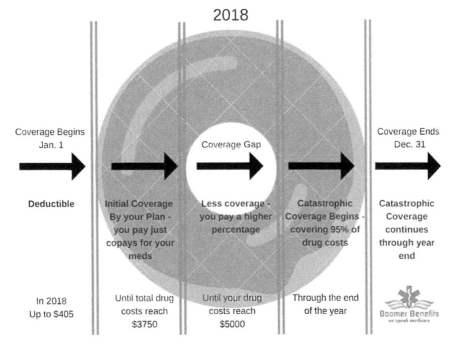

FIGURE 6-4 Medicare Donut Hole.

Medicare 24 months after the disability determination is made. About 3 months before the 2-year period is completed, Social Security will contact them. As noted, ALS is a special case. Individuals with ALS may begin receiving Medicare upon the diagnosis, without waiting.

There are several decisions that need to be made. Individuals will need to decide if they want to receive original Medicare (Parts A and B) or receive their coverage through a Part C Medicare Advantage Plan (Parts A, B, and usually D). Then, older adults will have to decide if they need to include prescription drug coverage (Part D). If they receive the original Medicare, individuals need to determine if they want a Medicare supplemental insurance or Medigap policy (U.S. Department of Health and Human Services, 2017). Individuals with a Medicare Advantage Plan are not eligible for a Medigap policy. The easiest time to purchase a Medigap policy is during the Medigap open enrollment period, which is the 6-month period that begins when an elder is 65 years or older and enrolled in Part B. Medicare beneficiaries under the age of 65 years may not be able to purchase a Medigap policy, depending on the state.

For the Medicare Savings Programs (see QMB, SLMB, QI, and QDWI programs discussed earlier), individuals with low income and low resources can contact their state Medicaid office for assistance with the application process and to determine eligibility.

Medicaid

Medicaid is a public assistance program that provides health care to individuals of all ages with low incomes, including individuals with disabilities. Medicaid is a federal and state partnership, whereas Medicare is the responsibility of the federal government. Medicaid is a voluntary program for each state, although all 50 states currently participate. To participate, a state must agree to cover certain services (discussed further in this section) and follow Medicaid regulations.

History (Paradise, Lyons, & Rowland, 2015) Medicaid was enacted at the same time as Medicare, in 1965. It is Title XIX of the Social Security Act. As a voluntary federal–state program, states choose whether or not to participate. It was only in 1982 that all states chose Medicaid, when Arizona created its Arizona Health Care Cost Containment System. In the years since Medicaid was created, coverage and eligibility requirements and options have expanded. Other changes have been enacted to allow states to better control costs (such as the Medicaid Drug Rebate Program created by the Omnibus Reconciliation Act of 1990) and to allow additional flexibility in meeting the needs of beneficiaries (such as Medicaid waivers). Still, other changes have made it easier for certain Medicaid beneficiaries with disabilities to work without losing all Medicare and Medicaid benefits (Ticket to Work and Work Incentives Improvement Act of 1999).

The federal government "matches" a percentage of the costs of the Medicaid program in each state. This percentage is known as the Federal Medical Assistance Percentage (FMAP). The FMAP ranges from 50% (for wealthier states) up to 75% (for poorer states). FMAPs are determined by financial criteria for each state and are published for each federal fiscal year (U.S. Department of Health and Human Services, 2015a).

Whom It Covers (Henry J. Kaiser Family Foundation, 2017c) Medicaid's eligibility requirements differ by state. There are mandatory eligibility groups that include children, elderly adults, parents/caretaker relatives of children up to 18 years old, and people with disabilities who meet specified minimum income levels. The ACA offers states the opportunity to expand eligibility to include all individuals meeting 138% of the federal poverty level. Some states are more expansive in their eligibility criteria than others, because Medicaid law allows for flexibility in determining which groups are covered. In 2014, approximately 80 million individuals were covered by Medicaid, with older adults accounting for 9% of the Medicaid population (Henry J. Kaiser Family Foundation, 2017c).

Each state has specific income levels and resource amounts for qualification for Medicaid. There are limits to how much an individual may own and also limits to how much an individual can transfer to another person in the previous 5 years if he or she is trying to qualify for Medicaid (the 5-year look back period for transfer of assets). These limits are in place to ensure that Medicaid benefits are given to individuals with lower incomes and few resources, not to individuals who are trying to appear to have lower incomes and few resources but in fact have access to such funds. Individuals can, however, spend down their resources and income through paying for health care to qualify for Medicaid. Spouses of individuals qualifying for Medicaid have protections, known as Spousal Impoverishment standards, to allow them to keep income, resources, and home equity.

Benefits   (Henry J. Kaiser Family Foundation, 2017c) Medicaid programs in each participating state must provide the following medically necessary services (medical necessity is determined by each state's requirements):

- Physician services
- Inpatient/outpatient hospital services
- Laboratory and X-ray services
- Early and periodic screening, diagnostic, and treatment services for people under the age of 21
- Federally qualified health center and rural health clinic services
- Family planning
- Nurse practitioner services
- Nurse midwife
- Nursing facilities for adults (age 21 and older)
- Home health care for nursing facility–eligible individuals
- Medically necessary transportation

Each state may provide additional optional services (e.g., prescription drugs, personal care services, dental services, respiratory care, and intermediate care facility services for individuals with intellectual or developmental disabilities). The services that a state's Medicaid program covers are described in the State Medicaid Plan, a document that must be approved by the Centers for Medicare and Medicaid Services (CMS). States can change what is in their State Medicaid Plan at any time through the State Plan Amendment (SPA) process. Amendments can be based on new data, changes in state or federal law, or a court order, and must be approved by CMS (Centers for Medicare and Medicaid Services, 2017c).

How to Access   Each state operates its own Medicaid program. Each program has local eligibility offices where an older adult can apply. Information also is available online and can be viewed by searching for the state's Medical Assistance Office. State Medicaid programs may be known as Medicaid or another name (see **TABLE 6-2** for some examples).

To apply for Medicaid, an older adult will need to complete an application form and provide documentation about finances and functional level.

TABLE 6-2 State Medicaid Program Names (Examples)

State	Name of Medicaid Program
California	Medi-CAL
Massachusetts	MassHealth
Oklahoma	SoonerCare
Tennessee	TennCare

Older Adults and Disabilities Policies

The Aging Network

The Aging Network is the name of the collaboration of the AoA, state units on aging, **area agencies on aging**, tribal and native organizations, service providers, and volunteers. From the most recently published report to Congress, the AoA in the Executive Summary noted:

> AoA's core programs, authorized under the Older Americans Act (OAA), help people choose to remain in their homes and communities for as long as possible. These services complement efforts of the nation's public health networks, as well as existing medical and healthcare systems, and support some of life's most basic functions, such as bathing and preparing meals. These programs also support family caregivers; address issues of exploitation, neglect, and abuse of older adults; and adapt services to the needs of Native Americans. The most recent data available show that, in FY 2015, AoA and the national aging services network rendered direct services to nearly 11 million individuals age 60 and over (one out of every six older adults), including nearly three million clients who received intensive in-home services. Critical supports, such as respite care and a peer support network, were provided to over 700,000 caregivers (U.S. Department of Health and Human Services, 2015b).

The AoA, funded through the Older Americans Act, provides block grants for services through state and territorial units on aging, designated by the governor or legislature of each state/territory. These units then procure services through area agencies on aging and their network of service providers and volunteers (Gelfand, 2006).

History (Administration for Community Living, 2017a) The OAA was signed into law in 1965, following the first White House Conference on Aging in 1961. The OAA established the AoA. Originally, the OAA designated its population as anyone 65 years or older. However, in subsequent amendments and reauthorizations, the age was changed to 60 years and older to allow individuals approaching "elderhood" to benefit from information and referral resources as part of their preretirement planning.

In addition, as elder policies evolved, OAA amendments have established the Aging Network framework through area agencies on aging (1974), added funding for senior centers (1974), created the Long-Term Care Ombudsman program for nursing facilities (1978; and later board and care homes and other residential options in 1981), added services related to elder abuse (1992), and focused interventions on caregivers (1992, 2000). Some of the amendments and reauthorizations have emphasized the role of the Aging Network in providing supportive services for older adults in the community so that they can remain at home (1984, 2006). Bearing this emphasis in mind, in 2012, the U.S. Department of Health and Human Services brought together the AoA, the Administration on Developmental Disabilities, and the Office on Disability to create the Administration for Community Living to further strengthen federal efforts to respond to the community living needs and preferences of people with disabilities of all ages, including older adults (Administration for Community Living, 2017b).

Whom It Covers The Aging Network and the OAA define an older American as being 60 years or older. Caregivers of older individuals are also covered.

Benefits (Gelfand, 2006) The AoA provides funds to state units on aging and tribal organizations to provide specific services as mandated by the OAA. State units on aging then fund area agencies on aging to provide these services to local older adults through service providers. The specific services include nutritional services (Title IIIc of the OAA), which involves both congregate meals (group dining) and home-delivered meals (Meals on Wheels); supportive services, which includes transportation, in-home care/personal care, adult day care, and information and referral; preventive health services; elder rights services, including the Long-Term Care Ombudsman program; and the National Family Caregiver Support Program, which offers counseling, training, and respite care to caregivers.

How to Access   Area agencies on aging are the primary access point for the Aging Network. To find an area agency on aging or a specific service provider at the local level, an older adult, family member, or healthcare professional can contact the Eldercare Locator. This resource is maintained by the AoA and consists of a telephonic and web-based database of resources at the state and local level. To contact the Eldercare Locator, call 1-800-677-1116 or visit the website www.eldercare.gov.

Americans with Disabilities Act

Thirty-five percent of older adults report some type of disability in terms of hearing, vision, cognition, ambulation, self-care, or independent living (Administration on Aging, n.d.). This rate increases with age. Some older adults have disabilities or functional limitations that prevent them from performing activities and fully integrating into community living. The ADA is an important policy for all individuals with disabilities, including older people. The main aim of the ADA is to integrate individuals with disabilities into all aspects of living in the United States. The ADA prohibits discrimination of individuals with a disability in all areas of everyday life, including employment, transportation, public facilities, healthcare, and telecommunications (Americans with Disabilities Act Home Page, n.d.).

History   (U.S. Department of Justice, 2017) The ADA was signed into law by President George H. W. Bush in 1990. This law represented a culmination of decades of work by people with disabilities and other advocates to have official recognition of discrimination due to disability as a civil rights issue (Frieden, 2005). Just as the civil rights movement demanded equal treatment under the law for people of all races, so did the ADA for people with disabilities (Frieden, 2004).

The ADA has provided tremendous gains in accessibility in many areas for individuals with disabilities (Frieden, 2005). These gains occurred despite several Supreme Court decisions in the 1990s that limited the ADA. However, the ADA was amended in 2008 (Americans with Disabilities Act Amendments Act [ADAAA]). These amendments have sought to broaden and strengthen the ADA and its mandate of equal treatment regardless of disability (Americans with Disabilities Act Home Page, n.d.).

Whom It Covers   (U.S. Department of Justice, 2017) The ADA covers anyone who has a disability, which the ADA defines as "a physical or mental impairment that substantially limits a major life activity." The ADAAA further provided examples of life activities that include caring for one's self, eating, sleeping, walking, standing, and communicating. Thus, many older people with self-described disabilities are covered under the ADA.

Benefits   Importantly, for older adults, the ADA provides accessibility for health care and healthcare facilities. For example, hospitals and doctor's offices must be physically accessible to individuals with disabilities (**FIGURE 6-5**). Accessibility comes in many forms and may involve architectural access as well as specific access to medical equipment.

How to Access   In general, the ADA is not a policy that individuals access; rather, it is a

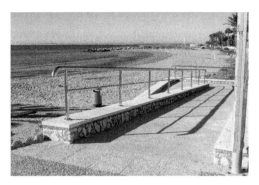

FIGURE 6-5 Thanks to the Americans with Disabilities Act, ramps (built to ADA specifications) are required so that people can access public spaces without difficulty.

© SoniaBonet/iStock/Getty Images Plus

policy that provides access to individuals with disabilities. Individuals with disabilities can bring complaints and/or lawsuits under the ADA if they believe that an organization (e.g., doctor's office, provider, or hospital) is discriminating against them due to their disability. Healthcare professionals can access additional ADA information and training through their professional organization or www.ada.gov.

Long-Term Services and Supports

Long-term services and supports are those services that individuals, including older adults, need when their ability to take care of themselves is limited due to disability or chronic disease. As the name suggests, these services are often needed for long spans of time—years for older people and perhaps decades for individuals with disabilities. About 60% of adults who need long-term services and supports are 65 years or older (Nguyen, 2017). These services may involve healthcare services such as skilled nursing, physical or occupational therapy services, which are required for the ongoing treatment of a condition or the maintenance of functioning or more personal care services like bathing assistance or meal preparation. Long-term services and supports are available in both facility

(e.g., nursing facilities or assisted living facilities) and community settings (e.g., at home).

In 1999, a Supreme Court decision (*Olmstead v. L.C.*) impacted long-term services and supports in the United States. The *Olmstead* decision supported the belief that institutionalization was discrimination based on disability and was against the ADA. Under the *Olmstead* decision and the ADA, states were required to make modifications to programs to avoid institutionalization and provide services in the most community-integrated setting possible. It is within this policy background that current long-term services and supports are provided (U.S. Department of Justice, Civil Rights Division, 2017).

Other trends have also impacted long-term service and support delivery for older adults and individuals with disabilities: independent living, consumer or self-direction, and family or person-centered care. Independent living is a philosophy and advocacy position of people with disabilities, who strongly support and demand that people with disabilities have the right to live independently and make their own decisions about their lives (Gibson, 2003). "Nothing about us without us" is one mantra of this group, which advocates for long-term supports and services in the setting of one's choice (typically, home and community). Consumer or self-direction is about the organization and management of long-term services and supports that allow individuals receiving care or their chosen surrogates/representatives to plan and implement their own services through a variety of mechanisms. Self-direction may include the ability to hire and fire personal care workers, set the specific schedule of workers, buy equipment to take the place of workers, or buy different services chosen by the individual. Family or person-centered care could include self-direction, but is more about how service providers are oriented to individuals needing care and their families (Feinberg, 2012). These types of long-term services and supports take an individual's needs, preferences, goals, and desires into account as the organizing framework around which all care is to be provided. For older adults, often the term used is *family centered care* to underscore the prominence of the family in caring for older adults needing care.

In spite of the *Olmstead* decision and the ADA, there is still an institutional bias in many policies and programs. Policymakers, advocates, and other stakeholders have been working over the last two decades to balance long-term supports and services so that more services are provided in the community and fewer services are provided in facility settings. This is particularly true for Medicaid. Medicaid pays for a large portion of long-term services and supports, both in facilities and at home and community-based settings. In 2013, HCBS accounted for 53% of all Medicaid long-term care spending (Nguyen, 2017). However, among services for older adults, home- and community-based spending accounted for 27% of Medicaid spending (Henry J. Kaiser Family Foundation, 2016).

Long-term services and supports can be quite expensive. In facilities, the cost of a semiprivate room can average $82,000 a year or more. For personal care services in the community, costs reported in 2016 averaged $31,000 a year; home health services bill an average of $20 an hour. Depending on the types of services an individual needs, typically community-based care will be less expensive than facility-based care. In 2013, the total formal long-term services and supports expenses were $339 billion (Nguyen, 2017).

Medicare

Many older people and their families mistakenly believe that Medicare covers long-term services and supports. It is true that Medicare funds some long-term services and supports, with about 22% paid for through Medicare (Nguyen, 2017). Specifically, Part A funds skilled nursing facility care, rehabilitation, and home health care; however, this coverage is limited and not intended for long-term stays or custodial care. Medicare can cover certain types of nursing facility stays, but only for 100 days and only if certain conditions are met. Personal care in the community is never covered through Medicare.

Medicaid

The largest payer of long-term services and supports in the United States is Medicaid. This includes both nursing facility care and HCBS. About 43% of the $339 billion spent on long-term services and supports is paid for through Medicaid (Nguyen, 2017). In fact, nursing facility care is one of the mandatory services covered by Medicaid in all states. This institutional bias is being addressed, but at present, HCBS are not mandated as Medicaid requirements. Community Medicaid services are provided through mandatory home health services, through any optional services that a state chooses to provide as part of its state plan (including but not limited to personal care attendant services), and through a specific regulatory device called a Medicaid waiver (discussed in the following section). For all Medicaid services, individuals must meet the eligibility requirements for their state's Medicaid program to qualify for any long-term services and supports, even if they do need long-term assistance. Often, even if they do not initially qualify financially for Medicaid at the beginning of the need for long-term services, they soon use their resources and "spend down" their assets and income to the point where they then do qualify for Medicaid.

Medicaid HCBS Waivers and Special Programs

Medicaid services that states provide must meet certain requirements. For example, states cannot limit or deny services because of specific conditions or diagnoses: the comparability requirement. States must fund services that are in effect throughout the state: the statewideness requirement. However, because of certain amendments to the Medicaid Act, states can "waive" specific requirements and provide services in alternative ways. Notably, **Medicaid waivers** are available for states to provide HCBS (long-term services and supports available in nonfacility settings) (O'Keeffe et al., 2010). Many of these waivers are called either 1915(c) waivers, named after the section of the Social Security Act that authorizes them, or HCBS waivers. These HCBS waivers allow states to provide services to Medicaid recipients who would otherwise be in a nursing facility.

Medicaid also funded the Money Follows the Person (MFP) demonstration program currently wrapping up in 43 states and the District of Columbia. This program was expanded as part of the ACA. MFP programs have helped more than 63,000 people transition from facilities into the community from 2008 to December 2015 (Centers for Medicare and Medicaid Services, 2017b). In each of the MFP states, enhanced Medicaid funding is available to the state (through a higher FMAP amount) for certain services designed to assist individuals with Medicaid currently residing in a nursing facility or other long-term care facility to transition into the community with a menu of services, including state-specific State Plan services, MFP demonstration services, and/or HCBS waiver services. With this enhanced funding, states are expected to strengthen the HCBS system for these individuals transitioning out of facilities as well as individuals already in the community who require home- and community-based long-term services, to allow them to be diverted from an admission into a nursing facility. Each state's MFP program is unique, with specific requirements and criteria approved by CMS.

In addition to MFP demonstration expansions, additional ACA benefits include a greater flexibility for states to offer HCBS through a state plan amendment. Another program, the Balancing Incentive program (2011–2015), provided enhanced Medicaid funds to states that had less than half of their long-term services and supports spending in HCBS to make these community services more accessible and understandable (Centers for Medicare and Medicaid Services, 2017a).

The Aging Network

About 7% of long-term services and supports expenses are funded through other public funding, including OAA funding and the Aging Network (Nguyen, 2017). The Aging Network provides supportive services and nutritional services that can make up part of an older adult's long-term services and supports requirements (Gelfand, 2006). These services can include personal care and homemaker services (FIGURE 6-6), Meals on Wheels/dining options, transportation, and respite care. The Aging Network can also provide help through case management and information and referral programs. Benefits counseling, available through local Aging Network service providers, may also be of value to older adults needing long-term services and supports. In contrast to Medicaid, these services are available to all older adults age 60 years and older regardless of income, but are generally targeted towards low income, minority, or rural older adults, persons with frailty and or other disabilities.

Private Funding

Some of the long-term services and supports that older adults need in the United States are provided either through private pay or by informal caregivers (family or friends) (Nguyen, 2017). About 17% (or almost $1 out of every $5) of long-term services and support expenses are paid out of pocket. Older adults often have savings, income, or other resources to pay for services. As noted earlier, some older adults will need to spend their savings and other resources before they can

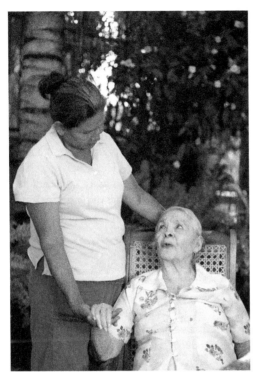

FIGURE 6-6 The Aging Network provides supportive services such as personal care and homemaker services.

© Pixieme/Shutterstock

qualify for Medicaid long-term care. Families of older adults may also pay for services. A certified elder law attorney or financial planner can assist older adults and their families in determining the most appropriate long-term services and supports financing options. Benefits counseling through the Aging Network may also be of assistance.

Informal caregivers perform all types of caregiving activities, including activities of daily living (ADLs) and instrumental activities of daily living (IADLs) to the tune of an annual economic value of $470 billion (in 2013), which dwarfs formal (i.e., paid) caregiving expenses. ADLs include eating, toileting, transferring, dressing, and bathing activities. IADLs include using the telephone, laundry, housekeeping, transportation, shopping, managing medications, and handling finances.

These caregivers are more likely to be women and typically spend about 18 hours per week providing unpaid care. One study found that most (more than half) older adults who receive long-term services and supports in the home receive only informal care, with no publicly funded services (Houser, Gibson, & Redfoot, 2010). These informal caregivers are often at risk for a decline in their own physical and emotional health, with resulting depressive symptoms, stress, anxiety, and other chronic conditions.

Long-Term Care Insurance

Some older adults may have **long-term care insurance**. There are about 7–8 million private long-term care policies in force (Gleckman, 2017). Taken together, these policies currently fund about 6% of long-term services and supports expenditures in the United States. (Nguyen, 2017).

Depending on the policy and its coverage, the policy may cover HCBS (such as home health care, personal attendant services, assisted living, and adult day care) as well as nursing facility care. Each policy will have different eligibility criteria and service requirements. Typically, a policy holder will qualify for benefits when he or she requires help with ADLs. Policies can be expensive, and premiums usually rise with age.

▶ Summary

Policy issues can affect every aspect of an older adult's life, from how much money he or she receives each month, to what health care he or she receives, to the types of medications he or she can afford. This chapter has presented several specific policies healthcare professionals working with older adults should understand to better assist older individuals with these aspects of life.

The policies and programs covered in this chapter include:

- Social Security, a policy impacting retired workers, spouses, dependents, and individuals with disabilities.
- SSI, a program providing resources for lower income individuals, including older adults and people with disabilities.
- Medicare, health insurance for older adults and certain people with disabilities.
- Medicaid, a program providing health care for people with lower incomes and few resources.

- The Aging Network through the OAA, which provides social, nutritional, and supportive services to older adults and their caregivers.
- The ADA, a law providing civil rights protection to people with disabilities, including older adults.

Each policy affects different aspects of life, with a variety of eligibility criteria and covered benefits or programs. Healthcare professionals and organizations can assist older adults in determining which policies or programs impact them and how to access specific benefits.

🔍 CASE STUDIES

Case 1: Ben was born in 1960 and has remained steadily employed since getting his first job at age 17. For the last 28 years, he has been a long-haul driver for a trucking company. He enrolled in a defined benefit pension plan when he was hired, and once he reaches the 30-year employment mark, he can retire with full benefits. After many years of working away from home for weeks at a time, Ben is looking forward to spending more time with his family. Yet, he worries that he might be in a bad accident someday, leaving his wife, who just turned 61, in dire financial straits. His manager has told him that if he wants to continue working after 30 years, he could switch to a local delivery route or a desk job in the office. With those options, he can keep working until he is able to claim his full Social Security benefit. Ben is glad that he has options, but does not know what he wants to do. He thinks that maybe he will work for a few years after giving up his job as a long-haul driver, but is not sure that he wants to work at a desk job until he reaches his Social Security retirement age.

1. **If Ben continues working until he reaches age 64, would he be able to claim Social Security benefits, and if so, what percentage of his full benefit would he receive?**
2. **If Ben was in an accident and passed away before retiring and claiming his benefit, would his wife receive any Social Security benefits? Why or why not?**
3. **Ben is enrolled in a defined benefit pension plan with his employer. How does that plan differ from a defined contribution program?**

Case 2: Amelia is a single 63-year-old woman in semiretirement. She worked full time as a nurse at a hospital for 35 years, and now works part-time at a private practice. Although she is relatively healthy, she is not in perfect health. She is slightly obese, takes medication to control her hypertension, and has had cataracts removed from both eyes. She is also starting to feel the first twinges of arthritis and the cartilage in her left knee is deteriorating, which will eventually necessitate knee replacement surgery. Amelia has been able to maintain her health insurance, but it is expensive, and she will not be able to afford it when she retires. She would like to apply for Medicare as soon as she is able to do so.

1. **Does Amelia qualify for Medicare now? Why or why not? If not, when will she qualify?**
2. **Based on Ameila's circumstances, which version of Medicare do you think would be the best option for her and why?**
3. **What programs, if any, are available to help Amelia pay for her Medicare plan when she enrolls if her income is too low for her to afford it?**

TEST YOUR KNOWLEDGE

Review Questions

1. Match the policy or program to the characteristic.
   1. Social Security
   2. Supplemental Security Income
   3. Medicare
   4. Medicaid
   5. Americans with Disabilities Act
   6. Older Americans Act

   a. Created the Aging Network
   b. Designed during the Great Depression
   c. Civil rights law
   d. Health insurance funded through payroll taxes
   e. Federal–state partnership providing health care
   f. Can be administered by the state or by the federal government

2. The "doughnut hole" of Part D of Medicare refers to the gap
   a. in prescription drug coverage.
   b. in coverage for emergency room visits.
   c. in rehabilitation coverage after 30 days.
   d. in coverage for nursing home care.

3. If an older adult who has worked for 40 years wants to retire with full Social Security benefits, what is the most important factor to consider?
   a. Date of birth
   b. Length of work history after 40 years
   c. Marital status
   d. Availability of a 401(k)

4. What is the name of the federal agency that provides funding for aging services?
   a. Social Security Administration
   b. Centers for Medicare and Medicaid Services
   c. White House Conference on Aging
   d. Administration on Aging in connection with the Administration for Community Living

5. _____ is the social insurance program for older adults and certain younger people with disabilities.
   a. Medicare
   b. Medicaid
   c. Medigap
   d. Social Security

Learning Activities

1. People often get the Medicare and Medicaid programs confused. Compare and contrast Medicare and Medicaid in terms of eligibility, services, and funding. Develop a simple way to present this information (e.g., PowerPoint presentation, table, notes, or illustrations). Ask someone to review it for clarity.

2. An older woman needs long-term services and supports and wants to stay in her home. She receives Medicare and Medicaid, and a modest Social Security benefits. What other resources would you pursue to assist her?

3. Think about a situation in which you might need to identify resources for an older adult (maybe a family member needs long-term services and supports or a friend is nearing retirement or someone close to you has to make a healthcare decision). Check out the websites listed under "Resources."
   a. Which websites or resources were the most helpful to you? Why? What kinds of information were

available, accessible, and most interesting to you? Were you able to find out what you needed or wanted to know?

b. Based on your experiences and knowledge, develop your own pamphlet or resource for older adults and their families/caregivers.

4. The year 1965 comes up several times in this chapter. Why was 1965 such an important year for policy issues? Conduct some research online and uncover what was going on in the

United States at that time. Talk to an older person to learn about their perspectives on the policies that helped shape the futures of older adults.

5. Conduct a research project on how another country funds long-term services and supports. Compare and contrast that country to the United States in terms of public versus private funding, the balance between institutional and home and community-based services, and informal caregiving.

Resources

Social Security
www.ssa.gov
Supplemental Security Income
www.ssa.gov/pgm/ssi.htm
Pensions
www.pensionrights.org/find-help
Medicare
www.medicare.gov
Medicaid
www.medicaid.gov
Aging Network
www.eldercare.gov
www.acl.gov
www.n4a.org
www.longtermcare.acl.gov
Americans with Disabilities Act
www.ada.gov
www.ncd.gov

References

Administration for Community Living. (2017a). Older Americans Act. Retrieved from https://www.acl.gov/about-acl/authorizing-statutes/older-americans-act

Administration for Community Living. (2017b). Organizational History. Retrieved from https://www.acl.gov/about-acl/history

Administration on Aging. (n.d.). Profile of Older Americans 2016 (AoA). Retrieved from https://www.acl.gov/aging-and-disability-in-america/data-and-research/profile-older-americans

Administration on Community Living. (n.d.). Older Americans Act: Historical Evolution of Programs for Older Americans. Retrieved from: www.acl.gov/about-acl/authorizing-statutes/older-americans-act

Americans with Disabilities Act Home Page. (n.d.). Retrieved from https://www.ada.gov/

Centers for Medicare and Medicaid Services. (2017a). Balancing Incentive Program. Retrieved from https://www.medicaid.gov/medicaid/ltss/balancing/incentive/index.html

Centers for Medicare and Medicaid Services. (2017b). Money Follows the Person. Retrieved from https://www.medicaid.gov/medicaid/ltss/money-follows-the-person/index.html

Centers for Medicare and Medicaid Services. (2017c). Medicaid State Plan Amendments. Retrieved from https://www.medicaid.gov/state-resource-center/medicaid-state-plan-amendments/medicaid-state-plan-amendments.html

Centers for Medicare and Medicaid Services. (n.d.). What's Medicare? Retrieved from https://www.medicare.gov/sign-up-change-plans/decide-how-to-get-medicare/whats-medicare/what-is-medicare.html

Committee on Social Insurance of the American Academy of Actuaries. (1998). Social Insurance (Do. No. 062). Actuarial Standards Board. Retrieved from http://www.actuarialstandardsboard.org/wp-content/uploads/2014/07/asop032_062.pdf

Cubanski, J., & Neuman, T. (2017). The facts on Medicare spending and financing. San Francisco, CA: Henry J. Kaiser Family Foundation.

Federal Interagency Forum on Aging-Related Statistics (2016). *Older Americans 2016: Key indicators of well-being.* Washington, DC: U.S. Government Printing Office.

Feinberg, L. (2012). *Moving toward person- and family-centered care* (Indights on the Issues 60). Washington,

DC: AARP Public Policy Institute. Retrieved from https://www.aarp.org/content/dam/aarp/livable-communities/old-learn/health/moving-toward-person-and-family-centered-care-aarp.pdf

Frieden, L. (2004). Righting ADA. National Council on Disability. Retrieved from https://ncd.gov/rawmedia_repository/b6fbb02a_34f3_4bfb_a048_3385cbb184f8.pdf

Frieden, L. (2005). NCD and the Americans with Disabilities Act: 15 Years of Progress. National Council on Disability. Retrieved from https://ncd.gov/rawmedia_repository/578d6d94_2d35_4d21_b0c6_d71a5a86a86a.pdf

Gelfand, D. (2006). The Aging Network: Programs and Services. New York: Springer.

Gibson, M. (2003). Beyond 50.03: A Report to the Nation on Independent Living and Disability: Executive Summary. AARP. Retrieved from https://www.aarp.org/health/doctors-hospitals/info-11-2003/aresearch-import-753.html

Gleckman, H. (2017). Who Owns Long-Term Care Insurance (2016). Retrieved from Forbes https://www.forbes.com/sites/howardgleckman/2016/08/18/who-owns-long-term-care-insurance/#131071ca2f05

Henry J. Kaiser Family Foundation. (2013). Summary of the Affordable Care Act. Retrieved from https://www.kff.org/health-reform/fact-sheet/summary-of-the-affordable-care-act/

Henry J. Kaiser Family Foundation. (2015). Medicare Timeline. Retrieved from https://www.kff.org/medicare/timeline/medicare-timeline/

Henry J. Kaiser Family Foundation. (2016). Medicaid's Role in Meeting Seniors' Long-Term Services and Support Needs. author. Retrieved from http://files.kff.org/attachment/Fact-Sheet-Medicaids-Role-in-Meeting-Seniors-Long-Term-Services-and-Supports-Needs

Henry J. Kaiser Family Foundation. (2017a). An Overview of Medicare. author. Retrieved from http://files.kff.org/attachment/issue-brief-an-overview-of-medicare

Henry J. Kaiser Family Foundation. (2017b). Medicare Advantage. Retrieved from http://files.kff.org/attachment/Fact-Sheet-Medicare-Advantage

Henry J. Kaiser Family Foundation. (2017c). Medicaid Pocket Primer. author. Retrieved from http://files.kff.org/attachment/Fact-Sheet-Medicaid-Pocket-Primer

Henry J. Kaiser Family Foundation. (2018, April 3). Poll: Survey of the Non-Group Market Finds Most Say the Individual Mandate Was Not a Major Reason They Got Coverage in 2018, And Most Plan to Continue Buying Insurance Despite Recent Repeal of the Mandate Penalty. Retrieved from https://www.kff.org/health-reform/press-release/poll-most-non-group-enrollees-plan-to-buy-insurance-despite-repeal-of-individual-mandate-penalty/

Houser, A., Gibson, M., & Redfoot, D. (2010). *Trends in family caregiving and Paif home care for older people with disabilities in the community: Data from the national long-term care survey.* Washington, DC: AARP Public Institute. Retrieved from https://assets.aarp.org/rgcenter/ppi/ltc/2010-09-caregiving.pdf

Medicare.gov. (n.d.). The Affordable Care Act and Medicare. Retrieved from https://www.medicare.gov/about-us/affordable-care-act/affordable-care-act.html

National Law Review. (2011). HHS Halts Implementation of the CLASS Program. Retrieved from https://www.natlawreview.com/article/hhs-halts-implementation-class-program

Nguyen, V. (2017). *Long-term support and services.* Washington, DC: AARP Public Policy Institute. Retrieved from https://www.aarp.org/content/dam/aarp/ppi/2017-01/Fact%20Sheet%20Long-Term%20Support%20and%20Services.pdf

O'Keeffe, J., Saucier, P., Jackson, B., Cooper, R., McKenney, E., Crisp, S., & Charles, M. (2010). *Understanding Medicaid home and community services: A primer.* Washington, DC: U.S. Department of Health and Human Services Office of the Assistant Secretary for Planning and Evaluation.

Paradise, J., Lyons, B., & Rowland, D. (2015). *Medicaid at 50.* San Francsico, CA: Henry J. Kaiser Family Foundation.

Romig, K., & Sherman, A. (2016). Social Security Keeps 22 Million Americans Out of Poverty: A State by State Analysis. Center on Budget and Policy Priorities. Retrieved from https://www.cbpp.org/research/social-security/social-security-keeps-22-million-americans-out-of-poverty-a-state-by-state

Social Security Administration. (2005). Social Security: A Brief History (SSA Publication No. 21-059). Washington, DC: U.S. Government Printing Office.

Social Security Administration. (2017a). *How work affects your benefits* (SSA Publication No. 05-10069). Washington, DC: U.S. Government Printing Office.

Social Security Administration. (2017b). *Understanding the benefits* (SSA Publication No. 05-10024). Washington, DC: U.S. Government Printing Office.

Social Security Administration. (2017c). *What you need to know when you get Supplemental Security Income (SSI)* (SSA Publication No. 05-11011). Washington, DC: U.S. Government Printing Office.

The Boards of Trustees, F. H. (2017). *2017 annual report.* Washington, DC: The Board of Trustees.

U.S. Department of Health and Human Services. (2015a). ASPE FMAP 2017 REPORT. author. Retrieved from https://aspe.hhs.gov/basic-report/fy2017-federal-medical-assistance-percentages

U.S. Department of Health and Human Services. (2015b). FY2015 Report to Congress: Older Americans Act. author. Retrieved from https://www.acl.gov/about-acl/reports-congress-and-president

U.S. Department of Health and Human Services. (2017). *Choosing a Medigap policy: A guide to health insurance for people with Medicare.* Baltimore, MD: U.S. Government Printing Office.

U.S. Department of Health and Human Services, C. f. (2014). *Medicare basics.* Baltimore, MD: U.S. Government Printing Office.

U.S. Department of Justice, Civil Rights Division. (2017). Olmstead: Community Integration for Everyone. Retrieved from https://www.ada.gov/olmstead/

U.S. Department of Justice. (2017). Americans with Disabilities Act. Retrieved from https://www.ada.gov/2010_regs.htm

Van De Water, P. (2017). *Medicare is not "bankrupt": Health care reform has improved program's financing.* Washington, DC: Center on Budget and Policy Priorities.

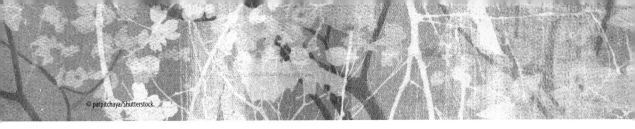

CHAPTER 7

The Physiology and Pathology of Aging

Kimberly Wilson, DNP, RN

CHAPTER OUTLINE

BEHAVIORAL OBJECTIVES

Upon completion of this chapter, the reader will be able to:

1. Differentiate between average life expectancy and maximum life span.
2. Compare and contrast the genetic and environmental theories of aging.
3. Explain the possible role of free radical formation in the aging process.
4. Identify common age-related changes related to the cardiovascular, respiratory, gastrointestinal, genitourinary, musculoskeletal, nervous, sensory, endocrine, immune, and integumentary systems.
5. Discuss health promotion for the aging process in relation to prevalent chronic diseases.

KEY TERMS

Atherosclerosis	Fecal incontinence	Osteoporosis
Average life expectancy	Free radical	Peptic ulcers
Cataract	Gastritis	Presbycusis
Chronic bronchitis	Hyposmia	Presbyopia
Chronic obstructive pulmonary disease	Hypothalamus	Sarcopenia
	Kyphosis	Senescence
Diabetes mellitus	Maximum life span	Urinary incontinence
Diaphragm	Metastasize	Xerostomia
Diverticulosis	Myocardial infarction	
Dysphagia	Osteoarthritis	

▶ Introduction

For hundreds of years, people have sought ways to live longer and slow down the aging process. Remedies have been promoted through abundant advertising and have included therapies such as special diets, vitamin supplements, cosmetic measures, and various other aids to help reduce the impact of aging. Even though researchers may study specific aspects of aging associated with their particular fields, a commonly held opinion is that the aging process is not linear, but multifaceted and influenced by individual biopsychosocial factors as well as external factors such as context, environment, and technology.

The **average life expectancy** (**TABLE 7-1**) in the United States has risen from about 47.3 years in 1900 to 78.8 years in 2015 (National Center for Health Statistics, 2017). This increase can largely be attributed to improvement in water supplies, sanitation, health technology, disease control, health promotion, and lower infant mortality rates (Forsberg & Fichtenberg, 2013). However, during the same period, there has been no change in the **maximum life span** (MLS), that is, the oldest age reached by an individual in a population, which is estimated to be about 120 years (Hayflick, 1997; Schneider, 1985). Although improvements in our standard of living have helped spare us from several causes of premature death, such as cholera, tuberculosis, and influenza, changes have done nothing to slow down the inherent aging process. In fact, any medical intervention that claims to slow down human aging must be shown to increase the MLS potential. But, to date, none have done so.

TABLE 7-1 Life Expectancy at Selected Ages, by Sex: United States 1900, 1950, 2014, and 2015

| | Life Expectancy at Exact Age (Years) | | | | | |
| | At Birth | | | At Age 65 | | |
Year	Both Sexes	Male	Female	Both Sexes	Male	Female
1900[1,2]	47.3	46.3	48.3			
1950[2]	68.2	65.6	71.1	13.9	12.8	15.0
2014[3]	78.9	76.5	81.3	19.4	18.0	20.6
2015[3]	78.8	76.3	81.2	19.4	18.0	20.6

[1] Death registration area only. The death registration area increased from 10 states and the District of Columbia (DC) in 1900 to the coterminous United States in 1933. See Appendix II, Registration area.

[2] Includes deaths of persons who were not residents of the 50 states and DC.

[3] Life expectancy estimates for 2013 are based on final Medicare data. Life expectancy estimates for 2014 and 2015 are based on preliminary Medicare data.

Data from National Center for Health Statistics. (2017). *Health, United States, 2016: With chartbook on long-term trends in health*. Hyattsville, MD: Centers for Disease Control and Prevention.

An unchanging MLS coupled with increasing life expectancy suggests two dimensions to the aging process. First, it supports the notion of distinguishing disease from aging. To illustrate, one of the most important chapters in the history of medicine has been the eradication of smallpox from the face of the earth through the use of vaccines. Although children who are immunized against smallpox have been spared a devastating infectious disease, they are not likely to age more slowly than nonimmunized children. Second, a MLS that has not likely changed in centuries points to the existence of a "biological clock" that predetermines humans' length of life. No such clock has been discovered, and it is perhaps an oversimplification of human physiology to suggest that one single mechanism in the body is responsible for aging. Nonetheless, it certainly appears that there are relatively fixed limits on how long the human body lasts.

A fixed life span, however, does not necessarily sentence adults to pain and suffering as they get older. Many of the physiologic changes associated with aging can be slowed to some extent with a healthy diet and consistent regimen of moderate exercise. Moreover, many of the chronic diseases prevalent in older adults are either preventable or modifiable with healthy lifestyle habits (**TABLE 7-2**). Reduction of dietary fat (especially saturated fats and cholesterol) lowers one's risk of coronary artery disease and stroke (i.e., occlusion or rupture of a cerebral artery) as well as breast and colon cancer (Spence, 2007; Tufts University, 2012). A program of increased physical activity increases one's resting and maximum cardiac output (the amount of blood pumped out of the heart per minute) while decreasing the chance of developing hypertension (American Heart Association, 2014). To the extent that exercise helps prevent obesity, it also

TABLE 7-2 Common Chronic Diseases of Aging Potentially Modifiable in Middle Age Through Personal Changes in Lifestyle

Disorder	Preventive Strategy
Hypertension (high blood pressure)	Reduction of dietary sodium and alcohol Reduction of body weight Develop a daily exercise program Monitor blood pressure Stress management
High cholesterol	Smoking cessation Reduction of alcohol consumption Develop a daily exercise program Eat a heart-healthy diet
Arthritis	Smoking cessation Stress management Develop a daily exercise program (stretching/strength building) Maintain healthy weight
Ischemic heart disease (coronary heart disease)	Smoking cessation Stress management Develop a daily exercise program (including cardio) Avoid saturated and trans fat in diet Reduce intake of sugar and sodium Develop healthy sleep patterns
Diabetes mellitus (Type 2)	Monitor carbohydrates and calories Discuss alcohol consumption with physician Develop a daily exercise program Maintain a healthy weight
Chronic kidney disease	Risk factors for kidney damage: diabetes and high blood pressure Maintain regular healthcare screenings
Heart failure	Eat a heart-healthy diet Maintain regular healthcare screenings Develop a daily exercise program with help from physician
Depression	Develop a daily exercise program Maintain a healthy weight Stress management Maintain a healthy diet—limit alcohol, caffeine, and processed foods

Disorder	Preventive Strategy
Alzheimer's disease and dementia	Develop a daily exercise program Develop healthy sleep patterns Maintain a healthy diet
Chronic obstructive pulmonary disease (COPD)	Smoking cessation Develop a daily exercise program Avoid secondhand smoke and other irritants Ask physician about flu and pneumonia vaccines

Modified from National Council on Aging. (2017). *Top 10 chronic conditions in adults 65+ and what you can do to prevent or manage them.* Retrieved from www.ncoa.org/blog/10-common-chronic-diseases-prevention-tips/

decreases the likelihood that an individual will develop **osteoarthritis** and non-insulin-dependent **diabetes mellitus** (DM; a disease that affects the body's ability to produce or use insulin) or suffer from a heart attack (American Diabetes Association, 2014; National Osteoporosis Foundation, 2017). Regular exercise, coupled with sufficient dietary calcium intake, lowers the risk of **osteoporosis** and its complications such as broken hips and slipped intervertebral disks (National Osteoporosis Foundation, 2017). In addition to these physical benefits, exercise appears to have psychological benefits as well. Exercise can lift one's spirits and alleviate loneliness and depression (Ruuskanen & Ruoppila, 1995). Conversely, sedentary lifestyles and, in particular, extended bed rest increase the chances of thromboembolic disease, respiratory infection, and decubitus ulcers (bed sores; Biswas et al., 2015).

Perhaps, the most important lifestyle choice an individual can make is to not smoke cigarettes or use tobacco products. Indeed, cigarette smoking is the most common preventable cause of disease and death in the United States. It leads to **chronic obstructive pulmonary disease** (COPD; e.g., emphysema, chronic bronchitis), lung cancer, and is a major cause of other cancers of the upper respiratory and digestive tracts (Li et al., 2014). Cigarette smoking also increases a user's chance of developing **atherosclerosis** and its complications—heart attacks and strokes. Ultimately, cigarette smoking has been shown to decrease life expectancy by 7 years and disease-free years by 14 years (Bernhard, Moser, Backovic, & Wick, 2007).

▶ Theories of Aging

Although research on the aging process has continued for decades, we continue to seek to understand it and find the fountain of youth! Aging, or **senescence**, needs to be conceptualized as a multifactorial process with a rate dependent on both genetic (programmed) and environmental (damage or error) phenomena (Jin, 2010; Weinert & Timiras, 2003; Tosato, Zamboni, & Ferrini, 2007). Senescence is characterized as decreased human functioning due to the inability of cells within the body to reproduce over time (Timiras, 1994). Although many theories have been proposed to explain the aging process, no single theory has yet to fully explain the phenomenon. Aging is a complex process influenced by multiple factors occurring at several organizational levels in the body. The following sections highlight a few of these incomplete theories of aging.

Programmed Theories of Aging

Because the stages of cellular, tissue, organ, and body development are, for the most part, controlled by our genetic machinery and thus programmed, some theories of aging have focused on the role of DNA (deoxyribonucleic acid), RNA (ribonucleic acid), and the proteins made from nucleic acid "blueprints." One such theory is that senescence results from the gradual accumulation of random mutations (alterations in the DNA) in somatic cells of the body (Ziegler, Wiley, & Velarde, 2015). According to this somatic mutation theory, radiation and other environmental mutagens alter the structure of the genetic code and thus change the sequence of amino acids found in enzymes and other proteins. Over time, such minor alterations accumulate and have damaging effects on protein functioning and thus on body functions. The varying rates of mutagenesis and proficiencies of DNA repair may affect longevity. Research findings have suggested that longer lived species tend to have more effective mechanisms for repairing molecular damage than shorter lived species (Burkle et al., 2002; Ogburn, et al., 2001). Although the number of DNA mutations increases with age, proving that such changes is the cause rather than the result of aging has been more difficult (Ziegler et al., 2015). Two other program-based theories, endocrine and immunological, focus on a gradual biological decline over time. In the former, biological clocks and hormone regulation control the rate of aging. In the latter, the immune system is "coded" to erode over time, thus enhancing the body's susceptibility to disease and death.

Environmental Theories of Aging

The wear and tear theory of aging proposes that aging is inevitable as cells, tissues, and organs, much like machines, wear out from continued use. The machine analogy is not a perfect fit because cells, unlike machines, have several mechanisms to repair their injuries. However, with the passage of time, the damage resulting from wear and tear might accumulate to a point at which the body's capacity for maintenance and repair is slowed and halted. Cells (and therefore organisms) with higher rates of metabolism might "wear out" more quickly than do those with lower metabolic rates, thus aging more quickly and dying sooner.

The inverse correlation between basal metabolic rate and longevity (across a wide number of species) has led some experimental gerontology researchers to reformulate the wear and tear hypothesis into a rate-of-living theory of aging. This reconceptualized approach attributes variation in life span to varying metabolic rates per gram of metabolizing tissue across species (Kirkwood, 2002). Every organism, then, is endowed with the ability to burn a fixed number of calories in its lifetime, after which the accumulation of wear and tear results in the organism's death. Members of a species with a high metabolic rate burn up their fixed number of total calories more quickly, sustain accumulated wear and tear more rapidly, and die sooner than species with low metabolic rates.

On the surface, the well-documented effect of caloric restriction (i.e., limiting food intake) to increase average life expectancy seems to support the rate-of-living theory of aging (Bishop & Guarente, 2007; Dilova, Easlon, & Lin, 2007). Many studies have consistently shown that caloric restriction not only increases average life expectancy, but also diminishes many of the physiologic changes associated with increasing age such as rising serum cholesterol levels, decreasing bone mass, and deteriorating immune system function (Yamada, et al., 2017). Nonetheless, it does not appear that caloric restriction has a significant effect on an organism's specific basal metabolic rate (Ravussin et al., 2015). The basis for its effect must, therefore, lie elsewhere. However, the rate-of-living theory has been challenged by researchers who have identified exceptions to the underlying assumption that animals with lower metabolic rates live longer than those with higher metabolic rates (Austad & Fischer, 1991; de Magalhaes, Costa, & Church, 2007).

Still, the rate-of-living theory of aging has helped focus experimental gerontology on another promising theory, the **free radical** theory of aging, which is a specific version of the wear and tear theory. The free radical theory attributes cellular (and therefore organismal) aging to the highly reactive accumulating by-products of oxidative metabolism known as free radicals (Harman, 2002). Free radicals are molecules that contain at least one unpaired electron in their outer valence shells. Free radicals most notably form in the mitochondria of cells, the site of aerobic respiration (where food is "burned up" for energy) and where electrons are stripped from temporary carrier molecules and passed down a chain of membrane-bound protein carriers to be accepted by oxygen (Lippman, 1981; Nohl & Hegner, 1978). Free radicals are relatively rare in nature because they are chemically unstable. When formed, they usually bind with other free radicals to create more stable molecules. However, when free radicals form in cells, they can initiate chain reactions that consume oxygen and randomly damage lipid molecules, enzymes, and nucleic acids.

One part of a cell's structure that is particularly vulnerable to chemical attack by free radicals is the cell membrane and organelles, including the mitochondria. The lipids embedded in these membranes are major targets for free radicals. But cells have specific defenses against attacks, including vitamin E (alphatocopherol), vitamin C (ascorbic acid), and several enzymes that stop free radical chain reactions (Leibovitz & Siegel, 1980).

If the levels of free radical "scavengers" such as vitamins E and C are depleted, damage to lipid membranes may be more permanent. Repeated peroxidation (oxidation of lipids) of unsaturated lipids can cause inappropriate cross-linking of lipids to proteins and nucleic acids (Pryor, 1978) and lead to the formation of lipofuscin (pronounced lip-uh-*fuhs*-en; also known as age pigment). Granules of this yellowish-brown pigment are found in the cytoplasm of aged cells. Slow, predictable accumulation of lipofuscin is the most reliable marker of chronological age in cells and has been found in nearly every organism with cells with nuclei (Brunk & Terman, 2002; Sohal, 1981).

Evidence for the age-related accumulation of lipofuscin and other types of free radical-mediated cell damage is widespread; however, proving that free radical damage is the primary determinant of aging has been more difficult. Lipofuscin accumulation appears to be a consequence rather than a cause of aging (Timiras, 2007a). Although studies in which organisms were given supplements of vitamin E throughout life revealed that the rate of lipofuscin accumulation decreased, none showed vitamin E to be a greatly beneficial change in the MLS potential (Brunk & Terman, 2002; Ernst et al., 2013).

Nonetheless, the potential importance of free radical-mediated destruction in aging cells should not be ignored, especially in its relationship with diseases. Consider cigarette smoking, the most common preventable cause of disease and death in the United States. The smoke from cigarettes contains free radicals whose presence can alter or destroy important biological molecules such as DNA and enzymes (Church & Pryor, 1985; Nakayama, Kodama, & Nagata, 1984). Damage to DNA, in turn, may play a role in the etiology of lung cancer, whereas damage to enzymes such as alpha-1 antitrypsin may cause the progressive and irreversible destruction of lung tissue in patients with emphysema (see the section "Respiratory System" later in this chapter). Thus, smoking may accelerate the aging process by accelerating the free radical mechanism, a process that some researchers claim is at the heart of the natural aging process (de Magalhaes et al., 2007).

Clearly, the distinction between disease and pure aging becomes less clear at the cellular level and no single explanation of the aging process is completely satisfactory. Aging is a complex phenomenon orchestrated by events at several organizational levels in the body. Any efforts aimed at limiting the effects of aging will also likely have to occur on multiple levels. Although the causes of aging remain elusive, the effects of aging are more readily apparent as disease processes occur more frequently as one ages.

▶ Physiological Changes of Aging

Cardiovascular System

The cardiovascular system (consisting of the heart and blood vessels) is responsible for the circulation of blood that delivers oxygen and nutrients to, and removal of waste products from, all parts of the body. Damage to this system can have negative implications for the entire body. The *ventricles* of the heart generate pressure that propels blood through arteries, arterioles, capillaries (the site of nutrient and waste exchange), venules, and finally veins, the blood vessels that return blood to the atria of the heart. The left ventricle has the thickest muscular wall and pumps blood out to the body systems (via higher pressure systemic circulation) while the right ventricle pumps blood to the lungs (via lower pressure pulmonic circulation; FIGURE 7-1).

The significance of cardiovascular disease (CVD) in middle-aged and older adults cannot be overemphasized. CVD continues to be one of the leading causes of death (World Health Organization, 2017a). Public health initiatives have contributed to reduction the prevalence of risk factors related to CVD such as smoking, hypertension, and other related factors (Centers for Disease Control and Prevention, 2017b).

The predominant change that occurs in blood vessels with age is atherosclerosis, defined as the development of fatty plaques

and proliferation of connective tissue in the walls of arteries. Slow destruction of the arterial wall can lead to blockage of the artery, particularly when a blood clot develops on its damaged surface. This condition is so prevalent that one might argue it is an inevitable phenomenon of aging. Although the clinical consequences of atherosclerosis are often sudden and life-threatening (e.g., heart attacks and strokes) and come toward the end of life, it has become clear in recent years that the earliest evidence of fatty accumulation is detectable in the first decade of life and that lesions progress throughout life (Alpert, 2012). Muscles within the heart become less efficient and lose strength causing cardiac output to decrease and place more demand on the heart. As a result, the heart needs additional time to perform basic functions and due to decreased elasticity and sensitivity, has more difficulty regulating blood pressure. Cardiovascular conditions affected by those changes are shown in **TABLE 7-3**.

Complications resulting from atherosclerosis begin as early as the fourth decade of life and increase in frequency with each succeeding decade. Particular consequences of the disease depend on the artery or arteries involved. Blockage of coronary arteries can cause **myocardial infarction** (heart attack), whereas occlusion or rupture of a cerebral artery can result in a stroke. The development of fatty plaques in the renal arteries can cause hypertension and kidney failure, whereas blockage of an artery in the leg can cause peripheral vascular disease marked by severe pain (called claudication) deep vein thrombosis (DVT) and ulcerations of the skin.

Although nearly everyone is prone to some degree of atherosclerosis, there are several risk factors that seem to accelerate the disease process. They include older age, genetic predisposition, hypertension, DM, high blood cholesterol level, cigarette smoking, obesity, poor physical fitness, and "type A" personality (e.g., aggressive, competitive, ambitious).

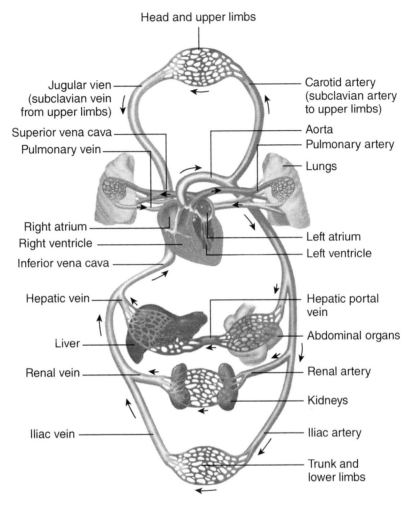

Head and upper limbs

Jugular vien (subclavian vein from upper limbs)

Carotid artery (subclavian artery to upper limbs)

Superior vena cava
Pulmonary vein

Aorta
Pulmonary artery

Lungs

Right atrium
Right ventricle
Inferior vena cava

Left atrium
Left ventricle

Hepatic vein

Liver

Hepatic portal vein

Abdominal organs

Renal vein

Renal artery

Kidneys

Iliac vein

Iliac artery

Trunk and lower limbs

FIGURE 7-1 The cardiovascular system. Note: The arrows indicate the direction of blood.

The confluence of many of these risk factors in older adults makes complications of atherosclerosis more prevalent in this age group (Alpert, 2012).

Heart attacks are more common in individuals older than age 50, and coronary artery disease leading to heart attack is the number one killer of people in the United States (Johnson & Sandmire, 2004). Worldwide, CVD accounts for about 37% of all deaths (World Health Organization, 2017a).

The warning signs of an impending heart attack are not always obvious in older adults and individuals with DM, sometimes making quick response and treatment unlikely. Common signs of an impending heart attack could be chest pain/pressure, discomfort in the arms, back, neck jaw, or stomach, shortness of breath (with or without discomfort in chest), lightheadedness, nausea, and sweating (American Heart Association, 2016). Women may experience a heart attack without experiencing chest pain or pressure (American Heart Association, 2016).

Given the increased risk of CVD in late life, it makes sense for everyone, regardless of

TABLE 7-3 Cardiovascular Conditions

Disease	Description
Coronary heart disease	Disease of the blood vessels supplying the heart muscle
Cerebrovascular disease	Disease of the blood vessels supplying the brain
Peripheral arterial disease	Disease of blood vessels supplying the arms and legs
Rheumatic heart disease	Damage to the heart muscle and heart valves from rheumatic fever caused by streptococcal bacteria
Congenital heart disease	Malformations of heart structure existing at birth
Deep vein thrombosis and pulmonary embolism	Blood clots in the leg veins, which can dislodge and move to the heart and lungs

Reprinted from World Health Organization. (2017a). Cardiovascular diseases fact sheet. Retrieved from www.who.int/mediacentre/factsheets/fs317/en/.

age, to maintain a proper diet, exercise regularly, maintain a healthy weight, manage stress, avoid cigarettes, and schedule annual physicals. Nearly all people know this information about what is good for them, but carrying through on these recommendations takes motivation and commitment, and often the assistance of a caring health care professional.

As health care professionals, it is important to provide education to all clients or patients. Prevention should be the priority for helping older people avoid the onset of disease. For individuals already diagnosed with cardiovascular problems, it is prudent for health care professionals to still engage them in education to prevent further complications. Encouragement through effective intervention more likely will lead to a pathway of success.

Respiratory System

The function of the respiratory system is to transport oxygen to and remove carbon dioxide from the bloodstream. The air breathed in is warmed, humidified, and cleansed as it passes successively through the mouth and nasal cavities, pharynx, larynx, trachea, and bronchi to reach the lungs (**FIGURE 7-2**). In the lungs, inhaled air continues through smaller bronchi, bronchioles, and alveolar ducts to finally reach alveoli, the tiny, thin-walled air sacs covered by capillaries that are the major site of gas exchange between air and the bloodstream. The 300 million alveoli in the lungs provide about 75 square meters of surface area for gas transport to and from the blood. The lungs, located in the thoracic cavity (or thorax) are enclosed by the rib cage and **diaphragm**, a dome-shaped skeletal muscle located beneath the lungs. During inhalation, the diaphragm contracts, lowering the floor of the thorax while external intercostal muscles between the ribs contract to swing the ribs forward and upward. Both these actions help expand the thorax, creating a vacuum-like effect that draws air into the respiratory tract and lungs. The lungs expand passively during this process because of their adherence to the inner thorax

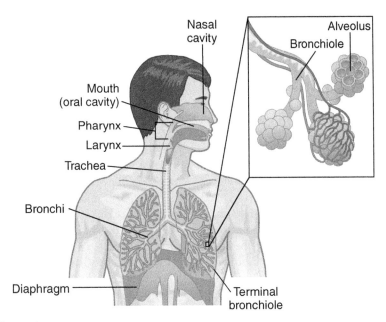

Nasal cavity

Alveolus

Bronchiole

Mouth (oral cavity)

Pharynx

Larynx

Trachea

Bronchi

Diaphragm

Terminal bronchiole

FIGURE 7-2 The respiratory system.

wall. Exhalation is normally a passive process, whereby the relaxation of breathing muscles causes the thorax to contract down to a smaller volume, largely by elastic recoiling of the rib cage and lung tissue.

Changes in mechanical properties of the thorax wall are coupled with changes in lung tissue as we age. Moreover, the rib cage stiffens over time due to calcification of cartilage between the ribs and vertebrae, and the exaggerated curvature of the thoracic spine (i.e., **kyphosis**). These skeletal changes limit mobility of the rib cage, making it difficult for external intercostal muscles to expand the rib cage. Thus, it is not surprising that older adults experience shortness of breath (dyspnea) more quickly during exercise than do younger individuals. Additionally, although a healthy older adult might breathe adequately to meet the body's needs at rest, the changes (described earlier) may limit his or her tolerance for exercise, especially when coupled with the age-related decrease in cardiac output (also described earlier).

Superimposed on the normal age-related changes to the respiratory system are diseases and conditions that increase in frequency after age 50. Respiratory health problems include emphysema, **chronic bronchitis**, pneumonia, and lung cancer. Together, the first two are referred to as COPD, and these along with lung cancer are caused primarily by cigarette smoking or chronic exposure to unhealthy air.

The steps leading to emphysema begin when cigarette smoke (or other pollutants in the air) irritates the respiratory tract, stimulating proliferation of white blood cells (WBCs) called macrophages. These macrophages release chemicals that attract large numbers of neutrophils, another type of WBC, to the inflamed area. Neutrophils release protease enzymes, one of which is elastase that can damage elastin proteins found in elastic the tissue of the lungs. The effects of elastase are limited by a protective enzyme called alpha-1 antitrypsin, which inactivates elastase. However, alpha-1 antitrypsin can be damaged by the free radicals produced from cigarette smoke. Thus, elastase is free to destroy the lung tissue. The stage is then set for a slow, irreversible loss of functional elastic tissue in the lungs, resulting in the loss of alveolar wall surface area and premature collapsing of small bronchioles during exhalation (hence, the "obstructive" in COPD) (Janoff, 1985; Pryor, Dooley, & Church, 1986; Travis & Salvesen, 1983; Weiss, 1989).

As more air gets "trapped" distal to the bronchiolar obstruction, the lung volume increases, creating the classic "barrel chest" appearance. In the end stages of emphysema, destruction of alveolar walls can be so extreme that large, visible air pockets form in the lungs. Collapsed bronchiolar airways are more difficult to reopen upon inhalation. Thus, emphysema increases the work demand of breathing, so that an individual must use the accessory muscles of inhalation to supplement the activity of the diaphragm and external intercostal muscles. Because of the diminished rate of gas transport and increased work of breathing, persons with emphysema are often short of breath and cannot tolerate rigorous exercise well.

Chronic bronchitis, like emphysema, is more common in older adults, especially in individuals with a long history of cigarette smoking. It is clinically defined as chronic cough ("smoker's cough"), producing sputum and occurring on most days for at least a 3 month duration over at least 2 consecutive years. Whereas emphysema primarily affects the smallest airways, chronic bronchitis involves inflammation of the larger bronchi, due to the irritating effects of cigarette smoke or other environmental inhalants. The inflammatory process causes excessive mucus production, which is difficult to clear from the lungs. Further difficulties arise because the tiny, beating cilia covering the bronchi that normally help move the mucus upward are also damaged by smoking. The pooling of excessive mucus can block bronchi (the additional "obstructive" in COPD) and provide a nutrient-rich environment for bacterial infection.

Considering that an older immune system is not as efficient as it once was, and the cough reflex that helps clear excess mucus and aspirated food from the respiratory tract does not work as well, one can easily understand why an older smoker with chronic bronchitis is at increased risk for spreading inflammation and infection to the bronchioles and alveoli, which can lead to the development of pneumonia.

Collectively, the number of people who die each year of respiratory illnesses is considerable. COPD and other chronic lower respiratory tract diseases (e.g., asthma) represent the fourth leading cause of death in the United States; pneumonia and influenza collectively rank eighth on the list (National Center for Health Statistics, 2017). The World Health Organization estimates that 235 million people worldwide have been diagnosed with asthma and 383,000 deaths were attributed to asthma in 2015 (World Health Organization, 2017b). In 2015, COPD was the cause of three million deaths globally (World Health Organization, 2017c).

Gastrointestinal System

One major function of the gastrointestinal system is to process incoming food so that nutrients can be absorbed into the body. The primary structural feature of this system is the digestive tract made up of the mouth, pharynx, stomach, small intestine, large intestine (or colon), rectum, and anus (**FIGURE 7-3**). This canal works like an assembly line, with each part having a specialized function in digestion. Attached to the digestive tract are exocrine glands, such as salivary glands, pancreas, and liver, which secrete substances to aid in digestion and absorption. Although aging in an otherwise healthy individual has minimal effects on the digestive system, many specific diseases of this system increase in frequency with advancing years. The age-related alterations in structure and function are discussed in descending order, starting with the mouth and proceeding to the rectum.

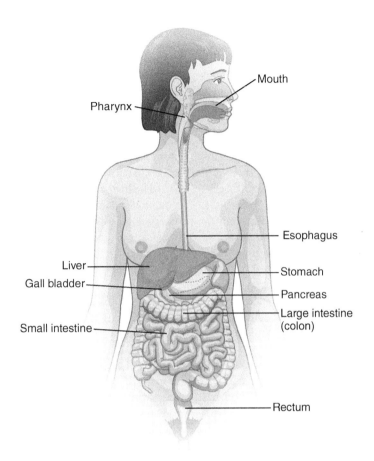

FIGURE 7-3 The digestive system.

Food entering the mouth undergoes the initial stages of mechanical digestion (via chewing) and chemical digestion (via release of salivary amylase enzyme). In the mouth, teeth undergo perhaps the most visible changes with age, becoming yellowish-brown (because of exposure to coffee, cigarette smoke, and other staining agents) and worn on the surface (because of years of chewing, night grinding, and jaw clenching). **Xerostomia** or dry mouth, is a problem reported in old age and has several causes: decreased saliva production (often causing complications such as chewing, swallowing, and tasting), radiation therapy, adverse effects of medications, hormonal changes, and diabetes (American Dental Association, 2017). For more information about oral health issues in late life, see Chapter 12.

Once sufficiently chewed, food is swallowed through the complex coordination of muscles in the tongue, palate, pharynx, and esophagus. A common problem faced by older adults is **dysphagia** or difficulty swallowing, which often occurs as the result of a stroke. Dysphagia may be caused by weakness of tongue muscles, poor control of the swallowing reflex, or a lack of coordinated muscular action of the pharynx or esophagus. Severe dysphagia can cause aspiration of food into the larynx and farther down the respiratory tract, which can place a person at risk for indigestion and aspiration pneumonia. Treatment of severe cases of dysphagia often requires the expertise of a team consisting of a physician and speech and language pathologist.

In the stomach, the swallowed food is chemically digested by virtue of hydrochloric acid (gastric acid) and pepsin enzyme secretion, and is mechanically digested by the stomach's muscular churning action. In old age, the rate of gastric acid secretion decreases and incidence of **peptic ulcers** and **gastritis** (i.e., inflammation of the stomach lining) increases. These gastric problems in older adults may be a result of *Helicobacter pylori*, (or *H. pylori*, a bacterial infection), drug ingestion (e.g., aspirin, caffeine, alcohol), or genetically programmed changes that may occur with age. Chronic bleeding from a peptic ulcer or gastritis can result in iron-deficiency anemia and acute bleeding can place severe stress on the cardiovascular system.

The initial section of the small intestine, called the duodenum, receives partially digested food (or chyme) from the stomach and continues the process of digestion with the help of secretions from the liver and gallbladder (bile) and from the pancreas (digestive enzymes and bicarbonate-rich fluid). As chyme is further digested, nutrient molecules become small enough to be absorbed through the small intestine wall, a process that occurs primarily in the more distal parts of the small intestine (the jejunum and the ileum). Movement of chyme through the small intestine by peristaltic contractions of the muscular wall is fairly slow to allow sufficient time for nutrient absorption. Aging has surprisingly little effect on the small intestine's digestive function and smooth muscle contractility. With the possible exceptions of calcium, vitamin D, and iron, most nutrients are absorbed efficiently in the small intestine in healthy older adults.

The *liver* has several functions, some related to digestion and others not. It produces bile that is stored below in the gallbladder until its release into the duodenum. Bile is required for emulsification of fats in chyme. Without bile, fats would pass through the digestive tract without being absorbed. Storage of bile in the gallbladder can lead to its precipitation into solid stones or *gallstones*, a phenomenon that is increasingly likely as we age. Gallstones, in turn, can get lodged in the ducts that normally convey the bile to the duodenum, resulting at times in obstructive jaundice and inflammation of the gallbladder (cholecystitis) or pancreas (pancreatitis).

The liver also detoxifies many foreign and potentially damaging chemicals that enter or are produced within the body. Indeed, many medications given for disease and illness are broken down by the liver and are released either through the bile or in the bloodstream to be eliminated by the kidneys in urine. But, in old age, this detoxifying ability is diminished. This is particularly important to realize because it means that many drugs given to older adults remain in the body for longer periods of time. Thus, recommended dosages of many drugs for older adults are smaller than they would be for younger individuals. Failure to consider this leads to dangerous overdosing of medications for older adults. For more information on medication challenges in late life, see Chapter 10.

The remainder of the small intestinal contents (largely water and indigestible fiber) enters the *large intestine* or *colon*, an area of the digestive tract that is heavily colonized by a normal bacterial flora. The large intestine reabsorbs much of the remaining water and stores the feces until defecation. One common problem seen in older adults is **diverticulosis**, which is a development of small sacs where the large intestinal lining has herniated through the intestinal muscular wall. These herniations usually result from muscular spasms and increased intracolonic pressure associated with long-term diets low in fiber. These pockets or diverticuli can become impacted with feces, resulting in ulceration and inflammation of the mucosal lining (diverticulitis).

With age also comes decreased motility of smooth muscle in the large intestinal wall, which prolongs the time that feces are stored in the colon and rectum. This, in turn, causes excessive water reabsorption and hardening of feces, leading to constipation and, in extreme cases, intestinal obstruction. Conversely, some older adults experience **fecal incontinence** (the inability to control defecation), often due to the weakening of the external anal sphincter muscle and possibly due to lack of awareness (e.g., in late stage dementia). Fecal incontinence can be exacerbated when there is increased intrarectal pressure during episodes of diarrhea.

The small and large intestines, like most other parts of the body, are vulnerable to the ravaging effects of atherosclerosis. Blockage of arteries supplying the intestines with blood can result in ischemia (reversible tissue damage caused by oxygen depletion) and ultimately infarction (tissue death and breakdown). When infarction occurs, perforations can develop in the intestinal wall, allowing bacteria-laden feces to spill out into the normally sterile peritoneal cavity, causing severe inflammation (peritonitis), a life-threatening condition.

Finally, the large intestine is susceptible to cancer as well. In the late 1940s, colorectal cancer was the most common form of cancer in the United States (Siegel, DeSantis, & Jemal, 2014). The prevention, screening, and treatment of this type of cancer has substantially reduced both incidence and mortality rates. Colorectal cancer is now the third leading cancer leading to death in the United States (Siegel et al., 2017).

Genitourinary System

The genitourinary system consists of the kidneys and the complete urinary tract. The paired *kidneys* serve two principal yet overlapping functions:

- Excretion of waste products from the body
- Maintenance of homeostasis (stability) in the fluid compartments of the body such as plasma and interstitial fluid

Excretion of Waste

Remarkably, each kidney only weighs about 5 ounces, yet jointly receive about 20% of the cardiac output, which illustrates their importance in carrying out these clean-up tasks. If they fail to function, nitrogenous waste products (e.g., urea) build up in the bloodstream leading to imbalanced levels of water, electrolytes, or acids, which alter normal physiologic processes. One would expect organs of such importance to have considerable functional reserve so that they could make necessary compensations when damaged in any way; and for the most part, this is true. Consider the nephrons, the microscopically sized functional units of the kidneys that filter blood and then "choose" which substances of the filtered fluid to excrete and which substances to place back in the bloodstream. Researchers have studied nephrons in the aging population and have only determined that the loss of nephrons is associated with a decreased kidney filtration rate (Aleksandar et al., 2016).

Nonetheless, the kidneys of older adults have a more difficult time responding to any added metabolic stressor on the body when nephrons become less efficient and fewer in numbers. Like the other organs discussed, older kidneys work well under normal conditions but have reduced tolerance for disease, whether originating from the kidneys themselves or from other organs. This is why older adults are more likely to experience acute and chronic renal failure (conditions in which toxic metabolites build up in the body because of an inability of the kidneys to remove them at a sufficient rate) than younger individuals.

Like the liver, the kidneys help eliminate medications and their by-products from the body. The decreased functional reserve capacity that comes with age makes it more difficult for kidneys to excrete drugs efficiently. Thus, to prevent overdosing medications, older adults typically require smaller drug dosages than do younger individuals.

Maintaining Homeostasis in Fluid Compartments

One of the major roles of the kidneys is to maintain water balance in the body. Indeed, the amount of water in bodily fluids such as the blood, the interstitial fluid, and the intracellular fluid determines the concentrations of all substances dissolved in those fluid compartments. Therefore, to maintain levels of elements (e.g., sodium, potassium, calcium) and other vital components within the required (i.e., healthy) ranges of concentration, the kidneys must regulate the rate of water removal from the body.

Severe water loss or dehydration can result from excessive sweating or inadequate fluid intake. Prolonged dehydration can cause increased concentration of bodily substances to dangerously high levels, if not for the ability of the kidneys to respond by producing smaller volumes of highly concentrated urine, thus minimizing the amount of water lost. On the other hand, when someone is overhydrated, the kidneys respond by producing large volumes of diluted urine.

The ability of the kidneys to regulate the concentration of bodily substances according to need diminishes with age. For this reason, older adults are more likely to become dehydrated, especially when confusion, immobility, or fear of **urinary incontinence** prevents them from drinking adequate amounts of liquids. Dehydration may be further exacerbated by the overuse of diuretics, which are medications used for congestive heart failure and hypertension to increase urinary output.

Other age-related changes in the genitourinary system pertain to the structures required for urinary collection and removal, that is, the ureters, urinary bladder, and urethra (**FIGURE 7-4**). Normally, urine produced by the kidneys flows through the ureters to be temporarily stored in the urinary bladder. As the bladder fills with urine, its walls stretch out. The expanding bladder compresses the ureteral openings, preventing a reflux of urine in the bladder back into the ureters. In addition, a smooth muscle sphincter at the urethral opening prevents urine in the bladder from entering the urethra. As fluid pressure in the bladder rises, the internal urethral sphincter opens up and urine enters the proximal urethra. However, another more distal and voluntary muscle sphincter located in the pelvic floor must relax before urine can exit through the urethra. Thus, although the release of urine, called micturition, is made possible by an involuntary reflex, we nonetheless have voluntary control over it under normal conditions.

The loss of control of micturition, or urinary incontinence, is not uncommon among older adults. Indeed, 59% of individuals living in institutions may experience this embarrassing and distressing condition (Jerez-Roig, Santos, Souza, Amaral, & Lima, 2016). Postmenopausal women are prone to urinary incontinence because lowered estrogen levels cause the skeletal muscles of the pelvic floor and smooth muscles of the urethra to weaken. Women who have had multiple pregnancies are particularly susceptible to incontinence and may involuntarily urinate whenever intra-abdominal pressure rises, such as when coughing, sneezing, or laughing, a common condition known as stress incontinence.

In older men, urinary incontinence is often caused by an enlarged prostate gland. The prostate gland, which produces some components of semen, is wrapped around the beginning section of the urethra. It enlarges as a man ages, which in turn can partially or completely obstruct the urethra. This enlargement is either benign (noncancerous) or malignant (cancerous) resulting in prostate cancer. In either case, the urinary bladder must contract more forcefully to eliminate urine. Over time, the bladder can become distended (expanded) and its muscular wall can weaken, ultimately leading to incontinence. As a result, distention increases the chance of urinary tract infection and kidney damage due to a buildup of fluid pressure. To avoid such complications, surgery is often

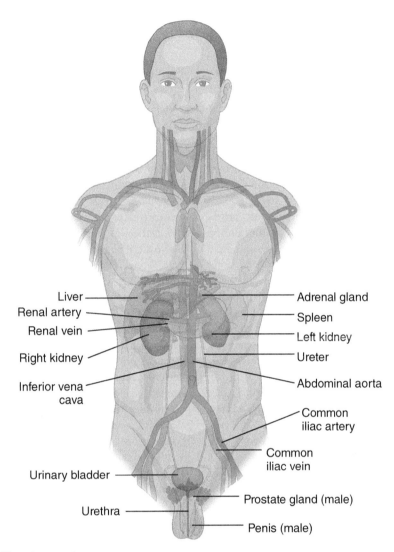

Liver
Renal artery
Renal vein
Right kidney
Inferior vena cava
Adrenal gland
Spleen
Left kidney
Ureter
Abdominal aorta
Common iliac artery
Common iliac vein
Urinary bladder
Urethra
Prostate gland (male)
Penis (male)

FIGURE 7-4 The urinary system.

performed to remove the part of the prostate gland blocking the urethra.

In addition to incontinence, nocturia, or frequent urination at night, is a problem for older adults. Individuals having to get up frequently at night to urinate should be evaluated for urinary problems. Contributing factors are known to include adverse effects of medications and chronic conditions (e.g., cardiac disease, diabetes, obesity, sleep disorders; Burgio et al., 2010).

Musculoskeletal System

Musculoskeletal dysfunction is a major cause of disability in older adults altering mobility, fine motor control, and the mechanics of respiration. It occurs as a result of a decline in muscle mass (**sarcopenia**), which causes overall strength to deteriorate. Other changes that take place within the musculoskeletal system include decreased reflexes, loss of cartilage and thinning of the vertebrae, decreased calcium absorption, joint cartilage deterioration, and deterioration of the extrapyramidal system. As a result of these changes, older adults are more prone to falls (and thus fractures), respiratory infections, and the general physiologic decline that accompanies an increasingly sedentary lifestyle, which can be the result of fear of falling (again).

One of the most significant changes in the aging skeleton is osteoporosis. Defined as a reduction in bone mass and bone density, this condition predisposes an individual to fractures, especially in the vertebrae, proximal femur, and distal radius. In the United States, an estimated 10 million people have osteoporosis and 44 million have lower bone mass thus increasing risk of fractures (National Osteoporosis Foundation, 2015). Osteoporosis is responsible for approximately two million fractures per year, which accounts for approximately $19 billion in healthcare costs annually (National Osteoporosis Foundation, 2015). Osteoporosis-related fractures are predicted to increase to three million fractures by 2025, with annual healthcare costs rising to $25.3 billion (National Osteoporosis Foundation, 2015).

Important risk factors for osteoporosis include estrogen depletion (in postmenopausal women), calcium deficiency (exacerbated in older adults because of decreased intestinal absorption of calcium), decreased bone mass, physical inactivity, testosterone depletion (in males), alcohol dependence, cigarette smoking, and tobacco use (International Osteoporosis Foundation, 2015). The loss of bone mass, combined with fluid loss within the intervertebral discs, and reduction of cartilage causing stiffening of the vertebrae results in decreased height (Vergroesen et al., 2015). Collapse or severe wedging of the vertebrae causes the characteristic appearance of kyphosis, an exaggerated convex curvature of the upper spine leading to a "hunchbacked" posture. A concomitant deformity of the rib cage can alter the normal mechanics of breathing.

Osteoarthritis, also called degenerative joint disease (DJD), is the most common chronic joint condition, affecting more than 30.8 million Americans (Cisternas et al., 2016). Its prevalence increases with age, affecting about 2% of adults under the age of 45, but up to 80% of people older than age 75 (Berger, Hartrick, Edelsber, Sadosky, & Oster, 2011). The disease is so common in older adults that for many years it was believed to be a normal aspect of aging. However, histological studies have revealed clear differences in joint and cartilage structure between persons with osteoarthritis and individuals with healthy joints. Osteoarthritis is marked by ulceration and destruction of joint cartilage, eventually leading to exposure and destruction of the underlying bone. The normal cushioning effect of cartilage is lost, causing bone to rub on bone. As might be expected, weight-bearing joints are the most commonly affected (e.g., knee and hip joints), with obesity being a primary contributing risk factor. Osteoarthritis is the most common cause of the need for total knee and hip replacements, but other frequently used movable joints such as the proximal and distal interphalangeal joints of the fingers are also commonly affected by DJD (Arthritis Foundation, 2017).

Inflamed joints are marked by pain, swelling, and decreased range of motion. Other less common forms of arthritis that occur more frequently with age include rheumatoid arthritis and gout. Rheumatoid arthritis is an autoimmune disease process where antibodies attack healthy joint tissue causing inflamed joints (Arthritis Foundation, 2017). Gout is a condition where uric acid crystals build up in joint spaces as well as in the connective tissue causing pain and swelling in the joint (Arthritis Foundation, 2017). With these disease processes, it is critical to differentiate and diagnose correctly as treatment varies.

Skeletal muscle undergoes changes as well. The number of skeletal muscle fibers (cells) decreases with age, although the rate of decline varies from muscle to muscle (Brunner et al., 2007). For example, little change is noted in the diaphragm, the primary breathing muscle that never relaxes for more than a few seconds, whereas muscles used less frequently such as those of the lower extremities exhibit greater rates of muscle fiber loss. Other changes in skeletal muscle are microscopic, including a decrease in muscle fiber size (atrophy) and capillary supply, an increase in the deposition of lipofuscin and adipose (fat) cells, and a spotty loss of the motor neuron innervation (muscle stretching). Microscopic changes create a gradual decline in muscle strength and efficiency over time, although change may vary among muscle groups. It cannot be overemphasized that regular physical training can improve muscle strength and endurance, even in very old adults (Mian, Baltzopoulos, Minetti, & Narici, 2012). This fact, coupled with the benefits of exercise in maintaining bone strength and cardiovascular fitness, argues for a physician-approved exercise regimen for almost everyone.

Nervous System

The central nervous system (CNS) is the principal regulatory system of the body and is dependent on other systems to function effectively, just as these other systems depend on the CNS for oversight. For example, cerebral blood flow declines with age and can cause complications with the circulatory system, which can lead to blood pressure problems and potentially a stroke (Timiras, 2007b).

The CNS consists of the brain, brain stem, and spinal cord. It regulates and monitors peripheral activities via the cranial nerves, which are the communication networks that form the peripheral nervous system (PNS). The neuron is the basic functional unit of the nervous system, capable of transmitting electrochemical impulses (or messages) over its cell body and cell extensions (the axon and dendrites). Neurons form functional boundaries, or synapse, with other neurons and with target structures such as muscles and glands.

The nervous system of an older adult loses nerve cell mass and shows some brain atrophy. Nerve cells and dendrites decline in number, which slows transformation of information, shortens reaction times, and weakens reflexes. Brain weight is said to decrease with age, but this does not seem to interfere with individual thought processes (Erickson, Gildengers, & Butters, 2013).

The nervous system utilizes several different neurotransmitters to transfer signals from neurons through synapses. Some neurotransmitters are characterized as excitatory (e.g., stimulates signals in neurons) and some are inhibitory (e.g., slows down signals in neurons). The well-characterized neurotransmitters include acetylcholine, dopamine, gamma-aminobutyric acid (GABA), and serotonin. Acetylcholine is mainly responsible for the contraction of skeletal muscles, regulating cardiac rhythms, and encoding new memories. Dopamine is responsible for regulating emotional responses as well as movement. GABA is an inhibitory neurotransmitter that aids in reducing activity with neurons during stressful events. Serotonin is a chemical neurotransmitter that regulates mood, appetite and digestion, memory, and behavior such as depression. Individual neurons may store and release more than one type of neurotransmitter. The smooth functioning of the nervous system relies on balanced activity among the various neurotransmitters. In later life, neurotransmitter dysfunction has likely more to do with a loss of this delicate balance than with an absolute loss of any one particular neurotransmitter. Neurotransmitters play a role in various disease processes such as depression (GABA and serotonin), Parkinson's disease (dopamine), and Alzheimer's disease (serotonin), where there is an increase or decrease responses within the neurons.

Memory

Memory loss associated with dementia is different from age-associated memory loss. Although most mental functions do not decline with age, mild loss of memory and recall for recent events is quite common, whereas long-term memory generally remains intact. Early stages of dementia commonly mimic normal aging in relation to memory loss (Caddell & Clare, 2013). Decline in memory loss varies with each individual as the disease process progresses. For more information on memory, see Chapter 8.

Intelligence

Some aspects of intelligence change with age. Specifically, crystallized intelligence (the ability to apply previously learned concepts to new tasks) can continue to increase as we age, perhaps because a lifetime of experiences and exposures provide a broader knowledge and skill base to apply to problems. In contrast, fluid intelligence (the ability to organize information in new ways and generate novel ideas or hypotheses about phenomena) decreases with age. Older adults frequently score lower on timed tests of cognitive performance because they require more decision-making time and favor a slow, deliberate approach to tasks (Szwabo, 2006). Although components of intelligence change with age, overall intelligence measured by an intelligence quotient (IQ) remains fairly stable throughout adult life in well elders. For more information on intelligence, see Chapter 8.

Motor Function

Gradual impairment of locomotor function (physical activity) greatly contributes to disability in older adults. Chief symptoms include the slowing of fine motor tasks, diminished postural reflexes, and decreased gross motor skills. Fine motor skills consist of movement in the smaller muscle movements such as buttoning clothing and other simple tasks conducted by the hands and fingers. Postural reflexes are related to maintaining posture through balancing during movement. Gross motor skills consist of the action of larger muscles to make

movement, such as walking or lifting something. The confident, long stride of youth morphs into a more hesitant, broad-based gait as people age. Such deficiencies in motor skills are attributed primarily to decreased functioning in the motor control centers of the brain such as the basal nuclei, cerebellum, and cerebral cortex. However, motor control is also influenced by diminished sensory input, including diminished proprioception (sense of body position), vestibular sensation (sense of head movement), and kinesthetic sensation (sense of body movement) as well as the five commonly known senses. These functions decrease slightly in typical aging. Interestingly, many of the characteristics of the stride of a frail elder such as tentative, shuffling steps, and stooped posture are similar to characteristics experienced by individuals with Parkinson's disease. The only difference is that individuals with the disease show more severe impairments. These changes in balance and movement place older adults at risk for falls. Notable is that motoric decline may be more significantly associated with decreased activity level rather than aging per se (Buchman, Boyle, Wilson, Bienias, & Bennett, 2006). For more information about functional performance, see Chapter 9.

Sleep

The aging process brings about notable changes in pattern and quality of sleep. Approximately, half of the older adult population report difficulty with falling or staying asleep (Crowley, 2011). The total amount of time spent sleeping changes little over the course of a lifetime, but as one ages, episodes of sleep (especially deep sleep) are shorter and more frequent. Feeling tired during the day and napping is a constant reminder that quality of sleep is declining. Causes of sleep disturbances experienced by older adults include insomnia, neurological conditions such as restless leg syndrome, breathing disorders, pain, medical diagnosis, and possibly medications (Crowley, 2011).

Disturbances tend to affect the deepest levels of sleep (the most rejuvenating forms of slumber) among older adults. For more information about sleep performance, see Chapter 9.

Endocrine System

Like the nervous system, the endocrine system is a principal regulatory system in the body. It helps control several aspects of physiology, such as body temperature; basal metabolic rate; growth rate; carbohydrate, lipid, and protein metabolism; stress responses; and reproduction. Dysfunction within this system could have widespread ramifications for health and well-being. A few of the many age-related changes to the endocrine system are highlighted in this section.

The endocrine system is a collection of glands spread throughout the body that produce and secrete chemical messengers called hormones into the bloodstream. Hormones have physiologic effects on specific target organs throughout the body. The cells of target organs have protein receptors that bind to a specific hormone. This binding initiates a cascade of metabolic events within the target cell that mediate the hormone's effects. That is, when released in the bloodstream, receptors in the target cell will receive and activate the hormone by binding to the receptor protein of the cell or diffusing hormones through plasma membranes.

There is a hierarchical control of the release of most hormones, which begins in the CNS (**FIGURE 7-5**). Neural activity from higher centers in the CNS is relayed to the **hypothalamus**, a small but extremely important structure that, in turn, controls activity of the pituitary gland by releasing hormones that stimulate or inhibit its hormonal production and release. The pituitary gland, under the influence of these higher control centers, releases a battery of hormones that have selective stimulatory effects on glands such as the thyroid, adrenal gland, and gonads (ovaries and testes). However, it should be emphasized that even the structures at the top of this

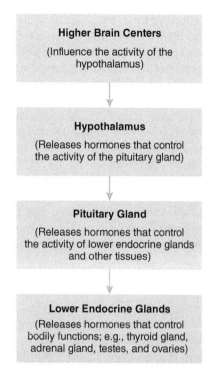

FIGURE 7-5 The hierarchy of control over the endocrine system.

endocrine hierarchy are influenced by "lower" events. For example, the thyroid gland is stimulated to release thyroid hormone in response to the sequential release of thyrotropin-releasing hormone (TRH) from the hypothalamus and thyroid-stimulating hormone (TSH) from the pituitary gland. But, as its level in the blood increases, the thyroid hormone "turns off" further production of TRH and TSH in the higher centers. In effect, the endocrine system operates under a system of checks and balances so that under normal conditions the appropriate levels of all hormones are maintained.

The thyroid hormone released from the thyroid gland has many physiologic effects, such as regulation of tissue growth and development (particularly of the skeletal and nervous systems), regulation of the basal metabolic rate (BMR) by promoting oxygen consumption and heat production in most tissues (i.e., a calorigenic effect), enhancement of the effects of the sympathetic nervous system (or fight-or-flight response), increased mental alertness, and possibly regulation of cholesterol metabolism. As one ages, the level of thyroid hormone secretion declines. However, this decrease is matched by a decline in its rate of removal from the bloodstream so that, overall, levels change little over the years. Furthermore, aging per se does not appreciably affect the increased release of TRH, TSH, or thyroid hormone required in times of greater need. However, several characteristics of older adults such as a reduced metabolic rate, suboptimal regulation of body temperature, decreased effectiveness of the fight-or-flight response, reduced mental alertness, and increased incidence of cholesterol-related atherosclerosis are also symptoms of reduced thyroid activity (hypothyroidism). Thus, it is possible that the age-related changes in thyroid function could result from inadequate responses of target cells to the thyroid hormone rather than from direct damage to the thyroid gland.

The paired adrenal glands consist of an outer layer called the adrenal cortex and an inner section called the adrenal medulla (which, from a functional standpoint, is more aptly considered part of the sympathetic nervous system, and thus is not discussed here). The adrenal cortex produces a number of corticosteroid hormones such as cortisol, which helps the body adapt to stress; aldosterone, which helps the body conserve sodium and thus water; androgens, which have masculinizing effects; and estrogens, which have feminizing effects. The latter two hormones, whose levels decline with age, supplement the action of testosterone and estrogen released from the testes and ovaries, respectively. The loss of estrogen production from postmenopausal ovaries appears to upset the androgen–estrogen balance in favor of androgens produced in the adrenal gland. This might explain the mild masculinization of both sexes.

Aldosterone is a hormone that stimulates the reabsorption of sodium ions from renal tubules back into the bloodstream, which osmotically draws water back in as well, thus increasing blood volume, and therefore regulating blood pressure when needed. Aldosterone levels fall as one ages, impairing an important component of blood pressure regulation. Although the aldosterone mechanism is just one of many ways that increase blood pressure, its loss may bring the body one step closer to disruption of homeostasis.

Cortisol, the quintessential stress hormone, is released into the bloodstream during prolonged periods of physical or psychological stress. It is a catabolic hormone whose function is to mobilize the body's energy reserves, increasing blood levels of glucose, fats, and amino acids during times of illness, physical injury, or emotional distress. In addition, baseline cortisol release (in conjunction with release of the hormone glucagon from the pancreas) in the absence of stress helps prevent blood glucose levels from falling dangerously low during sleep and in between meals. High levels of cortisol can place older adults at higher risk for CVD, diabetes, weight gain, and sleep issues (Manenschijn et al., 2013). Low levels of cortisol place older adults at risk for insomnia, weight loss, inflammation, and various other disease processes (Cohen et al., 2012).

As was true of thyroid hormone, cortisol levels remain normal well into old age, because of a balance between the hormone's decreased production and its decreased excretion. In addition, stress-induced increases in cortisol release are not affected by aging. However, it appears to take older adults longer to reestablish normal blood cortisol levels following a stressful event. A persistently elevated cortisol level may actually have a negative impact on the health of older adults. Some of the well-documented effects of chronically high blood cortisol levels include hyperglycemia (excessively high blood glucose level), hypertension (high blood pressure caused by the aldosterone-like effects of cortisol), and immunosuppression (increased susceptibility to infection and cancer). It is plausible that elevated cortisol responses to stress might also exacerbate concomitant DM, hypertension, and infectious disease in older adults (Manenschijn et al., 2013).

Unlike in the thyroid gland, adrenal cortex, and gonads, hormone release from the endocrine cells of the *pancreas* is not controlled by the hypothalamus and pituitary gland. Instead, the two major hormones produced by the pancreas, *insulin* (which decreases the blood glucose level) and *glucagon* (which increases the blood glucose level), are released at various rates based on blood glucose levels. Deficient insulin action causes diabetes mellitus (DM), a systemic condition marked by hyperglycemia and long-term complications such as diabetic retinopathy, renal failure, nerve damage, atherosclerosis, and gangrenous infection—a peripheral vascular disease often necessitating amputation of all or part of the leg.

Non-insulin-dependent diabetes mellitus (NIDDM) or type II diabetes is a type of diabetes mellitus that increases in frequency with age and accounts for about 90–95% of all cases of diabetes. It appears to be caused by deficient target organ responses to the effects of insulin—the level of insulin itself is actually decrease or increased (Wilcox, 2005).

In 2015, the prevalence of diabetes in the United States was 30.3 million people (9.4% of the total population). Among Americans aged 65+, 12% are both diagnosed and undiagnosed. Diabetes is so prevalent that in 2015, it was the seventh leading cause of death in the United States (American Diabetes Association, 2015). Risk factors that increase complications with diabetes consist of high blood pressure, physical inactivity, high cholesterol, smoking, obesity (Centers for Disease Control and Prevention, 2017a). Individuals diagnosed with diabetes and hospitalized in 2014 were discharged with more serious diagnosis such as strokes, CVD, and lower extremity amputations (Centers for Disease Control and Prevention, 2017b).

Immune System

The ability of our bodies to remain free of infections and cancer requires that the WBCs in our immune system are able to distinguish "self" cells (i.e., our own healthy cells) from "nonself" cells (i.e., invading microorganisms and parasites or structurally altered cancer cells). To appreciate the enormity of this task, think about the thousands of different types of organisms that can invade the body, each of which must be specifically recognized by the immune system as foreign and destroyed without damaging the integrity of our own tissues in the process. Similarly, imagine the countless number of precancerous cell types, each of which may differ from normal cells in only subtle ways that need to be recognized and destroyed by the immune system on a regular basis. Indeed, when it is working well, the immune system is to be marveled at for its accuracy. But, as is true of most systems, age can take its toll. A discussion of the most important aspects of the immune response is followed by a review of those age-related changes in immunity that have implications for health and well-being.

To be immune to an infection implies being protected from it. The development of immunity to a particular infectious organism, however, usually requires initial exposure to it, which in turn often causes mild illness. Nonetheless, on recovery from the sickness, the individual is immune to subsequent infection and illness from that organism; the body has developed an "immunological memory" (sometimes called adaptive immunity) so that it can act more swiftly and effectively the next time it is exposed to the same invader (Iwasaki & Medzhitov, 2010).

The development of this immunological memory occurs by one of two general processes: the humoral- and cell-mediated immune responses. The former process produces proteins called antibodies, which circulate through the blood (or "humor") and specifically bind to the foreign organism, and the latter process activates WBCs called T-lymphocyte "killer cells," which directly destroy the invading organism. Lymphocytes play a critical role in the development of immunity to infections and cancer. Unfortunately, it is these lymphocytes whose function most noticeably diminishes with age. During the aging process, individuals have a slower inflammatory response due to the decline of killer cell function to fight off bacteria or fungal infections (Hazeldine & Lord, 2013).

The age-related decline of immune system functioning gives rise to three general categories of illness that preferentially afflict older adults: infections, cancer, and autoimmune disease. The overall incidence of infectious disease rises in late adulthood. Infectious diseases, particularly prevalent among the older adults, are influenza, pneumonia, tuberculosis, meningitis, and urinary tract infections. Cancer increases in prevalence with age, as well. Leukemia, lung, prostate, breast, stomach, and pancreatic cancer occur most frequently (American Cancer Society, 2017). The increase with age may be caused in part by altered immune surveillance of precancerous and cancer cells that also comes with age. Several components of the immune system play roles in cancer protection, including natural killer cells. Both the number and function of natural killer cells in animal studies decline with age, which may partly explain the rising incidence of cancer in older adults (Hazeldine & Lord, 2013).

Autoimmune diseases are also more common as people age. These diseases are marked by the mistaken immunological destruction of the body's own cells. Prominent examples of autoimmune diseases affecting older adults include rheumatoid arthritis, Hashimoto's thyroiditis, lupus, and chronic hepatitis. In autoimmune diseases, the body loses the ability to distinguish "self" (body's own cells) from "non-self" (foreign cells). Tolerance to our own tissues develops early in life (during development of the immune system), when the thymus gland selects out and eliminates those clones of T cells programmed to destroy our own tissues—a process called clonal deletion. However, with the slow, age-related destruction of the thymus gland, the body may lose the ability to detect and destroy these potentially self-harming T cells. Indeed, with aging comes an increased level of autoantibodies which target the body causing autoimmune disorders (Elkon & Casali, 2009).

Integumentary System

The integumentary system consists of the skin and all of its accessory structures such as hair, nails, sebaceous (oil) glands, and eccrine (sweat) glands. Because skin covers the body, changes in its appearance are the most visibly noticeable of all the changes occurring in the aging body. Skin consists of three major layers: the epidermis, dermis, and subcutaneous layers. This section focuses on changes in the layers due to age and the consequences of those changes for the structure and function of the integumentary system (**FIGURE 7-6**).

The epidermis is a multilayered sheet of cells called keratinocytes, which are named for their production of keratin, a fibrous protein that gives the epidermis strength. Interspersed among the keratinocytes are melanocytes, which produce the melanin pigment that browns the skin, and dendritic (or Langerhans) cells, which prevent the development of skin cancers, ingest microorganisms, and stimulate WBCs called lymphocytes (Romani et al., 2006). The epidermal cells rest on a thin membrane, which separates the epidermis from the underlying dermis. This membrane is normally undulated (wavelike movement), which helps hold the two layers together. However, with age, the membrane flattens out, making the skin more vulnerable to shearing forces, abrasion, and blister formation (**FIGURE 7-7**; Tobin, 2017). Due to everyday wear and tear on the skin, epidermal cells must be continuously replaced with new cells that divide by mitosis in the deepest layers of the skin. The new cells slowly get pushed up through

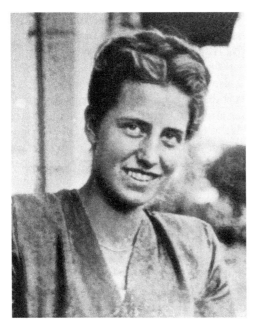
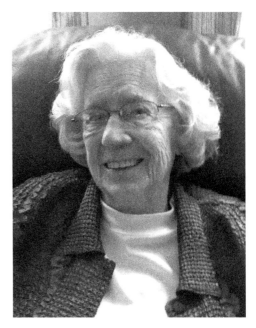

FIGURE 7-6 Change in appearance of skin with aging. The same woman is shown at (left) age 19 and (right) age 95.

the epidermis and ultimately are shed from the skin, a process that takes about 28 days.

Thus, our epidermis is completely replaced every month. The skin regenerations, however, decrease by 50% between ages 30 and 70, which increases the time during which individ-ual epidermal cells are exposed to carcinogens (i.e., cancer-causing agents) such as ultraviolet light from the sun (Tobin, 2017). Furthermore, the number of melanocytes (and therefore the amount of protective melanin pigment) decreases with age, making ultraviolet light

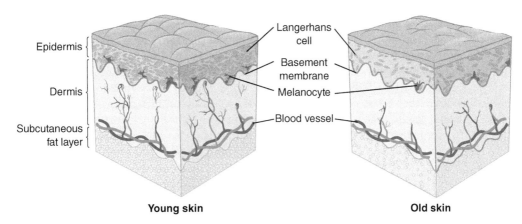

FIGURE 7-7 Changes in the structure of skin with aging. Note that older skin has (1) a thinner epidermis, (2) a flatter basement membrane, (3) fewer melanocytes and Langerhans cells, (4) a diminished dermal blood supply, and (5) a thinner subcutaneous fat layer.

more dangerous. The combination of fewer macrophage-like dendritic cells with fewer melanocytes helps explain why older adults are particularly prone to developing skin cancer.

The dermis is a thick layer of loose connective tissue well supplied with blood vessels, lymphatic vessels, nerves, and accessory organs such as sweat glands, sebaceous glands, and hair follicles. The predominant cells found in the dermis are fibroblasts, mast cells, and macrophages. Fibroblasts produce and release collagen and elastin, which gives skin its strength and elasticity. Mast cells release substances that mediate the inflammatory response following injury to the skin.

The rich supply of blood vessels in the dermis provides oxygen and nutrients as well as an efficient mechanism for regulating body temperature. When the body is overheated, blood flow to the dermis increases so that heat can be radiated through the skin. This mechanism, together with the action of sweat glands, allows for the release of large amounts of heat in a short period of time.

The amount of collagen and elastin in the dermis decreases with age, accounting for the thinning and wrinkling of skin on older adults. Loss of collagen makes the skin more susceptible to wear and tear, while loss of elastin causes skin to lose its resilience. The density of the dermal blood supply also decreases with age, blunting outward signs of inflammation in aging skin. This is noteworthy because older adults often lack some of the early warning signs of tissue injury (e.g., redness and swelling) from, for example, sunburn, bacterial infection, or skin cancer. The diminished blood flow to the dermis also impairs wound healing and, together with poorly functioning sweat glands, makes older adults especially vulnerable to overheating syndromes such as heat stroke.

The dermis also contains sensory receptors, which make the skin sensitive to vibration, pressure, and light touch. The gradual loss of these receptors due to age decreases the tactile sensitivity of the skin and increases the threshold for pain stimuli.

The subcutaneous layer of the skin is largely adipose (i.e., fat) and loose connective tissue. This fat layer provides cushioning and thus protection to the underlying tissues. It also serves to insulate the body from rapid heat loss or gain. With age comes a thinning (or atrophy) of this layer, particularly noticeable in the face and on the backs of the hands. Loss of the fat pad on the sole of the foot can increase trauma when walking and exacerbate other foot conditions.

Chronic overexposure to sunlight is the biggest scourge of aging skin, as it is directly correlated with wrinkling, coarseness, and irregular pigmentation of the skin. It also contributes to the development of lesions such as skin tags (loose fibrous tissue), and seborrheic keratoses (precancerous skin growths). More important, the ultraviolet component of sunlight predisposes people to three major forms of skin cancer: basal cell carcinoma, squamous cell carcinoma, and malignant melanoma.

Basal cell carcinoma (a localized lesion that generally does not spread) is the most common form of skin cancer in the United States (American Cancer Society, 2017), followed by squamous cell carcinoma (a lesion found in the epidermal layer of the skin; American Cancer Society, 2016). An estimated 5.4 million diagnoses for these treatable lesions occur each year (American Cancer Society, 2016). Malignant melanoma is one of the most common cancers diagnosed, making up about 1% of skin cancers and causing the most skin-related cancer deaths (American Cancer Society, 2017). In 2017, approximately 87,110 cases of melanoma were diagnosed (American Cancer Society, 2017). Unlike basal and squamous cell carcinomas, melanoma can **metastasize** (i.e., spread) if not treated. Clearly, sun-induced changes damage and accelerate the aging of skin. Thus, in order for skin to look great at age 80, consistent use of protective hats and clothing and sunscreens with a sun protection factor of 30 (SPF-30) or higher is required (Farberg, Glazer, Rigel, White, & Rigel, 2017).

Whereas excessive exposure to sunlight has adverse effects on the skin, some exposure is still needed to stimulate the production of vitamin D in the skin. Vitamin D is needed to stimulate sufficient absorption of calcium from the small intestines into the bloodstream. Approximately 5–30 minutes of sun exposure to the face, arms, legs, or back without sunscreen between 10 a.m. and 3 p.m. twice a week stimulates sufficient vitamin D production (Holick, 2007). However, UV-B light exposure decreases the farther a person lives from the equator. People living more than 42° of latitude north or south of the equator (e.g., northern states in the United States and Tasmania in the south) do not receive sufficient sunlight during the winter months to produce enough vitamin D (Holick, 2007). Although vitamin D can be stored in adipose tissue, individuals living far from the equator must nonetheless be sure that they have adequate dietary intake of vitamin D during those months. Scientists have not yet determined if there is a minimal amount of sun exposure that stimulates sufficient vitamin D production without increasing the risk of skin cancer (National Institutes of Health Office of Dietary Supplements, 2016).

Hair

Perhaps, the most striking changes to the integumentary system are the graying, thinning, and loss of hair. Hair follicles are specialized epidermal cells packed into cylinders rooted in the dermis. Hair growth is made possible by mitotic cell divisions at the base of the follicle. Hair color is based on the amount of melanin pigment located within the specialized cells. Blonde, brown, and black hairs have successively higher concentrations of melanin. With advancing years, the number of hair follicles decreases. The remaining follicles grow at slower rates than before and contain lower concentrations of melanin, which causes the hair to become thin and white. These changes have more than a cosmetic effect. They also reduce the hair's protective ability to screen the skin on the scalp from the damaging effects of sunlight.

Sensory Organs

Each of the five senses undergo age-related changes which may inhibit functioning.

Vision

Changes in vision are due to alterations to structural components of the visual system (**FIGURE 7-8**). The cornea and the lens are the principal focusing structures in the eye; they refract (or bend) incoming light rays so that images can be brought into focus on the retina in the back of the eye. Both the cornea and lens undergo predictable changes. A gradual loss of cones and rods are associated with the aging process, and with these losses, visual acuity decreases. The lens also becomes thicker and more opaque, resulting in blurry vision, night vision issues, and sensitivity to glare. These changes in the lens can lead to the development of **cataracts**, often described as a cloudy lens.

The lens is controlled by ciliary muscles which regulates curvature. The muscle contracts when focusing on near objects and adjusting to changes in lighting, causing the lens to become rounder (a process called accommodation). When the elasticity of the lens decreases and the muscles stiffen, the ability to focus on near objects becomes difficult (a condition called **presbyopia**). In response, corrective lenses are prescribed to aid in improving visual performance for daily tasks.

Several conditions of the eye are associated with old age. Cataracts are considered the condition most aligned with senescent changes (i.e., if people live long enough, they will get cataracts). Other visual impairments in old age include macular degeneration, glaucoma, and diabetic retinopathy. For more information on vision related to functional performance, see Chapter 9.

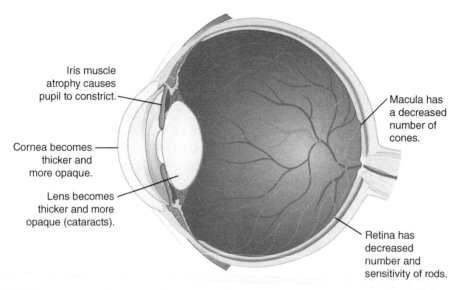

Iris muscle atrophy causes pupil to constrict.

Cornea becomes thicker and more opaque.

Lens becomes thicker and more opaque (cataracts).

Macula has a decreased number of cones.

Retina has decreased number and sensitivity of rods.

FIGURE 7-8 The structure of the eye and its age-related changes.

Hearing

Hearing impairment is the most common condition in older adults. It affects about one-third of adults 65–70 years old and half of adults over 70 years old (National Institute on Deafness and other Communication Disorders, n.d.). Hearing and interpreting sounds is a multistep process that converts sound waves (air pressure) into nerve impulses (**FIGURE 7-9**).

Progressive hearing loss experienced by older adults is called **presbycusis**, the most common form of sensorineural hearing loss. Men are affected more than women, and urban dwellers sustain greater losses than persons living in rural areas (suggesting significant effects from chronic exposure to environmental noise). The type and degree of loss is more severe for high-frequency sounds than for low-frequency sounds. Specifically, the loss of high-frequency hearing makes it more difficult to hear consonants. Vowel sounds, on the other hand, are lower pitched and can still be heard fairly well. This selectivity suggests that the origin of the problem is in the inner ear and/or the nerve pathways to and through the brain.

Overall, changes in hearing can cause speech to sound muffled. To compensate, some people resort to lip reading; this is easier to do for consonant sounds than for vowel sounds. Hearing conversations in a crowded room can also be difficult for older adults, not only because of the presbycusis, but also because older adults have a diminished ability to localize sound and to ignore those sounds that are deemed less important. For more information on hearing related to functional performance, see Chapter 9.

Taste

Sensitivity to taste declines with age, as well. The ability to taste occurs with the activation of taste cells, which are clustered together in taste buds on the tongue and in other regions of the oral cavity. Nerves transmit information about taste to the brain stem and higher centers in the brain.

The perception of taste can be affected by many factors such as medications, an increase or decrease in saliva production, oral disorders, and chronic disease (Boyce & Shone, 2006). Decreased taste has been assumed to be linked to a decrease in taste buds with age, but studies have discovered no such correlation (e.g., Feng, Huang, & Wang, 2014). However, it

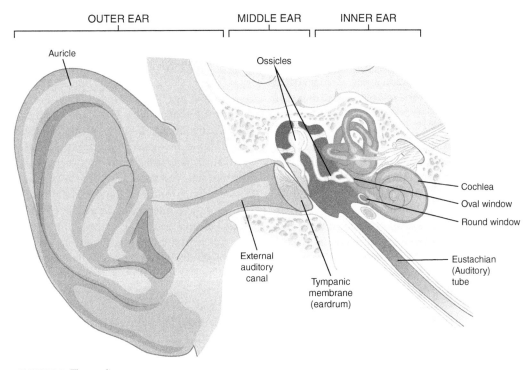

FIGURE 7-9 The auditory system.

is clear that older adults experience difficulty gauging the intensities of tastes and identifying specific tastes, such as salty, when in a mixture of flavors. Taste sensations undergo different changes during the aging process as the ability to distinguish salty foods decreases but tasting sweets is maintained (Methven, Allen, Withers, & Gosney, 2012). For more information on taste related to functional performance and oral health, see Chapters 9 and 12.

Smell

Another functional decline with important ramifications on overall functioning is the ability to smell, a condition known as **hyposmia** (decrease in smell sensation) or anosmia (complete loss of smell sensation). Similar to taste, the degree of impairment varies with the particular odor, and the ability to identify individual odors in a mixture is more difficult with age. Men are more affected by loss of smell than women.

Smell is made possible by the activation of sensory cells in the upper mucosal surface of the nasal cavity, which pass the sensory information through the bony roof into the olfactory bulb at the base of the frontal lobe. From there, the information is processed and relayed through the olfactory tract to higher brain centers. The decline in the numbers of mucosal sensory cells and olfactory bulb relay cells in later life account for the decreased sensitivity to smell.

Because of the crucial role played by smell in distinguishing the tastes of different foods, hyposmia makes foods less desirable, causing a decreased appetite and irregular eating habits. As a result, older adults can experience weight loss and malnutrition (Leopold, Cairns, Holbrook, & Noell, 2016). Moreover, the inability to smell can place an individual at risk by impairing the ability to detect noxious or toxic odors, spoiled food, or a fire within the home (Leopold et al., 2016). For more information on smell related to functional performance and oral health, see Chapters 9 and 12.

Driving becomes a concern as individuals age. As discussed throughout this chapter, various disease processes and bodily changes occur in older adults. For example, impairments in vision, hearing, reaction time (motor function), and strength can create obstacles in maintaining the ability to drive. Although everyone ages differently, driving can be a difficult discussion for older adults and their families as they note declines in themselves, their family member, or friend. Careful review of all aspects of an individual's abilities to drive needs to be taken into consideration when deciding whether an older adult should continue driving. Safety is the top concern for all. For more information on driving, see Chapter 9.

▶ Summary

Clearly our health and well-being depends on the degree to which our organ systems can successfully work together to maintain homeostasis. Diminished function in one system can be minimized by appropriate compensatory mechanisms in other systems. The linear decline that seems to characterize many physiologic functions challenges and impedes the body's ability to maintain

homeostasis over time. The gradual loss of functional reserve capacity in the organ systems is clearly associated with age. A physiologic disturbance that is easily correctable at age 30 may cause significant illness at age 60 or death at age 90. Perhaps, it should not be surprising that the linear decline in physiologic functioning directly correlates with a logarithmic increase in mortality (Timiras, 2007a). Our bodies tend to function well during younger years, despite the accumulation of environmental and genetic insults. However, at some point, we reach a "critical mass" of impairment, a point beyond which our homeostatic correction mechanisms are no longer able to keep pace. When this point is reached, the likelihood of illness, disease, and death rises exponentially (Caughey & Roughead, 2011).

We may take comfort in the fact that much of the illness and suffering that tends to come with old age can be delayed or at least modified by taking proper care of ourselves. The hallmarks of preventive medicine, such as eating right, exercising, and avoiding cigarettes, are most effective when initiated early in life and practiced habitually throughout life. Although there may be wisdom in the adage "live for the day," it is equally wise, from a health perspective, to "live for tomorrow."

🔍 CASE STUDIES

Case 1: Mrs. Winnie Smith is a 74-year-old who participates in a local adult day care program. Mrs. Smith has been participating for the last 2 years at the facility with little decline noted. She is a retired teacher and enjoys talking with other residents that attend activities at the facility. Her intake record lists her medical history as having mild hypertension and osteoporosis. Recently, one of the staff at the facility notices that Mrs. Smith has been having difficulty swallowing during meals and snacks. She mentions it to her manager, who places a call to Mrs. Smith's son, Phillip, her primary caretaker. Phillip asks, "Is this something I should take her to the doctor for, or is it normal?"

1. **What is Mrs. Smith's condition called?**
2. **What could be causing this problem?**
3. **Would you recommend that Phillip take his mother to the doctor? Why or why not?**

Case 2: Mrs. Chewning is a 78-year-old recently admitted to the hospital for respiratory distress. She has a history of asthma, hypertension, and diabetes. Mrs. Chewning lives with her husband in a two story home with little support from other family members. She retired after working 30 years at a paper mill, and smoked a half pack of cigarettes a day for 30 years. She finally quit when her husband was diagnosed with COPD. After numerous tests at the hospital, she was diagnosed with chronic bronchitis.

1. **In addition to her emphysema and chronic bronchitis, what age-related changes are likely affecting Mrs. Chewning's ability to breathe?**
2. **What is causing Mrs. Chewning's difficulty with clearing her lungs?**
3. **Is Mrs. Chewning facing an increased risk of developing pneumonia? Why or why not?**

TEST YOUR KNOWLEDGE

Review Questions

1. Aging results from accumulating damage to cells caused by molecules that have unpaired electrons in their outermost valence shells describes _____.
   a. Rate of living theory
   b. Free radical theory
   c. Somatic mutation theory
   d. Wear-and-tear theory

2. Match the following cardiovascular conditions to the most appropriate descriptions.
   _____ Coronary heart disease
   _____ Peripheral arterial disease
   _____ Congenital heart disease
   _____ Deep Vein Thrombosis
   _____ Cerebrovascular disease
   a. Changes in the blood vessels that supply oxygen to the brain
   b. Narrowing of the blood vessels that supply oxygen rich blood to the heart
   c. Defects of the heart present at birth
   d. The disease process arteries narrow and circulation to extremities is reduced
   e. The formation of blood clots commonly in the leg veins

3. When working with an older adult that has a pathological fracture of the leg, what is most likely the cause of the fracture?
   a. Osteoarthritis
   b. Kyphosis
   c. Osteoporosis
   d. Sarcopenia

4. Visual problems related to the aging process include all the following except:
   a. Presbyopia
   b. Cataracts
   c. Presbycusis
   d. Macular degeneration

5. When blood flow is diminished to the _____, wound healing is impaired.
   a. Connective tissue
   b. Epidermis
   c. Fibroblasts
   d. Dermis

Learning Activities

1. Develop a concept map that highlights concepts of the age-related changes of the organ systems.

2. Identify age-related changes that you see in an individual (family member or client/patient) and describe the impact these changes have had on the individual.

3. Develop a teaching module on health promotion through the life span in order to encourage healthy aging.

4. Discuss the various physiological changes of aging to which smoking contributes.

5. Describe effects of aging with regard to the cardiovascular system.

6. Describe why older adults are more likely to develop acute or chronic renal failure.

7. Discuss factors that decrease mobility in the musculoskeletal system.

8. Explain the controls of the endocrine system and how it relates to aging.

References

Aleksandar, D., Lieske, J., Chakkera, H., Poggio, E., Alexander, M., Singh, P., … Rule, A. (2016). The substantial loss of nephrons in healthy human kidney with aging. *Journal of American Society of Nephrology, 28*, 313–320. doi:10.1681/ASN.2016020154

Alpert, J. (2012). A few unpleasant facts about atherosclerotic arterial disease in the United States and the world. *The American Journal of Medicine, 125*(9), 839–840. doi:10/1016/j.amjmed.2012.04.031

American Cancer Society. (2016). *Key statistics for basal and squamous cell skin cancers.* Retrieved from http://www.cancer.org/cancer/skincancer-basalandsquamouscell/detailedguide/skin-cancer-basal-and-squamous-cell-what-is-basal-and-squamous-cell

American Cancer Society. (2017). *Cancer facts and figures 2017.* Retrieved from https://www.cancer.org/.../cancer.../cancer-facts...statistics/...cancer-facts.../cancer-facts

American Dental Association. (2017). *Oral health topics: Zerostoma.* Retrieved from http://www.ada.org/en/member-center/oral-health-topics/xerostomia

American Diabetes Association. (2014). *The obesity paradox—Does excess weight improve survival.* Retrieved from http://www.diabetes.org/research-and-practice/we-are-research-leaders/recent-advances/archive/the-obesity-paradox.html

American Diabetes Association. (2015). Statistics about diabetes. Retrieved from http://www.diabetes.org/diabetes-basics/statistics/

American Heart Association. (2014). *High fitness level reduces chance of developing hypertension.* Retrieved from http://newsroom.heart.org/news/high-fitness-level-reduces-chance-of-developing-hypertension

American Heart Association. (2016). *Heart attack symptoms.* Retrieved from http://www.heart.org/HEARTORG/Conditions/HeartAttack/WarningSignsofaHeartAttack/Warning-Signs-of-a-Heart-Attack_UCM_002039_Article.jsp#.Wjqr2GefZXp

Arthritis Foundation. (2017). *Osteoarthritis.* Retrieved from http://www.arthritis.org/about-arthritis/types/osteoarthritis/treatment.php

Austad, S., & Fischer, K. (1991). Mammalian aging, metabolism, and ecology: Evidence from the bats and marsupials. *Journal of Gerontology: Biological Sciences, 46*, B47–B53.

Berger A., Hartrick, C., Edelsber, J., Sadosky, A., & Oster, G. (2011). Direct and indirect economic costs among private-sector employees with osteoarthritis. *Journal of Occupational and Environmental Medicine, 53*, 1228–1235. doi:10.1097/JOM.0b013e3182337620

Bernhard, D, Moser, C., Backovic, A., & Wick, G. (2007). Cigarette smoke: An aging accelerator? *Experimental Gerontology, 42*, 160–165. doi:10.1016/j.exger.2006.09.016

Bishop, N., & Guarente, L. (2007) Genetic links between diet and lifespan: Shared mechanisms from yeast to humans. *Nature Reviews Genetics, 8*, 835–844.

Biswas, A., Oh, P. I., Faulkner, G. E., Bajaj, R., R., Silver, M. A., Mitchell, M. S., & Alter, D. A. (2015). Sedentary time and its association with risk for disease incidence, mortality, and hospitalization in adults: A systematic review and meta-analysis. *Annuals of Internal Medicine, 162*, 123–132. doi:10.7326/M14-1651

Boyce, J., & Shone, G. (2006). Effects of ageing on smell and taste. *Postgraduate Medication Journal, 82*(966), 239–241. doi:10.1136/pgmj.2005.039453

Brunk, U., & Terman, A. (2002). Lipofuscin: Mechanisms of age-related accumulation and influence on cell function. *Free Radical Biology and Medicine, 33*, 611–619. doi:10.1016/S0891-5849(02)00959-0

Brunner, F., Schmid, A., Sheikhzadeh, A., Nordin, M., Yoon, J., & Frankel, V. (2007). Effects of aging on type II muscle fibers: A systematic review of the literature. *Journal of Aging and Physical Activity, 15*, 336–348. doi:10.1123/japa.15.3.336

Buchman, A., Boyle, P., Wilson, R., Bienias, J., & Bennett, D. (2006). Physical activity and motor decline in older persons. *Muscle & Nerve, 35*, 354–362. doi:10.1002/mus.20702

Burgio, K., Johnson, T., Goode, P., Markland, A., Richter, H., Roth, D., … Allman, R. (2010). Prevalence and correlates of nocturia in community-dwelling older adults. *Journal of the American Geriatrics Society, 58*(5), 861–866. doi:10.1111/j.1532-5415.2010.02822.x

Burkle, A., Beneke, S., Brabeck, C., Leake, A., Meyer, R., Muiras, M., & Pfeiffer, R. (2002). Poly (ADP-ribose) polymerase-1, DNA repair and mammalian longevity. *Experimental Gerontology, 37*, 1203–1205. doi:10.1016/S0531-5565(02)00144-4

Caddell, L., & Clare, L. (2013). A profile of identity in early-stage dementia and a comparison with healthy older people. *Aging & Mental Health, 17*, 319–327. doi:10.1080/13607863.2012.742489

Caughey, G., & Roughead, E. (2011). Multimorbidity research challenges: Where to go from here? *Journal of Comorbidity, 1*, 8–10.

Centers for Disease Control and Prevention. (2017a). *National Diabetes Statistics Report, 2017*. Retrieved from http://www.diabetes.org/assets/pdfs/basics/cdc-statistics-report-2017.pdf

Centers for Disease Control and Prevention. (2017b). *Heart disease facts*. Retrieved from https://www.cdc.gov/heartdisease/facts.htm

Church, D., & Pryor, W. (1985). Free radical chemistry of cigarette smoke and its toxicological implications. *Environmental Health Perspectives, 64*, 111–126.

Cisternas M., Murphy, L., Sacks, J., Solomon, D., Pasta, D., & Helmick, C. (2016) Alternative methods for defining osteoarthritis and the impact on estimating prevalence in a U.S. population-based survey. *Arthritis Care Research, 68*, 574–580. doi:10.1002/acr.22721

Cohen, S., Janicki-Deverts, D., Doyle, W., Miller, G., Frank, E., Rabin, B., & Turner, R. (2012). Chronic stress, glucocorticoid receptor resistance, inflammation, and disease risk. *Proceedings of the National Academy of Sciences, 109*, 5995–5999. doi:10.1073/pnas.1118355109

Crowley, K. (2011). Sleep and sleep disorders in older adults. *Neuropsychology Review, 21*, 41–53. doi:10.1007/s11065-010-9154-6

de Magalhaes, J. P., Costa, J., & Church, G. M. (2007). An analysis of the relationship between metabolism, developmental schedules, and longevity using phylogenetic independent contrasts. *Journals of Gerontology A, Biological Sciences and Medical Sciences, 62*, 149–160.

Dilova, I., Easlon, E., & Lin, S. (2007). Calorie restriction and the nutrient signaling pathways. *Cellular and Molecular Life Sciences, 64*, 752–767. doi:10.1007/s00018-007-6381-y

Elkon, K., & Casali, P. (2009). Nature and functions of autoantibodies. *Nature Clinical Practice Rheumatology, 4*, 491–498. doi:10.1038/ncprheum0895

Erickson, K., Gildengers, A., & Butters, M. (2013). Physical activity and brain plasticity in late adulthood. *Dialogues in clinical neuroscience, 15*, 99–108.

Ernst, I., Pallauf, K., Bendall, J., Paulsen, L., Nikolai, S., Huebbe, P., … Rimbach, G. (2013). Vitamin E supplementation and lifespan in model organisms. *Ageing Research Reviews, 12*, 365–375. doi:10.1016/j.arr.2012.10.002

Farberg, A., Glazer, A., Rigel, A., White, R., & Rigel, D. (2017). Dermatologists' perceptions, recommendations and use of sunscreen. *Journal of American Medical Association Dermatology, 153*, 99–101. doi:10.1001/JAMADERMATOL.2016.3698

Feng, P., Huang, L., & Wang, H. (2014). Taste bud homeostasis in health, disease and aging. *Chemical Senses, 39*, 3–16. doi:10.1093/chemse/bjt059

Forsberg, V., & Fichtenberg, C. (2013). The prevention and public health fund: A critical investment in our nation's physical and fiscal health: 2012. Retrieved from http://www.apha.org/NR/rdonlyres/D1708E4607E9-43E7-AB99-94A29437E4AF/0/Prev-PubHealth2012_web.pdf

Harman, D. (2002). Aging: A theory based on free radical and radiation chemistry. *Science Science's SAGE KE, 37*. Retrieved from http://sageke.sciencemag.org/cgi/content/abstract/sageke;2002/37/cp14

Hayflick, L. (1997). Myths of aging. *Scientific American, 276*, 110.

Hazeldine, J., & Lord, J. (2013). The impact of ageing on natural killer cell function and potential consequences for health in older adults. *Ageing Research Reviews, 12*, 1069–1078. doi:10.1016/j.arr.2013.04.003

Holick, M. (2007). Vitamin D deficiency. *New England Journal of Medicine, 357*(3), 266–281. doi:10.1056/NEJMra070553

International Osteoporosis Foundation. (2015). Smoking is a real danger to your bone health. Retrieved from https://www.iofbonehealth.org/news/smoking-real-danger-your-bone-health

Iwasaki, A., & Medzhitov, R. (2010). Regulation of adaptive immunity by the innate immune system. *Science, 327*(5963), 291–295. doi:10.1126/science.1183021

Janoff, A. (1985). Elastase in tissue injury. *Annual Review of Medicine, 36*, 207–216.

Jerez-Roig, J., Santos, M., Souza, D., Amaral, F., & Lima, K. (2016). Prevalence of urinary incontinence and associated factors in nursing home residents. *Neurourology Urodynamics, 35*, 102–107. doi:10.1002/nau.22675

Jin, K. (2010). Modern biological theories of aging. *Aging and Disease, 35*, 102–107. doi:10.1002/nau.22675

Johnson, D., & Sandmire, D. (2004). *Medical tests that can save your life: 21 tests your doctor won't order unless you know to ask* (p. 68). New York: Rodale and St. Martin's Press.

Kirkwood, T. (2002). Evolution of ageing. *Mechanisms of Ageing and Development, 123,* 737–745. doi:10.1016 /S0047-6374(01)00419-5

Leibovitz, B., & Siegel, B. (1980). Aspects of free radical reactions in biological systems: Aging. *Journal of Gerontology, 35,* 45–56.

Leopold, D., Cairns, C., Holbrook, E., & Noell, C. (2016). Disorders of taste and smell. *Medscape.* Retrieved from: http://emedicine.medscape.com /article/861242-overview

Li, L., Chan, L., Shen, J., Zhang, L., Wu, W., Wang, L., … Cho, C. (2014). Cigarette smoking and gastro-intestinal diseases: The causal relationship and underlying molecular mechanisms (Review). *International Journal of Molecular Medicine.* doi: 10.3892 /ijmm.2014.1786

Lippman, R. (1981). The prolongation of life: A comparison of antioxidants and geroprotectors versus superoxide in human mitochondria. *Journal of Gerontology, 36,* 550–557. doi:10.1093/geronj/36.5.550

Manenschijn, L., Schaap, L., van Schoor, M., van der Pas, S., Peeters, M., Lips, P., …. van Rossum, E. (2013). High long-term cortisol levels, measured in scalp hair, are associated with a history of cardiovascular disease. *The Journal of Clinical Endocrinology & Metabolism, 98,* 2078–2083. doi:10.1210/jc.2012.3663

Methven, L., Allen, V., Withers, C., & Gosney, M. (2012). Aging and taste. *Proceedings of the Nutrition Society, 71,* 556–565. doi:10.1017/S0029665112000742

Mian, O., Baltzopoulos, V., Minetti, A., & Narici, M. (2012). The impact of physical training on locomotor function in older people. *Sports Medicine, 37,* 683–701.

Nakayama, T., Kodama, M., & Nagata, C. (1984). Generation of hydrogen peroxide and superoxide anion radical from cigarette smoke. *Gann Japanese Journal of Cancer Research, 75,* 95–98. doi:10.20772/ cancersci1959.75.2_95

National Center for Health Statistics. (2017). *Health, United States, 2016: With chartbook on long-term trends in health.* Hyattsville, MD: Centers for Disease Control and Prevention. Retrieved from https://www.cdc.gov/nchs /data/hus/hus16.pdf

National Council on Aging. (2017). *Top 10 chronic conditions in adults 65+ and what you can do to prevent or manage them.* Retrieved from https://www.ncoa.org /blog/10-common-chronic-diseases-prevention-tips/

National Institute on Deafness and other Communication Disorders. (n.d.). *Hearing loss and older adults.* Retrieved from https://www.nidcd.nih.gov/health /hearing-loss-older-adults

National Institutes of Health Office of Dietary Supplements. (2016). Vitamin D fact sheet for health professionals. Retrieved from https://ods.od.nih.gov /factsheets/VitaminD-HealthProfessional/

National Osteoporosis Foundation. (2015). *Osteoporosis facts and statistics.* Retrieved from https://cdn .nof.org/wp-content/uploads/2015/12/Osteoporosis -Fast-Facts.pdf

National Osteoporosis Foundation. (2017). *Preventing fractures.* Retrieved from https://www.nof.org /preventing-fractures/exercise-to-stay-healthy/

Nohl, H., & Hegner, D. (1978). Do mitochondria produce oxygen radicals in vivo? *European Journal of Biochemistry, 82,* 563–567. doi:10.1111/j.1432-1033.1978 .tb12051.x

Ogburn, C., Carlberg, K., Ottinger, M., Holmes, D., Martin, G., & Austad, S. (2001). Exceptional cellular resistance to oxidative damage in long-lived birds requires active gene expression. *Journals of Gerontology. Series A, Biological Sciences and Medical Sciences, 56,* B468–B474. doi:10.1093/gerona/56.11.B468

Pryor, W. (1978). The formation of free radicals and the consequences of their reactions in vivo. *Photochemistry and Photobiology, 28,* 787. doi:10.1111/j.1751-1097.1978.tb07020.x

Pryor, W., Dooley, M., & Church, D. (1986). The inactivation of alpha-1-proteinase inhibitor by gas-phase cigarette smoke: Protection by antioxidants and reducing species. *Biochemical and Biophysical Research Communications, 122,* 676–681. doi:10.1016/S0006-291X(84)80086-8

Ravussin, E., Redman, L., Rochon, J., Das, S., Fontana, L., Kraus, W., … Kritchevsky, S. (2015). A 2-year randomized controlled trial of human caloric restriction: Feasibility and effects on predictors of health span and longevity. *The Journals of Gerontology: Series A, 70*(9), 1097–1104. https://doi.org/10.1093/gerona/glv057

Romani, N., Ebner, S., Trip, C., Flacher, V., Koch, F., & Stoitzner, P. (2006). Epidermal Langerhans cells—changing views on their function in vivo. *Immunology Letters, 106,* 119–125. doi:10.1016/j .imlet.2006.05.010

Ruuskanen, J., & Ruoppila, I. (1995). Physical activity and psychological well-being among people aged 65 to 84 years. *Age and Ageing, 24,* 292–296.

Schneider, E. L. (1985). Aging research: Challenge of the twenty-first century. In A. D. Woodhead, A.D. Blackett, & A. Hollaender (Eds.), *Molecular biology of aging* (pp. 1–11). New York: Plenum Press.

Siegel, R., DeSantis, C., & Jemal, A. (2014). Colorectal cancer statistic, 2014. *CA: A Cancer Journal for Clinicians, 64,* 104–117. doi:10.3322/caac.21220

Siegel, R., Miller, K., Fedewa, S., Ahnen, D., Meester, R., Barzi, A., & Jemal, A. (2017). Colorectal cancer statistics, 2017. *CA: A Cancer Journal for Clinicians, 67*, 177–193. doi:10.3322/caac.21395

Sohal, R. (1981). *Age pigments*. Amsterdam: Elsevier/North-Holland.

Spence, J. (2007). Stroke prevention in the high-risk patient. *Expert Opinion on Pharmacotherapy, 8*, 1851–1859. doi:10.1517/14656566.8.12.1851

Szwabo, P. A. (2006). Psychological aspects of aging. In J. Pathy, A. J. Sinclair, & J. E. Morley (Eds.), *Principles and practice of geriatric medicine* (4th ed.) (pp. 53–57). Chichester, England: Jon Wiley and Sons.

Timiras, P. S. (1994). Aging of respiration: Erythrocytes, and the hematopoietic system. In P. S. Timiras (Ed.), *Physiological basis of aging and geriatrics* (2nd ed.) (p. 226). Boca Raton, FL: CRC Press.

Timiras, P. S. (2007a). Aging and disease. *Physiological basis of aging and geriatrics* (4th ed.). Boca Raton, FL: CRC Press.

Timiras, P. S. (2007b). The nervous system: Structural, biochemical, metabolic, and circulatory changes. *Physiological basis of aging and geriatrics* (4th ed.). Boca Raton, FL: CRC Press.

Tobin, D. (2017). Introduction to skin aging. *Journal of Tissue Viability, 26*, 37–46. doi:10.1016/j.jtv.2016.03.002

Tosato, M., Zamboni, V., & Ferrini, A. (2007). The aging process and potential interventions to extend life expectancy. *Clinical Interventions in Aging, 2*, 401–412.

Travis, J., & Salvesen, J. (1983). Human plasma protease inhibitors. *Annual Review of Biochemistry, 52*, 655–709. doi:10.1146/annurev.bi.52.070183.003255

Tufts University (2012). *My plate for older adults*. Retrieved from http://www.nutrition.tufts.edu/myplate

Vergroesen, P., Kingma, I., Emanuel, K., Hoogendoorn, R., Welting, T., Van Royen, B., … Smit, T. (2015). Mechanics and biology in intervertebral disc degeneration: A vicious circle. *Osteoarthritis and Cartilage, 23*, 1057–1070. doi:10.1016/j.joca.2015.03.028

Weinert, B., & Timiras, P. (2003). Invited review: Theories of aging. *Journal of Applied Physiology, 95*, 1706–1716. doi:10.1152/japplphysiol.00288.2003

Weiss, S. (1989). Tissue destruction by neutrophils. *New England Journal of Medicine, 320*, 365–376. doi:10.1056/NEJM198902093200606

Wilcox, G. (2005). Insulin and insulin resistance. *The Clinical Biochemist Reviews, 26*, 19–39.

World Health Organization. (2017a). *Cardiovascular diseases fact sheet*. Retrieved from http://www.who.int/mediacentre/factsheets/fs317/en/

World Health Organization. (2017b). *Chronic respiratory diseases fact sheet*. Retrieved from http://www.who.int/respiratory/en/

World Health Organization. (2017c). *Chronic obstructive pulmonary disease (COPD) fact sheet*. Retrieved from http://www.who.int/mediacentre/factsheets/fs315/en/

Yamada, Y., Kemnitz, J., Weindruch, R., Anderson, R., Schoeller, D., & Colman, R. (2017). Caloric restriction and healthy life span: Frail phenotype of nonhuman primates in the Wisconsin National Primate Research Center Caloric Restriction Study. *The Journals of Gerontology: Series A*. doi:10.1093/gerona/glx059

Ziegler, D., Wiley, C., & Velarde, M. (2015). Mitochondrial effectors of cellular senescence: Beyond the free radical theory of aging. *Aging Cell, 14*, 1–7. doi:10.1111/acel.12287

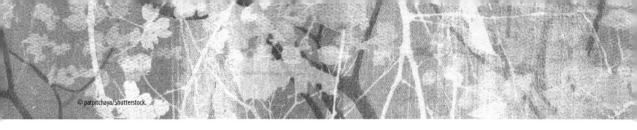
© patpitchaya/Shutterstock.

CHAPTER 8

Cognitive and Psychological Changes Related to Aging

Regula H. Robnett, PhD, OTR/L, FAOTA

CHAPTER OUTLINE

BEHAVIORAL OBJECTIVES

Upon completion of this chapter, the reader will be able to:

1. Describe the three basic factors that cause cognitive impairments in older adults.
2. Describe how general (fluid and crystallized intelligence) and specific aspects of cognition (attention, orientation, memory, executive functioning, and learning) may change with the aging process.
3. Describe compensatory measures which could be used for persons with decreased or changed cognitive functioning.
4. List possible screens for use in detecting cognitive changes.
5. Compare and contrast signs of delirium, depression, and dementia.
6. Complete a screen for depression to make a referral for assistance.
7. List general guidelines for working with people to enhance performance of people with all cognitive levels.
8. Understand conditions that may mimic dementia (but that are often reversible).
9. Differentiate aspects of personality that may tend to change over time from those that may not, based on current research.
10. Discuss aspects of behavioral change as these relate to older adults.
11. Describe factors believed to contribute to a positive quality of life in older people.

KEY TERMS

Age-associated memory
 impairment
Alzheimer's disease
Attention
Behavior change
Bereavement
Cerebrovascular accident
Cognition
Crystallized intelligence
Delirium
Dementia

Depression
Episodic memory
Failure to thrive
Fluid intelligence
Gerotranscendence
Heterogeneous
Learned helplessness
Long-term memory
Malnutrition
Mild cognitive impairment
Motivational interviewing

Orientation
Personality
Primary memory
Procedural memory
Prospective memory
Quality of life
Semantic memory
Short-term memory
Stereotypes
Suicide
Working memory

▶ Introduction

Stereotypes of aging depict a steady decline of **cognition** and most aspects of functioning despite evidence to the contrary, which shows that the majority of older adults are able to care for themselves and maintain independence throughout most of their lives. The Centers for Disease Control and Prevention (CDC), estimated using 2003–2007 data that 82% of older people, 85+, do not have any limitations in activities of daily living (ADLs) and 65% have no limitations in the more complex instrumental activities of daily living (IADLs; Arias, 2007). In other words, the majority of older adults perform adequately to be able to complete both basic and complex daily tasks.

Human cognition develops into adulthood, including the finishing touches on the frontal lobes, which take place in one's mid-20s. Development is described as a positive emerging state, whereas aging, especially in the latter third of expected life span, is viewed as a negative state moving toward the inevitable end of life (Perlmutter, 1988). Yet, individuals who are aging typically do continue to develop throughout life. They learn new skills and continue to make lifestyle changes as life progresses. Well older adults (the vast majority of all of a certain age) work at making life better (and in the process often enjoy it more).

This chapter explores cognitive human development throughout life in the typical aging process and juxtaposes it with the atypical or abnormal aging process with which it is sometimes confused. Although change is a constant in our lives and the aging process inevitably entails change, not all age-related changes are negative. Adverse physical and cognitive changes that do occur in older people may be the result of disease, the accumulation of poor lifestyle choices, the simple aging process alone (including genetics), the expectations of decline, disuse of the body and/or the mind or a combination of these detrimental forces.

When working with older people, knowledge of the typical aging processes needs to be combined with an understanding of the predominance of individuality within this **heterogeneous** population. This chapter demonstrates that chronological age is less a predictor of cognitive performance than other factors such as subjective and objective health status, personality traits, and lifestyle choices, especially as the impact of these choices accumulates over decades of time.

▶ Typical Cognitive Changes of Aging

The simple statement "cognition decreases with age," although widely accepted as hardcore fact, needs to be fully scrutinized because the state of cognition in old age offers many facets of complexity. Due to the cumulative nature of lifestyle choices (e.g., in the realms of nutrition, self-neglect, or substance use or abuse) and the impact that disabling conditions have on some older people but not others, elders tend to become more and more different from one another over time—they become a more heterogeneous group (in this case, in the realm of cognitive performance), even though people beyond a certain age (60–65+) tend to be lumped together into a single group, as if they were all alike. Older people, who have inherited the right genes, have made positive choices throughout life (e.g., regarding exercise, nutrition, and managing stress), and perhaps have garnered a little luck, may be able to function as well as or even better than when they were young, whereas others succumb to disease or functional decline. As caring healthcare professionals, we can help older people enhance their brain health, live their best possible lives, and promote the compression of the period of infirmity that may occur at the end of our natural life span (an idea first proposed by Fries, 2005).

Typical Cognition Overview

Cognition or mental processing includes thinking, learning, and memory. Our brains control everything we do intentionally and much of our unintentional behavior as well. A well-known assertion posits that cognition declines with older age. This premise is only partially true. Zec (1995) asserted that cognitive impairments in older adults primarily are caused by three factors: disease, disuse, and the aging process. Although we cannot turn back the clock and will inevitably get older, we do have some control over the other two factors.

Several disease processes affect cognition, and these conditions are more common in older people than in persons who are younger. Diseases related to cognitive performance include the minor and major neurocognitive disorders (NCDs; American Psychiatric Association [APA], 2013), as well as diabetes mellitus and cardiac and cerebrovascular diseases. Individuals with an interest in the problems of aging related to specific diseases are encouraged to investigate these. This chapter focuses on a few of the most prevalent thieves of brain power or cognition.

We explore optimal brain functioning later in the chapter. First, we delve into various aspects of cognition and how each aspect may change over the course of typical (i.e., healthy) aging. To simplify the presentation, cognition is divided into several sections. However, keep in mind that these cognitive components rarely have distinct boundaries. Given the vast interconnecting networks in the brain, each aspect of cognition influences other aspects as we perform our daily tasks. In fact, it is rare for a person to have an isolated cognitive deficit because the human brain tends to work in a highly integrated fashion.

Crystallized and Fluid Intelligence

Crystallized intelligence tends to remain strong in persons who are aging typically, and includes skills such as language comprehension, educational qualifications, and life and occupational skills. Baltes (1993) compared this type of intelligence with what we term wisdom or "an expert knowledge system in the fundamental pragmatics of life permitting excellent judgment and advice involving important and uncertain matters of life." Older adults, especially persons known as wise elders, may become more skilled at making decisions, perhaps because of their ability to take life's ambiguities into account (Kim & Hasher, 2005).

In spite of a strong perceived link between wisdom and aging, even highly intellectual older individuals in our society are not necessarily revered for their level of understanding of life's complexities. In certain cultures, especially ancient ones, elders are expected to share historical stories, songs, rituals, and traditions with future generations. They are considered the sages of the community. Yet, in our modern Western society, older people rarely have such important societal roles, and therefore the wisdom of aging may often get lost in favor of individualism, materialism, and the quest for eternal youth, thus losing "our sense of history and real wisdom" (do Rozario, 1998, p. 121). Schachter-Shalomi and Miller (1995), in their book *From Ageing to Sageing: A Profound New Vision of Growing Older*, put forward the idea that older people who work on expanding their consciousness and promoting their spiritual growth may demonstrate wisdom in their actions, thereby attaining "the crowning achievement of life" (p. 17). Rather than lamenting a "silver tsunami" of older adults that will burden the system, we could view this turn of events as a "silver windfall." Perspectives and words do matter (as discussed later).

Fluid intelligence includes the speed and accuracy of information processing such as item discrimination, comparison, and categorization. This type of intelligence has been deemed to be largely evolutionarily and genetically based. Baltes (1993), who has extensively researched the two types of intelligences in young and old subjects, found that only fluid intelligence showed a significant decline in older adults. Even though many studies (e.g., Schaie, Willis, Knight, Levy & Park, 2016) have shown that the human mind has limitations in old age, Baltes, Staudinger, Maercker, and Smith (1995) pointed out that these limits often are not apparent because the brain is generally not used to its full potential. They drew an interesting analogy of a young and an old person strolling together. Walking together works out well until the couple approaches a hill; the steeper the hill, the more difficult it may be for the older person to keep up. This is true not only with physical performance, but also with mental functioning, especially processing speed.

Processing Speed

A decrease in speed of processing information has been demonstrated consistently as people age (Anderson & Craik, 2017). Lichtenberger and Kaufman (2012) proposed that this decrease in processing speed is strongly associated with higher level cognitive performance. However, cognitive processing may be heavily influenced by physical motor speed, which also declines with age (Ebaid, Crewther, MacCalman, Brown, & Crewther, 2017). Impaired sensory functioning (e.g., vision and/or hearing) may also contribute to slowed processing speed (perhaps due to associated neuronal atrophy due to disuse; Valentijn et al., 2005).

Learning in Late Life

The ability to learn new information can change as people age (**FIGURE 8-1**). Certainly, the old (and we hope outdated) adage that "an old dog can't learn new tricks" does not apply to older people who are aging well. Ongoing research, such as that cited by Curlik and Shors (2013) and taking place at the Salk Institute, has unequivocally demonstrated that even older (middle aged and beyond) brain cells can regenerate, an exciting finding with huge implications for stroke rehabilitation and medicine in general. Older individuals indeed may need more practice sessions than their younger counterparts to

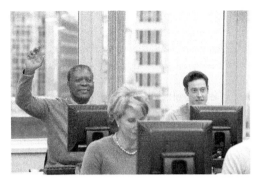

FIGURE 8-1 The saying "old dogs can't learn new tricks" could not be farther from the truth. While older adults may take longer to learn and need accommodations, they are still capable of absorbing new information.
© Noel Hendrickson/Digital Vision/Getty Images

master a task. They also may need to have the instructions presented in a variety of ways (e.g., verbal, written, or demonstrated) and perhaps geared toward their sensory capacities (e.g., larger print) before learning can occur.

Specific Factors Impacting Cognition

A number of factors, both intrinsic and extrinsic to each individual, affect each person's cognitive performance. Innate intelligence provides the foundation of capacity for learning throughout life. For example, we cannot expect someone of average intelligence to perform at the capacity of a neurobiologist. Along with individual innate intelligence, the constructs of neuroplasticity and cognitive reserve are pertinent for the topic of aging and cognition.

Neuroplasticity

Within the relatively small mass of each brain (approximately three pounds for the average adult) lies a marvelously plastic organism that stays dynamic throughout a healthy life. While it is generally easier to learn and adapt at younger ages (e.g., think of the speed with which a toddler or young child learns a new language compared to an adult), nonetheless older brains can adapt and engage in new learning. An example is that of London taxi drivers who have larger hippocampi (where topographical orientation processing takes place) compared to others (even bus drivers; Maguire, Woolett, & Spiers, 2006). A study by Draganski et al. (2004) found that the experience of learning to juggle in adults (although these subjects were young adults) increased gray matter mass of part of the brain within one week of intense training, a finding that replicated earlier animal studies. This outcome is suggestive of the plasticity of mature human brains, although additional research is needed to substantiate these results. Motor skill training may not only enhance learning, but it could also change the brain for improved learning in the future.

Cognitive Reserve

Cognitive reserve is akin to a cognitive savings bank. People who have substantial reserves may be able to use readily available or alternative brain structures to maximize performance on cognitive tasks even after sustaining a brain injury or illness. An example is effectively using environmental cues to compensate for decreased memory performance (perhaps in people who are in an early stage of dementia). Technology (e.g., a computer or smart phone) may be helpful to maintain outward cognitive performance (e.g., quickly looking at the phone to determine what day it is). A high level of cognitive reserve is often associated with higher levels of education, higher IQ levels, and more engagement in complex occupations and leisure pursuits (Stern, 2009). Cognitive reserve levels clarify (at least to a degree) why essentially similar structural brain damage in two people (e.g., through a stroke) may have very different behavioral manifestations or outcomes of impairment. Interestingly, in various studies, up to 25% of people who tested "normal" on cognitive testing were found to have brain pathology commensurate with AD (Stern, 2009).

What has not been determined is if people can build up their cognitive reserve (as they can build muscle strength). As noted earlier and explored later in the chapter, engaging in learning (education), and complex leisure, and work occupations (Reed et al., 2011) as well as positive and frequent social interactions may promote cognitive reserve and forestall at least the cognitive and behavioral manifestations of brain disease (Stern, 2006; Xu, Yu, Tan, & Tan, 2015).

Sensory Issues (Sensory Decline and Sensory Deprivation)

Yet another associated factor of cognitive performance to be considered is that of sensory functioning, such as hearing and vision. Decreases in these two realms can impact cognition indirectly, in that due to not hearing/seeing properly the person may demonstrate behaviors that outwardly give the appearance that they have decreased cognition. People who cannot hear may tend to miss important incoming auditory input and subsequently not answer questions correctly. Similarly, people who cannot see to read important information cannot properly process that information. Not surprisingly, decreased visual skills (after correction) and presbycusis (decreased hearing associated with older age) are both associated with lower cognitive performance (Li & Lindenberger, 2002; Anderson & Craik, 2017). Hearing and vision performance (after correction) accounted for more of the variability in cognitive outcome scores (including memory) than speed of processing or age in older adults (Herzog & Wallace, 1997; Humes, Busey, Craig, & Kewley-Port, 2013). Taking into account sensory awareness levels of older clients is important, especially since there are compensatory measures that can be taken to enhance sensory input and level of understanding. At the very least, someone who needs corrective lenses and/or hearing aids should be encouraged to wear them, and the practitioner should ensure that they are in working order.

Environmental Factors

The context or environment surrounding the older adult can either support or hinder the learning process and overall cognitive performance. Keeping in mind that most people have individual preferences regarding favored environmental features, a few examples of how this influence might work are:

- *Physical environment*: For example, in a noisy environment many find it difficult to concentrate.
- *Internal environment*: Discomfort of any kind (including pain, feeling tired, chilled, too hot) is not conducive to optimal performance.
- *Cultural aspects of the tasks to be completed*: For example, if the person has always deferred money management to a partner, the task may not be meaningful for the person currently.
- *Social context*: Some would rather work alone, while others prefer group work.

In a therapeutic situation, any cognitive task to be completed needs to be presented at the level of "the just-right challenge" (Rebeiro & Polgar, 1999). Tasks that are too easy will quickly lead to boredom, while tasks that are too challenging will lead to frustration on the part of the participant. Neither facilitates optimal cognitive performance.

A complication related to mostly social context that has received little attention as a problem of aging is **learned helplessness**, which is a condition that develops when living beings "learn that their responses are independent of desired outcomes" (Fincham & Cain, 1986). Consequently, they adapt to the situation by losing the initiative to respond to stimulation. For example, in experiments when dogs learned that they could not control the onset of electric shocks, they eventually gave up and became helpless and apathetic. Similar results can occur in human beings, especially older people who may receive (too much) care from others. If you hear a caregiver say "Let me

do that for you," this instance may offer an opportunity for a discussion. Every time we do something for older adults that they could do for themselves, we may be making it more difficult for them to do this task next time when no one is there to help.

Stereotypes of Aging

Most of the stereotypes about aging adults seem to be negative (e.g., frail, forgetful, and slow to move and learn). Bennett and Gaines (2010) reported that while aging stereotypes can be both negative and positive, in the United States, they tend to be negative. Levy (2003, 2009), through her noteworthy research on the stereotypes associated with aging, concluded that aging stereotypes may become self-fulfilling prophecies that actually may lead to poorer performance among elders. As people age, these stereotypes become ingrained in a people's self-perceptions, with a resulting negative impact on their cognitive and functional well-being. Levy (2009) suggested that we need to restructure our deep-seated views by focusing more on the positive changes of aging. Ageist stereotypes can send messages that result in giving in to the "infirmities of old age," while more effective, positive messages (such as "it's never too late to learn" or "entering old age is like opening a door to an exciting new chapter of life") could potentially boost elders' self-esteem, and subsequently their ability to remain vital and productive (Joslyn, 2016). By busting negative stereotypes (which is more difficult than it sounds) and increasing societal awareness of the strong impact of these negative preconceived notions (i.e., not the actual changes of aging, but merely the expectations), we can begin to promote a more realistic image of aging, improved health, and better performance over time (Levy, 2003, 2009).

Many of the common stereotypes of aging (e.g., decreased cognition, less capable) do, however, relate to **dementia**, which does become more prevalent as people age, but recall that dementia is not considered part of the typical or normal aging process. Dementia is an umbrella term that describes a number of conditions that cause a decline in cognition and everyday performance (as described later).

An important factor contributing to the current less than rosy outlook on the aging process is the prospect of cognitive decline, which many consider scarier than death. Garrett (2013) describes a new societal phenomenon titled "dementiaphobia"; he describes this fear as "the idea of losing who we are—becoming a stranger in an unfamiliar body" (Garrett, 2013, para 8). According to a study out of the United Kingdom, one-third of individuals aged 55+ feared getting dementia more than they feared cancer, stroke, or heart disease (Davies, 2015).

Specific Aspects of Cognition

This section explores different aspects of cognition. While these are divided into separate sections for ease of understanding, the way the brain works, one rarely has deficits in one lone area. The brain contains so many interconnections that distinct divisions of cognitive skills are difficult to discern.

Orientation

People who are aging are generally alert and oriented; they fully understand who they are, where they are, and the aspects of time and the situation they are in. This is referred to as being A&O × 3 (alert and oriented times three; **TABLE 8-1**). However, the flexible schedule of retirement rather than a specific disease process may contribute more to apparent disorientation to exact date or time of day. Therefore, when determining someone's level of **orientation**, allow a little flexibility and consider the potential influence of an unstructured lifestyle. A psychiatric disturbance is indicated when a person is alert but is not oriented at least to him- or herself. This is not a common occurrence among older people,

except for persons with severe dementia, another psychiatric or severe illness, or perhaps due to the influence of strong medication.

Attention

Attention, that is the ability to focus or concentrate on an activity, does not seem to be affected specifically by age (Zec, 1995; Blazer, Yaffe, & Liverman, 2015). Simple, overlearned, or automatic tasks do not usually become more difficult for older people. However, in a study by Tun and Wingfield (1995), older adults were questioned about their perceptions of their own abilities to complete 16 different divided attention tasks, such as walking and talking or driving and planning a schedule. The researchers found that the older participants did not perceive routine tasks and tasks involving speech processing to become more challenging over time. However, relative to younger adults, the older respondents reported increasing difficulties with simultaneous dual task performance on more demanding tasks. Therefore, it may be more difficult for older adults to divide their attention between two activities (e.g., driving and talking; cooking multiple courses at the same time). Older people do tend to have more difficulty with divided attention tasks, especially when the two or more tasks are complex (e.g., not automatic or overlearned; Verhaeghen & Cerella, 2002; Blazer et al., 2015).

Memory

Memory is not a simple, unidimensional construct; it is rather multifactorial and extremely complex, and much about the workings of memory in the brain remain elusive (Park & Festini, 2017). Although overall memory performance does decline with age, it is worth taking the time to qualify exactly what the construct of memory entails and to explore the different aspects of memory in relation to the aging process. Recalling something out of the blue is a more complex task and is affected to a greater extent by age rather than recognition (e.g., in which one is given hints about the potential answer with multiple-choice answers). Recognition, which is simpler, may be retained to a high level throughout life (Parkin & Java, 2000). Other basic memory tasks such as those requiring procedural memory (i.e., remembering motor patterns), basic cognitive skills (mathematics or use of vocabulary), or remembering facts that have been well-learned are usually preserved throughout the typical aging process.

Several types of memory are described here, although these categories are not an exhaustive list. The description includes how

TABLE 8-1 The Cognitive Changes of Aging

Aspect of Cognition	Changes of Aging	Helpful Hints
Orientation: Knowing who one is (A&O × 1), where one is (A&O × 2), and having an adequate understanding of time (A&O × 3). A&O × 4 includes an awareness of the situation as well (not always addressed).	In the typical aging process, orientation usually remains largely intact as part of crystallized intelligence.[a] As a result of retirement lifestyle, older adults may have more difficulty remembering the exact date or day.	Use calendars and orient person as needed. If the older adult is in an institution, be sure that the orienting information available is up-to-date. Questioning people about orienting information may be intimidating.
Attention: Includes being able to *sustain* attention or focus on one task, *alternating* attention between two tasks, or *dividing* attention between two or more tasks (simultaneously). *Selective* attention involves paying attention to relevant stimuli while filtering out unimportant information.	Ability to sustain attention without distractions remains intact, although older adults tend to be less able to ignore distractions during tasks. Alternating and divided attention tasks may become more difficult, for example, in the task of driving which often involves competing tasks.[b]	Limit distractions, especially when older adults are completing difficult or multifaceted tasks (such as driving) or when they are attending to crucial information (such as healthcare instructions). For example, if a stroke patient is concentrating on walking, the practitioner should not be chattering about unimportant topics.
Memory: The different types of memory are defined in the chapter.	A decline in memory acuity at older ages has been corroborated by a number of cross-sectional studies.[c] Older people tend to have more difficulty with short-term memory and remembering more recent episodes in their lives, including the source of information or the episode (e.g., where it happened, whom they already told).[d]	Repetition is important for learning. Writing lists and other memory aids can be helpful (and may be used more spontaneously by older adults than by younger people).[e] Do not assume just by telling someone something that he or she will remember and incorporate what you said.

(continues)

TABLE 8-1 The Cognitive Changes of Aging (*continued*)

Aspect of Cognition	Changes of Aging	Helpful Hints
Crystallized intelligence: Includes both basic knowledge and skills that accumulate over the course of life.	In typical aging, this remains intact or may even continue to improve, especially for overlearned material and individual work-related skills. Reading comprehension, for example, is maintained well into old age, at least until age 75+.[f] Elders may see themselves as more open-minded or able to better differentiate shades of gray (i.e., ambiguity) rather than just accepting concrete black/white "facts" as truth.[g]	This is related to the construct known as wisdom, and may relate to the ninth stage of life, "gerotranscendence."[h] Well older adults have the potential to gain wisdom through life experience and an increased universal knowledge base.[i] Plenty of older people have wisdom to share with others, including their healthcare providers.
Fluid intelligence: "The ability to find meaning in confusion and solve new problems . . . [and] to draw inferences and understand the relationships of various concepts, independent of acquired knowledge."[j] Includes executive skills that involve judgment, awareness, and problem-solving.	Declines with age to a degree; older adults tend to have more difficulty with more complex, multiple-step tasks.[k] Because fluid intelligence is crucial to the learning process,[l] learning may slow down but does not stop in typical older adults.	Fluid intelligence may improve through practice of tasks requiring executive skills such as self-monitoring performance, completing two tasks simultaneously, and inhibiting irrelevant stimulation. However, this finding was based on respondents mostly in their 20s.[l] Challenging (not frustrating) tasks, especially novel ones, may be crucial for maintaining brain health.[m]
Executive skills: High-level cognitive skills (including working memory). These skills enable us to plan, organize, socialize, and complete complex management and interaction tasks.	Declines do occur even in typical agers, who tend to begin using both sides of the prefrontal cortex for working memory tasks (younger adults activate only one side). Decreased selective attention also interferes with working memory performance.[n]	The typical older adult naturally compensates by recruiting more neuronal resources. Maximize performance by limiting distractions and keeping the number of prompts (or steps) within the person's ability (usually four or fewer).[n]

Data from Robnett (2008). [a] Perlmutter (1988). [b] Tun & Wingfield (1995); West (1999); Verhaeghen & Cerella (2002); Anderson & Craik (2017). [c] Colsher & Wallace (1991); Hultsch, Hertzog, Small, McDonald-Miszcak, & Dixon (1991); Wheeler (2000). [d] Hoyer & Verhaeghen (2006). [e] Baddeley (1995). [f] Schaie (1996); Salthouse (1999). [g] Erikson, Erikson, & Kivnick (1994). [h] Erikson & Erikson (1998). [i] Ardelt (2008). [j] Cavanaugh & Blanchard-Fields (2006). [k] West (1999). [l] Jaeggi, Buschkuehl, Jonides, & Perrig (2008). [m] Nussbaum (2003). [n] Kirova et al. (2015).

aging is associated with the type of memory in question.

The following types of memory are based on *temporal* aspects of remembering:

- **Primary memory** has limited capacity and is based on incoming information that is either used or generally forgotten in a matter of seconds. Immediate recall of seven digits (plus or minus two) has been considered normal for adults since Miller's research in the 1950s (reported in Connor, 2001). Primary memory does not seem to be affected by aging. This type of memory involves sustained attention and is of extremely short duration (unless rehearsal takes place).

- **Short-term memory** involves remembering information for a short duration of time. For example, normal short-term memory is being able to recall a few items or a seven-digit number (e.g., a telephone number) for a few minutes. Older people do show a decline in this type of memory, and the decline is more pronounced as the information increases in length or complexity (Lustig & Lin, 2016).

- **Working memory** refers to being able to actively use or manipulate information from the brain's short-term storage base during a task. For example, it involves recalling a telephone number while dialing the number or retaining the steps of a new recipe while cooking (both without looking up the information mid-task). Age-related deficits such as decreases in reading and listening span (especially for later use) have been consistently significant (Lustig & Lin, 2016).

- **Prospective memory** enables a person to remember to do something in the future (e.g., appointments, taking medications, chores). With regard to aging, older people may be better at spontaneously compensating for losses in prospective memory as they learn to adjust to memory losses gradually over the course of their lives. In naturalistic or real-life settings, older people often outperform their younger counterparts by incorporating compensatory strategies such as list making (Baddeley, 1995; Hoyer & Verhaeghen, 2006).

- **Long-term memory** is permanent or long-term storage, for example, autobiographical information, early life experiences, or repetitive information that involves "more durable encoding and storage systems" (Birren & Schroots, 2006, p. 479). For well-learned knowledge, this type of memory is the least affected by age, although it may be difficult to conjure up the exact facts when needed.

Rather than being time based, the following types of memory are based on the *type* of information to be encoded:

- **Episodic memory** is oriented toward the past and is what most people think of when they think of the global term *memory*. Specifically, this type of declarative or conscious memory involves remembering episodes or experiences in our lives (e.g., what we ate for lunch, our last birthday party; Bäckman, Small, & Wahlin, 2001). Episodic memory can be either short term, such as remembering that you just turned on the stove, or long term, such as remembering the very first day of school. Episodic memory is particularly vulnerable to the effects of aging (Lustig & Lin, 2016; Hultsch, Hertzog, Dixon, & Small, 1998). When tested simultaneously, younger age groups tend to consistently outperform older age groups on tests of episodic memory (Hultsch et al., 1998; Lustig & Lin, 2016).

An analogy involving episodic memory could be to imagine a bucket (i.e., the brain) that holds just a certain amount of information. As time goes by, the bucket gets filled with memories of life's events. As the bucket nears capacity, more of the potential memories get sloshed out; only memories that are intensely emotional go deep enough to be retained. Although this analogy has limited direct scientific evidence, it can explain the increased difficulty of retaining additional information as we grow older. Another explanation for declining episodic memory skills could be disuse caused by less environmental stimulation (e.g., less contact with the outside world) or decreased sensory awareness (e.g., due to poor vision or hearing).

- **Semantic memory** involves a cumulative knowledge base about the world in general (e.g., language, including the meaning of words and the relationship of words, mathematical facts, symbols and formulas, vocational information learned during one's career, and recall of history and worldly facts). This "internal lexicon" is the buildup of information over the course of one's life (as part of crystallized intelligence; Bäckman, Small, & Wahlin, 2001, p. 352). Semantic memory changes over time portray a complex picture, in that elders have more word-finding problems (such as the tip of the tongue phenomenon), but overall vocabulary may even improve well into old age (Schaie, 1996; Lustig & Lin, 2016).
- **Procedural memory** is performance based, for example, remembering how to ride a bicycle or the motoric steps to completing a recipe or self-care task. Because repetitive daily tasks are often overlearned and have become automatic, this type of memory is often maintained into old age. This situation can be problematic at times, for example, when a person with dementia remembers the procedure of driving (e.g., inserting the key, turning the wheel, pushing on the gas pedal) but has forgotten how to manage the more cognitively challenging aspects of driving (e.g., problem-solving in the midst of traffic or navigating in unfamiliar territory).

A great number of studies have been completed on memory and aging (for a review, see Park & Festini, 2017). What is noteworthy is that not all types of memory are affected equally by the typical aging process. Critical differences have been found among the various memory systems. Research in the areas of episodic versus semantic memory has often demonstrated a more severe decline in memory for events (episodic memory tasks), whereas verbal memory such as vocabulary (semantic memory) tends to be better preserved (Lustig & Lin, 2016). Working memory tends to decline more sharply with age than immediate or primary memory. Most older people were able to retain 7-digit telephone numbers just as well as their younger counterparts (primary memory task); however, when a 10-digit number was used (e.g., a long-distance telephone number), the older participants did not perform as well (Gorman & Campbell, 1995). Studies showing a memory decline with age have often involved more complicated tasks (Hoyer & Verhaeghen, 2006; Lustig & Lin, 2016). Older people also seem to have more difficulty ignoring distractions during working memory tasks and less able to ignore irrelevant thoughts (Gazzaley, Sheridan, & Cooney, 2007).

Memory remediation may be possible for persons who are motivated to improve their ability to remember. Results have been mixed, with some promising results, but also with an ongoing concern about the limited transfer of the training to improvement in everyday working memory performance (Hering, Meuleman, Bürki, Borella, & Kliegel, 2017). Compensating for rather than trying to improve decreased memory performance seems to work best for most older people who have learned to adapt over the ensuing years. Sometimes, elders get creative in their approaches to remind themselves. For example, putting car keys in the refrigerator as a reminder to bring lunch with them or keeping pill boxes at the dinner table as a reminder to take medications can both be helpful.

Compensatory techniques and adaptive measures may be necessary to maintain **quality of life** if memory skills start to diminish significantly. Self-help books and online sites on this subject are readily available. For the healthcare professional, several tactics may be helpful when working with people who tend to be forgetful:

- Make the material to be learned interesting (applicable to the client's life). A story, an anecdote, or even a song may more easily catch and hold the client's attention.
- Use multimodal sensory input (e.g., let the person hear and read the information, as well as use other senses to interact with the material as appropriate).
- Use repetition, but not to the point of boredom or becoming condescending as if you are testing the person.
- Use cuing, but only as needed.
- Have clients engage with or manipulate the information if possible (e.g., have them write out or input their own schedule rather than just giving them the printed schedule; **FIGURE 8-2**).
- Information that the older person perceives to be important will more likely be able to find a place in memory storage banks.
- Immediately following an instruction session, have clients paraphrase what was just conveyed or show-and-tell the information they just encountered; both can be effective techniques to enhance the learning process, applying the adage that one learns best by teaching. (This is an example of the teach-back method found in Chapter 5.)

Following are some tips to stimulate remembering (or compensate for decreased memory), adapted from Straus (2009). These may be especially helpful for older adults.

- *Concentrate on paying attention*: Usually, information can be remembered only if it is initially acknowledged.
- *Repeat what you want to remember by rehearsing aloud*: If you meet someone and want to remember his or her name, be sure to use the name in conversation within the next few minutes.
- *Make lists or use a date book (or electronic calendar)*: Write down what you want to

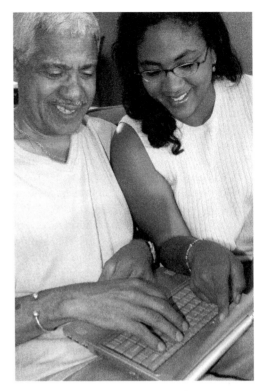

FIGURE 8-2 Allowing clients to actively engage in obtaining information helps them remember the material.
© Rob Marmion/Shutterstock

remember (but then practice remembering without the list).

- *Establish habits*: For example, always put your keys on the hook beside the door or always park in the same section of the parking lot at the mall. Healthy habits of proper diet and exercise may improve not only physical, but also cognitive well-being.
- *Relax*: Relaxation may allow the mind to clear itself of problems, which may help to facilitate recall, whereas excess stress can hinder learning and memory.
- *Use self- and environmental cues*: These cues can be invaluable for stimulating memory skills. Environmental cues can be as diverse as signs, kitchen timers, or alarm clocks. Use memory triggers; look over photos to provoke memories.

Problems with memory tasks, both subjective (memory complaints) and objective (actual losses), are probably the most commonly acknowledged types of age-related cognitive decline (Bartrés-Faz et al., 2001). Displaying poor memory skills does not mean that a person has dementia. Mild forgetfulness, when it is an isolated cognitive impairment, is not cause for alarm and is often experienced by the young and old alike. Decreased memory or **age-associated memory impairment (AAMI)** is widespread and simply refers to memory skills that are lower than average. AAMI by itself may not be a serious condition. Everyone forgets names, events, and factual information. A red flag needs to be raised when one forgets crucial well-learned information (e.g., how to toast bread or how to find a familiar destination).

Executive Functioning

An agreed-upon definition of executive functioning (EF), aptly named to describe the cognitive skills used by an executive on the job, is not readily found. The "central executives," also known as the frontal lobes of the brain, are key to performance of EF skills in the realms of working memory, mental flexibility, and self-control. Another way of viewing EF is thinking of the frontal lobes as our own personal "air traffic controllers" (Center for the Developing Child, Harvard University, 2011). A person who has deficits in EF has difficulty organizing multistep tasks such as managing multiple medications or financial management. This person may also have difficulty appropriately responding to social cues and demonstrates decreases in working memory, which is the ability to remember information for retrieval as needed during a task (e.g., the steps to a recipe while cooking or the cards already played during a poker game).

Typically, older adults show some declines in EF. Specifically, working memory has been studied extensively. Kirova, Bays, and Lagalwar (2015) reviewed the expected changes that occur in working memory in older adults.

Aspects that change with age include cognition-related biological markers such as decreased brain mass and less dense neuronal connections (Drag & Bieliauskas, 2009). As these changes occur in the frontal lobes, high-level cognitive skills such as EF decreases, and thus, younger adults consistently outperform older adults in working memory tasks such as recalling if a stimulus was just presented previously (Kirova et al., 2015). Older adults also tend to be more susceptible to extraneous interference (e.g., distractions while completing EF tasks; Kirova et al., 2015). These findings support the recommendation to provide a supportive environment to enhance learning and memory tasks for older adults.

Table 8-1 gives a brief overview of the cognitive changes associated with advanced age, along with a few helpful hints for healthcare providers. An important caveat is that these hints just barely scratch the surface. People need individualized (client centered) care, and these shared ideas may occasionally help. A few areas are described in more depth in the body of the text.

Assessing Cognition

One way to assess whether older people have memory or other cognitive impairments is simply to ask them. Yet, it is worth noting that people, in general, do not have a good sense of how well they can remember, and individuals with other cognitive deficits (e.g., decreased insight or judgment) likely have difficulty accurately judging their own cognitive performance. Although self-assessments are efficient and easy to use, their usefulness can be questionable. Studies have shown that the correlation, between level of memory impairment per self-report and level determined through objective neuropsychological testing, has typically been insignificant or low (Ryan, 1992; Craik, Anderson, Kerr, & Li, 1995; Knight & Godfrey, 1995). Keep in mind that we would be asking persons with less than perfect memory capabilities to make judgments about their

TABLE 8-2 Tools for Assessing Cognition

Name	Tool Description
Montreal Cognition Assessment (MoCA)[a]	Rapid screening tool for mild cognitive dysfunction that assesses attention and concentration, executive functions, memory, language, visuoconstructional skills, conceptual thinking, calculations, and orientation.
The Saint Louis University Mental Status (SLUMS)[b]	Examination with oral and written content for detecting mild cognitive impairment (MCI) and dementia; results can help a doctor determine if further diagnostics are needed if dementia is suspected. May be more sensitive than the MMSE for persons who are mildly impaired.[b]
Mini Mental State Exam (MMSE) and the MMSE-2™[c]	Common screening tool that provides quantitative measure of cognitive impairment. New version takes about 15 minutes to administer and is available in 10 languages.
Short Blessed Test (SBT)[d]	Sensitive screen used to detect early cognitive changes associated with AD. Low score is best.
Executive Function Performance Test (EFPT)[e]	Top-down functional assessment that assesses executive cognitive function in an environmental context by way of task initiation, execution, and completion.
Confusion Assessment Method (CAM)[f]	A quick screen designed specifically for clinicians to quickly assess for delirium signs and symptoms; this is especially important because delirium is so common in older hospitalized patients.

Data from [a]Nasreddine et al. (2005); http://www.mocatest.org. [b]Tariq, Tumosa, Chibnall, Perry & Morley, (2006); http://medschool.slu.edu/agingsuccessfully/pdfsurveys/slumsexam_05.pdf. [c]MMSE: Folstein, Folstein, & McHugh (1975); MMSE-2™: Folstein & Folstein (2010); www.parinc.com/WebUploads/samplerpts/Fact%20Sheet%20MMSE-2.pdf. [d]Katzman et al. (1983); http://alzheimer.wustl.edu/adrc2/Images/SBT.pdf. [e]Baum et al. (2008); www.ot.wustl.edu/about/resources/executive-function-performance-test-efpt-308. [f]Waszynski (2003).

ability to *remember*. A more objective measure would be observing functional memory performance, for example, noting whether the person has left the stove on, has had difficulty with medication routines, or has forgotten important appointments.

Healthcare practitioners can use various screens to assess cognitive function. The results can influence the approach to rehabilitation, offer suggestions for caregivers, and provide strategies for managing cognitive decline. A team approach seems to work best for assessing and treating cognitive perfor-

mance deficits. **TABLE 8-2** provides a brief list of a few available tools.

Interventions to Maintain or Enhance Cognition in Older Adults

Performing well in the realm of cognitive performance (e.g., being able to effectively think, remember, and problem solve) is often viewed as a key aspect of "successful aging." The best time to start exercising our brain muscles was yesterday or as young as possible (and on a consistent basis), but as a common adage also implies "it may never be too late for improvements." This brain health program is offered in the chapter section on typical cognitive changes, because prevention of significant decline may be easier to accomplish than returning to high performance levels once the roll downhill has begun.

The PACES Program to Promote Brain Health

The PACES program or the idea of "Running through the PACES" can guide older adults (or adults of any age) to promote cognitive performance through the use of evidence-based guidelines to promote positive outcomes in the realms of thinking, memory, and learning. Most of the suggestions work best for typically aging elders, while individuals with **mild cognitive impairments** (MCIs) often see positive results as well. Once cognitive disease has rooted itself, the most successful approach often seems to be compensatory (discussed later). While the PACES program offers something for everyone, it should be individualized to meet the desires or the goals of the elder. The program is not prescriptive, but rather simply offers suggestions, based on substantial evidence, for factors to consider.

PACES stands for:

- Purpose
- Activity
- Cognitive (pursuits)
- Emotional (health)
- Socialization (and sleep; Robnett, 2015)

Purpose

The "P" in PACES stands for *purpose* or finding meaning in life. This purpose may be work related or it can be whatever the individual decides. Pasricha (2016), in his book on quality of life, describes the distinctive nature of the Okinawans who live on islands in the East

China Sea. They tend to be healthy, long-lived people (seven years longer on average than persons in the United States), but the most important feature of these islanders is their lack of a word for "retirement." They simply do not retire from life, because they have "ikigai" roughly translated as the reason to get up in the morning or the drive to live a full life. In a longitudinal study that spanned seven years done in Japan, people who had "ikigai" were reported to have higher levels of education, lower levels of stress, and were more likely to still be engaged in productive activity at the end of the study. They were also more likely to be alive (95% were still living versus 83% of people without "ikigai"; Pasricha, 2016). In a recent longitudinal study using the national Health and Retirement Study data, Kim, Kawachi, Chen, and Kubzansky, (2017) examine the correlation of a sense of purpose in life with physical measures (grip strength and walking speed). They found that a higher purpose in life was associated with better physical outcomes, and they reminded us that having a sense of purpose is a modifiable factor—one that can be cultivated and encouraged, perhaps to improve the overall aging process. In a related study, Allen, Mejía, and Hooker (2015) examined the sense of usefulness among a group of older adults and found that a high degree of self-perceived usefulness (or productivity), which could be viewed as a sense of purpose, was associated with lower levels of neuroticism. By potentially reshaping older adults' self-perceptions of cognitive functioning and making these more positive (e.g., increasing their personal sense of purpose), more "optimal aging" could result (Allen et al., 2015).

Active/Activity

The "A" in the PACES program relates to activity or remaining active and engaged in life. These meaningful activities, in which we engage, are our daily occupations. The recommendation to remain active may be self-evident, but when working with elders, too often one hears the excuse "I'm too old for that." If the person wants to do the activity, and it can be adapted if necessary, age should not be a factor. While television offers wonderful opportunities for learning and entertainment, too much of this passive activity can be detrimental to health. Depp, Schkade, Thompson, and Jeste (2010), by assessing a national sample of adults, found that older adults watched television on average three times more than younger adults, and this level of increased television time was statistically associated with lower levels of life satisfaction. The bottom line is: "Our bodies are meant to move. And our brains are built for novelty" (Span, 2010), or as we shared recently in a wellness group for older adults: "If you can, do it; if not, do something else." Movement and regular physical activity are important to brain health. In a recent article on training the brain, Curlik and Shors (2013), using rodent models, found evidence that aerobic physical exercise helped the brain produce new neurons in the hippocampus, while mental stimulation such as learning novel tasks helped those new neurons survive. Making and sustaining positive lifestyle choices can have lasting effects well into old age. While the relationship between exercise and cognitive performance in older adults has not been firmly established, the results of study reviews are suggestive of a significant positive relationship (Young, Angevaren, Rusted, & Tabet, 2015). However, the answer to whether healthier people just exercise more or if exercise truly is brain protective remains to be determined (Gow et al., 2012). Nonetheless, evidence touting the benefits of exercise is easy to find. The Mayo Clinic (2016) cites several advantages of exercising regularly, including better health (also brain health), weight control, better mood, better sleep patterns, more energy, and potentially, improved socialization and an improved sex life. An additional note: exercise does not need to take place at a gym. Sports (e.g., pickle ball, golf, swimming) and activities such as dancing (Burzynska, Finc, Taylor, Knecht, & Kramer, 2017) may even serve to enhance interest levels over rote

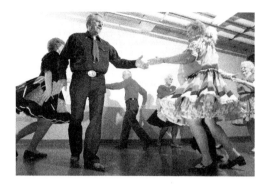

FIGURE 8-3 Exercise has many health benefits, from weight control to improved socialization and an improved sex life. One form of exercise, dancing, has even been found to help slow the decline of brain white matter.

© Jupiter Images/Stockbyte/ Getty Images

exercise. A research team out of Colorado State University, (Burzynska et al., 2017) found that dancing seemed to stave off decline of brain white matter, which is the brain's wiring system, associated with speed of processing and memory performance (**FIGURE 8-3**). Perhaps, we all need to dance into old age.

Cognitive Pursuits

The "C" in the PACES program refers to cognitive stimulation, which is as important as physical stimulation. The Curlik and Shors (2013) study reminds us that while physical activity is important, mental stimulation may be just as important in assuring that the newly formed neurons survive.

People often believe that simply engaging in thinking tasks such as crossword puzzles or card games will be enough to promote optimal cognitive functioning. However, once these activities are no longer challenging, they may not offer enough cognitive stimulation. Neuropsychologist Dr. Paul Nussbaum, in his book *Brain Health and Wellness*, promotes the idea that learning should no longer be considered merely a means to an end, but that learning *for its own sake* is crucial to maintaining health, both physical and cognitive (Nussbaum, 2003).

He expands on the adage "use it or lose it" by suggesting that we not only need to use our brains to maintain brain health, but also that we must stimulate our brains to a greater degree by engaging in activities both "novel and complex" on a regular basis (Nussbaum, 2003, p. 162). By consistently challenging our brains to learn new skills and/or gain new knowledge, we can enhance our thinking processes and potentially create brain reserve throughout life. Additionally, energizing environments that engage participants in socialization, physical activity, and mental stimulation help to create a healthy brain, one that may be able to delay the onset of disease (Nussbaum, 2003, 2011; Metz & Robnett, 2011).

One recommendation heard often and worth repeating is that of the idea of lifelong learning. We are never too old to learn something new, as long as the new learning is enticing to the learner. Myriad opportunities for lifelong learning exist online, through volunteer and work experiences, as well as through programs such as senior colleges and community learning opportunities. The Road Scholar provides one such opportunity; the program is a not-for-profit global program that provides learning experiences for older adults on various topics, including history, culture, nature, music, outdoor activities, crafts, and study cruises (see www.roadscholar.org/). Participants explore their interests with leading scholars and researchers share their knowledge while sailing on cruises, walking through national parks, and visiting culturally diverse areas. Our world is resplendent with opportunities for exploration; no one of any age has an excuse to not participate in some sort of learning pursuit. (See "Learning Activity.")

A relatively recent development has been the proliferation of computer-based programs for cognitive training. Through a meta-analysis on cognitive training and mental stimulation, Kelly et al. (2014) found that the training programs often did improve certain aspects of cognition such as recall, working memory, and processing speed. However,

transfer of learning, that is, to improve performance on everyday cognitive tasks, was not always evident, although offering 10 or more sessions and long-term follow-up sessions did help. Kelly et al. (2014) could not find enough rigorous studies in this realm to make definitive recommendations. More research on cognitive training is clearly needed.

Emotional Health

The next letter in PACES is "E," which involves taking care of emotional health to promote cognitive health in old age. People may not have control over the traumatic events that occur in our lives, but experts such as psychologist Viktor Frankl (1963) would maintain that we do have control over our attitude or how we *respond* to these life events. Our emotional health can influence our brain health in different ways. Older adults tend to focus more on the positive (known as the "positivity effect") and seek to avoid negative people and interactions (Reed, Chan, & Mikels, 2014; Scheibe & Carstensen, 2010). However, due to this tendency toward optimism and the avoidance of negativity, they may also be more trusting and less able to detect scams or other deceitful actions (Scheibe & Carstensen, 2010). Even positivity, when it is oversubscribed, has its downside.

On the other hand, **depression**, especially when it progresses beyond an occasional blue mood, is a common disorder among all ages of adults (described in more depth in the atypical changes of aging section). Clinical depression tends to have a negative impact on general health as well as cognition. Jeste, Depp, and Vahia (2010) found that individuals with the diagnosis of clinical depression tended to exercise less, become more socially isolated, and neglect eating in a healthy manner. The good news of this scenario though is that clinical depression is one of the disorders that often can be treated successfully. Both antidepressant medications and psychotherapy have been shown to be helpful (CDC, 2016a, 2016b;

Chand & Grossberg, 2013). At least one study demonstrated that Cognitive Behavioral Therapy, which helps people reframe their negative or destructive thoughts, when adapted to the needs of older adults, worked even better than the standard treatment (Chand & Grossberg, 2013). Emotionally well older adults tend to be more active, more optimistic, more resilient, more socially engaged, and tend to self-perceive themselves as being healthier (Jeste et al., 2010). There is also evidence that persons who consider themselves optimistic, tend to live happier and longer lives (Adams, 2016; DuBois et al., 2015).

Socialization and Sleep

The last aspect of the PACES program is "S," which stands for two important brain health promoters: social engagement and sleep. Human beings are not meant to be isolated on their own; they are social beings who do best when they have at least one significant and positive relationship with another being (Cacioppo & Cacioppo, 2014). Currently, one may wonder if online communication and relationships are just as effective as face-to-face encounters. A study conducted by Teo et al. (2015), using the Health and Retirement national data set, found that face-to-face social interactions were preferred, and such encounters with family and friends played a significant role in preventing depression. Physical limitations, sensory declines, and the loss of colleagues may make getting out socially more problematic. Healthcare professionals can assist their older clients to engage with others in a positive way rather than isolating themselves. Isolation is associated with loneliness, depression, poor health behaviors, and overall worse health with shorter life spans. Furthermore, executive cognitive skills are more likely to be impaired in individuals who are lonely and isolated (Cacioppo & Cacioppo, 2014). Assistance for these elders may involve finding and procuring resources (such as transportation or available local activities) or

helping to set and meet personal goals related to socialization.

Historically, sleep has been viewed as a passive activity and sometimes considered a waste of potentially productive time. More recently, the evidence has been mounting that adequate sleep is essential for day-to-day functioning, and even more important for optimal cognitive functioning (Malhotra & Desai, 2010). Wilckens, Woo, Kirk, Erickson, and Wheeler (2014) found that consistent and healthy sleep patterns are needed for the consolidation of memories (thus improving memory performance). Adequate sleep promotes brain plasticity and helps the person work through any unresolved daily conflicts. People who do not get adequate sleep do not learn as well or as quickly, and demonstrate decreased insight, memory, and problem-solving (Malhotra & Desai, 2010). Sleep disorders and interventions are considered in more depth in Chapter 9. The relationship between positive sleep patterns and better cognitive performance has been established. However, the causal relationship remains muddled: One wonders, do conditions associated with cognitive impairment (such as dementia) cause one to have poor sleep patterns or do poor sleep patterns contribute to the disease process? (Mattis & Sehgal, 2016).

Following the PACES program does not guarantee high levels of cognitive performance, but the evidence provided does suggest that consistently following a general holistic health plan can certainly decrease the risk factor for the onset of atypical cognitive decline.

▶ Atypical Changes of Cognitive Aging

Mild cognitive changes that do not significantly interfere with daily performance are typical as people age. Speed of processing does tend to decline, along with decreases in certain aspects of memory (such as working, short-term, or episodic memory), and more difficulty tends to occur tuning out distractions, especially during more complex tasks. These changes are normal. Atypical changes of cognitive performance start at one end of a continuum with mild changes (minor neurocognitive disorders), which only subtly impact daily performance and end for some at the other end of the continuum with major debilitating cognitive changes (major neurocognitive disorders). Dementia or major neurocognitive disorders are not a normal or typical part of the aging process. (The continuum, related specifically to cognition, is explored later.)

Risk Factors for Cognitive Decline

Risk factors for cognitive decline in old age include diabetes, smoking, hypertension, sedentary lifestyle, lack of engagement in cognitively challenging tasks, high cholesterol levels, and depression (Mayo Clinic, 2013), whereas higher levels of education, innate intelligence, and intact sensory abilities are associated with better cognitive performance in old age (Zec, 1995; Wilson et al., 2009). These factors associated with worse or better performance over time tend to be either fixed or modifiable. While the genetic factors (e.g., race, gender, innate intelligence) cannot be changed, people can influence many factors related to cognitive performance, as described through the PACES program earlier.

Minor Neurocognitive Disorders (Mild Cognitive Impairment [MCI])

The Diagnostic and Statistical Manual, 5th edition (DSM-5; APA, 2013), defines what is commonly known as MCI as the diagnosis of minor neurocognitive disorder (NCD). People with MCI can complete their ADLs, but might note decreases in memory or optimal performance in complex tasks such as IADLs (e.g., home management, taking care of finances). Approximately, 1–2% of persons age 65+ develop MCI every year. While it is difficult to determine the exact prevalence of MCI (due to it often not being formally diagnosed), the range for persons age 65+ is 5–40% (Roberts & Knopman, 2013). Langa and Levine (2014) estimate the prevalence at 10–20%, with men seemingly more impacted than women. Not only does the risk of developing MCI increase with age, but individuals with the most common type of MCI (which includes decreased memory performance) also are more likely to have their cognitive impairment convert to dementia. The risk factor is 8.5 times higher for persons with MCI compared to their peers without cognitive impairments (Alegret et al., 2014). One estimate of the conversion rate of MCI progressing to dementia is approximately 10–15% per year (Roberts & Knopman, 2013). Despite this dire fact, the good news is that a meta-analysis of various cohort studies conducted by Mitchell and Shiri-Feshki (2009) found that over a 10-year period, the majority (69%) of individuals diagnosed with MCI had not progressed to having the diagnosis of dementia. An even rosier prognosis is that a significant portion of persons with MCI (about one-third of persons diagnosed) converted back to typical cognitive functioning (Sachdev et al., 2013; Gao et al., 2014).

Malek-Ahmadi et al. (2012) determined that four questions were most predictive of amnestic MCI (involving memory impairments; **FIGURE 8-4**). These are:

1. Does the person have trouble remembering the date, year, and time? (most predictive)
2. Does the person repeat questions/statements in the same day?
3. Does the person have difficulty managing finances?
4. Does the person have a decreased sense of direction?

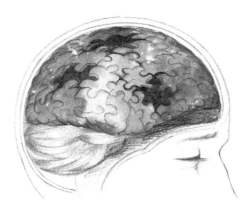

FIGURE 8-4 Mild cognitive impairment disorders are often compared to missing puzzle pieces, which represent cognitive impairments such as memory loss.

© Carla Francesca Castagno/Shutterstock

Overview of DSM-V Major Neurocognitive Disorders

Cognitive decline is occurring more frequently, primarily because people around the globe are living longer. Cognitive deficits can be described on a continuum from mild (minor NCDs, which entail slight forgetfulness and slight slowing of mental processing, both of which do not interfere significantly with routine day-to-day activities) to late stage dementia (major NCDs, which in the end can rob the affected persons of their will and capacity to stay alive). In the following sections, we will explore this cognitive continuum.

As stated in the segment on minor NCD, older adults with this diagnosis are more likely to convert to more serious major NCD (e.g., dementia), but also many will not decline further and may even revert back to typical cognition. Since intact cognition plays a major role in human functioning, generally the major NCDs affect life relatively more than the mild disorders. The major disorders, often commonly referred to as dementia, relate to several different diagnoses.

Alzheimer's Disease

Alzheimer's disease (AD) is the most frequent diagnosis under the umbrella of major NCDs. AD involves a significant decline in learning and memory as well as a continuing decline in cognition (sometimes with periods of plateaus). Most with AD also display behavioral and psychological changes (APA, 2013, pp. 611–612). Approximately, 5.5 million people in the United States (most of whom are over age 65) are living with AD, and worldwide 47 million people are affected (Alzheimer's Disease Association, 2017). While overall one out of nine people over the age of 65 (approximately 11% of the population) have the diagnosis of AD, the level of prevalence rises to one out of three (approximately 32%) after the age of 85 (Alzheimer's Disease Association, 2016; Gardner, Valcour, & Yaffe, 2013). However, it is crucial to understand that AD is not a part of typical aging, even though 59% of people mistakenly think that it is (Alzheimer's Disease Association, 2017). Ironically, AD and several other NCDs are unintended gifts associated with the vast scientific progress that has occurred over the past century. As more people live longer, more of these older people are getting dementia. While the prevalence does increase with advancing age, it never becomes an inevitable diagnosis for the majority of older adults even among the oldest-old.

Some key characteristics are outlined in **TABLE 8-3**, although each individual is different and will not display all the characteristics, any set pattern, or any specific level of traits.

AD progresses through three stages: mild, moderate, and severe. Because there is no cure, and medications are only marginally effective, the current emphasis of medical providers is to prolong the first two stages while the person generally is still physically capable and still the same person. Reisberg (1988), who developed the stage theory of AD, demonstrated that the stages often emulate a reverse developmental pattern (**TABLE 8-4**).

TABLE 8-3 Alzheimer's Disease Symptom Progression

	Initial	End-Stage
General behavior	Indifferent; may be delusional or depressed; may deny problems	Withdrawn, agitated, mood may change abruptly
Language	Normal or mild word finding difficulties	Severe impairment, words may be meaningless, "word-salad"
Memory	Mild short-term deficits	Unable to test
Orientation	Fully oriented (A&O × 3 or 4)	Oriented to self only (A&O × 1)
Reasoning	Decreased abstract reasoning and problem-solving; decreased executive functioning[a]	Unable to test
Personal care/ADL skills[b]	Inattention to detail, but able to complete basic personal care	Dependency, may show fear of bathing
Instrumental ADLs[c]	Slight impairment, carelessness, decreased safety awareness, may need supervision	Unable to complete
Mobility	Normal	Impaired, may not be able to walk or transfer independently
Posture	Normal	Flexed, often preferring a fetal position
Range of motion/movement	Normal or within functional limits	Increased muscle tonus; contractures[d] are common
Visuospatial skills	Slight visual perceptual changes (e.g., decreases in navigation skills and visual memory[e]	May have hallucinations and delusions; poor visual memory and topographical orientation

[a]APA (2013).
[b]ADLs (activities of daily living) include bathing, dressing, self-feeding, grooming, and basic self-care.
[c]IADLs (instrumental activities of daily living) include home management, money management, care of others, and meal preparation.
[d]A contracture is defined as a decrease of 50% or more of normal passive range of motion. It is a painful condition affecting many in long-term care settings, including more than three-quarters of patients who can no longer walk (Souren, Frensses, & Reisberg, 1995).
[e](Possin, 2010).
Data from Ham (1995); Morris (1993); Cole (1995).

TABLE 8-4 Overview of the Functional Assessment Staging for AD

Stage (AD)	Skill Level/Behavioral Manifestations	Helpful Hints
1 (Typical Aging)	Normal adult behavior and cognition	Preventative care (such as the PACES program)
2	Minor memory problems	Prevention; engage in new learning
3	Performance on the job declining; may get lost easily; more disorganized	Reminders may be helpful; begin to simplify routines; stress management
4	Difficulty with IADLs (e.g., finances, complex meal management, driving)	Build set routines; family and friend support is needed; build the person's legacy
5	Can do ADLs but may have difficulty with judgment (e.g., choosing proper clothing)	Support what person can do; simplify routine; allow more time; review photo albums (reminisce)
6	Difficulty with ADLs such as dressing, bathing, and toileting	Promoting strengths—what the person can do (e.g., eating finger foods, even if this takes longer)
7 (End-stage AD)	Incontinence, limited communication, physical decline, may prefer fetal position	Engage senses; gentle touch; music; movement (though not forced)

Frontotemporal NCD

Frontotemporal NCD, similar to AD, is also insidious in its onset and has behavioral or language variants. Although not nearly as common (only 2–10 people per 100,000), frontotemporal NCD when it does occur, is more frequently found among individuals under age 65. Only 20–25% of cases are older. The behavior that is commonly seen may be manifested as disinhibition, apathy, loss of social skills such as empathy for others, perseverative behaviors, and/or hyperorality (e.g., changes/increases in food intake or substance misuse). The language variant, while demonstrating general features of dementia as

well, also involves decreases in language skills (APA, 2013, pp. 614–615).

Dementia with Lewy Bodies

Dementia with Lewy Bodies (now named Neurocognitive Disorder with Lewy Bodies [NCDLB]; APA, 2013) also has a gradual onset and course. Cognitive performance may fluctuate more with this diagnosis, even seemingly normal at times, and people with NCDLB tend to have more perceptual disturbances (such as visual hallucinations), especially if comparing diagnoses early in the disease process. NCDLB may account for up to 30% of all the dementias. Prior to being diagnosed, the person may display times of confusion or **delirium** (APA, 2013, p. 619).

Parkinson's Disease with Dementia

Yet another NCD is due to Parkinson's disease (PD), which can be either minor (mild) or major (serious). Major NCD due to PD is explored here in juxtaposition to the other dementias. Parkinsonian dementia (as it is often known) also tends to have an insidious onset, but one primary difference between this and AD is that the cognitive impairments in the PD variation take place after the physical symptoms of PD have been well established. PD impacts proportionately more men than women and has been diagnosed in approximately 3% of individuals age 85+ (APA, 2013, pp. 636–637). A common feature of PD is hallucinations, experienced by 30–60% of persons with PD (Llorca et al., 2016). Although visual hallucinations (especially the feeling that there is someone just to the side or behind the person) are the most prevalent type of hallucination, up to 30% of individuals with PD have multimodal hallucinations (combination of visual, auditory, olfactory, etc.). According to Llorca et al. (2016), who analyzed the repercussions of these hallucinations on PD patients, these symptoms have less impact on quality of life than for people with schizophrenia.

Working with Persons Who Have Major NCD

Some general guidelines may be helpful to follow when working with persons who have major NCD (dementia). Again, remember that these are suggestions only; what works for one may have the opposite impact on another.

- Caring and respect are essential, even when the person cannot reciprocate.
- Healthcare professionals (or anyone) should never speak about persons with dementia in front of them while ignoring them as if they were not there.

- The behavior of persons with AD and other NCDs may try your patience even as a professional, but controlling your emotions is crucial. Remember that the person is not intentionally trying to provoke you.
- Soothing music may defuse the intensity of an uncomfortable situation and foster relaxation.
- A sense of humor, so that you can laugh together, also can be extremely helpful, although it is important for the person not to feel that you are laughing at him or her.
- Diversion (or engagement in occupation) may help to calm a stressful situation, including:
  - Involvement in simple (not childish) activities (some favorites are doing arts together—making cards, bird feeders, and terrariums)
  - Playing games, playing or enjoying music, and singing songs they have enjoyed formerly (**FIGURE 8-5**)
  - Drawing, writing, or painting (providing assistance, but only as needed; perfection is not the goal)
  - Looking through old photograph albums; creating albums or scrapbooks for the future

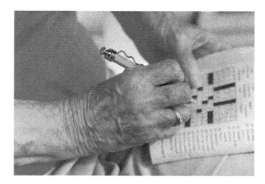

FIGURE 8-5 Games that make a person think and strategize may have a positive effect on cognitive performance.
© Plamens Art/Shutterstock

- Reminiscing ("Tell me about …"; Tamura-Lis, 2017)
- Involving them in tasks or parts of tasks they enjoy, for example, helping with meal preparation or taking care of or just interacting with a pet

A method that has been recently adapted to work with persons who have AD (and other major NCDs) is improvisation, using techniques such as meeting people with AD where they are at, entering their world, and "going with the flow" rather than trying to have individuals with AD enter your world. A helpful TEdMed talk that may assist healthcare professionals in developing their Improv skills can be found at www.youtube.com/watch?v=GciWItvLo_s (Stobbe & Carter, 2016).

Several books are available for individuals who want to improve their ability to work with older people who have dementia. A few examples are *Creating Moments of Joy Along the Alzheimer's Journey: A Guide for Families and Caregivers* by Brackey (2017); *A Dignified Life: The Best Friends Approach to Alzheimer's Care* by Bell and Troxel (2002); *The Best Friends Book of Alzheimer's Activities* (Volumes I and II; Bell, Troxel, Cox, & Hamon [2008]); and *Talking to Alzheimer's* by Strauss and Khachaturian (2002). **TABLE 8-5** offers some more specific, though not prescriptive, suggestions as well.

TABLE 8-5 Major NCDs: Problems and Potential Solutions

Functional Problem Area	Potential Solutions
Decreased self-care skills (ADLs)	▪ Offer supervision ▪ Simplify clothing/environment ▪ Gently encourage person to do as much as possible without nagging ▪ Remove safety hazards ▪ Obtain an occupational therapy referral
Decreased involvement in daily activities	▪ Encourage involvement in what person can still do well ▪ Praise successes and have patience ▪ Try safe, simple repetitive chores (especially together) ▪ Offer items of interest ▪ Referral for occupational therapy
Wandering	▪ Take walks together in safe areas ▪ Purchase identification bracelet or GPS device ▪ Alert neighbors ▪ Remove obstacles indoors ▪ If balance is decreased, obtain physical therapy referral
Impaired communication	▪ Speak slowly and calmly; do not yell ▪ Give simple directions, one step at a time ▪ Use repetition as needed ▪ Remain nonconfrontational; arguing will not help ▪ Obtain speech therapy referral

(continues)

TABLE 8-5 Major NCDs: Problems and Potential Solutions (*continued*)

Functional Problem Area	Potential Solutions
Sleep disturbance	▪ Establish a bedtime routine ▪ Make sure person gets enough exercise/activity during the day ▪ Limit liquid before bedtime ▪ Encourage toileting immediately before bedtime ▪ Omit obstacles in bedroom to bathroom route or purchase bedside commode ▪ A back rub may promote restful sleep

Problem Behavior	Possible Solutions
Inappropriate behavior	▪ Always treat person with dignity and respect ▪ Divert person to another activity ▪ Watch for signs of overstimulation and try to avoid these situations ▪ Listen and respond to the feeling behind the words being said rather than the words themselves ▪ Ask for help (e.g., from team, doctors, support group, adult day care) ▪ Use humor ▪ Do not ignore requests for assistance ▪ Use improvisation ("yes, and")
Anxiety and/or agitation	▪ Structure environment ▪ Establish daily routine with lots of opportunity for structured activities ▪ Promote the feeling of security ▪ Sensory issues, refer to occupational therapy ▪ Consider referral to social work/counseling
Anger	▪ Offer a drink, a snack, or a favorite item ▪ Do not confront, tease, or argue with the person ▪ Listen and divert to new topic if possible ▪ Limit stimulation (or overstimulation) ▪ Remove from disruptive environment ▪ Take care of your own safety

Data from Cole (1995); Colorado State University (1989); Gwyther (1998).

Comparing Dementia with Depression and Delirium

Both clinical depression and delirium are sometimes confused with dementia, even though both tend to have more rapid onset, especially delirium. Often, one condition can be superimposed on another. These conditions are described later. **TABLE 8-6** describes some of the contrasting features.

Depression

Clinical depression impacts adolescents and adults of all ages. Overall, reported depression

TABLE 8-6 Comparing and Contrasting Dementia, Depression, and Delirium

Characteristic	Dementia	Depression	Delirium
Onset	Insidious, gradual	Abrupt or with major life change	Abrupt; sudden over hours or days
Course	Long; years, may plateau	Situational fluctuations; may wax and wane	Fluctuates; may be worse late in day or upon awakening; can clear or last
Duration	Years; irreversible	Six weeks to months to years	Hours to a month; can last longer
Awareness	Decreasing over time	Generally OK	Decreased; fluctuating mental status
Alertness	Generally OK	Normal	Fluctuates; lethargy or hypervigilance
Attention	Generally OK (focus)	Mild decrease; easily distracted	Decreased; fluctuates
Orientation	Decreases over time A&O × 3,2,1	Generally OK	Decreased
Memory	Decreased STM	Selective; may be OK	Decreased, especially STM, and immediate
Thinking	Decreased abstract thought and judgment	Intact; may feel helpless or hopeless	Disorganized; incoherent speech
Language	Word finding difficulties	Intact	Slow, incoherent, or inappropriate language
Perception	Occasional misperception (paranoia)	Intact	Distortions; delusions; hallucinations; decreased sense of reality
Psychomotor performance	OK initially; apraxia later	OK; some agitation or slowness of movement	Hyper or hypokinetic or mixed
Sleep	Decreased, fragmented	Decreased; may awaken early; insomnia	Decreased, may be reversed

(continues)

TABLE 8-6 Comparing and Contrasting Dementia, Depression, and Delirium (*continued*)

Characteristic	Dementia	Depression	Delirium
Assessment	Errors, poor performance highlighted by others such as family	Errors more likely highlighted by person, or person may not care, may seem indifferent	Numerous errors, may not be able to test

Modified from Foreman, Fletcher, Mion, Simon, & Faculty (1996). Table 1, p. 229; Beers & Berkow (2000).

occurs in 6% of males and 10% age12+ (CDC, 2012). Perhaps, surprisingly the percentage of people who report depression is higher among middle aged adults (7% of males and 12% of females 40–59 years old), compared to persons over age 60 (5% of males and 7% of females; CDC, 2012). One consideration for the lower apparent prevalence of (reported) depression among older adults may be due to the cohort effect of being members of the stoic generation that as a cohort may believe in taking care of themselves and not wanting to admit (or report) the negative feelings associated with depression. Depression is most prevalent in women (1.5–3-fold higher than men), minority groups, persons with less than a high school education, previously married people, individuals unable to work or who are unemployed, and persons without health insurance (CDC, 2016a; APA, 2013, p. 165).

While major depressive disorder (clinical depression) is not a normal part of growing old, it is a common co-morbid condition in individuals diagnosed with dementia (up to 69%), and potentially can be viewed as both a consequence of having, as well as a risk factor for getting dementia (Muliyala & Varghese, 2010). The number of people with depression rises sharply in hospitals and long-term care facilities, where the prevalence of clinical depression reaches up to 35% (Thakur & Blazer, 2008). Despite this high prevalence of depression in vulnerable older adults, depression as a clinical condition often goes

unnoticed and therefore undiagnosed. This is an especially heart-wrenching fact considering that depression is often amenable to treatment (APA, 2013; Mayo Clinic, n.d.).

The DSM-V (APA, 2013) offers the following as common signs and symptoms of a major depressive disorder, especially when these occur at least over a 2-week period and indicate a change from the person's typical functioning and demeanor. (For a full and detailed list, see APA, 2013, pp. 160–168.)

- Subjective report of a "depressed mood most of the day, nearly every day" (APA, 2013, p. 160). The person may feel sad or appear tearful. The person may complain of feeling hopeless. (This may be the easiest symptom to recognize, but because we all have "off" days, it may go unnoticed.)
- Sleep disturbances.
- Disinterest in former valued activities.
- Agitation, listlessness, loss of energy (enough to negatively impact daily occupations).
- Feelings of worthlessness or guilt.
- Thoughts of death or suicidal ideation.
- Decreased cognition such as indecisiveness (APA, 2013, p. 161). Related to depression, Thomas and O'Brien (2008), also include potential changes in cognition such as impaired episodic and working memory, decreased language processing, decreased executive skills, and delayed processing speed.

If the symptoms are severe enough to be concerning, a referral to the person's physician is in order. As a healthcare professional, you may need to confer with the doctor and/or healthcare team to let them know of your concern while being careful not to violate patient confidentiality. A crucial point to keep in mind is that older people do not tend to "fake" the signs and symptoms of depression (Juratovac, 1996).

Suicide in Older Adults

Despite societal beliefs to the contrary, feeling down and depressed is not a natural or normal consequence of the aging process. Unusual mood disturbances must be taken seriously. **Suicide** has generally been listed in the top 10 leading causes of death in the United States. The highest suicide rate (19.6 per 100,000 in 2015) was among persons aged 45–64 years, but nearly the same rate occurred in people age 85+ (19.4 per 100,000; American Foundation for Suicide Prevention, 2017). Specifically, White males age 65 and over comprise over 80% of all suicides in late life. No demographic is immune to the devastating effects of suicide or suicide ideation (National Institute for Mental Health, 2017). Fixed risk factors for suicide in the United States include being male (currently 4–1 ratio), single, older, and having a family history of suicide (CDC, 2015). Besides major depressive disorders, other risk factors for suicide include psychiatric illness (schizophrenia, schizoaffective illness, and delusion disorder as well as anxiety disorders and substance abuse), chronic physical illness and pain, decreased functional capacity, and social disconnectedness of the older person from his or her family, friends, and community (Conwell, Van Orden, & Caine, 2011; Cukrowicz, Cheavens, Van Orden, Ragain, & Cook, 2011).

Healthcare professionals need to be aware of the potential for suicide and give serious consideration to *any* indication that the person may be thinking about it. Indicators of potential suicide include not only past history of attempts, but also threats of suicide, substance misuse, sudden feelings of euphoria (especially after feeling depressed), giving away possessions, bodily complaints, and persistent **bereavement** (APA, 2013, pp. 789–790; Welton, 2007). Older adults may be less likely to seek mental health services, but when they seek medical care, they may report only somatic symptoms related to depression and suicidal ideation (e.g., insomnia, loss of appetite, or gastrointestinal symptoms; Neufeld & O'Rourke, 2009).

Although it is beyond the scope of this text to discuss the ethical issues raised by suicide undertaken to escape excruciating, irreversible pain, and/or terminal illness, it suffices to reiterate that depression, which often precedes a suicide attempt, is generally amenable to treatment through medication management, psychotherapy, and/or electroconvulsive shock therapy. Our job as healthcare professionals is to be on guard for signs and symptoms of depression and potential suicide, to support and educate the person about basic treatments, and to refer the person to an expert who can begin the treatment protocol. A toll-free hotline available 24/7 is offered by the National Suicide Prevention Lifeline at 1-800-273-TALK (8255); (NIMH, 2017).

Delirium

Delirium is a common occurrence for older adults who have been hospitalized, have undergone major surgery, or who are overmedicated, but it is not commonplace in a healthy aging population. However, up to 30% of people admitted to the hospital without delirium will develop it during their hospital stay (Vasilevskis, Jan, Hughes, & Ely, 2012). Generally, delirium is a transient state of fluctuating cognitive abilities often characterized by hallucinations, decreased ability to focus, increased confusion, and poor memory performance. The symptoms of delirium can be difficult to recognize and can be mistaken for dementia or depression (Flinn, Diehl, Seyfried, & Malani, 2009).

A healthcare professional may be able to ease the tense situation experienced by families by explaining that the state of being delirious is *generally* temporary in nature and by educating the family about the side effects of the patient's current medical procedure or medication. Nonetheless, the development of delirium is associated with increased mortality, increased length of stay in the hospital, increased rate of discharge to long-term care facilities, and increased medical complications. Cognitive decline is also a risk for people who have experienced delirium (Flinn et al., 2009).

Risk factors for delirium include age greater than 70 years, self-reported alcohol abuse, poor cognitive status, visual impairment, depression, poor functional status, **malnutrition**, metabolic abnormalities, infections, noncardiac thoracic surgery, or abdominal aneurysm surgery (Vasilevskis et al., 2012; Flinn et al., 2009). Any change in mental status should be reported to and addressed by the healthcare team. Post-operation delirium research is ongoing. Medical teams are looking for ways to reduce the incidence of delirium by developing better post-operation clinical pathways and to ensure that the specific medications used are appropriate for older adults. In addition, adequate sleep patterns while in the hospital are encouraged. Also, the healthcare professional should ensure that sensory equipment (e.g., hearing aids and/or glasses) are clean and available and provide desired level of appropriate sensory stimulation and activities (Flinn et al., 2009). Furthermore, family collaboration is crucial if delirium is suspected, because the family can provide information regarding the older adult's baseline behavior/cognition and may be the first to detect a change (Keyser, Buchanan, & Edge, 2012). Prevention, detection, and management are the solutions for delirium, with prevention being the best first line of defense. See Table 8-2 for information about the CAM tool to assess for delirium. Delirium may be concurrent with either or both dementia and depression. A person may have one, two, or all three of these conditions simultaneously. Agitation may be present in all three (Table 8-6).

Related Potentially Reversible Disorders

Sometimes, what appears to be dementia is actually another medical disorder in disguise. Gaining a basic understanding of some of these common disorders may help healthcare professionals decide when to make referrals. Some of the more common ailments with signs and symptoms similar to dementia are briefly described here.

Malnutrition

Deficiencies of the B-complex vitamins, vitamin C, zinc, magnesium, folic acid, and protein, or malnutrition can cause behavioral disturbances, including those implicated in the diagnosis of clinical depression and dementia (Patenaude, 1996). Vitamin B_{12} deficiency has been linked specifically to dementia symptoms. Eastley, Wilcock, and Bucks (2000) found that vitamin B_{12} treatment did not reverse dementia, but it did improve language and frontal lobe (executive) functioning to a degree.

Cerebrovascular Accident or Stroke

Cerebrovascular accident (CVA) or stroke, especially small infarcts with limited accompanying functional declines, may cause behavior disturbances much like those brought about by a major depressive disorder or AD. In fact, a rather common type of dementia (multi-infarct dementia) is caused by a series of small strokes.

Hypothyroidism

Hypothyroidism slows metabolic processes, which causes the affected person to respond slowly and to be lethargic.

Failure to Thrive

A related syndrome is described as **failure to thrive** (FTT). An insidious deterioration in functioning that is not related to a specific disease, FTT can be caused by depression, dementia, chronic conditions, or medication/drug reactions. Social isolation, low socioeconomic status, and functional dependency all are predisposing factors of FTT. Case examples are common; perhaps, we all know of someone who just seemed to wither away prior to dying. Common features of FTT include weight loss resulting from lack of appetite, social withdrawal, lack of concern about appearance, memory loss, impaired ambulation, and incontinence (common in nearly half the cases described; Palmer, 1990). People with this syndrome simply seem to be giving up on life. A referral to a geriatrician (a medical doctor who specializes in working with older adults) is usually appropriate for people with (potential) FTT.

Urinary Tract Infection

Urinary tract infections (UTI) are among the most frequently diagnosed infection in older adults, especially women. UTIs are the most common infection in the long-term care setting, accounting for one-third of all the infections there. About 10% of women age 65+ have had a UTI in the past year (Rowe & Juthani-Mehta, 2013). Symptoms include frequent, often painful voiding, potential back pain, and malaise (perhaps flu-like symptoms). UTIs occur more often in individuals who have diabetes or eat a high sugar diet, especially without adequate hydration. In older adults, particularly persons who are institutionalized or have other health issues, atypical symptoms of UTI such as mental status changes and confusion are also common (Rowe & Juthani-Mehta, 2013).

Lack of Oxygen

Certain disorders (e.g., lung disease, pneumonia) are associated with a lowered ability of the body to effectively complete oxygen uptake. *Hypoxemia* refers to insufficient oxygen levels in the blood. Oxygen saturation levels (O_2Sat) for most people should be 95%

or higher. The saturation level is measured by a pulse oximeter that is placed on the finger. Although a physician must determine what is abnormal for any one person, generally hypoxemia can lead to tissue damage as well as mental confusion, including impaired judgment and problem-solving ability. Therefore, older adults with low blood oxygen levels may appear confused, as if they might have the diagnosis of dementia. Fortunately, administering oxygen, often through a nasal cannula per physician's orders, may improve mental status quickly (**FIGURE 8-6**).

Substance Misuse and Abuse

Inadvertent misuse or deliberate abuse of substances (such as alcohol, prescriptions, and over-the-counter drugs) tends to be viewed as a problem of the young, but this is a growing issue among older adults (Bogunovic, 2012). Although older adults make up about 13% of the total U.S. population, they consume at least 25% of the prescribed medications, with 50% taking 5 or more medications and 20% taking 10 or more (Sparacino, 2013). Friedman and Williams (2015) estimate that 20–25% of older adults drink more than the recommended amount (one drink per day or less) and approximately 3–5% fall into the more serious category of heavy consumption

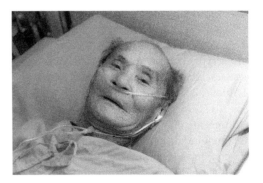

FIGURE 8-6 Oxygen being administered through a nasal cannula.
© Lidea Studio/Shutterstock

(i.e., alcoholic). This level of consumption leaves room for many drug-to-drug or drug-to-alcohol interactions which are often unreported or ignored. The problem with paying so little attention to this situation is that excess alcohol or drug use (including prescribed medications) can cause cognitive problems such as slurred speech, drowsiness, and confusion, as well as exacerbate the effects of any current cognitive impairments (such as those wrought by the minor or major NCDs) or impairments in hearing and vision (Sparacino, 2013). The Substance Abuse and Mental Health Services Administration (SAMHSA; samhsa.gov) recommends brief substance use/misuse screening for everyone (including older adults) through the SBIRT screening program using tools such as the AUDIT. (For more information, visit www.integration.samhsa.gov/clinical-practice/sbirt.)

▶ Personality Development

Personality is what makes a person a unique individual. Each of us has a set of character traits, attitudes, habits, and emotional tendencies that distinguish us from everyone else. These dispositions can be intimated by our appearance (e.g., tattoos, clothing styles, or level of care taken in grooming), but are essentially inner characteristics causing us to behave as we do. To a degree, one's personality also predicts life events such as quality of relationships, ability to accept change, employment choices and successes, happiness, and health and mortality (McAdams & Olson, 2012; O'Shea, Dotson, & Fieo, 2017). Many studies have explored the development of personality in youth and into young adulthood, whereas fewer studies have concentrated on personality evolvement during later adulthood. The question posed is whether significant personality change takes place during old age (in both healthy adults and individuals afflicted with disease).

There are many theories on personality, yet the well-known theorists (e.g., Maslow, Piaget, Freud) devoted little attention to the personality of older people. One theorist who may already be familiar to many readers is Erik Erikson, who initially proposed eight stages of psychosocial development (Erikson, Erikson, & Kivnick, 1994). Originally, the final stage was integrity versus despair. Erikson viewed people who were successful in this stage as being able to develop a sense of pride in their past accomplishments. They have a sense of satisfaction and judge that their lives have been worthwhile. Others, who do not successfully complete this stage, experience instead a feeling of despair not only about the course of their lives thus far, but also because they do not believe that they have enough time left to improve the course of their life. Overall, Erikson et al. (1994) proposed that this then-final stage of life was both a positive and integrating time for well older adults. In an updated version of personality development, Erikson and Erikson (1998) included a ninth stage in their theory: **gerotranscendence**, which is associated with wisdom and a moving away from early and midlife materialism. Ardelt (2008) described this "transcendence of the self" as a move toward selflessness, and increased compassion and reflection, all embodying the characteristics of a truly wise person.

Five-Factor Model of Personality

Social scientists are beginning to show more interest in the final years of life with regard to personality development. The trait theory espoused by McCrae and Costa (1990) is perhaps the most widely known with a continuum on five different aspects of personality. Their five-factor model of personality is as follows:

1. *Neuroticism*: Associated with hostility, depression, anxiety, and impulsiveness
2. *Extraversion*: Associated with a high level of energy and being outgoing in social situations

3. *Openness to experience*: Associated with open-mindedness, curiosity, and adjustment to change
4. *Agreeableness*: Associated with affection, compassion, and being altruistic
5. *Conscientiousness*: Associated with a strong commitment to goals and being a principled person

Personality Stability

When studying this model, there are three key questions that arise. One is whether these traits are stable over adulthood and into old age. Research conducted on these traits has determined they have the greatest instability between the ages of 17 and 35 years, and then they tend to become more fixed. When these traits were studied in older people over 3- and 6-year intervals, strong stability of all five traits was found using both self and spousal reports. Even when the intervals between testing increased to as much as 50 years, stability coefficients remained statistically significant, with life events exerting little overall influence for major change (Costa, Herbst, McCrae, & Siegler, 2000).

Other evidence also supports the relative permanence of personality traits in typically aging older adults. For example, test-retest correlations of optimism scores have been found to be high (over 0.7) over a 10-year period, even when considerable life change was occurring in the participants' lives (Carver, Scheier, & Segerstrom, 2010). Hayflick (1994), in citing the results of the Baltimore Longitudinal Study of Aging (BLSA), maintained that personality traits remain essentially the same throughout the life span in typically aging adults, although most people older than age 50 begin to prefer slower paced activities. This is a valuable piece of information for healthcare professionals who work with older people. Pacing healthcare intervention for the convenience of the older clients rather than the provider is essential for good care (and

perhaps, getting more difficult in these hectic times for health care).

Personality Differences by Cohort

The second key question that arises when examining personality is whether there are differences among groups of different aged individuals or how old age and gender might impact personality. Weiss et al. (2005) found few differences in the five traits based on age when looking at more than 1,000 Medicare patients from ages 65–100. In the Weiss study (2005), the older participants did show a higher level of agreeableness, which may have been the result of a cohort effect or due to higher death rates among adults with lower levels of this trait (individuals with an intense "type A" personality have proportionately more heart disease, which ultimately could lead to an earlier death).

Research has shown that men, as they get older, may become more nurturing and open about their feelings, whereas women may become more assertive, confident, and comfortable with themselves. Social scientists believe these changes could be influenced by hormonal fluctuations, perhaps causing a diminution of the character distinctions between the genders (Carver et al., 2010). Levels of agreeableness and conscientiousness also may tend to increase with age (at least until age 70) for both genders (*Harvard Mental Health Letter*, 2006).

In the longitudinal Lothian study out of Scotland, Mõttus, Johnson, and Deary (2012) reviewed the five-factor traits in people in their 70s and 80s extensively. They found that women's emotional stability declined in their 70s, and that there was a gender differential for the trait of agreeableness. The level of agreeableness tended to decline in older women, whereas for men there was an increase of agreeableness in their 70s and no change in persons in their 80s. Mõttus et al. (2012) suggested that mean level changes (of the five-factor model traits) accelerate in old age resulting in "pronounced changes in the ninth decade" (p. 14) not seen in previous decades. More research that examines personality in older adults, especially the old-old, is clearly needed.

In a pivotal study done by Erikson et al. (1994), older people described themselves as more tolerant, patient, open-minded, understanding, compassionate, and less critical than when they were younger. However, many study participants viewed both themselves and the other older adults in the study as more set in their ways. This seeming contradiction was explained by the suggestion that as people age, they not only increasingly integrate their own personal style, but they also can gain a new understanding and tolerance of others' behavioral styles.

Malleability of Personality Traits

The third, and perhaps most important, question for healthcare providers and elders as well is: Can people change their personality traits? Although overall the five factors show stability, nonetheless personality changes can and do occur; but, often study results are not definitive. Wood and Roberts (2006) suggested that personality traits are open systems that are plastic and can be influenced throughout life. Representations of the self, such as one's goals, values, coping styles, and control beliefs, are likely to change over the course of one's lifetime.

Some older adults' personalities change due to disease processes. In these cases, it is crucial to remember that these people are not necessarily still "themselves" and may be acting out due to an illness rather than the behavior being self-directed. Disease processes, especially the major NCDs such as AD, absolutely can rob a person of their essential personality, leaving someone quite different in their wake. A helpful maxim to remember is: "Don't blame

the person, blame the disease." Even when working with people who have challenging personality types, compassion is the path of least resistance and the most fulfillment when all things are considered at the end of the day. Demonstrating respect is never out of place, even if acting respectful does not match how you may be feeling toward the person.

Personality Summary

Personalities come in myriad flavors, and not all are compatible with one another. As healthcare professionals, we need to make a concerted effort to provide excellent health care or service to all our clients of any age (and personality style). We now have substantial evidence that several aspects of personality seem to improve with age for people who are aging well. Yet, old age, as a stage of life, does not equate with any specific personality traits, especially those often heard on the street (e.g., grumpy [old men], doddering [old woman], stubborn, disagreeable, closed-minded, etc.). Some people may have been this way their whole lives, whereas others become "better with age" (Kersting, 2003, p. 14). Overall, in the realm of personality, there are no definitive answers regarding aging. People who go through typical life development adhere to their personhood throughout life: they remain unique individuals with distinct features, and if they are determined, they can change for the better.

Behavior Change

Aging or just continuing to live life does entail inevitable changes, but when people age well, they become more aware of and more determined to take advantage of the positive changes they encounter (e.g., wisdom, maturity, increased self-esteem, increased level of confidence, increased ability to appreciate ambiguity; Carstensen, Fung, & Charles, 2003; Erikson & Erikson, 1998). Well elders also take actions to counteract the negative changes that are often associated with the aging process (potential declines in physical and cognitive realms). Older people deserve healthcare professionals who are hopeful, caring, and have a positive attitude that will promote an optimal, individualized aging process.

One is never "too old" to make a positive change in behavior. If a person has the cognitive capacity to set positive health goals, chronological age will not interfere. The naysayers tend to believe that being old is an excuse not to change, but clinical experience has shown that even the "old-old" can make positive health choices, including improving nutrition, exercising to get stronger, improving balance to prevent falls, and quitting smoking to feel better. While sometimes these positive behavior changes do come about through a **behavior change** strategy known as "dramatic relief" (an intense emotional event such as having a stroke or getting a dreaded diagnosis causes one to immediately reassess current unhealthy behavior; Burbank, Padula, & Nigg, 2000), older adults may decide to embark on change just for the sake of improving their lives.

Healthcare professionals may be familiar with the well-known behavior change theories: the Transtheoretical Model (TTM; for an overview, see Prochaska, Norcross, & DiClemente, 1995) and the Health Belief Model (HBM; Rosenstock, 1974; Jones et al., 2015). Both provide methods of thinking about behavior change and techniques to promote movement toward positive outcomes. In the TTM, behavior change is divided into several steps: from precontemplation, during which the person has not even considered making a change, all the way to termination when the attempted successful behavior change has been integrated into the person's everyday life (Prochaska et al., 1995). Each stage offers the healthcare professional the opportunity to assist the person to move on to the next stage of change. For example, in the second or contemplation stage, the healthcare

professional may help the older person to examine the benefits and barriers to making a change (or not). Many strategies (such as stimulus control, self-reevaluation, and consciousness raising; Burbank et al., 2000) can be utilized for people of all ages who may need or want to make positive life changes.

The HBM was developed in the 1950s and 1960s to explain the reasoning behind why people did not readily embrace the preventative measures offered by the public health service (e.g., vaccinations; Rosenstock, 1974). The HBM sets out to predict health behaviors by assessing the person's self-perceived views on the severity, susceptibility, benefits, and barriers to change (in this case, taking a preventative health measure). The healthcare professional can then work with the client to explore and potentially modify the individual factors that would impact behavior change (i.e., the perceived severity, susceptibility, benefits, and barriers to making the change). For example, the older adult may get the diagnosis of diabetes, and may need assistance weighing the benefits and barriers to changing one's diet. Certainly, the healthcare provider may provide education and support to help the client set healthy goals and embark on more healthy eating patterns.

Recently, improving life satisfaction, as a potential behavior change outcome in old age, has been explored by a number of researchers who have offered community programs. For example, Turner et al. (2017) designed an innovative, eight-week community program based on positive psychology titled "The Art of Happiness," during which the older participants from a senior center attended group sessions on humor, mindfulness, positive relationships, happiness, and stress management. Outcomes included decreased tension, increased happiness, and decreased symptoms of depression. A related and larger program also involved a novel intervention titled "Lighten up!," during which the group of elders worked on changing perspectives, also over an eight-week period, with similar encouraging results. The participants learned to recognize their emotions and savor positive experiences (Friedman et al., 2017). As a final example, McCarthy, Hall, Crawford, and Connelly (2017) conducted a randomized controlled trial of an eight-week psychoeducational group with community-dwelling older women with the intention of increasing self-transcendence. The groups included mindfulness, creative activities, and homework.

These types of quality of life-based interventions, based on changing attitudes and perceptions of well-being, are not limited to older adults who are community dwelling. For example, Cesetti, Vescovelli, and Ruini (2017) offered a positive narrative intervention group based on fairy tales to nursing home residents, and they also found positive results for improved perceptions of well-being and sleep patterns. These engaging group options offer promise as effective interventions to promote higher life quality and positive behavior change for community dwelling as well as more dependent older adults, although all agree that more research is needed before definitive protocols can be recommended.

Motivational Interviewing

One evidence-based technique to support positive behavior change is the use of **motivational interviewing** (MI). Helping professionals use this approach of communicating to assist clients in becoming experts to manage their own behavior changes in meeting their objectives in their quest toward better health (Miller & Rollnick, 2013). Key concepts include collaboration and compassion, and the use of the primary skills of asking open-ended questions, along with affirmations, reflections, and summary statements. While traditional medicine employs education and advice giving to promote new and healthier patterns of living, MI promotes conversations about

ambiguity ("change talk") and may involve clients of any age setting goals and making self-motivated changes to promote healthy living patterns for themselves. MI practitioners guide and follow rather than direct (Miller & Rollnick, 2013).

Healthcare professionals can appropriately help clients set and fulfill behavior change goals and engage older adults in programs intended to improve well-being. These interventions may help promote an optimal level of life satisfaction in the latter part of life (also see Chapter 1).

As healthcare professionals, our contributions to clients' life quality may be minimal, or by using keen listening skills, client-centered approaches, and creative problem-solving, and/or by making referrals to others who may be able to provide this direct assistance, our input may be invaluable and much appreciated. Healthcare professionals can do their part to promote wellness for people of every age, as all ought to have the opportunity to live their best lives (or as is the motto in occupational therapy: everyone deserves to "live life to its fullest").

▶ Summary

Although change is inevitable throughout life, the essential core of the human being is not likely to be altered by the aging process alone. As people age, if they experience typical aging, they *tend* to exhibit the following characteristics:

- Take longer to learn new tasks and process information a little more slowly
- Become more forgetful, especially of short-term information
- Prefer somewhat slower paced activities
- Retain essential personhood

Many cognitive, psychological, and personality changes can and do occur over time. These changes can be positive, such as when someone makes an effort toward self-improvement by making significant adjustments in lifestyle patterns. Other times, disease, misfortune, or injurious lifestyle choices impose detrimental influences on cognitive functioning, personality, and thus quality of life. Each age cohort becomes more diverse as their ages increase. Although as a group the members tend to show the signs of aging already mentioned, within each age group there are individuals who continue to perform essentially as well as they ever did (or even better) and persons who have succumbed to the "ravages of old age."

Although no one is guaranteed a long life that includes success or happiness throughout the aging process, everyone can take steps to improve their odds of living *well* into old age. The PACES program reminds us of the value of having a life purpose, partaking in physical and mental exercise, maintaining close human connections, and pursuing ongoing involvement in challenging and desirable occupations, including the essential and often overlooked occupation of sleep.

By being good listeners, who are supportive and considerate, and by promoting a personal level of independence and desired life change (if the client is motivated), and by making referrals as appropriate, we can help older persons promote healthy brain aging, and remain as productive or engaged as they choose. Our goal, as a caring, highly developed society, should be to promote meaningful involvement in life endeavors at a level of challenge fitting the person throughout life, right up until his or her final days.

🔍 CASE STUDIES

Case 1: Emma is an 85-year-old African American female who was recently widowed. She lives independently in her small home in a large city. She is fairly active in her community—she likes to attend church, weekly exercise classes, and social outings with her friends. Recently, she has found little interest or joy with leaving her home; this began after a bout of the flu where she was hospitalized for 3 days. She was happy enough with her medical care and was glad to be feeling well enough to return home. However, she finds she has little energy to manage her home, let alone socialize with friends. Her visiting nurse asks her often about her mood, appetite, and sleep patterns. Emma is vague with her responses and says she is "fine." The nurse requests a social worker to speak with Emma to see if any community services would help her recover and get back to her former routine.

1. **What condition does Emma likely have and how can you tell?**
2. **What risk factors does Emma have for this condition?**
3. **The visiting nurse requested that a social worker meet with Emma to discuss community services. Who else should Emma meet with and why?**

Case 2: Mr. Means was referred to the skilled nursing facility rehabilitation center after his primary care physician noted a decline in functioning since his last visit, even though the only medical issue involved was rather minor surgery. While being evaluated, Mr. Means was unable to complete his self-care skills, even though he had no medical or physical reason not to (other than deconditioning). It turned out that his home health aides, provided by his well-intentioned family, had taken over doing everything for him, even the most basic self-care tasks such as dressing.

1. **What might be transpiring for Mr. Means and why?**
2. **What might need to happen to get Mr. Means back on track?**

TEST YOUR KNOWLEDGE

Review Questions

1. What is the primary accomplishment of the ninth stage added to Erikson's theory of psychological development?
   a. Developing a sense of pride in your past accomplishments
   b. Discovering yourself and finding meaning to your personhood
   c. Moving toward selflessness, compassion, and reflection
   d. Feeling that you contribute something meaningful to society

2. Alzheimer's disease always involves:
   a. Memory impairment
   b. A strong attention to detail
   c. Language disturbances
   d. Decreased muscle tonus

3. Rebecca's client, a 75-year-old woman named Gail, tends to be forgetful. Rebecca has been using cuing to help Gail try to recall information during their instruction sessions, but she can see that it is starting to annoy Gail.

   What is another strategy Rebecca can use to help Gail remember during their sessions?
   a. Limiting the presentation of information to verbal instruction
   b. Being careful not to be repetitive
   c. Making the material applicable to Gail's life
   d. Focusing on information Gail would consider trivial

4. Which is a component of fluid intelligence?
   a. Language comprehension
   b. Occupational skills
   c. Categorization
   d. Educational qualifications

5. Which of the following is NOT a component of the PACES program?
   a. Purpose
   b. Activity
   c. Commitment
   d. Sleep

Learning Activities

1. Think of the role models you know who are at least 65 years old. What personality traits do you appreciate in these older people? How can you ensure that you will have some of these traits when you are older? Do you think one can develop these traits? Why or why not?

2. It may be interesting to interview a few older people. Ask them how they think their personalities and thinking skills have changed over the course of years. How does this compare with the research data? How do you think you will change as you get older?

3. Brainstorm 10 things you want to learn before you die. The list needs to include new learning—you may say travel and that is fine, but what do you intend to learn in your travels? New learning is the most important (e.g., a new sport, dance, language, learning to play an instrument, any skill, etc.). Discuss *why* new learning is important.

4. Generally speaking, the level of cognition declines as one gets older. How can you ensure that this decline will be minimal? List five things that you can personally do to improve your cognitive level.

5. Discuss wisdom. What is it and what makes someone wise? Do you equate being wise with being older? Why or why not? In the United States, how do we view wisdom compared to other world cultures?

6. Discuss depression in older adults. What are some of the reasons that older

people become depressed? (Include life events and changes that tend to occur.) What is the prognosis for individuals with clinical depression? How can you (in your own profession) help?

References

Adams, J. M. (2016). The pessimist's guide to being optimistic. *Prevention*. Retrieved from: http://www.prevention.com/mind-body/the-pessimists-guide-to-being-optimistic

Alegret, M., Cuberas-Borrós, G., Espinosa, A., Valero, S., Hernández, I., Ruíz, A., ... Castell-Conesa, J. (2014). Cognitive, genetic, and brain perfusion factors associated with four year incidence of Alzheimer's disease from mild cognitive impairment. *Journal of Alzheimer's Disease, 41*(3), 739–748.

Allen, P. M., Mejía, S. T., & Hooker, K. (2015). Personality, self-perceptions, and daily variability in perceived usefulness among older adults. *Psychology and Aging, 30*(3), 534.

Alzheimer's Disease Association. (2016). *Alzheimer's disease facts and figures*. Washington DC: author.

Alzheimer's Disease Association. (2017). Alzheimer's disease is a global epidemic. Retrieved from https://alz.org/global/.

American Foundation for Suicide Prevention. (2017). Suicide statistics. Retrieved Dec 19, 2017, from https://afsp.org/about-suicide/suicide-statistics/

American Psychiatric Association (APA). (2013). *Diagnostic and statistical manual of mental disorders. (DSM-5)*. Washington, DC: American Psychiatric Association.

Anderson, N. D., & Craik, F. I. (2017). 50 years of cognitive aging theory. *The Journals of Gerontology: Series B, 72*(1), 1–6.

Ardelt, M. (2008). Self-development through selflessness: The paradoxical process of growing wiser. In H. A. Wayment & J. J. Bauer (Eds.), *Transcending self-interest: Psychological explorations of the quiet ego*. pp. 221–223. Washington, DC: American Psychological Association.

Arias, E. (2007*). National vital statistics reports, 4*(14). Centers for Disease Control, Division of Vital statistics.

Bäckman, L., Small, B. J., & Wahlin, A. (2001). Aging and memory: Cognitive and biological perspectives. In J. E. Birren & K. W. Schaie (Eds.), *Handbook of the psychology of aging*. San Diego: Academic Press.

Baddeley, A. D. (1995). The Psychology of memory. In A. D. Baddeley, B. A. Wilson, & F. N. Watts (Eds.), *The handbook of memory disorders*. Chichester, UK: John Wiley and Sons.

Baltes, P. B. (1993). The aging mind: Potential and limits. *The Gerontologist, 33*, 580–594.

Baltes, P. B., Staudinger, U. M., Maercker, A., & Smith, J. (1995). People nominated as wise: A comparative study of wisdom-related knowledge. *Psychology and Aging, 10*(2), 155.

Bartrés-Faz, D., Junque, C., López-Alomar, A., Valveny, N., Moral, P., Casamayor, R., ... Clemente, I. C. (2001). Neuropsychological and genetic differences between age-associated memory impairment and mild cognitive impairment entities. *Journal of the American Geriatrics Society, 49*(7), 985–990.

Baum, C. M., Connor, L. T., Morrison, T., Hahn, M., Dromerick, A. W., & Edwards, D. F. (2008). Reliability, validity, and clinical utility of the Executive Function Performance Test: A measure of executive function in a sample of people with stroke. *American Journal of Occupational Therapy, 62*(4), 446–455.

Beers, M. H., & Berkow, R. (Eds.). (2000). *The Merck manual of geriatrics*. Whitehouse Station, NJ: Merck Research Laboratories.

Bell, V., & Troxel, D. (2002). *A dignified life: The best friends approach to Alzheimer's care*. Deerfield Beach, FL: Health Communications.

Bell, V., Troxel, D., Cox, T. M., Hamon, R. (2008). *The best friends book of Alzheimer's activities* (Vol. I and II). Baltimore, MD: Health Professions Press.

Bennett, T., & Gaines, J. (2010). Believing what you hear: The impact of aging stereotypes upon the old. *Educational Gerontology, 36*(5), 435–445. doi:10.1080/03601270903212336

Birren, J. E., & Schroots, J. J. F. (2006). Autobiographical memory and the narrative self over the life span. In J. E. Birren & K. W. Schaie (Eds.), *Handbook of the psychology of aging* (pp. 477–498). Burlington, MA: Elsevier.

Blazer, D. G., Yaffe, K., & Liverman, C. T. (2015). *Cognitive aging: Progress in understanding and opportunities for *action*. Washington, DC: Institute of Medicine of the National Academies.

Bogunovic, O. (2012). Substance abuse in aging and elderly adults: New issues for psychiatrists. *Psychiatric Times, 29*(8), 39.

Brackey, J. (2017). *Creating moments of joy along the Alzheimer's journey: A guide for families and caregivers* (5th ed.). West Lafayette, IN: Purdue University Press

Burbank, P. M., Padula, C. A., & Nigg, C. R. (2000). Changing health behaviors of older adults. *Journal of Gerontological Nursing, 26*(3), 26–33.

Burzynska, A. Z., Finc, K., Taylor, B. K., Knecht, A. M., & Kramer, A. F. (2017). The dancing brain: Structural and functional signatures of expert dance training. *Frontiers in Human Neuroscience, 11*(566), 1–15.

Cacioppo, J. T., & Cacioppo, S. (2014). Social relationships and health: The toxic effects of perceived social isolation. *Social and Personality Psychology Compass, 8*(2), 58–72.

Carstensen, L. L., Fung, H. H., & Charles, S. T. (2003). Socioemotional selectivity theory and the regulation of emotion in the second half of life. *Motivation and Emotion, 27*(2), 103–123.

Carver, C. S., Scheier, M. F., & Segerstrom, S. C. (2010). Optimism. *Clinical Psychology Review, 30*, 879–889.

Cavanaugh, J. C., & Blanchard-Fields, F. (2006). *Adult development and aging* (5th ed.). Belmont, CA: Wadsworth Publishing/Thomson Learning.

Center on the Developing Child, Harvard University. (2011). Building the brain's "air traffic control" system: How early experiences shape the development of executive function. Working Paper No. 11. Retrieved from www.developingchild.harvard.edu.

Centers for Disease Control and Prevention. (2012). QuickStats: Prevalence of Current Depression Among Persons Aged ≥12 Years, by Age Group and Sex — United States, National Health and Nutrition Examination Survey, 2007–2010. *Weekly Morbidity and Mortality Weekly Report, 60*(51), 1747. Retrieved from https://www.cdc.gov/mmwr/preview/mmwrhtml/mm6051a7.htm

Centers for Disease Control and Prevention. (2015). Suicide: Facts at a glance. Retrieved from https://www.cdc.gov/violenceprevention/pdf/suicide-datasheet-a.pdf

Centers for Disease Control and Prevention. (2016a). Depression. National Center for Health Statistics. Retrieved from https://www.cdc.gov/nchs/fastats/depression.htm

Centers for Disease Control and Prevention. (2016b). Depression is not a normal part of growing older. Retrieved from https://www.cdc.gov/aging/mental health/depression.htm

Cesetti, G., Vescovelli, F., & Ruini, C. (2017). The promotion of well-being in aging individuals living in nursing homes: A controlled pilot intervention with narrative strategies. *Clinical Gerontologist, 40*(5), 380–391.

Chand, S. P., & Grossberg, G. T. (2013). How to adapt cognitive-behavioral therapy for older adults. *Current Psychiatry, 12*, 10–15.

Cole, S. A. (1995). Behavioral disturbances in Alzheimer's disease. *Patient Care, 29*(11), 120–130.

Colorado State University (1989). *Guidelines for working with people with Alzheimer's disease* [class handout]. Fort Collins, CO: Alzheimer's Disease and Aging Research, Department of Psychology.

Colsher, P., & Wallace, R. (1991). Longitudinal application of cognitive function measures in a defined population of community-dwelling elders. *Annals of Epidemiology, 1*, 215–230.

Connor, L. T. (2001). Memory in old age: Patterns of decline and preservation. *Seminars in Speech and Language, 22*(2), 117–125.

Conwell, Y., Van Orden, K., & Caine, E. D. (2011). Suicide and older adults. *Psychiatric Clinics of North America, 34*(2), 451–468. doi:10.1016/j.psc.2011.02.002

Costa, P. T., Herbst, J. H., McCrae, R. R., & Siegler, I. C. (2000). Personality at midlife: Stability, intrinsic maturation, and response to life events. *Assessment, 7*(4), 365–378.

Craik, F. I. M., Anderson, N. D., Kerr, S. A., & Li, K. Z. H. (1995). Memory changes in normal aging. In A. D. Baddeley, B. A. Wilson, & F. N. Watts (Eds.), *Handbook of memory disorders*. pp. 211–241. Chichester, UK: John Wiley and Sons.

Cukrowicz, K., Cheavens, J. S., Van Orden, K. A., Ragain, R. M., & Cook, R. L. (2011). Perceived burdensomeness and suicide ideation in older adults. *Psychology and Aging, 26*(2), 331–338. doi:10.1037/a0021836

Curlik, D. M., & Shors, T. J. (2013). Training your brain: Do mental and physical (MAP) training enhance cognition through the process of neurogenesis in the hippocampus? *Neuropharmacology, 64*, 506–514.

Davies, M. (2015). We're more scared of getting dementia in old age than any other disease such as stroke, cancer and heart disease. *Daily Mail*. Retrieved from http://www.dailymail.co.uk/health/article-2947718/We-scared-getting-dementia-old-age-disease.html

Depp, C. A., Schkade, D. A., Thompson, W. K., & Jeste, D. V. (2010). Age, affective experience, and television use. *American Journal of Preventive Medicine, 39*(2), 173–178.

do Rozario, L. (1998). From ageing to sageing: Eldering and the art of being as occupation. *Journal of Occupational Science, 5*(3), 119–126.

Draganski, B., Gaser, C., Busch, V., Schuierer, G., Bogdahn, U., & May, A. (2004). Neuroplasticity: Changes in grey matter induced by training. *Nature, 427*(6972), 311–312. doi:10.1038/427311a

DuBois, C. M., Lopez, O. V., Beale, E. E., Healy, B. C., Boehm, J. K., & Huffman, J. C. (2015). Relationships between positive psychological constructs and health outcomes in patients with cardiovascular disease: A systematic review. *International Journal of Cardiology, 195*, 265–280.

Eastley, R., Wilcock, G. K., & Bucks, R. S. (2000). Vitamin B12 deficiency in dementia and cognitive impairment: the effects of treatment on neuropsychological function. *International Journal of Geriatric Psychiatry, 15*(3), 226–233.

Ebaid, D., Crewther, S. G., MacCalman, K., Brown, A., & Crewther, D. P. (2017). Cognitive processing speed across the lifespan: Beyond the influence of motor speed. *Frontiers in Aging Neuroscience, 9,* 62. doi:10.3389/fnagi.2017.00062

Erikson, E. H., & Erikson, J. M. (1998). *The life cycle completed: Extended version with new chapters on the ninth stage of development.* New York: W. W. Norton.

Erikson, E. H., Erikson, J. M., & Kivnick, H. Q. (1994). *Vital involvement in old age.* New York: W. W. Norton & Company.

Fincham, F. D., & Cain, C. M. (1986). Learned helplessness in humans: A developmental analysis. *Developmental Review, 6,* 301–333.

Flinn, D. R., Diehl, K. M., Seyfried, L. S., & Malani, P. N. (2009). Prevention, diagnosis, and management of postoperative delirium in older adults. *Journal of the American College of Surgeons, 209*(2), 261–268. doi:10.1016/j.jamcollsurg.2009.03.008

Folstein, M. F., & Folstein, S. E. (2010). Mini Mental State Exam, 2nd ed. Psychological Assessment Resources. Retrieved from https://www.parinc.com/Products/Pkey/238

Folstein, M. F., Folstein, S. E., & McHugh, P. R. (1975). Mini-mental status: A practical method for grading the cognitive state of patients for the clinician. *Journal of Psychiatric Research, 12*(3), 189–198. doi:10.1016/0022-3956(75)90026-6

Foreman, M. D., Fletcher, K., Mion, L. C., Simon, L., & Faculty, N. (1996). Assessing cognitive function: The complexities of assessment of an individual's cognitive status are important in making an accurate and comprehensive evaluation. *Geriatric Nursing, 17*(5), 228–232.

Frankl, V. (1963). *Man's search for meaning.* Boston, MA: Beacon Press (reprint Simon & Schuster, 1984).

Friedman, E. M., Ruini, C., Foy, R., Jaros, L., Sampson, H., & Ryff, C. D. (2017). Lighten UP! A community-based group intervention to promote psychological well-being in older adults. *Aging & Mental Health, 21*(2), 199–205.

Friedman, M. B. & Williams, K. A. (2015). Substance abuse and misuse in older adults. *Behavioral Health News.* Retrieved from https://pdfs.semanticscholar.org/aacf/372b3e82f47ca1f7d2e43833f7593d72bb16.pdf

Fries, J. F. (2005). The compression of morbidity. *The Milbank Quarterly, 83*(4), 801–823.

Gao, S., Unverzagt, F. W., Hall, K. S., Lane, K. A., Murrell, J. R., Hake, A. M., ... Hendrie, H. C. (2014). Mild cognitive impairment, incidence, progression, and reversion: Findings from a community-based cohort of elderly African Americans. *The American Journal of Geriatric Psychiatry, 22*(7), 670–681.

Gardner, R. C., Valcour, V., & Yaffe, K. (2013). Dementia in the oldest old: A multi-factorial and growing public health issue. *Alzheimer's Research & Therapy, 5*(4), 27. doi:10.1186/alzrt181

Garrett, M. D. (2013). Fear of dementia: The emerging fear in America. *Psychology Today.* Retrieved from https://www.psychologytoday.com/blog/iage/201305/fear-dementia

Gazzaley, A., Sheridan, M. A., & Cooney, J. W. (2007). Age-related deficits in component processes of working memory. *Neuropsychology, 21*(5), 532–539.

Gorman, W. F., & Campbell, C. D. (1995). Mental acuity of the normal elderly. *Journal of the Oklahoma State Medical Association, 88,* 119–123.

Gow, A. J., Bastin, M. E., Maniega, S. M., Hernández, M. C. V., Morris, Z., Murray, C., ... Wardlaw, J. M. (2012). Neuroprotective lifestyles and the aging brain: Activity, atrophy, and white matter integrity. *Neurology, 79*(17), 1802–1808.

Gwyther, L. P. (1998). Social issues of the Alzheimer's patient and family. *The American Journal of Medicine, 104*(4), 17S-21S.

Ham, R. J. (1995). Making the diagnosis of Alzheimer's disease. *Patient Care, 29*(11), 104–120.

Harvard Mental Health Letter (2006). As a man (or woman) grows older. Retrieved from https://www.health.harvard.edu/newsletter_article/In_Brief_As_a_man_or_woman_grows_older

Hayflick, L. (1994). *How and why we age.* New York, NY: Ballantine.

Hering, A., Meuleman, B., Bürki, C., Borella, E., & Kliegel, M. (2017). Improving older adults' working memory: The influence of age and crystallized intelligence on training outcomes. *Journal of Cognitive Enhancement, 1*(4), 358–373.

Herzog, A. R., & Wallace, R. B. (1997). Measures of cognitive functioning in the AHEAD study. *The Journals of Gerontology, Series B, 52B,* 37–48.

Hoyer, W. J., & Verhaeghen, P. (2006). Memory aging. In J. E. Birren & K. W. Schaie (Eds.), *Handbook of the psychology of aging* (pp. 209–232). Burlington, MA: Elsevier.

Hultsch, D. F., Hertzog, C., Dixon, R. A., & Small, B. J. (1998). *Memory change in the aged.* Cambridge, UK: Cambridge University Press.

Hultsch, D., Hertzog, C., Small, B., McDonald-Miszcak, L., & Dixon, R. (1991). Short-term longitudinal change in cognitive performance in later life. *Psychology and Aging, 7,* 571–584.

Humes, L. E, Busey, T. A., Craig, J., & Kewley-Port, D. (2013). Are age-related changes in cognitive function driven by age-related changes in sensory processing? *Attention, Perception, & Psychophysics, 75*(3), 508–524.

Jaeggi, S. M., Buschkuehl, M., Jonides, J., & Perrig, W. J. (2008). Improving fluid intelligence with training on working memory. *Proceedings of the National Academy of Sciences, 105*(19), 6829–6833.

Jeste, D. V., Depp, C. A., & Vahia, I. V. (2010). Successful cognitive and emotional aging. *World Psychiatry, 9*(2), 78–84.

Jones, C. L., Jensen, J. D., Scherr, C. L., Brown, N. R., Christy, K., & Weaver, J. (2015). The Health Belief Model as an explanatory framework in communication research: Exploring parallel, serial, and moderated mediation. *Health Communication, 30*(6), 566–576.

Joslyn, H. (2016, September). Words that change minds. *Chronicle of Philanthropy,* 20–24.

Juratovac, E. (1996). The Ohio Nurses Association presents "Anxiety and depression in older adults": An independent study. *Ohio Nurses Review, 71*(3), 4–13.

Katzman, R., Brown, T., Fuld, P., Peck. A., Schechter, R., & Schimmel, H. (1983). Validation of a short orientation-memory concentration test of cognitive impairment. *American Journal of Psychiatry, 140,* 734–739.

Kelly, M. E., Loughrey, D., Lawlor, B. A., Robertson, I. H., Walsh, C., & Brennan, S. (2014). The impact of cognitive training and mental stimulation on cognitive and everyday functioning of healthy older adults: A systematic review and meta-analysis. *Ageing Research Reviews, 15,* 28–43.

Kersting, K. (2003). Personality changes for the better with age. *Monitor on Psychology. In Brief. American Psychological Association, 34*(7), 14.

Keyser, S. E., Buchanan, D., & Edge, D. (2012). Providing delirium education for family caregivers of older adults. *Journal of Gerontological Nursing, 38*(8), 24–31.

Kim, E. S., Kawachi, I., Chen, Y., & Kubzansky, L. D. (2017). Association between purpose in life and objective measures of physical function in older adults. *Journal of the American Medical Association Psychiatry, 74*(10), 1039–1045.

Kim, S., & Hasher, L. (2005). The attraction effect in decision making: Superior performance by older adults. *Quarterly Journal of Experimental Psychology, 58A*(1), 120–133.

Kirova, A. M., Bays, R. B., & Lagalwar, S. (2015). Working memory and executive function decline across normal aging, mild cognitive impairment, and Alzheimer's disease. *BioMed Research International,* 2015. doi:10.1155/2015/748212

Knight, R. G., & Godfrey, H. P. D. (1995). Behavioral and self-report methods. In A. D. Baddeley, B. A. Wilson, & F. N. Watts (Eds.), *The handbook of memory disorders.* Chichester, UK: John Wiley and Sons.

Langa, K. M., & Levine, D. A. (2014). The diagnosis and management of mild cognitive impairment: A clinical review. *Journal of the American Medical Association, 312*(23), 2551–2561.

Levy, B. R. (2003). Mind matters: Cognitive and physical effects of aging self-stereotypes. *Journals of Gerontology, Series B: Psychological Sciences and Social Sciences, 58B*(4), P203–P211.

Levy, B. R. (2009). Stereotype embodiment: A psychosocial approach to aging. *Current Directions in Psychological Science, 18*(6), 332–336.

Li, K. Z., & Lindenberger, U. (2002). Relations between aging sensory/sensorimotor and cognitive functions. *Neuroscience & Biobehavioral Reviews, 26*(7), 777–783.

Lichtenberger, E. O., & Kaufman, A. S. (2012). *Essentials of WAIS-IV Assessment.* Hoboken, NJ: Wiley.

Llorca, P. M., Pereira, B., Jardri, R., Chereau-Boudet, I., Brousse, G., Misdrahi, D., … Marques, A. (2016). Hallucinations in schizophrenia and Parkinson's disease: An analysis of sensory modalities involved and the repercussion on patients. *Scientific Reports,* 6, 38152. doi:10.1038/srep38152. Retrieved from https://www.nature.com/articles/srep38152

Lustig, C., & Lin, Z. (2016). Memory: Behavior and neural basis. In K. W. Schaie, S. Willis, B. G. Knight, B. Levy & D. C. Park (Eds.), *Handbook of the psychology of aging,* 8th ed. (pp. 147–164). Amsterdam: Elsevier.

Maguire, E. A., Woollett, K., & Spiers, H. J. (2006). London taxi drivers and bus drivers: A structural MRI and neuropsychological analysis. *Hippocampus,* 16, 1091–1101.

Malek-Ahmadi, M., Davis, K., Belden, C. M., Jacobson, S., Sabbagh, M. N. (2012). Informant-reported cognitive symptoms that predict amnestic mild cognitive impairment. *BMC Geriatrics,* 12, 3. doi:10.1186/1471-2318-12-3.

Malhotra, R. K., & Desai, A. K. (2010). Healthy brain aging: What has sleep got to do with it? *Clinics in Geriatric Medicine, 26*(1), 45–56.

Mattis, J., & Sehgal, A. (2016). Circadian rhythms, sleep, and disorders of aging. *Trends in Endocrinology & Metabolism, 27*(4), 192–203.

Mayo Clinic. (2013). Mild Cognitive Impairment. Retrieved from http://www.mayoclinic.com/health/mildcognitive-impairment/DS00553

Mayo Clinic. (2016). Exercise: Seven benefits of regular exercise. Retrieved 1/23/2017 from http://www.mayoclinic.org/healthy-lifestyle/fitness/in-depth/exercise/art-20048389

Mayo Clinic. (n.d.). Depression: Major depressive disorder. Retrieved 12/17/2017 from https://www.mayoclinic.org/diseases-conditions/depression/diagnosis-treatment/drc-20356013

McAdams, D. P., & Olson, B. D. (2012). Personality development: Continuity and change over the life course. *Annual Review of Psychology, 61,* 517–542. doi:10.1146/annurev.psych.093008.100507

McCarthy, V. L., Hall, L. A., Crawford, T. N., & Connelly, J. (2017, February). Facilitating self-transcendence: An intervention to enhance well-being in late life. *Western Journal of Nursing Research.* doi: 0193945917690731.

McCrae, R. R., & Costa, P. T. (1990). *Personality in adulthood.* New York: Guilford Press.

Metz, A. E., & Robnett, R. (2011). Engaging in mentally challenging occupations promotes cognitive health throughout life. *Gerontology Special Interest Section Quarterly, 34*(2), 1–4.

Miller, W. R., & Rollnick, S. (2013). *Motivational interviewing: Helping people change* (3rd ed.). New York: Guilford.

Morris, J. C. (1993, November). The Clinical Dementia Rating (CDR): Current version and scoring rules. *Neurology, 43*(11), 2412–2414.

Mõttus, R., Johnson, W., & Deary, I. J. (2012). Personality traits in old age: Measurement and rank-order stability and some mean-level change. *Psychology and Aging, 27*(1), 243.

Muliyala, K. P., & Varghese, M. (2010). The complex relationship between depression and dementia. *Annals of Indian Academy of Neurology, 13*(Suppl. 2), S69.

Mitchell, A. J., & Shiri-Feshki, M. (2009). Rate of progression of mild cognitive impairment to dementia–meta-analysis of 41 robust inception cohort studies. *Acta Psychiatrica Scandinavica, 119*(4), 252–265.

Nasreddine, Z. S., Phillips, N. A., Bédirian, V., Charbonneau, S., Whitehead, V., Collin, I., ... Chertkow, H. (2005). The Montreal Cognitive Assessment, MoCA: A brief screening tool for mild cognitive impairment. *Journal of the American Geriatrics Society, 53*(4), 695–699.

National Institute for Mental Health. (2017). Suicide prevention. Retrieved from https://www.nimh.nih.gov/health/topics/suicide-prevention/index.shtml

Neufeld, E., & O'Rourke, N. (2009). Impulsivity and hopelessness as predictors of suicide-related ideation among older adults. *Canadian Journal of Psychiatry, 54*(10), 684–692.

Nussbaum, P. D. (2003). *Brain health and wellness.* Tarentum, PA: Word Association.

Nussbaum, P. D. (2011). Brain health: Bridging neuroscience to consumer application. *Generations, 35*(2), 6–12.

O'Shea, D. M., Dotson, V. M., & Fieo, R. A. (2017). Aging perceptions and self-efficacy mediate the association between personality traits and depressive symptoms in older adults. *International Journal of Geriatric Psychiatry, 32*(12), 1217–1225. doi: 10.1002/gps.4584.

Palmer, R. M. (1990). "Failure to thrive" in the elderly: Diagnosis and management. *Geriatrics, 45*(9), 47–55.

Park, D. C., & Festini, S. B. (2017). Theories of memory and aging: A look at the past and a glimpse of the future. *The Journals of Gerontology: Series B, 72*(1), 82–90.

Parkin, A. J., & Java, R. I. (2000). Determinants of age-related memory loss. In T. J. Perfect & E. A. Maylor (Eds.), *Models of cognitive aging* (pp. 188–203). Oxford, UK: Oxford University Press.

Pasricha, N. (2016). *The happiness equation: Want nothing + do anything = have everything.* New York, NY: Putnam.

Patenaude, J. (1996). Nutrient deficiency-related depression and mental changes in elderly persons. *Home Health Care Management and Practice, 9*(1), 29–39.

Perlmutter, M. (1988). Cognitive potential throughout life. In J. E. Birren & V. L. Bengston (Eds.), *Emergent theories of aging* (pp. 247–268). New York, NY: Springer.

Possin, K. L. (2010). Visual spatial cognition in neurodegenerative disease. *Neurocase, 16*(6), 466–487.

Prochaska, J. O., Norcross, J. C., & DiClemente, C. C. (1995). *Changing for good.* New York, NY: Avon Books.

Rebeiro, K. L., & Polgar, J. M. (1999). Enabling occupational performance: Optimal experiences in therapy. *Canadian Journal of Occupational Therapy, 66*(1), 14–22.

Reed, A. E., Chan, L., & Mikels, J. A. (2014). Meta-analysis of the age-related positivity effect: Age differences in preferences for positive over negative information. *Psychology and Aging, 29*(1), 1–15.

Reed, B. R., Dowling, M., Farias, S. T., Sonnen, J., Strauss, M., Schneider, J. A., ... Mungas, D. (2011). Cognitive activities during adulthood are more important than education in building reserve. *Journal of the International Neuropsychological Society, 17*(4), 615–624.

Reisberg, B. (1988). Functional Assessment Staging (FAST). *Psychopharmacology Bulletin, 24*, 653–659.

Roberts, R., & Knopman, D. S. (2013). Classification and epidemiology of MCI. *Clinics in Geriatric Medicine, 29*(4), 753–772.

Robnett, R. (2015). Staying Sharp: The Cutting Edge of Research on Cognition and Aging. Maine Geriatrics Society presentation. Retrieved from http://dune.une.edu/ot_facpres/2/

Robnett, R. H. (2008). Client factors and their effect on occupational performance in late life. In S. Coppola, S. J. Elliott, & P .E. Toto (Eds.), *Strategies to advance gerontology excellence* (pp. 163–197). Bethesda, MD: AOTA Press.

Rosenstock, I. M. (1974). Historical origins of the health belief model. *Health Education Monographs, 2*(4), 328–335.

Rowe, T. A., & Juthani-Mehta, M. (2013). Urinary tract infection in older adults. *Aging Health, 9*(5), 519–528.

Ryan, E. B. (1992). Beliefs about memory changes across the adult lifespan. *Journal of Gerontology: Psychological Sciences, 47*, 41–46.

Sachdev, P. S., Lipnicki, D. M., Crawford, J., Reppermund, S., Kochan, N. A., Troller, J. N, ... Kang, K. (2013). Factors predicting reversion from mild cognitive impairment to normal cognitive functioning: A population-based study. *PLoS ONE, 8*(3), e59649, 1–10. doi:10.1371/journal.pone.0059649

Salthouse, T. A. (1999). Pressing issues in cognitive aging. In D.C. Park and N. Schwartz, (Eds.), *Cognitive aging: A primer* (Chapter 3). Philadelphia: Psychology Press.

Schachter-Shalomi, Z., & Miller, R. (1995). *From age-ing to sage-ing: A profound new vision of growing older.* New York: Warner.

Schaie, K. W. (1996). *Intellectual development in adulthood: The Seattle Longitudinal Study.* New York: Cambridge University Press.

Schaie, G. W., Willis, S., Knight, B. G., Levy, B., & Park, D. C. (2016). *Handbook on the psychology of aging* (8th ed.). Amsterdam: Elsevier.

Scheibe, S., & Carstensen, L. L. (2010). Emotional aging: Recent findings and future trends. *The Journals of Gerontology Series B: Psychological Sciences and Social Sciences, 65*(2), 135–144.

Souren, L. E., Frensses, E. H., & Reisberg, B. (1995). Contractures and loss of function in patients with Alzheimer's disease. *Journal of the American Geriatrics Society, 43*(6), 650–655.

Span, P. (2010). Schooling the aging brain. *New York Times.* Retrieved from https://newoldage.blogs.nytimes.com/2010/01/26/using-it-or-losing-it/

Sparacino, B. (2013). Substance use and abuse in older adults. MAGEC Mental Health Module. Retrieved from http://www.centeronaging.med.miami.edu/documents/substanceuseandabuseamongolderadults.pdf

Stern, Y. (2006). Cognitive reserve and Alzheimer disease. *Alzheimer Disease & Associated Disorders, 20*(2), 112–117.

Stern, Y. (2009). Cognitive reserve. *Neuropsychologia, 47*(10), 2015–2028.

Stobbe, K., & Carter, M. (2016). Using improv to improve life with Alzheimer's. Retrieved from https://www.youtube.com/watch?v=GciWItvLo_s

Straus, C. (2009). Strategies for Improving Memory. Retrieved from http://psychcentral.com/lib/2009/strategies-for-improving-memory/

Strauss, C. J. & Khachaturian, Z. S. (2002). *Talking to Alzheimer's: Simple ways to connect when you visit with a family member or friend.* Oakland, CA: New Harbinger Publications.

Substance Abuse and Mental Health Services Administration. (SAMHSA, n.d.). Retrieved from https://www.integration.samhsa.gov/clinical-practice/sbirt

Tamura-Lis, W. (2017). Reminiscing—A tool for excellent elder care and improved quality of life. *Urologic Nursing, 37*(3), 151–158.

Tariq, S. H., Tumosa, N., Chibnall, J. T., Perry III, H. M., & Morley, J. E. (2006). The Saint Louis University Mental Status (SLUMS) examination for detecting mild cognitive impairment and dementia is more sensitive than the mini-mental status examination (MMSE)—A pilot study. *American Journal of Geriatric Psychiatry, 14*(11), 900–910.

Teo, A. R., Choi, H., Andrea, S. B., Valenstein, M., Newsom, J. T., Dobscha, S. K., & Zivin, K. (2015). Does mode of contact with different types of social relationships predict depression in older adults? Evidence from a nationally representative survey. *Journal of the American Geriatrics Society, 63*(10), 2014–2022.

Thakur, M., & Blazer, D. G. (2008). Depression in long-term care. *Journal of the American Medical Directors Association, 9*(2), 82–87.

Thomas, A. J., & O'Brien, J. T. (2008). Depression and cognition in older adults. *Current Opinion in Psychiatry, 21*(1), 8–13.

Tun, P. A., & Wingfield, A. (1995). Does dividing attention become harder with age? Findings for the divided attention questionnaire. *Aging and Cognition, 2*(1), 39–66.

Turner, J., Greenawalt, K., Goodwin, S., Rathie, E., & Orsega-Smith, E. (2017). The development and implementation of the Art of Happiness intervention for community-dwelling older adults. *Educational Gerontology, 43*(12), 630–640.

Valentijn, S. A., van Boxtel, M. P., van Hooren, S. A., Bosma, H., Beckers, H. J., Ponds, R. W., & Jolles, J. (2005). Change in sensory functioning predicts change in cognitive functioning: Results from a 6-year follow-up in the Maastricht Aging Study. *Journal of the American Geriatric Society, 53*, 374–380. doi:10.1111/j.1532-5415.2005.53152.x

Vasilevskis, E. E., Jan, J. H., Hughes, C. G., & Ely, E. W. (2012). Epidemiology and risk factors for delirium across hospital settings. *Best Practice and Research in Clinical Anaesthesiology, 26*, 277–287. doi:10.1016/j.bpa.2012.07.003

Verhaeghen, P., & Cerella, J. (2002). Aging, executive control, and attention: A review of meta-analyses. *Neuroscience and Biobehavioral Reviews, 26*(7), 849–857.

Waszynski, C. M. (2003). The Confusion Assessment Method (CAM). *Annals of Internal Medicine, 113*(12), 941–948. Retrieved from https://www.nhqualitycampaign.org/files/CAM_Confusion_Assessment_Instrument.pdf

Weiss, A., Costa, P. T., Karuza, J., Duberstein, P. R., Friedman, B., & McCrae, R. R. (2005). Cross sectional age differences in personality among Medicare patients aged 65 to 100. *Psychology and Aging, 20*(1), 182–185.

Welton, R. S. (2007). The management of suicidality: Assessment and intervention. *Psychiatry (Edgmont), 4*(5), 24.

West, R. (1999). Visual distraction, working memory, and aging. *Memory and Cognition, 27*(6), 1064–1072.

Wheeler, M. A. (2000). A comparison of forgetting rates in older and younger adults. *Aging, Neuropsychology, and Cognition, 7*(3), 179–193.

Wilckens, K. A., Woo, S. G., Kirk, A. R., Erickson, K. I., & Wheeler, M. E. (2014). Role of sleep continuity and total sleep time in executive function across the adult lifespan. *Psychology and Aging, 29*(3), 658.

Wilson, R. S., Hebert, L. E., Scherr, P. A., Barnes, L. L., De Leon, C. M., & Evans, D. A. (2009). Educational attainment and cognitive decline in old age. *Neurology, 72*(5), 460–465.

Wood, D., & Roberts, B.W. (2006). The effect of age and role information on expectations for big five personality traits. *Personality and Social Psychology Bulletin, 32*(11), 1482–1496.

Xu, W., Yu, J. T., Tan, M. S., & Tan, L. (2015). Cognitive reserve and Alzheimer's disease. *Molecular Neurobiology, 51*(1), 187–208.

Young, J., Angevaren, M., Rusted, J., & Tabet, N. (2015). Aerobic exercise to improve cognitive function in older people without known cognitive impairment. *Cochrane Database of Systematic Reviews, 4*, CD005381. doi:10.1002/14651858.CD005381.pub4

Zec, R. F. (1995). The neuropsychology of aging. *Experimental Gerontology, 30*, 431–442.

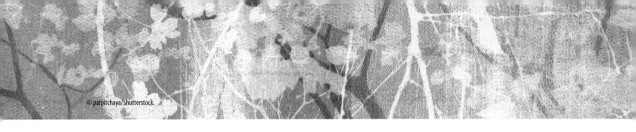

CHAPTER 9

Functional Performance in Later Life: Basic Sensory, Perceptual, and Physical Changes Associated With Aging

Jessica J. Bolduc, DrOT, MS, OTR/L

CHAPTER OUTLINE

BEHAVIORAL OBJECTIVES

Upon completion of this chapter, the reader will be able to:

1. List at least four recommendations for healthcare professionals who work with people who have diminished visual skills.
2. Define visual perception and describe how perceptual skills may change as one ages.
3. Describe compensatory measures related to decreased visual perceptual functioning.
4. Describe how sensory systems tend to change over the course of aging, impacting function.
5. List compensatory measures for each of the sensory changes related to aging.
6. List at least four recommendations for healthcare professionals who work with people who are hard of hearing.
7. Describe the basic physical changes of aging related to range of motion, strength, motor control, and endurance.
8. Discuss how physical changes affect performance in various life skills, including self-care and work.
9. Describe how sleep patterns change with age.
10. Describe the components of interventions related to sleep disorders, including cognitive behavioral therapy.

KEY TERMS

Agnosia	Insomnia	Range of motion
Anosmia	Maximum muscle strength	Reaction time
Apraxia	Motor coordination	Restless leg syndrome
Cognitive behavioral therapy	Obstructive sleep apnea	Scotoma
Contracture	Olfaction	Senescence
Dyspraxia	Perception	Sleep hygiene
Endurance	Praxis	Sleep restriction
Hyposmia	Presbycusis	Stimulus control

▶ Introduction

Ironically, change may be the only constant in our lives. This chapter explores the sensory, perceptual, and physical changes associated with the aging process. The intent of the chapter is to provide a brief overview of these potential changes and to provide suggestions that may help the healthcare professional in assisting older adults who have experienced these age-related changes in these realms.

Healthcare professionals who are rehabilitation specialists, such as occupational and physical therapists and speech-language pathologists, are the experts in the realm of sensory, perceptual, and physical changes, including how to remediate dysfunction or how to compensate for the problems not amenable to restoration. These professionals are skilled at in-depth interventions to improve functional performance based on extensive professional theories and evidence-based research and practice. Although intended to be helpful to rehabilitation specialists and other healthcare professionals, including students, this chapter is not a comprehensive manual for intervention. Each of the mentioned professions has textbooks focusing precisely on the topics in this chapter. The interested reader can view this chapter as an introduction or review; readers with the skill and motivation can go for more in-depth information through additional reading and education.

In this chapter, the focus is on the typical physical, sensory, and perceptual changes taking place within the aging body, especially as these changes relate to function. **Senescence** or the process of physical decline due to aging does occur, but often at a slower and more variable rate than is customarily believed.

An important aspect to consider, along with these physical and sensory changes related to aging, is associated performance levels. Even though the described changes are rarely outwardly encouraging, nonetheless daily functioning throughout life can remain adequate or even good given enough determination, good fortune, the right genes, as well as the absence of disease. Regardless, it is important to remember that within our growing aging population, approximately 63% of adults aged 65–75, 78% of adults aged 75–84, and 83% of adults 85 and 85+ have multiple chronic health conditions (Centers for Disease Control and Prevention [CDC], 2015). The most common chronic conditions now facing Americans are heart disease, cancer, and diabetes (CDC, 2015). Yet, most persons with chronic conditions are still able to live well and are able to improve their functioning with a little assistance or a bit of education to promote small changes. This chapter starts with an overview of sensation, including vision, hearing, **olfaction**, and taste followed by an overview of physical changes, physical performance, and sleep. Emphasis is placed on what a healthcare professional needs to know when working with older adults in various capacities.

▶ Vision

Vision typically begins to deteriorate around age 30 although older adults typically are able to maintain an acuity level close to unimpaired vision (20/20) with corrective lenses until about age 88 (**FIGURE 9-1**; Schieber, 2006). In addition to loss in acuity, the aging eye is vulnerable to diseases that can permanently damage the ability to see. For an overview of common visual conditions that occur in older adults, see **TABLE 9-1**.

While diseases can rob people of perfect vision, other visual skills known to show a decline with advancing age are:

- Visual processing speed
- Sensitivity to light
- Ability to see well in dim light
- Near vision, especially problematic for reading small print
- Upward gaze without moving head
- Contrast sensitivity, separate from visual acuity
- Color sensitivity, especially along the blue–yellow axis of color
- Dynamic vision, which includes:
  - Smooth visual pursuits of a moving target (such as watching the movement of a tennis ball), especially with distractions or with increased velocity of targets.

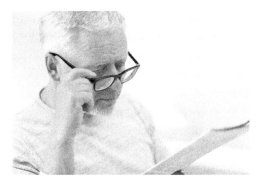

FIGURE 9-1 Corrective lenses often allow older adults to maintain their vision well into their 80s and beyond.
© Syda Productions/Shutterstock

TABLE 9-1 Common Visual Diagnoses and Functional Implications in Older Adults

Disease of the Eye	Prevalence by Age	Functional Implications
Cataracts	50–54 (5%)[a] 80+ (68%)[a]	World appears dull, as if seeing through dusty or cloudy lens; readily amenable to treatment, usually on an outpatient basis
Age-related macular degeneration (AMD)	50–54 (<0.05%)[a] 80+ (<12%)[a]	Central field vision is impaired, affecting reading and other fine detail work. Reading skills are especially impaired compared to controls when the wording is out of context[b]
Glaucoma	50–54 (<1%)[a] 80+ (<8%)[a]	Loss of peripheral vision, usually gradually; may lead to tunnel vision or total blindness
Diabetic retinopathy (DR)[c]	40–49 (7–31%) 75+ (12–23%)	The person with diabetes and DR has **scotomas** (i.e., blind spots); visual skills may fluctuate; may be associated with depressed mood
Retinal detachment	10–12.5 of 100,000 population annually (approximately 0.001%), typically between ages 40 and 70[d]	Tearing or separation of retina from underlying tissue that can be caused by trauma or illness[e]
Dry eyes	48–91 (14%)[f]	Poor lubrication of the eye due to poor tear production[e]

Data from [a] Schieber (2006). [b] Lott, Schneck, Haegerstrom-Portnoy, Hewlett, & Brabyn (2017). [c] Eye Diseases Prevalence Research Group, Diabetic Retinopathy Subsection (2004). [d] Larkin (2009). [e] American Optometric Association (2013). [f] Gayton (2009).

- Visual tracking or saccades, the small ballistic eye movements needed for reading (although decline with age is less than for pursuits; Schieber, 2006). In fact, older adults use anticipatory saccades (or predictive visual tracking) to maintain their tracking skills well into old age (Maruta, Spielman, Rajashekar, & Ghajar, 2017).

Visual skills that tend to be preserved with age include basic color vision and the ability to maintain fixation on a target. After age 70, remaining visually fixated on an object decreases with age (Wolters Kluwer Health, 2014). The healthcare professional working with older persons may offer several simple compensatory measures to mitigate the effects of decreased eyesight. **TABLE 9-2** outlines some of these measures. Although the measures can be helpful, it is not an inclusive list nor can it be expected to address the needs of all clients. If the older person is having difficulty with daily tasks because of impaired visual skills, a certified low vision therapist (CLVT; i.e., a person who works exclusively with blind persons and persons with visual impairment), a behavioral optometrist, or an occupational therapist may be of assistance.

TABLE 9-2 Selected Compensatory Measures Related to Specific Visual Impairments

Visual Impairment	Compensatory Measures
Decreased visual acuity	▪ Corrective lenses (clean and in good repair) ▪ Larger print—font size 12–14 points ▪ Larger images/signs ▪ Magnifiers ▪ Closed-circuit television (a device to magnify objects or written material) ▪ Tactile cues for phone, oven, or microwave dials/buttons
Central vision loss	▪ Visual scanning training and eccentric viewing
Increased sensitivity to light	▪ Use nonreflective materials on walls, floors, and ceilings (environmental modifications) ▪ Use yellow film to reduce glare ▪ Wear protective lenses ▪ Shield eyes from bright lightbulbs ▪ Provide overhangs on windows
Decreased ability to see in dim light	▪ Use task lighting directed at work area and/or overhead lighting to also reduce glare (environmental modification) ▪ Use nightlights ▪ Avoid driving at night, dawn, or dusk
Decreased ability to see contrasts	▪ Use black with white or yellow contrasts ▪ Highlight obstacles or changes in floor surface levels (environmental modification) ▪ Avoid difficult color discriminations, such as blue/green when safety is a concern (otherwise, a safety pin on the waistband of a blue pair of pants can distinguish them from a similar green or black pair) ▪ Avoid moving from dark to/from light areas too quickly, give the eyes time to adjust

Data from American Occupational Therapy Association; Charness & Bosman (1990); Zoltan (1996); Pizzimenti & Roberts (2005); Warren (2013).

Visual Perception

Perception refers to the brain's ability to make sense of incoming sensory information. Typically, perception not only refers to being able to interpret visual data, but it can also refer to auditory, olfactory, and gustatory sensation as well. One must have the foundation of adequate visual acuity for visual perception to be intact. Unlike visual acuity, visual perceptual skills do not show a uniform decline with aging. Kim and colleagues (2014) studied the visual perceptual skills of an aging population and found that poor visual perception skills were related to aging, but were more likely a correlate or symptom of cognitive decline. However, in reverse, impaired memory may also impact visual perceptual skills

(James & Kooy, 2011). In a study by Lindfield, Wingfield, and Bowles (1994), the older adult participants actually were able to identify fragmented pictures more accurately than their younger counterparts, perhaps because of their vast sensory experience perceiving the world. Even with decreased sensory functioning, older adults may become more proficient at inferring meanings from less sensory input, but they may have difficulty distinguishing novel items (James & Kooy, 2011; Lindfield et al., 1994). Older adults also tend to be slower at processing the information and take in less visual information per unit of time.

Decreases in perceptual skills such as **agnosia** (i.e., not understanding what common objects are used for), loss of spatial awareness (e.g., right/left, back/front), and impaired visual constructional abilities (e.g., completing puzzles, assembling common objects) are not usually associated with typical aging to any notable degree. When perception goes awry, the problem is usually related to a disease process such as dementia, stroke (cerebrovascular accident), or a psychiatric disorder. Intact perceptual skills generally are necessary for typical or normal everyday living. For example, imagine if a toothbrush and comb were indistinguishable. After a stroke, those with decreased visual perception (form recognition) may reach for the toothbrush to brush their hair. Rehabilitation specialists such as occupational therapists can work with individuals who have perceptual difficulties in adapting the environment (e.g., decreasing clutter) and adapting daily tasks (e.g., using simpler clothing) to promote functional performance.

▶ Hearing

Hearing is another sensory modality with a tendency to decline with age. **Presbycusis** (i.e., hearing loss) occurs in both genders, but men especially tend to lose the ability to hear higher frequencies. Older adults have more difficulty distinguishing higher pitched consonant sounds, although understanding lower pitched vowel sounds tends to remain intact. Additionally, older adults tend not to be able to recall earlier conversations when the number of words spoken per minute is high (Glyde, Hickson, Cameron, & Dillon, 2011). Persons of all ages are able to recall more verbal information if the words are spoken in the context of normal sentences rather than in random word strings. However, older adults' accuracy decreased more dramatically than did the younger participants with unrelated words (Fozard, 1990).

Older women are more likely than older men to report hearing loss and compensate by searching for nonverbal cues during conversation. They are also more likely than men to seek treatment as it relates to their ability to communicate and relate to others (**FIGURE 9-2**). In contrast, older men, who are actually more likely to have hearing loss than women, are more likely to deny a problem and not seek treatment as it could be perceived as a sign of weakness or denial that there are problems (Bainbridge & Wallhagen, 2014).

Mild hearing loss doubles for every decade past the age of 50 and is often worsened by repeated or on-going exposure to high-intensity sound (Bainbridge & Wallhagen, 2014). Older

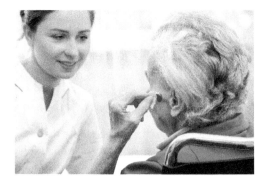

FIGURE 9-2 More women than men are likely to seek treatment for hearing loss, including getting assessed for a hearing aid.
© Alexander Raths/Shutterstock

adults also tend to have more difficulty tuning out background noise (Glyde et al., 2011), which often leads to discomfort or frustration during noisy social gatherings and may deter them from engaging with people in their surroundings. Consequently, having a hearing impairment may lead to social isolation. In large-scale longitudinal studies, researchers found that older adults with hearing impairments reported feelings of loneliness and anxiety due to social isolation caused by hearing loss (Contrera et al., 2017; Pronk et al., 2014). Not surprisingly, individuals with hearing loss had fewer people in their social network. Also, if they were widowed, they were even more at risk for social isolation than their married counterparts, as they had fewer social connections.

Being socially isolated can lead to mental decline due to the lack of cognitive stimulation. During conversations, people with hearing loss tend to rely on their cognitive reserve (i.e., ability to improvise or compensate for loss). Hearing loss is associated with a higher risk factor for being diagnosed with dementia. However, whether the hearing loss is associated with cognitive decline as a cause or whether it is a potentially modifiable risk factor (e.g., through surgery to correct hearing loss) still has not been definitively determined (Golub et al., 2017; Lin et al., 2011).

Scientific findings coupled with professional expertise suggest the following recommendations for healthcare professionals working with older adults with hearing loss:

■ Speak in a tone that can be heard. Although some older individuals may need you to increase your volume or decibel level, do not assume this is needed. More likely, the person who has difficulty hearing will need you to lower the pitch of your voice. Therefore, ask each person what works best for him or her.

■ Whenever possible, face people so they can see your lips when you speak. Begin conversations by saying their name to get their attention. Make and maintain normal eye contact, and keep your hands away from your face and mouth to enable lip reading. Speak in a clear and natural manner (Cleveland Clinic Foundation, 2012c).

■ Be sure your rate of speech is not too fast, but not so slow as to sound condescending. When necessary, rephrase what you have just said rather than repeat.

■ Avoid elderspeak, which is described as baby talk for older adults (e.g., use of more diminutives, slower speech, more repetition, and simpler words with fewer syllables; AARP, 2017). Even though older adults may have difficulty hearing, they should not be talked to as if they have lost their cognitive capacity.

■ Whenever possible, keep background noise to a minimum.

■ Do not jump from one idea to the next too quickly in conversation. Older adults are more likely to rely on the context of what is being said in order to understand the conversation.

▶ Smell

Other sensory perceptions that change over time include olfaction (i.e., smell) and taste. Declines in these closely related senses can have psychological implications. The ability to detect smells in general and correctly identify discrete odors decreases with age. Thus, older adults age 65 and older experience a high prevalence of **hyposmia** (i.e., decreased smell sensation) and **anosmia** (i.e., complete loss of smell) and most people older than age 80 have some level of impaired olfaction (Attems, Walker, & Jellinger, 2015). A large study by Mullol and colleagues (2012) found that nearly 20% of adults in the general population experienced impairment in smell, with women outperforming men in smell tasks across all age groups.

As people age, the sense of smell tends to decline insidiously, and therefore go unnoticed for some time. Such limited awareness of decline can constitute a serious safety issue for persons wishing to remain independent in their own homes. Hyposmia or anosmia have been consistently linked to decreased safety, poor nutrition, and decreased quality of life. Both conditions are also predictive of mortality. Moreover, olfactory impairments are also believed to be a prodromal symptom for Parkinson's and Alzheimer's diseases (Dong et al., 2017). Compensatory strategies to reduce risk to health and safety include installing natural gas/smoke detectors and having someone else with a normal sense of smell routinely check for spoilage of food. Loss of smell is also associated with depressive symptoms and lower quality of life, and can negatively impact enjoyment of food, drink, and socialization (Gopinath, Kaarin, Sue, Kifley, & Mitchell, 2011). Olfaction also informs taste sensation. A decreased sense of smell can decrease pleasure in eating, which over time can increase the potential for malnutrition.

▶ Taste

As people age, their ability to detect salty, bitter, and sour tastes decreases, and the threshold of salty flavor needed for detection increases however, the ability to taste sweets does not appear to change with age (Methven, Allen, Withers, & Gosney, 2012). These sensory changes may contribute to an overreliance on sweets and the oversalting of food.

Adequate hydration is needed for fluid and electrolyte balance and proper body function throughout life, yet thirst sensation declines as one ages (Goldberg et al., 2014). Other factors, besides advanced age that increase the risk of dehydration, include memory impairments, Parkinson's disease, Alzheimer's disease, stroke, or any other health condition that can cause dysphagia (i.e., difficulty swallowing; Goldberg et al., 2014).

A limited diet and inadequate dietary intake may actually cause losses in taste perception as the number of taste buds decreases due to malnutrition or as a side effect of medication. Appetite can also decrease due to the sense of fullness and early satiation caused by age or disease-related changes in the gastrointestinal tract (Ahmed & Haboubi, 2010). Collectively, these factors point to the extreme importance of maintaining an adequate diet, especially as we age. (For more details on nutrition see Chapter 11).

▶ Physical Changes

Not surprisingly, physical changes also take place as we age. This section introduces the reader to some of the primary changes that occur. While not always the consequence of living a long life, these changes occur more frequently in old age.

Range of Motion

Range of motion (ROM) refers to the ability of a joint to move through its natural pattern of movement. For example, the shoulder of a typical healthy person can flex up (toward the sky) nearly straight (about 170°; Soucie et al., 2011). This amount of movement is considered normal for that joint. In fact, every joint in the body has a typical range of movement.

Declines in joint ROM in the shoulder, hip, and wrist are known to occur with age, up to 5–6 degrees per decade after age 55 (Stathokostas, McDonald, Little, & Paterson, 2013). However, chronological age alone is not as likely to affect ROM as much as some age-related conditions, which can restrict smooth movements and limit maximum ROM. Specifically, arthritis; joint or muscle disuse, misuse, or overuse; injuries; stroke; Parkinson's disease; and dementia are associated with less than optimal movement patterns. Arthritis is the most common cause of disability in the United States, with more than 50 million people (approximately 50% of adults over age 65) living with the functional limitations and losses associated with its various forms (CDC, 2012).

Nonresistive, repetitive ROM exercises can be useful in maintaining or improving current range of movement, or may slow down the progression of disease processes as in the case of osteoarthritis (Mayo Clinic, 2016). Physicians and other professionals who are experts in movement (e.g., physical and occupational therapists) can help older persons work toward their best possible performance by developing personal movement programs suited to their needs (**FIGURE 9-3**). These prescribed exercise programs can potentially stave off loss of motion secondary to simple disuse or disease, maintain current range, or even increase ROM and increase strength. Regardless of a client's life situation, regular movement (especially through engagement in meaningful life tasks) can contribute to better health if the individual is able.

People who tend to be sedentary or immobile, including individuals who are bedridden for a prolonged period in the hospital or in long-term care facilities, are especially at high risk of sustaining joint contractures (i.e., stiffening of muscles and tissues leading to rigidity of joints). **Contractures** are generally caused by joint immobilization and result in decreased ROM, stiffening and subsequent structural changes, and pain upon movement at one or more joints. The joints typically affected are the hips, shoulders, fingers, and knees. The best treatment approach is to prevent contractures from occurring through regular movement and exercise/stretching. However, if remedial treatment is needed, the focus of intervention is to increase joint mobility through the use of a passive, active-assisted, or an active ROM program established by a rehabilitation specialist. If contractures are not resolved, surgical intervention may be required to reduce pain or immobility that is interrupting daily functioning (e.g., bathing, dressing, and eating).

Strength

Maximum muscle strength tends to occur in early adulthood; middle age is generally a time of only slight decline. After age 50, there is a reduction in strength, with losses tending to occur at a 15% loss in strength every 10 years (Keller & Engelhardt, 2013). However, not all individuals get progressively weaker with age. Physically capable older adults can still participate in and excel in sports requiring practice and skill such as tennis, golf, skiing, boating, and bowling (**FIGURE 9-4**). Research findings have indicated that older adults who exercise can reduce pain caused by arthritis, restore their balance and reduce the potential for falls, strengthen their bones, maintain their ideal weight, improve glucose control for diabetes management, and improve their heart health (CDC, 2011).

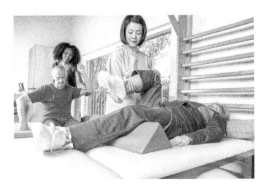

FIGURE 9-3 Physical and occupational therapists help clients improve mobility and strength.
© Gagliardi Images/Shutterstock

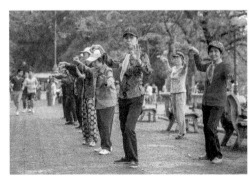

FIGURE 9-4 Practicing tai chi is a way to improve balance, strength, and agility.
© Alexander Mazurkevich/Shutterstock

By adding a prescribed exercise routine into daily life, people can improve their muscle strength. Encouraging physical activity is almost always appropriate, although the level of exertion and duration of activity needs to be determined by the person's primary healthcare provider(s), and goals related to physical fitness should be established collaboratively with the individual.

Endurance

Endurance is defined as the ability to sustain involvement in a physical activity. Lack of this physical reserve and ability to resist stressors can lead to frailty (Cadore, Pinto, Bottaro, & Izquierdo, 2014). Although not the same as strength, the two are closely intertwined. As muscle power decreases, frailty level increases (Cadore et al., 2014). The combination of endurance and strength training has been found to have a positive impact on heart and pulmonary function, improve muscle function, increase functional capacity, and improve cognition (Muscari et al., 2010; National Institutes of Health, 2012).

Physical Exercise

A meta-analysis of 13 aerobic exercise training programs for older adults demonstrated that long-term programs (more than 30 weeks in duration) were associated with improved physical endurance (Huang, Shi, Davis-Brezette, & Osness, 2005). An active lifestyle involving stretching, aerobic activity, and strength building can improve ROM, strength, and endurance. Participation in such a program may actually slow the course of physiologic aging (**FIGURE 9-5**).

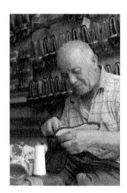
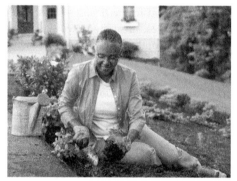
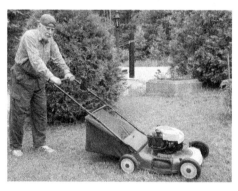

FIGURE 9-5 An active lifestyle involving activities that are mentally and physically stimulating, may actually slow the course of physiologic aging.

(top left) © asliuzunogu/Shutterstock; (top right) © Ariel Skelley/Digital Visions/Getty Images; (bottom) © Pierdelune/Shutterstock

In a recent review of both physical and mental training, Curlik and Shors (2013) found that physical exercise in rodents helped to build new brain cells, and therefore was also important for maintaining brain health. Even though aerobic activity fosters the production of new neurons in the hippocampus, it is brain activity associated with learning new skills (e.g., cognitive exercise) that helps the newly formed neurons survive over time (at least in the rodent models).

Praxis

Praxis is defined as the ability to carry out purposeful motor actions. **Dyspraxia** refers to a decreased ability to plan and/or execute purposeful movements, whereas **apraxia** is the complete inability to carry out these motor plans.

During most common routines, individuals do not need to think consciously about their performance. Simple tasks such as eating or dressing are completed automatically every day. Frequent repetition of routine goal-directed activities throughout the day (e.g., self-care, work, leisure, and housekeeping tasks) enables the conversion of once novel actions into established habits and routines. Functional performance is not lost rapidly or suddenly one day because of the aging process. However, if the level of motor (or cognitive) performance significantly decreases for any reason (e.g., injury, aging, or disease), the ability to live independently may be threatened. Often, when there is a decline in function, an overarching rehabilitation goal is to help people regain lost skills and learn to work with their remaining abilities.

▶ Physical Performance

When reviewing studies that have explored the physical performance of older adults, we find cross-sectional differences between age groups (i.e., 20-year-olds versus 80-year-olds), as well

within individuals over time (e.g., from age 60 to age 80). Genetics, lifestyle, and the presence of illness or disease can impact the onset and severity of change in physical performance. Age-related performance can be measured in several domains: reaction time, gross motor coordination (including balance and mobility), strength, endurance, and work-related performance.

Reaction Time

Perhaps, the most straightforward trend when examining performance is the slowing of **reaction time** as people reach old age. One example of a situation when a quick reaction time is needed is while driving a car and suddenly needing to yield or brake in traffic. As people age, they are not able to react as quickly as they were in their younger years. A recent study by Sventina (2016) found that reaction time and timed performance do slow significantly with age. However, there is variability among older drivers. Yet, other aging factors also need to be considered to determine an older person's fitness to drive: physical strength, mobility, cognition, and visual perception. Collectively these age-related changes challenge driver safety and performance and should be recognized and routinely examined.

Motor Coordination

Intact gross **motor coordination** (i.e., mobility or ambulation) is another crucial prerequisite to completing daily tasks without assistance. Falls affect older adults more than any other age group. An estimated one in three adults age 65 and older has at least one fall yearly. Of these 2.3 million falls, more than 800,000 resulted in hospitalization as a result of head injuries and hip fractures (CDC, 2017). Between 20% and 30% of people who fall sustain injuries such as lacerations, hip fractures, or head traumas. Injuries form falls can make it hard to ambulate or live independently, and increase the risk of early death (CDC, 2017).

In 2014, over 55,000 older adults died as a result of an unintentional fall (CDC, 2017).

Unfortunately, falling once increases the risk of falling again (Ganz, Bao, Shekelle, & Rubenstein, 2007). Repeated falls are often associated with declines in balance, coordination, and/or strength, all of which have been well researched and determined to be correlated with increased age. However, it is important to emphasize that there is variability in old age and the vast majority of older adults still have adequate levels of strength and coordination to complete their daily tasks and the activities they want to do.

Impaired ambulation may be cause for a referral to a physical therapist, who may be able to help remediate physical skills or possibly recommend assistive devices for safe ambulation. Local Area Agencies on Aging may be able to recommend local programs designed for older adults who want to improve their sense of balance (e.g., the "A Matter of Balance" program started by rehabilitation specialists at Boston University; Maine Health, 2017). There are several ways to improve postural control (i.e., exercises, sports, yoga, or tai chi) to limit the number of potential falls, by challenging balance and improving strength and agility (Gillespie et al., 2006). In conjunction with exercise, it is vital to make sure the home or living environment is clutter free and that obstacles (i.e., loose rugs, cords, and pets) are reduced so as not to present hazards. Rehabilitation specialists such as physical and occupational therapists are good resources for developing person-centered balance-related treatment strategies.

Fine motor coordination refers to hand-based skills such as writing, self-feeding, buttoning, and working with tools. When fine motor skills are impaired, as they often are in old age, the culprit is more than likely arthritis, stroke, or another skill-robbing disease rather than typical aging. When considering age alone, there is little change in the ability to complete fine motor tasks. Older adults who age typically without limitations brought on by disease are just as capable as their younger counterparts in completing fine motor tasks such as typing, cooking, knitting, and card playing. This maintenance of motor skills has two potential explanations: (1) consistent practice over the years has maintained and/or improved skill level over time, and (2) with ongoing repetition these tasks become more automatic and therefore require less skill for completion.

Any significant decreases in level of functioning, occurring either suddenly or over the course of a few weeks or months, are not generally consistent with the typical aging process and should be addressed. Abrupt behavioral changes should also send up warning flags to the older person and their families and social networks warranting a call, and probably a visit, to the person's primary care provider. The physician can then make referrals for further medical care or for rehabilitation.

▶ Work Performance

In considering age-related losses in functioning with regard to cognition, balance, reaction time, and muscle strength, one might surmise that general work performance of older workers would be inferior to that of their younger counterparts. However, this does not seem to be the case. Having health issues and being older does not significantly interfere with the quality of work. Older adults are considered more dependable (Prenda & Stahl, 2001; Reade, 2015), are less likely to be absent from work, and have fewer proportionately workplace injuries than younger workers (Ng & Feldman, 2008). They also demonstrate less workplace aggression and substance misuse than their younger counterparts (Prenda & Stahl, 2001; Reade, 2015). Employers praised older workers' stronger work ethic while others laud the older employees' experience and sense of leadership and wisdom (**FIGURE 9-6**; Reade, 2015).

Although there do seem to be age-related declines in cognition, sensation, perception,

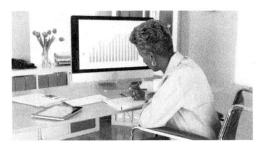

FIGURE 9-6 Some employers commend older adults on their work ethic, dependability, and leadership skills.

© Rocketclips, Inc./Shutterstock

and physical performance, for most typically aging older adults these changes do not make a substantial impact on either their comprehensive work performance or essential daily living skills. Being productive, as mentioned in Chapter 2, in a work environment can help keep older adults active and connected with their communities as well as foster a sense of well-being and self-esteem. As the aging population within the workplace grows, employers will be faced (if they are not already) with accommodating the needs of older workers. Most older adults can do very well in the workplace with minimal modifications for their health and safety (e.g., changes in workstation setup, improved lighting). These accommodations can also benefit younger workers (Kenny, Yardley, Martineau, & Jay, 2008).

According to a Sloan Center on Aging & Work report (2009), only about a third of employers had strategies to encourage workers to keep working past the traditional retirement age, even though nearly half of employers surveyed (46%) stated that retaining talented workers was essential to the future of their organizations.

The role of medical professionals in keeping older workers (and workers with disabilities) in the workforce was explored in a roundtable workshop supported by the U.S. Department of Labor (Heidkamp & Christian, 2013). The topic of supporting older workers is pertinent because older workers age 55 and

older will make up approximately 25% of the workforce in 2020. Moreover, the increase of workers age 65 and older is projected at 75%. Still, many older workers chose to retire instead of continuing to work after sustaining a disability, even though work overall is currently less physically demanding than it was in the past. Older workers are also more likely to stay unemployed (than prime-age workers) once they lose their jobs.

At the roundtable, participants discussed two cases of older workers who sustained the same medical condition ("bad" spinal cord disc, corrected by surgery) and both had "mediocre" work histories. In Case 1, the "weak" supervisor never followed up with the worker, work place teasing was expected, and the person's physician encouraged the person to stay home until he felt better; the result was the worker was placed on permanent disability. In Case 2, the "supportive" supervisor called to let the worker know that he was needed, the coworkers were supportive of the worker's return to work, the employer made workplace adaptations (i.e., adaptive equipment and transitional work); the result was that this worker returned to work after 6 weeks (Heidkamp & Christian, 2013, p. 7). Given that talented older workers are needed and that work (e.g., productive activity) can be good for one's physical and mental health, the conclusion of the roundtable discussion was that healthcare professionals need to help older workers remain on the job, even after incurring disabilities. They can support older workers efforts to return to work and remain employed by supporting accommodations and accepting partial absences instead of advocating for their permanent withdrawal from the workplace.

▶ Sleep

Sleep is an essential part of everyday life. This daily task is completely different from other activities, but we cannot live without doing it regularly. Sleep plays a central role in promoting good health and a high quality of life. Changes in sleep patterns, including lack of sleep quality, can occur with age due to difficulty falling and staying asleep (Yaffe, Falvey, & Hoang, 2014). Disturbance in sleep patterns caused by declines in memory and cognition are common for people with Alzheimer's disease and other dementias (Yaffe et al., 2014).

Lack of sleep contributes to how one feels and acts during the day. The National Sleep Foundation (2008) reported that nearly 20% of Americans representing all ages and socioeconomic statuses report sleep-related problems. Yet, older adults share more of this burden than other age groups. In a more recent study, the Foundation (2017) found that 39% of 65+ people reported sleep problems, such as waking up during the night. Still, 60% of older adults surveyed reported that they get refreshing sleep (National Sleep Foundation, 2017).

Normal Sleep

To discuss sleep disorders, it is important to have a basic understanding of sleep and the typical sleep cycle. People have a sleep–wake cycle that is known as the circadian rhythm—the 24-hour clock responsible for keeping most people awake during the day and allowing them to feel sleepy and go to sleep at night. The stimulating effects of light, through the retinohypothalamic tract, control this rhythm in the hypothalamus. The light causes alerting signals to help maintain wakefulness. As the day progresses, the sleep load increases and the alerting signals must get stronger for continued feelings of alertness. When darkness falls, evening/nighttime routines such as dinner and relaxation are associated with the decrease of alerting signals. Melatonin is released, causing further reduction in the alerting signals until the sleep load overtakes wakefulness and sleep ensues. For many individuals, this happens between 9 and 11 at night.

Once asleep, there is a rhythm to our sleep. Sleep is broken into two states: non-rapid eye movement (NREM) and rapid eye movement (REM) sleep. Non-REM sleep consists of three

stages: N1, N2, and N3 (and for younger people a fourth stage N4). N1 is the link between consciousness and unconsciousness. In this stage of sleep, we may have some awareness of surroundings and can easily be aroused. We spend about 5% of our time asleep in stage N1. In stage N2, we lose consciousness, but we are still in a light stage of sleep and still can be aroused fairly easily. Approximately 50% of our sleep time is spent in stage N2. Stage N3 is considered deep sleep. When we are in deep sleep, arousal is difficult. If aroused during deep sleep, we are usually somewhat disoriented. During this stage, growth hormone is released, which continues to be needed for tissue repair as we age. The N3 stage of sleep is when we experience the most restorative sleep that is essential to functional performance and feeling refreshed during the day. As we age, the N3 stage of deep sleep decreases and is replaced by the lighter stage N2 (**FIGURE 9-7**).

Stage R or REM sleep is when we dream. During this stage of sleep, the brain is more active than when we are awake. REM sleep is thought to be responsible for reorganization of our thoughts, similar to rebooting a computer. During stage R, we experience muscle atonia (i.e., extremely relaxed muscles), preventing us from acting out our dreams. We also lose a degree of autonomic control, which leads to heart rate variability, irregular respiration, and fluctuations in blood pressure. When all is well, stage R comprises about 25% of our sleep.

The sleep cycle consists of four to five periods of non-REM and REM sleep, each lasting about 90 minutes. The first part of the night consists of more deep sleep (N3) and shorter REM sleep, and the latter part of the night consists of longer REM periods and shorter deep sleep (N3) periods (Figure 9-7).

Impact of Sleep on Older Adults

Sleep requirements change over the lifespan. Infants need approximately 16 hours of sleep per day and adults need about 8 hours per day.

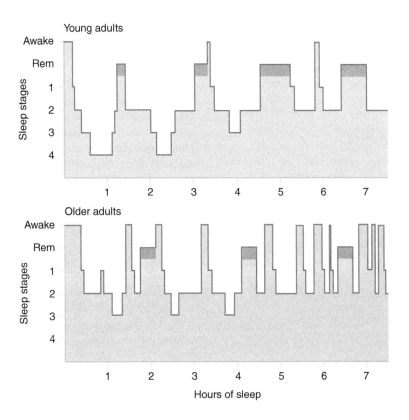

FIGURE 9-7 REM cycles of younger and older adults.

From the New England Journal of Medicine, Anthony Kales, M. D. and Joyce D. Kales, M. D., Sleep Disorders: Recent Findings in the Diagnosis and Treatment of Disturbed Sleep, 290, Page Nos. 487–499, Copyright © 1974 Massachusetts Medical Society. Reprinted with permission from Massachusetts Medical Society.

One long-standing misconception is that older adults need less sleep. They actually need the same amount of sleep as they get older, but getting enough of the refreshing type of sleep may become more difficult as less time is spent in deep sleep and more time is spent in lighter sleep stages. During lighter stages of sleep, individuals are more easily aroused and thus may be more susceptible to sleep disruptions caused by pain or discomfort associated with illness and disease. Older adults take more medications than any other age group and many of these medications can interfere with sleep (e.g., sedatives and benzodiazepines). Other health-related issues experienced in the second half of life, including depression, menopause, frequent need to urinate, heart disease, and stress, can also lead to **insomnia**

(i.e., inability to sleep; Smagula, Stone, Fabio, & Cauley, 2016). Although sleep requirements stay the same throughout adulthood, sleep efficiency (i.e., time asleep compared to time in bed) is reduced over time, requiring older adults to spend more time in bed just to get the required amount of sleep (Phillips, 2005).

Individuals' circadian rhythms also change as they age. The rhythm becomes phase advanced, which results in melatonin being released earlier in the evening. This may lead to moving bedtime up and early morning awakenings. Instead of getting sleepy between 9 and 11 p.m., sleepiness may occur as early as 7 p.m. This change leads to earlier wake-up times (usually between 4 and 5 a.m.). Although this change is considered normal, it can have a negative impact on one's work and social life. The easiest way to delay the hour of sleep is exposure to bright light (either natural sunlight or artificial light) later in the day. Artificial light of at least 2,500 lux (five times brighter than house lights) is recommended (Phillips, 2005).

Sleep Disorders

Common sleep problems or disorders (especially in older adults) include:

- Sleep-onset insomnia (i.e., difficulty falling asleep)
- Waking up often during the night (i.e., sleep maintenance insomnia)
- Waking up too early and not being able to get back to sleep (i.e., terminal insomnia)
- Waking up not feeling refreshed
- Snoring, which may be related to sleep apnea (i.e., temporary cessation in breathing)
- Unpleasant feelings in the legs (e.g., restless leg syndrome [RLS])

Insomnia

Insomnia is the most common symptom of more than 30 different sleep disorders, and approximately 30% of adults complain of insomnia (Phillips, 2005). Acute insomnia lasts fewer than 30 days, whereas chronic insomnia lasts longer than a month. The onset of insomnia may begin with an emotional event such as the loss of a loved one or a recent stay in the hospital. During the event, the normal rhythm of sleep is disrupted and an abnormal sleep cycle ensues. Once the new cycle becomes the norm, many people have difficulty resuming their previous sleep routine.

Although many people believe the most effective treatment for insomnia is in the form of a sleeping pill, that approach is not in the best interest of every person. Sleeping pills may be a good short-term solution, especially for people who have had a traumatic or emotional event that is interfering with sleep (e.g., death of a spouse or a forced move). However, in the long run, other techniques such as **sleep restriction**, **stimulus control**, **sleep hygiene**, and **cognitive behavioral therapy** can offer more sustainable and positive impacts on a person's overall quality of life (Phillips, 2005). Additionally, underlying health issues such as stress, illness, medication side effects, environmental interruptions (light or noise), depression, and/or pain should be fully addressed prior to considering sleep medications (Cleveland Clinic Foundation, 2012a).

Obstructive Sleep Apnea

Signs and symptoms of **obstructive sleep apnea** (OSA) include snoring and witnessed apnea (i.e., temporary cessation of breathing) during sleep and/or complaints of excessive sleepiness during the day. OSA occurs when the trachea is either totally or partially obstructed, causing the body's oxygen level to drop. This event signals the brain to wake up, which increases muscle tone and subsequently raises the oxygen level back to normal. The disruption of the sleep pattern can occur up to 60 times in an hour, so a person with OSA may need 10–12 hours of sleep each night just to get enough restorative sleep (National Sleep Foundation, 2013). Before age 50, twice as many men as women are afflicted with OSA, but after women reach menopause, differences in the prevalence of OSA diminishes between the sexes. Health conditions often attributed to the presence of OSA include high blood pressure, heart disease, stroke, diabetes, and poor brain oxygenation (National Heart, Lung, and Blood Institute, 2012). Loss of oxygen to the brain due to OSA or any other health condition can be life threatening and have serious consequences, including heart arrhythmias and mood and memory problems (National Sleep Foundation, 2013).

Maintaining a side-lying sleep pose may help reduce OSA as lying on one's back seems to exacerbate the problem. Also, the continuous positive airway pressure (CPAP) device is considered the leading therapy for OSA and

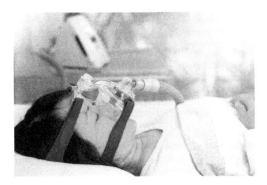

FIGURE 9-8 A woman wearing a CPAP device.

© sbw/Shutterstock

has helped millions of users overcome the negative impact of sleep apnea (**FIGURE 9-8**). A CPAP machine is often prescribed after a sleep study has been completed by a sleep specialist. During a study, aspects of sleep examined include sleep state, eye movement, muscle activity, heart rate, respiratory effort, airflow, and blood oxygen levels (National Sleep Foundation, 2013). Even though a temporary lack of oxygen underlies OSA, the CPAP device does not involve oxygen transmission. Rather, it works to keep the airway path unobstructed through air pressure (Berry & Sanders, 2005). CPAP hoses and masks require regular maintenance and cleaning. If not maintained, the buildup of bacteria can cause additional harm just by using the machine.

Restless Leg Syndrome/Periodic Leg Movements During Sleep

Restless leg syndrome (RLS) is a neurologic disorder that causes "creepy crawly feelings" or other unpleasant sensations in the legs and an irresistible urge to move the legs while in bed or at rest (National Institute of Neurological Disorders and Stroke [NINDS], 2017). These symptoms lead to periodic leg movements during sleep (PLMS), which hinder people from getting a good night's sleep. According to the NINDS (2017), PLMS may occur every 10–60 seconds and may last the entire night.

The constant need to move causes the brain to wake up, disrupting the sleep cycle (akin to sleep apnea). Parkinsonian-type medications (Levodopa), along with anticonvulsants, benzodiazepines, and narcotics, have been able to afford some relief to PLMS sufferers (Cleveland Clinic Foundation, 2012; NINDS, 2017). Individuals with PLMS are also advised to avoid stimulants such as alcohol, caffeine, chocolate, nicotine, tea, and soft drinks to lessen their symptoms (Cleveland Clinic Foundation, 2012b). Although there is no known cure, tips for managing RLS symptoms include exercise, leg messages, use of warm packs, and leg compression devices (NINDS, 2017).

Treatment of Sleep Disorders

Treating sleep disorders can be challenging. A systematic review and meta-analysis of treatments sought by 1,162 adults with sleep problems revealed that effective strategies included sleep restriction, stimulus control, sleep hygiene, cognitive behavioral therapy (CBT), and relaxation techniques (Trauer, Qian, Doyle, Rajaratnam, & Cunnington, 2015). Although the typical healthcare professional is not expected to help an older person overcome serious sleep disorders, understanding treatment approaches and being familiar with simple strategies can be useful in supporting an older adult's quest for regular restful nights of sleep.

Sleep restriction does not refer to actually restricting sleep, but rather to restricting one's time in bed. The goal is to be asleep 90% of the time that one spends in bed. Often, individuals who have insomnia will spend many hours in bed, but not sleeping. This leads to poor sleep habits whereby one learns (subconsciously) that a bed is not for sleeping. If people aim for the 90% rule, they can determine how long they would need to be in bed to get the desired number of hours of sleep. The first step is to rise out of bed at a designated time, whether or not enough sleep has been had. Then the goal is to stay awake (and out of bed) until it is time to go to sleep again. At a later date, additional time spent in bed can be gradually added back in.

Stimulus control also refers to the amount of time spent in bed, attempting to get to sleep or back to sleep. If a person cannot fall asleep within a half hour, it might be best to get out of bed and engage in a relaxing activity. When the person becomes sleepy, she or he should go back to bed and try to sleep. Rather than tossing and turning, consumed with worry that one will not get enough sleep, one gets out of the bedroom and does an activity. This activity should be soothing and tailored to personal interests such as reading, completing puzzles, or engaging in a craft.

Sleep hygiene involves those activities and habits that are conducive to sleeping soundly and are largely individualized. Most people find that a quiet, cool, dark room is helpful for inducing sleep, whereas eating, exercising, or listening to a blaring television are more likely to prevent sleep. When trying to promote sleep, exercise should take place at least 2–3 hours before bedtime and taking a hot bath can be helpful an hour or more before heading to bed. Some people find it helpful to write a to-do list for the next day to put the next day's demands into perspective before bedtime. It can be helpful for people experiencing sleep disturbances to spend time devising their own personal sleep hygiene "dos and don'ts" list so that they can work on promoting healthy, restful sleep patterns for themselves.

Last, CBT, an evidenced-based therapeutic approach used to change personal behaviors and thinking, has been found to be helpful for people having difficulty sleeping. A therapist who specializes in sleep disorders can teach a client about sleep and work with them to understand that it is not necessarily catastrophic if one does not get enough sleep, on occasion. Worrying about the lack of sleep only exacerbates the situation. A licensed therapist uses CBT to help an individual put sleep activities into perspective and reduce worries about

personal sleep patterns (Edinger, Wohlgemuth, Radke, Marsh, & Quillian, 2001; Morin, 2015).

One of the techniques mentioned may be all that is needed for a person to regain sound sleeping habits, or several strategies may be required. Fortunately, sleep disorders are usually treatable. Supporting older adults who report sleep problems is important because people with few sleep disturbances are more likely to age successfully (American Academy of Sleep Medicine, 2008).

▶ Summary

This chapter reviews some of the sensory and physical changes that accompany the aging process, especially with regard to day-to-day functioning. In reality, the vast majority of older adults manage their daily routines just fine. Persons who are affected by age-related health problems or who are living with the consequences of earlier poor lifestyle choices, are not likely to manage as well as their healthy counterparts. However, people with chronic health conditions or physical decline secondary to ill health can be surprisingly resilient and outperform the expectations placed upon them. As healthcare professionals, it is our responsibility to support them in making positive changes and to instill hope for their futures.

Highlights of the changes addressed in this chapter are as follows:

- Common visual diagnoses include decreased acuity, cataracts, macular degeneration, glaucoma, and diabetic retinopathy; yet, the majority of older adults are able to maintain adequate visual skills (with correction) for the successful completion of daily tasks.
- Visual perceptual skills or the ability to interpret incoming visual information is more affected by disease processes (such as stroke) than by the aging process alone.
- Physical skills such as joint ROM, strength, endurance, reaction time, and

motor coordination do change over the course of time, with older adults generally not performing as well as their younger counterparts. However, several measures can be taken to improve performance even among the oldest members of the population.

■ Perhaps surprisingly, for various reasons, older workers tend to perform as well as or better than their younger counterparts.

Retaining older workers is important for sustaining many organizations, yet relatively few organizations have strategies that encourage older workers to stay on the job.

■ Sleep disorders are common among older adults, and several treatment techniques for improving quality and quantity of sleep are available for individuals needing help in this realm.

⌕ CASE STUDIES

Case 1: Morton is an 88-year-old widowed male who lives with his daughter and her family in Virginia Beach, Virginia. Prior to retirement 18 years ago, Morton was an auto parts store manager and also worked as the town clerk. He describes himself as being social and enjoys reading and assembling model antique cars. He has managed to stay active, swimming daily and playing golf on the weekends with his former coworkers. He enjoys getting together with his golf buddies, even though they sometimes tease him about losing his hearing. But he denies that he has a problem, even though he often has to piece together what his friends are talking about based on the words and phrases he can make out. The only thing he does not like about these weekend meet-ups is lunch at the country club. Morton enjoyed the food there for decades, but in recent years none of his favorite dishes there taste like they used to. He has the same problem with the food his daughter prepares. "Jeez," he jokes with his friends, "Nobody knows how to cook anymore!" Morton enjoys staying active despite his advanced age.

1. **What are some ways in which regular exercise are benefitting him?**
2. **What can Morton's friends do during their weekly golf outings to help accommodate for his hearing loss?**
3. **Explain why Morton is likely complaining about the taste of food, including some possible root causes for this perception.**

Case 2: As a child, Susan was an excellent sleeper. She could fall asleep quickly, and typically slept straight through the night, often for as long as 10 hours. As a teenager, then as an adult, she did not sleep as long as she used to (usually about 8 hours), but still had no trouble falling or staying asleep at night. Today, Susan is 67 years old, and although she is relatively healthy, she just does not sleep the way she used to. Over the last few years, it has taken her longer and longer to fall asleep at night, to the point where she is often still awake after midnight. Regardless of how much sleep she ultimately gets, she still feels groggy throughout the day. A friend suggested that she might have sleep apnea and recommended that Susan talk to her doctor about having a sleep study done and possibly getting a CPAP machine. The way she is feeling, Susan is ready to try just about anything.

1. **What are some strategies Susan can try to combat her insomnia?**
2. **If Susan has a sleep study, what aspects of sleep will be evaluated?**
3. **If Susan does have sleep apnea, what is happening to her when she sleeps and how might a CPAP machine help her?**

TEST YOUR KNOWLEDGE

Review Questions

1. Velma has fallen in her home several times in the last few months. Luckily, she has not been seriously injured, but her daughter, Betty, is concerned that her mother might fall again and possibly break her hip. What can Betty do to help reduce the likelihood that Velma will fall again?
   a. Work with her to develop her fine motor skills
   b. Discourage her from engaging in any physical activity
   c. Remove any loose rugs from the house
   d. Have her tested for restless leg syndrome

2. A common sign of obstructive sleep apnea is:
   a. Snoring
   b. Dry mouth in the morning
   c. Sleeping on your back
   d. Numbness in the arm

3. Erin was recently diagnosed with restless leg syndrome, and her physician prescribed an anticonvulsant. In addition to taking her medication as prescribed, what else can Erin do to lessen the symptoms of her condition?
   a. Apply cold packs to her legs before bedtime
   b. Use a leg compression device
   c. Drink some brandy before bedtime
   d. Avoid exercising her legs

4. Which visual skill tends to be preserved with age?
   a. Ability to see well in dim light
   b. Contrast sensitivity
   c. Ability to maintain fixation on a target
   d. Visual processing speed

5. An active lifestyle involving stretching, aerobic activity, and strength building can:
   a. Improve hyposmia
   b. Reverse hearing loss
   c. Reduce the size of cataracts
   d. Improve range of motion

Learning Activities

1. (Complete the first part of this learning activity before reading the chapter.) On the left side of a piece of paper, make a list of the following: vision, visual perception, hearing, smell, taste, ROM, strength, endurance, work performance, and sleep. For each category, write down what you expect to happen with this factor as you get older. Then, read the chapter and compare what you expected with what you learned in the chapter. Were you surprised about any of the results?

2. Based on what you learned in the chapter, why are social gatherings more difficult with advancing age? What other life tasks may be more difficult for older adults and why?

3. Two, three, or four people should choose a card game they all know how to play. One player will wear glasses smeared with petroleum jelly; another player should wear earplugs

and heavy leather gloves; the third player must keep his or her hands in a fist and wear dark sunglasses. If there is a fourth player, he or she will cover one eye and can move her arms only by sliding them across the table due to arm weakness (although she can still move her fingers). Any time a player cheats, he or she will lose a point toward the total score. After

the game, discuss how the simulated age-related changes affected your ability to play the game.

4. Review the activity in item 3. How could you make it easier for the players to enjoy their game of cards? Come up with several suggestions.

5. Make a personal list of sleep hygiene "dos and don'ts" for yourself. Discuss with the group.

References

AARP. (2017). *Don't call me 'sweetie'!* Retrieved from https://www.aarp.org/caregiving/basics/info-2017/discouraging- elderspeak-from-caregivers-fd.html

Ahmed, T., & Haboubi, N. (2010). Assessment and management of nutrition in older people and its importance to health. *Clinical Interventions in Aging, 5,* 207–216.

American Academy of Sleep Medicine. (2008). *Normal sleep linked to successful aging.* Retrieved from http://www.aasmnet.org/articles.aspx?id=923

American Occupational Therapy Association. Living with low vision. Retrieved from https://www.aota.org/~/media/Corporate/Files/AboutOT/consumers/Adults/Low Vision/Low%20Vision%20Tip%20Sheet.ashx

American Optometric Association. (2013). Adult Vision: Over 60 Years of Age. Retrieved from http://www.aoa.org/x9454.xml

Attems, J., Walker, L., & Jellinger, K. A. (2015). Olfaction and aging: A mini-review. *Gerontology, 61,* 485–490.

Bainbridge, K. E., & Wallhagen, M. I. (2014). Hearing loss in an aging American population: Extent, impact, and management. *Annual Review of Public Health, 35,* 139–152.

Berry, R. B., & Sanders, M. H. (2005). Positive airway pressure treatment for sleep apnea. In P. R. Carney, R. B. Berry, & J. D. Geyer (Eds.), *Clinical Sleep Disorders* (pp. 290–310). Philadelphia, PA: Lippincott Williams & Wilkins.

Cadore, E. L., Pinto, R. S., Bottaro, M., & Izquierdo, M. (2014). Strength and endurance training prescription in healthy and frail elderly. *Aging and Disease, 5,* 183–195.

Charness, N., & Bosman, E. A. (1990). Human factors design for the older adult. In J. E. Birren, K. W. Schaie, M. Gatz, T. A. Salthouse, & C. Schooler (Eds.), *Handbook of the psychology of aging* (3rd ed.) (pp. 452–453). San Diego, CA: Academic Press:

Centers for Disease Control and Prevention. (2011). *Why strength training?* Retrieved from http://www.cdc.gov/physicalactivity/growingstronger/why/index.html

Centers for Disease Control and Prevention. (2012). *Arthritis-related statistics.* Retrieved from http://www.cdc.gov/arthritis/data_statistics/arthritis_related_stats.htm

Centers for Disease Control and Prevention. (2015). *Healthy aging helping older Americans achieve healthy and high-quality lives.* Retrieved from https://www.cdc.gov/chronicdisease/resources/publications/aag/pdf/2015/healthy-aging-aag.pdf

Centers for Disease Control and Prevention. (2017). *Falls among older adults: An overview.* 2017. Retrieved from http://www.cdc.gov/homeandrecreationalsafety/falls/adultfalls.html

Cleveland Clinic Foundation. (2012a). *Insomnia.* Retrieved from http://my.clevelandclinic.org/disorders/insomnia/hic_insomnia.aspx

Cleveland Clinic Foundation. (2012b). *Periodic limb movement disorder.* Retrieved from http://my.clevelandclinic.org/disorders/periodic_limb_movement_disorder/hic_periodic_limb_movement_disorder.aspx

Cleveland Clinic Foundation. (2012c). *Tips to improve communication when talking with someone with hearing loss.* Retrieved from http://my.clevelandclinic.org/disorders/hearing_loss/hic-tips-improve-communication-when-talking-someone-hearingloss.aspx

Contrera, K. J., Betz, J., Deal, J., Choi, J. S., Ayonayon, H. N, Harris, T., … Li, F. R. (2017). Association of hearing impairment and anxiety in older adults. *Journal of Aging and Health, 29,* 172–184.

Curlik, D. M., & Shors, T. J. (2013). Training your brain: Do mental and physical (MAP) training enhance cognition through the process of neurogenesis in the hippocampus? *Neuropharmacology, 64,* 506–514.

Dong, J., Pinto, J. M., Guo, X., Alonso, A., Tranah, G., Cauley, J. A. ... Chen, H. (2017). The prevalence of anosmia and associated factors among U.S. Black and White older adults. *Journals of Gerontology Series A: Biomedical Sciences and Medical Sciences, glx081, 72*(8), 1080–1086 .

Edinger, J. D., Wohlgemuth, W. K., Radke, R. A., Marsh, G. R., & Quillian, R. E. (2001). Cognitive behavioral therapy for treatment of primary chronic insomnia. *Journal of the American Medical Association, 285,* 1856–1864.

Eye Diseases Prevalence Research Group, Diabetic Retinopathy Subsection. (2004). The prevalence of diabetic retinopathy among adults in the United States. *Archives of Ophthalmology, 122,* 552–563.

Fozard, J. L. (1990). Vision and hearing in aging. In J. E. Birren, K. W. Schaie, M. Gatz, T. A. Salthouse, & C. Schooler (Eds.), *Handbook of the Psychology of Aging* (3rd ed.) (pp. 150–170). San Diego, CA: Academic Press.

Ganz, D. A., Bao, Y., Shekelle, P. G., & Rubenstein, L. Z. (2007). Will my patient fall? *Journal of the American Medical Association, 297,* 77–86.

Gayton, J. L. (2009). Etiology, prevalence, and treatment of dry eye disease. *Clinical Journal of Opthamalogy, 3,* 405–412.

Gillespie, L. D., Gillespie, W. J., Robertson, M. C., Lamb, S. E., Cumming, R. G., & Rowe, B. H. (2006). Interventions for preventing falls in elderly people. *The Cochrane Library, 1,* CD000340.

Glyde, H., Hickson, L., Cameron, S., & Dillon, H. (2011). Problems hearing in noise in older adults: A review of spatial processing disorder. *Trends in Amplification, 15*(3), 116–126.

Goldberg, L. R., Heiss, C. J., Parsons, S. D., Foley, A. S., Mefferd, A .S., Hollinger, D., ... Patterson, J. (2014). Hydration in older adults: The contribution of bio-electrical impedance analysis. *International Journal of Speech-Language Pathology, 16,* 273–281.

Golub, J. S., Luchsinger, J. A., Manly, J. J., Stern, Y., Mayeux, R., & Schupf, N. (2017). Observed hearing loss and incident dementia in a multiethnic cohort. *Journal of the American Geriatric Society, 65,* 1691–1697. doi:10.1111/jgs.14848

Gopinath, B., Kaarin, A., Sue, C. M., Kifley, A., & Mitchell, P. (2011). Olfactory impairment in older adults is associated with depressive symptoms and poorer quality of life scores. *American Journal of Geriatric Psychiatry, 19,* 830–834.

Heidkamp, M., & Christian, J. (2013). The aging workforce: The role of medical professionals in helping older workers and workers with disabilities to stay at work or return to work and remain employed. *NTAR Leadership Center,* 1–12. Retrieved from https://www.dol.gov/odep/pdf/NTAR-AgingMedical Professionals.pdf

Huang, G., Shi, X., Davis-Brezette, J. A., & Osness, W. H. (2005). Resting heart rate changes after endurance training in older adults: A meta-analysis. *Medicine and Science in Sports and Medicine, 37,* 1381–1386.

James, L. E., & Kooy, T. M. (2011). Aging and the detection of visual errors in scenes. *Journal of Aging Research,* 1–6. doi:10.4061/2011/984694.

Kim, E., Park, Y. K., Byun, Y. H., Park, M. S., & Kim, H. (2014). Influence of aging on visual perception and visual motor integration in Korean adults. *Journal of Exercise Rehabilitation, 10,* 245–250. doi:10.12965/jer.140147

Keller, K., & Engelhardt, M. (2013). Strength and muscle mass loss with aging process. Age and strength loss. *Muscles, Ligaments, and Tendons Journal, 3,* 346–350.

Kenny, G. P., Yardley, J. E., Martineau, L., & Jay, O. (2008). Physical work capacity in older adults: Implications for the aging worker. *American Journal of Industrial Medicine, 51,* 610–625.

Larkin, G. L. (2009). Retinal Detachment. Retrieved from http://emedicine.medscape.com/article/798501-overview

Lin, F. R., Metter, E. J., O'Brien, R. J., Resnick, S. M., Zonderman, A. B., & Ferrucci, L. (2011). Hearing loss and incident of dementia. *Archives of Neurology, 68,* 214–220.

Lindfield, K. C., Wingfield, A., & Bowles, N. L. (1994). Identification of fragmented pictures under ascending versus fixed presentation in young and elderly adults: Evidence for the inhibition-deficit hypothesis. *Aging and Cognition, 1,* 282–291.

Lott, L. A., Schneck, M. E., Haegerstrom-Portnoy, G., Hewlett, S., & Brabyn, J. A. (2017). Reading performance in intermediate age-related macular degeneration: Context effects. *Investigative Ophthalmology & Visual Science, 58*(8), 4701–4701.

Maine Health. (2017). *What is a matter of balance?* Retrieved from http://www.mmc.org/mh_body.cfm?id=432

Maruta, J., Spielman, L. A., Rajashekar, U., & Ghajar, J. (2017). Visual tracking in development and aging. *Frontiers in Neurology, 8,* 640. doi:10.3389/fneur.2017.00640

Mayo Clinic. (2016). Exercise helps ease arthritis pain and stiffness. Retrieved from https://www.mayoclinic.org/diseases-conditions/arthritis/in-depth/arthritis/art-20047971

Methven, L., Allen, V. J., Withers, C. A., & Gosney, M. A. (2012). Aging and taste. *Proceedings of the Nutrition Society, 71,* 556–565. doi:10.1017/S0029665112000742

Morin, C. M. (2015). Cognitive behavioral therapy for chronic insomnia: State of the science versus current clinical practices. *Annals of Internal Medicine, 163,* 236–237.

Mullol, J., Alobid, I., Mariño-Sánchez, F., Quintó, L., de Haro, J., Bernal-Sprekelsen, M., ... Marin, C. (2012). Furthering the understanding of olfaction, prevalence of loss of smell and risk factors: A population-based survey (OLFACAT study). *British Medical Journal Open, 2*(6), e001256.

Muscari, A., Giannoni, C., Pierpaoli, L., Berzigotti, A., Maietta., A, Foschi, E., … Zoli, M. (2010). Chronic endurance exercise training prevents aging-related cognitive decline in healthy older adults: A randomized controlled trial. *International Journal of Geriatric Psychiatry, 25,* 1055–1064. doi:10.1002/gps.2462

National Heart, Lung and Blood Institute. (2012). *How is sleep apnea treated?* Retrieved from https://www .nhlbi.nih.gov/health/health-topics/topics/sleepapnea /treatment

National Institutes of Health. (2012). *Exercise: Exercises to try.* Retrieved from http://nihseniorhealth.gov/exercise andphysicalactivityexercisestotry/enduranceexercises /01.html

National Institute of Neurological Disorders and Stroke. (2017). *Restless legs syndrome fact sheet: 2017.* Retrieved from https://www.ninds.nih.gov/Disorders /Patient-Caregiver-Education/Fact-Sheets/Restless -Legs-Syndrome-Fact-Sheet

National Sleep Foundation. (2008). *Sleep in America poll.* Retrieved from http://www.kintera.org/atf/cf/% 7BF6BF2668-A1B4-4FE8-8D1A-A5D39340D9CB %7D/2003SleepPollExecSumm.pdf

National Sleep Foundation. (2013). *Sleep apnea and sleep.* Retrieved from http://www.sleepfoundation.org /article/sleep-related-problems/obstructive-sleep-apnea -and-sleep

National Sleep Foundation. (2017). *Insomnia.* Retrieved from https://sleepfoundation.org/insomnia/content /insomnia-older-adults

Ng, T. W. H., & Feldman, D. C. (2008). The relationship of age to ten dimensions of job performance. *Journal of Applied Psychology, 93,* 392–423.

Phillips, B. (2005). Sleepiness. In P. R. Carney, R. B. Berry, & J. D. Geyer (Eds.), *Clinical sleep disorders* (pp. 101–112). Philadelphia, PA: Lippincott Williams & Wilkins.

Pizzimenti, J. J., & Roberts, E. (2005). The low vision rehabilitation service: Part two. Putting the program into practice. *Internet Journal of Allied Health Sciences and Practice, 3*(3), 1–11.

Prenda, K. M., & Stahl, S. M. (2001). The truth about older workers. *Business and Health, 19*(5), 30–38.

Pronk, M., Deeg, D. J. H., Smits, C., Twsk J. W., van Tilburg, T. G., Festen, J. M., & Kramer, S. E. (2014). Hearing loss in older persons: Does the rate of decline affect psychosocial health? *Journal of Aging and Health, 26,* 703–723.

Reade, N. (2015). *The surprising truth about older workers.* Retrieved from https://www.aarp.org/work/job -hunting/info-07-2013/older-workers-more-valuable .html

Schieber, F. (2006). Vision and aging. In J. E. Birren, K. W. Schaie (Eds.), *Handbook of the psychology of aging* (pp. 129–161). Burlington, MA: Elsevier.

Sloan Center on Aging & Work. (2009). Recruitment and retention of older workers. Fact sheet 21. Retrieved from http://www.bc.edu/content/dam/files/research _sites/agingandwork/pdf/publications/FS21_Recruit _Retain_OldrWrkrs.pdf

Smagula, S. F., Stone, K. L., Fabio, A., & Cauley, J. A. (2016). Risk factors for sleep disturbances in older adults: Evidence from prospective studies. *Sleep Medicine Reviews, 25,* 21–30.

Soucie, J. M., Wang, C., Forsyth, A., Funk, S., Denny, M., Roach, K. E., & Boone, D. (2011). Range of motion measurements: Reference values and a database for comparison studies. *Haemophilia, 17,* 500–507. doi: 10.1111/j.1365-2516.2010.02399.x

Stathokostas, L., McDonald, M. W., Little, R. M. D., & Paterson, D. H. (2013). Flexibility of older adults aged 55–86 years and the influence of physical activity. *Journal of Aging Research,* 1–8. Article ID 743843. doi:10.1155/2013/743843

Sventina, M. (2016). The reaction times of drivers aged 20 to 80 during a divided attention driving. *Traffic Injury Prevention, 17*(8), 810–814. doi: 10.1080/15389588.2016.1157590

Trauer J. M., Qian M. Y., Doyle J. S., Rajaratnam S. M., & Cunnington, D. (2015). Cognitive behavioral therapy for chronic insomnia: A systematic review and meta -analysis. *Annals of Internal Medicine, 163,* 191–204. doi:10.7326/M14-2841

Warren, M. (2013). Evaluation and treatment of visual deficits following brain injury. In H. M. Pendleton & W. Schultz-Krohn (Eds.). *Pedretti's occupational therapy* (7th ed.) (pp. 590–630). St. Louis, MO: Elsevier

Wolters Kluwer Health (2014). Color vision problems become more common with age, study shows. Retrieved from https://www.sciencedaily.com/releases/2014/02 /140220102614.htm

Yaffe, K., Falvey, C. M., & Hoang, T. (2014). Connections between sleep and cognition in older adults. *Lancet Neurology, 13,* 1017–1028.

Zoltan, B. (1996). *Vision, perception and cognition.* Thorofare, NJ: Slack.

CHAPTER 10

Drugs and the Older Adult

David J. Mokler, PhD

CHAPTER OUTLINE

BEHAVIORAL OBJECTIVES

Upon completion of this chapter, the reader will be able to:

1. Discuss the physiologic changes that occur as we age that affect our response to drug administration, including absorption, distribution, metabolism, and excretion.
2. Describe the symptoms of anticholinergic syndrome and identify classes of drugs with anticholinergic side effects.
3. Describe the symptoms of serotonin syndrome and identify classes of drugs that have serotonergic activity.
4. Identify classes of drugs that should be avoided in the older patient as outlined in Beer's criteria and STOPP.
5. Identify classes of drugs which are underutilized in the older patient, as described in START.
6. Discuss drug misuse/abuse in older adults.
7. Discuss the use of herbal therapy and supplements.

(continues)

(continued)

8. Describe the increase in drug side effects that occur as the result of taking an increased number of drugs.
9. Discuss how to manage polypharmacy.
10. Discuss the principle of Go Low–Go Slow in the use of drugs in older patients.

KEY TERMS

Dependence
Food and Drug Administration
Hydrophilicity
Inducibility

Lipophilicity
Pharmacodynamic
Pharmacogenomics
Pharmacokinetic

Physicochemical properties
Polypharmacy
Tolerance

▶ Introduction

Drug therapy continues to be the primary form of medical therapy for all age groups, especially within the older population. In this chapter, the term "drug" is used interchangeably with the term "medication," both of which are used to treat diseases. Although the focus will be on drug therapy, other medications such as herbals and supplements will be discussed as they are also used extensively to prevent disease.

Over the past 50 years, the use of pharmaceutical agents has exploded. Advances in medicine and technology have extended life expectancy, and with that, the numbers of drugs used by the average older patient has increased dramatically (**FIGURE 10-1**). According to the American Geriatrics Society, presently people aged 65 and older make up 13% of the U.S. population and buy 33% of the prescription drugs. By 2040, the figures are expected to increase; 25% of the older U.S. population will purchase approximately half of all prescription drugs (Medina-Walpole & Pacala, 2016). In a study looking at prescription, over-the-counter (OTC) and supplement use, Qato and colleagues (2016) found that 95% of the 70-year-old Americans studied reported to be using at least one medication and 68% are taking more than five.

Clearly, older Americans are heavy consumers of medications. A list of the most common medications and the percentage of older adults who use them is shown in **TABLE 10-1**.

The **Food and Drug Administration** (FDA) is responsible for the approval of prescription and nonprescription drugs. The FDA requires pharmaceutical companies to show that drugs are safe and effective by requiring them to use approved clinical trial protocols. The gold standard in clinical trials is a large double-blinded placebo controlled trial. In such trials, neither the researcher team nor the participants know who is taking the drug being

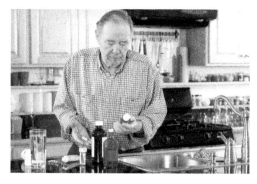

FIGURE 10-1 As advances in medicine and technology have emerged, the number of drugs used by older adults have increased. In the United States most older adults age 70+ take at least one medication.
© Jaren Jal Wicklund/Shutterstock

TABLE 10-1 Most Common Drugs Prescribed to Older Adults by Prevalence

Drug or Drug Class	Prevalence (percent)
Antihyperlipidemics (statins)	50.1
Simvistatin	22.5
Antihypertensives	65.1
ACE inhibitors	30.4
Diuretics	29.5
Anticoagulants (aspirin, warfarin, and related drugs)	47.6
Aspirin	40.2
Analgesics (includes aspirin)	54.3
NSAIDs (ibuprofen, naproxen, and related drugs)	13.7
Opiate analgesics (morphine, oxycodone, and related drugs)	6.7

Data from Qato, Wilder, Schumm, Gillet, & Alexander (2016).

tested and who is taking the placebo. This type of trial is difficult to accomplish well, which often leads to confusion about the value of pharmacotherapy due to nondefinitive results. As a result, views on the therapeutic values of different medications can continually change.

Examining the multiple stages of the FDA-required drug approval process is beyond the scope of this chapter. Of relevance to the present topic is that the FDA does not require drugs to be tested specifically in older populations. Therefore, we do not necessarily have information regarding how drugs affect aging physiology. Moreover, the FDA does not regulate the production of herbal medications and supplements; thus, the effects of both on older users are also unclear. Later in this chapter, there is a discussion of how healthcare practitioners can be informed of drugs which are relatively safe in the older patient and, importantly, drugs which are unsafe.

Many of the drug interactions that occur are due to both **pharmacokinetic** and **pharmacodynamic** interactions. Pharmacokinetics can be described as what the body does to a drug, while pharmacodynamics can be described by what the drug does to the body.

The four key phases of pharmacokinetics that are addressed in this chapter are drug absorption, distribution, metabolism, and excretion. Each area may overlap but all are affected by aging and administration with other drugs.

▶ Pharmacokinetics

Drug Absorption

How human physiology changes as we age is an important aspect in determining how the body handles drugs (i.e., pharmacokinetics). Drug absorption is dependent upon how a drug is administered. There are many different routes of administration: oral, sublingual (under the tongue), intranasal, intravenous, intramuscular, topical, subcutaneous, and inhaled. Each administration route could potentially be impacted by the aging process. Clinical studies tend to focus on the most common route of administration for a particular agent with oral administration being the most common route. Another common route of administration, which is affected by aging, is transdermal administration.

Oral Administration

Most drug absorption after oral administration occurs in the small intestine. Thus, the rate of gastric emptying needs to be considered. In the older patient, gut motility in general and gastric emptying in particular takes a longer amount of time (Cusack, 2004). However, research studies have resulted in mixed results as to the clinical relevance of these findings.

Generally, the slowed gastric emptying is reflected clinically in a time delay in attaining maximal drug concentrations in the blood without a change in maximal drug concentration. Studies on the absorption of drugs from the small intestine showed some changes in this parameter, but the changes uncovered were inconsistent and did not lend themselves to broad generalization. Thus, oral administration of drugs, in general, does not significantly affect the clinical response to drugs (Cusack, 2004; McLean & Le Couteur, 2004).

Transdermal Administration

Transdermal administration or medication administered through the skin, often through the use of a patch, is a convenient way to administer a steady amount of drug over a prolonged period (**FIGURE 10-2**). Examples of drugs administered though transdermal administration include estrogen (female hormone), fentanyl (an opioid painkiller), and scopolamine (treats motion sickness). Yet, as people age, they experience changes in the skin that can lead to changes in how drugs are absorbed through the skin. The outer layer or epidermis thins with age and becomes dryer, allowing for a decreased absorption of drug through the skin. Thus, use of transdermal medications in older adults may lead to lower concentrations in the blood.

Drug Distribution

The next phase of pharmacokinetics is distribution. Drugs distribute throughout the body based on their **physicochemical properties**, that is, the relationship between the chemical structure of the drug and its interactions with the body. The most important of these properties is the **hydrophilicity** or **lipophilicity** of the drug—is it more attracted to water or to fat, respectively? As people age, lean body mass decreases, which leads to increased fat content in the body. With fat content increased, a fat-soluble drug will show a larger volume of distribution, which will lower its concentration and lower its therapeutic efficacy. The effect of aging on distribution is very much dependent upon the specific drug, so there is no consensus on the general effect of all fat-soluble drugs.

Drug Metabolism

Drug metabolism is an area where the complexities of pharmacokinetics in older people are most apparent. The liver is the major organ of drug metabolism, although the intestines, lungs, and kidneys also have important drug metabolizing enzymes. Fortunately, in the absence of disease, drug metabolizing enzymes are not significantly affected by aging (McLean & Le Couteur, 2004). Other changes, however, are more significant. One factor that relates directly to drug metabolism is blood flow through the

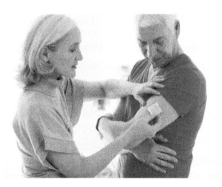

FIGURE 10-2 Transdermal patches administer drugs (e.g., fentanyl and nicotine) over a prolonged period through the skin.
© Image Point Fr/Shutterstock

TABLE 10-2 Hepatic Metabolism of Drugs in Older Patients

Decreased	Unchanged
Diltiazem	Alprazolam
Fluoxetine	Dolasetron
Citalopram	
Amlodipine	
Ondansetron	
Quinine	
Diphenhydramine	

liver. Studies consistently have shown that there is a reduction of blood flow through the liver that accompanies age. If blood flow is decreased, then the extraction of drugs from the blood is decreased and metabolism is slowed. This does vary according to the physicochemical properties of the drug. Some drugs have a high extraction from the blood, that is, a large portion of the drug in the blood is extracted by the liver; these medications are the most affected with age (see **TABLES 10-2** and **10-3**). Subsequently, the half-life of these drugs is increased. The half-life of a drug is the time it takes for half the administered dose

TABLE 10-3 Drugs with Low Oral Availability Due to Extensive Hepatic Metabolism

Cardiac Drugs	Antidepressants
Alprenolol	Amitriptyline
Metoprolol	Desipramine
Labetalol	Pain Medications
Diltiazem	Morphine
Propranolol	Pentazocine
Verapamil	
Nifedipine	
Nitroglycerine	

of a drug to be cleared from the blood. For example, the half-life of the antianxiety drug diazepam is 20 hours, meaning that if a person is given a 10 mg dose of diazepam, then 20 hours later there will be 5 mg left in the person's body. Diazepam is a good example of a drug that has a significant change in pharmacokinetics with aging. The half-life of 20 hours is for a person in her/his 20s. As a person grows older, this half-life of diazepam increases linearly. By the time a person is in her/his 80s, the half-life is around 80 hours, that is, it takes four times longer for a person in her/his 80s to metabolize the same dose of diazepam as a person in her/his 20s! This change needs to be taken into account when older adults are administered drugs which have significant hepatic metabolism.

One key aspect of drug metabolism is the metabolism of some drugs to active metabolites. That is, the drug breaks down but is transformed into another active drug. In general, the goal of drug metabolism is to inactivate a drug and make it more water soluble for easier extraction from the blood and excretion by the kidney. However, in some cases, after the drug has been metabolized, the resulting chemical is also active. Diazepam (Valium) is still a good example. Once ingested, it is metabolized to three active metabolites that also have half-lives. Although the half-life of diazepam is around 20 hours, a single dose with its active metabolites may continue to produce effects for up to six days. This adds a considerable length of time to how long active drugs remain in the body. If liver metabolism is slowed and if dosing is not adjusted, there will be a considerable buildup of drug in the older person leading to toxicity. Another lesson from this example is that in the older adult, the best benzodiazepine to use instead of diazepam or alprazolam (Xanax, which also has active metabolites) is oxazepam (Serax) which has no active metabolites.

Drugs are metabolized in the liver by a number of enzymes. The major group of drug metabolizing enzymes belongs to the class of cytochrome P450s. This group of enzymes has a number of subtypes. CYP3A4 (cytochrome P450 subtype 3A4) and CYP2D6 are two enzymes that together metabolize over 75% of prescription drugs in the liver. These enzymes vary considerably based on a person's genetic background, including their ethnic background, their previous exposure to drugs, and their current drug regimen. Although the amount of drug metabolizing enzymes in the body does not change with aging in the absence of liver pathology, the fact that the older patient will be on more drugs increases the risk of drug–drug interactions involving drug metabolism. Two drugs metabolized by the same enzyme will compete for the metabolism process, and this may slow their metabolism; although a more important clinical effect of drugs is in the inhibition or induction of these enzymes.

A number of therapeutically important drugs will inhibit the CYP450 enzymes. A list of some of these drugs can be found in **TABLE 10-4**. If a drug inhibits a P450 enzyme, the metabolism of other drugs will be slow and drug levels in the blood will increase, possibly leading to toxicity. This possibility should be considered in the event of unexpected toxicity of a drug (Lynch & Price, 2007).

Another property of the P450 enzymes is their **inducibility**. Enzyme induction occurs when the liver produces more of the metabolizing enzyme after exposure to the drug. This, then, leads to increased metabolism of drugs metabolized by this specific enzyme, lower blood levels of the drug, and thus decreased therapeutic efficacy. Some drugs which induce P450 enzymes are listed in Table 10-4.

Drug Excretion

The ability of the body to excrete drugs and metabolites is altered as a person ages. Most drugs and their metabolites are excreted in

TABLE 10-4 Drugs Which Inhibit or Induce Drug Metabolizing Enzymes

Drugs which inhibit drug metabolizing enzymes
St. John's Wort: herbal antidepressant
Fluvoxamine (Luvox): antidepressant
Cimetidine (Tagamet): antacid
Amiodarone (Cordarone): cardiac medication
Ciprofloxacin (Cipro): antibiotic
Diphenhydramine (Benadryl): antihistamine
Ketoconazole (Nizoral): antifungal
Metronidazole (Flagyl): antibiotic

Drugs which induce drug metabolizing enzymes
Fluoxetine (Prozac): antidepressant
Carbamazepine (Tegretol): anticonvulsant, mood stabilizer
Pentobarbital: sedative, anticonvulsant

Other substances that induce drug metabolism
Tobacco smoke
Alcohol (ethanol)
Grapefruit juice

the urine through the kidneys. Another route of drug excretion is through the bile into the intestines. The kidneys show a decline in blood flow in the older adult similar to that seen in the liver. In addition, the kidneys show a decrease in function with aging, which further decreases excretion of drugs (Weinstein & Anderson, 2010). The effect of this on drug excretion is again dependent upon the properties of the drug. To some extent, all drugs will be extracted by the kidney and excreted either unchanged or as a metabolite in the urine. A list of some important drugs whose excretion is affected by renal changes is shown in **TABLE 10-5**.

Thus, the changes in blood flow affect both drug metabolism and excretion. The organ

TABLE 10-5 Some Important Drugs
with Reduced Renal
Clearance in Older Patients

Methotrexate—Chemotherapy agent;
suppresses the immune system

Vancomycin—Antibacterial agents
Ampicillin/sulbactam—Antibacterial agents
Ciprofloxacin—Antibacterial agents
Azithromycin—Antibacterial agents

most involved will depend on the drug. Is it primarily metabolized by the liver or excreted by the kidney? These two factors are significant changes in pharmacokinetics that are affected by aging.

As noted in this section, many changes occur in the body as one ages and these changes affect how drugs are handled by the aging body. The most significant changes are in metabolism and excretion. While the liver continues to function well, blood flow to the liver is reduced. The kidneys are more affected with a decrease in function and blood flow. The healthcare practitioner needs to be aware of how individual drugs are affected by these changes; some more by the liver and others more by the kidneys. These changes make it important to consider that older patients may need to have decreased doses of many drugs to avoid high blood levels and toxic responses.

▶ Pharmacodynamics

Another aspect of pharmacology to consider in addition to pharmacokinetics is pharmacodynamics (i.e., what the drug does to the body). Pharmacodynamics involves examining how drug responses change based on changes in the cellular responses to drugs

over the life span. How this is altered as a person ages is dependent on the changes that occur in the drug's target(s), that is, the receptors or proteins in the body that interact with the drug to produce the effect. Given the considerable number of drugs that are used to treat chronic diseases and the increased number of chronic diseases that we are treating in older patients, the need for this research is critical. Because the FDA does not require testing in special populations of people, including older adults, the current understanding of pharmacodynamics in older patients is limited. However, studies are beginning to emerge that address this issue (e.g., Bowie & Slattum, 2007) with a goal to improve pharmacological treatment options for the older patient. Knowing more about why a person responds to specific medications is important information to have, as it can help a physician make decisions regarding the best drug to prescribe.

▶ Pharmacogenomics

Pharmacogenomics is the study of how a person's genetic background determines both the pharmacokinetic and pharmacodynamic responses to drugs. There is widespread variability in how older individuals metabolize drugs based on the levels of subtypes of cytochrome P450 enzymes (Ruscin & Linnebur, 2017). Currently, lab tests are available to clinicians that can determine the levels of these enzymes in a patient, so that prescribers can be informed as to which drugs can be used to treat a particular disease. As testing of this type becomes more widely available in terms of access and affordability, coupled with better understanding of the genetics that affect drug response, this approach will become standard practice in the pharmacy.

Advances are also being made in understanding how genetics change the response to drugs. For example, people differ in their response to selective serotonin reuptake inhibitor (SSRI) antidepressants such as fluoxetine (Prozac). This difference is because there are two variants of the gene that encodes for the protein that fluoxetine interacts with, the serotonin transporter. Patients with the long allele (variation) of the gene have a more effective transporter, hence fluoxetine is more effective in these patients. A blood test is available that would allow a physician to test for the presence of this allele, which would then inform the decision of which antidepressant would give the best response (**FIGURE 10-3**).

Another area that is being studied is precision dosing, often as a part of personalized medicine. Cancer therapy has been using precision dosing for some time. Because of the toxicity of cancer drugs, doses need to be determined precisely to give the patient the

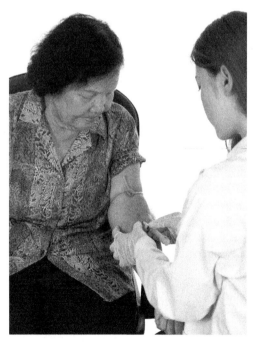

FIGURE 10-3 Physicians may use a blood test to determine the type of antidepressant to prescribe for a patient.
© BaLL LunLa/Shutterstock

right amount at the right time to minimize side effects while maximizing therapeutic response. Better attention to the exact doses given to the older patient would provide the same benefits. However, given the limited number of geriatricians (i.e., medical doctors specializing in working with older adults), this is very difficult to achieve, but may become possible with better training of primary care physicians.

A diagnosis of dementia can complicate precision dosing efforts. Patients with dementia have a more difficult time communicating if a drug is working and if they are experiencing side effects. So, it may take numerous attempts at communicating with them to elicit if they are experiencing drug effects or side effects. One of the most difficult areas to assess is pain. Since we have no noncognitive way of assessing a person's level of pain, we must rely on self-report. Because people with dementia may not be able to articulate about the pain they are experiencing, the practitioner might have to inquire repeatedly about the pain. Side effects may be apparent in noncognitive ways, such as falling asleep during a therapy session or signs of greater than normal confusion. Therefore, familiarity with a patient's baseline status and drug side effects are necessary to be able to raise concerns about over- or under-medication.

▶ Anticholinergic Syndrome

Anticholinergic syndrome refers to a collection of symptoms related to the effects of agents that block the neurotransmitter acetylcholine in the nervous system. The use of multiple drugs that have anticholinergic effects may result in a syndrome of symptoms that range from mild to severe. Anticholinergic syndrome may occur in a person at any age; yet, risk increases in older adults. A most important contributor is **polypharmacy** (i.e., taking more than one medications at a time).

The cholinergic system of the brain and the autonomic nervous system both use acetylcholine as a neurotransmitter. More specifically, acetylcholine is involved in learning and memory in the brain, and the central nervous system's influence on organs such as the heart, the bladder, and the gastrointestinal track. One type of acetylcholine receptor is the muscarinic receptor. This receptor is found throughout the brain, including areas involved in memory and cognition. General levels of arousal are also, in part, controlled by the cholinergic system. The parasympathetic nervous system also has acetylcholine as its neurotransmitter and muscarinic receptors as the primary receptors. Many organs are enervated by the parasympathetic nervous system, including the heart, intestines, salivary glands, and sweat glands. Activation of the parasympathetic nervous system decreases heart rate, increases the digestive system leading to increased intestinal motility, and increased salivation.

In the process of drug development, some classes of drugs have emerged from the large class of antihistamines. These include antipsychotics, such as chlorpromazine and haloperidol, and tricyclic antidepressants, such as imipramine and desipramine. In addition, the antihistamines have widespread usage. They are found in cold medications, sleep aids, and allergy medications. The antihistamines and other classes of drugs (Table 10-6) also act as antagonists at the muscarinic subtype of cholinergic receptors. That is, these drugs will block the physiologic action of acetylcholine at the muscarinic subtype of acetylcholine receptors. In addition, atropine-like drugs, which are also muscarinic receptor antagonists, are used in a variety of conditions, including motion sickness and diarrhea. Thus, it is possible to take multiple medications for multiple conditions that all have antagonist effects at the muscarinic cholinergic receptor.

TABLE 10-6 Anticholinergic Syndrome

Symptoms of Anticholinergic Syndrome

Forgetfulness	Tachycardia
Behavioral changes	Dry mouth
Motor incoordination	Constipation
Delirium	Urinary retention
Blurred vision	

Drugs with Anticholinergic Activity

Antihistamines	**Antipsychotics**
Chlorpheniramine	Chlorpromazine
Hydroxyzine	Haloperidol
Diphenhydramine	Olanzapine
Promethazine	Thioridazine

Antidepressants	**Antispasmotics**
Amitriptyline	Hyoscyamine
Desipramine	Dicyclomine
Doxepin	
Nortriptyline	

The symptoms of anticholinergic syndrome and drugs that produce these effects are shown in **TABLE 10-6**. A mnemonic used by medical students to remember the symptoms is shown in **TABLE 10-7**.

Because of multiple chronic conditions, an older patient may be taking many different medications, some of which may

TABLE 10-7 A Mnemonic for the Symptoms of Anticholinergic Syndrome

Red as a beet,
Dry as a bone,
Blind as a bat,
Mad as a hatter,
Hot as a hare,
Full as a flask

have anticholinergic effects. An important concern is the effects of this polypharmacy on cognition, through action on the cholinergic systems in the brain. Current evidence on aging in the brain across many species shows a slow and continuous decline in the cholinergic forebrain system, as well as other neurotransmitter systems (Mather, 2016). If there is a rapid decline of this system in the brain, a person may develop dementia at an early age as occurs with early onset of Alzheimer's disease. As age progresses, the risk of dementia increases. Symptoms are mild at first, often starting with forgetfulness. Then, they increase and intensify over time into more serious symptoms, including confusion, behavioral changes, and/or paranoia. If medications (i.e., anticholinergic drugs) are used that work against these same receptors in the brain, the patient will show a worsening of symptoms. Stopping these anticholinergic drugs will quickly reverse the drug-induced symptoms, although it will not reverse the underlying disease.

Other Syndromes

While anticholinergic syndrome may be common in older patients taking medications, another syndrome may also occur through the use of drugs that increase serotonin levels in the brain. The most commonly used drugs that increase serotonin in the brain are antidepressants and selective serotonin reuptake inhibitors (SSRIs) such as fluoxetine, sertraline, and citalopram (**TABLE 10-8**). Other drugs may also increase levels of serotonin in the brain, including some opioid pain relievers (e.g., meperidine), the antidepressant trazodone, which is often used to help induce sleep, and cold medications such as dextromethorphan.

Symptoms associated with serotonin syndrome vary from very mild to life threatening. Hyperreflexia and clonus, along with altered mental status (confusion) and hyperthermia,

TABLE 10-8 Serotonin Syndrome
Symptoms
Clonus
Hyperreflexia
Agitation
Hyperthermia
Tremor
Increased bowel sounds
Drugs with Serotonergic Activity
Antidepressants (all classes)
Migraine drugs (sumatriptan)
Trazadone
Opioids
Amphetamines
St. John's Wort
Anti-vomiting drugs: granisetron, ondansetron
Metaclopramide
Dextromethorphan
Cyclobenzaprine
L-DOPA, levodopa

are commonly seen. When the drugs are discontinued, the symptoms will resolve. This correlates with polypharmacy in older patients using different classes of medication that have effects on serotonin. These examples of syndromes associated with polypharmacy support the need for careful review of medications from many different perspectives, including the age of the patient.

▶ Drug Dependence, Misuse, and Addiction

Substance misuse and abuse is a current topic of considerable concern in modern medicine, affecting persons of all ages. Older adults have many chronic conditions involving pain. How we treat pain continues to be a significant challenge. Nonsteroidal anti-inflammatory drugs (NSAIDs) such as aspirin or ibuprofen (Advil) are the first line of therapy in the treatment of mild to moderate pain. These drugs are not without serious side effects, including gastrointestinal bleeding and renal toxicity, especially if these drugs are taken in high doses over prolonged periods of time. In persons who cannot tolerate these side effects or persons who are experiencing moderate or severe pain, the next level of pain relief is with opioids such as morphine or oxycodone (Oxycontin; FIGURE 10-4).

Difficulty sleeping is another symptom associated with chronic disease and aging. While need for sleep does not decrease, the ability to have productive sleep does, especially in older persons with chronic pain. Hence, individuals often are seeking pharmacological agents to help them sleep. Sleep medications can include benzodiazepines such as diazepam (Valium), alprazolam (Xanax), and oxazepam (Serax).

Unfortunately, both benzodiazepines and opioids are classes of drugs which can lead to tolerance and dependence. **Tolerance** means that as patients continue to use a drug the therapeutic effect declines, thus requiring an increased dose to maintain the therapeutic effect. **Dependence** occurs with

continued use of a drug and results in symptoms of withdrawal if the drug is discontinued. With opiates, discontinuation would result in increased pain, inability to sleep, and flu-like symptoms. With benzodiazepines, discontinuation may result in agitation, increased anxiety, and insomnia. Therefore, these drugs must be used only if absolutely needed and only for short periods. Alternatives, including nonpharmacologic solutions and other classes of drugs, should be considered first. In this regard, an interdisciplinary healthcare team can be useful in helping a person through such challenges. The most serious effect of long-term use of these drugs is addiction. If addicted, a person continues uncontrolled use of a drug despite experiencing adverse consequences.

If the use of medications with misuse potential is unavoidable, then strict limits should be placed on the use of the drugs. For example, the standard protocol for all patients is a written agreement between the prescriber and the patient that the patient will only take the medications as directed and will not give the medications to any other person. Some situations may require pill counts and limits on the number of pills prescribed. In the case of opiates, long-acting agents (i.e., drugs that are taken once a day as opposed to short-acting drugs which may need to be taken three to four times a day) are recommended. In the case of benzodiazepines, shorter acting agents with minimal active metabolites are recommended.

Alcohol misuse continues to be a problem for many people in late life. Continued use of moderate to high amounts of alcohol can lead to dependence and uncontrolled use. The health consequences of alcohol dependence cannot be covered adequately here, but can include decreased cognitive function, cardiomyopathy (damage to the heart), and hepatitis and cirrhosis of the liver. When combined with sedatives, alcohol use increases the risk of falls. Drinking alcohol can exacerbate the sedative side effects

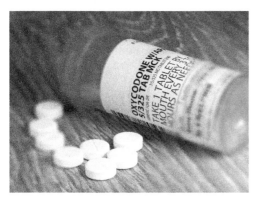

FIGURE 10-4 Oxycodone is the generic name for an opioid pain killing tablet.
© Steve Heap/Shutterstock

of many drugs, and thus should be avoided (Patton, 2002). Once again, polypharmacy places older adults at increased risk when alcohol is also used.

▶ Beers List and STOPP/START

Many drugs and drug groups have been mentioned that should be avoided (or only used after careful consideration) when treating older patients. Still, there are many more drug groups and drugs about which to be concerned. So, how do we know what drugs to avoid, and more importantly what drugs are safe to use in older patients?

In 1991, Beers and colleagues published a landmark study of inappropriate medications to be used for nursing home patients. Due to the lack of well-controlled clinical trials of medication effectiveness and toxicity in older patients, Beers and colleagues sought consensus from experts as to which medications should be avoided in frail, older patients. Some classes of drugs initially highlighted as inappropriate were sedative-hypnotics, antidepressants, antipsychotics, some antihypertensives, some analgesics, histamine-2 blockers, decongestants,

and muscle relaxants. Since this list was focused on the frail and sick older patient, Beers (1997) expanded his criteria to include all older patients. In his more recent recommendation, he not only included drug-disease interactions, but also drugs to avoid, independent of diagnoses. In 2003, Fick and colleagues, including Dr. Beers, updated the "Beers Criteria for Potentially Inappropriate Medication" even further, dropping 11 medications from the original list but adding 44 more! The change was a wake-up call to physicians and healthcare practitioners to consider all drug classes before prescribing for older populations.

In 2008, Gallagher and colleagues published the Screening Tool of Older People's Potentially Inappropriate Prescriptions (STOPP) for persons over 65 years of age. They divided findings into nine systems as well as indicated care with use of duplicate drug classes. Later, the team went one step further and created the Screening Tool to Alert doctors to Right (i.e., appropriate, indicated) Treatments (START) but retained the same nine systems as STOPP. Version 2 of STOPP/START was published by O'Mahoney and colleagues in 2015. Some examples of medications in the START list are shown in **TABLE 10-9**.

TABLE 10-9 Examples of START (Screening Tool to Alert doctors to Right Treatments) Medications

Drug Name	Diagnosis/Health Condition
Warfarin	Chronic atrial fibrillation
Statins	Documented history of vascular disease
ACE inhibitors	CHF and following acute MI
Regular inhaled B2 agonists and corticosteroids	Moderate to severe asthma or COPD
Metformin	Type 2 diabetes

▶ Herbal Medicines and Supplements

The use of herbal medicine and supplements has taken off during the past two decades. All age groups are using more nutraceuticals, a term that includes herbal medicines and supplements. Older adults consume more nutraceuticals than any other age group. In 2002, 30% of women and 24% of men over the age of 65 used nutraceuticals (Kelly et al., 2005). What nutraceuticals are used for varies considerably depending on current popular and medical opinion on its value. In a survey of over 2,000 older adults with a mean age of 71 years, 51.8% used dietary supplements in 2005–2006 and 62.7% used dietary supplements in 2010–2011 (Qato et al., 2016). More specifically, women used more dietary supplements than men. From 2005 to 2006, 4.7% of people studied used omega-3 fish oils. Usage jumped to 18.6% in 2010–2011, which is due in part to reports that suggested diets rich in omega-3 fish oils are cardio-protective (Eslick, Howe, Smith, Priest, & Bensoussan, 2009). A list of other nutraceuticals widely used by older adults is listed in **TABLE 10-10**.

A significant misconception about nutraceuticals is that they are safe and effective, although evidence indicates they may not be. The FDA does not regulate nutraceuticals unless they are shown to be a significant risk to public health. One such example is the herbal medicine ephedrine. Ephedrine is a component of Ma Huang tea, a Chinese herbal remedy. Taken correctly, it can be a mild stimulant which increases a feeling of well-being. In higher doses, it can cause significant increases in blood pressure and has caused strokes in some individuals (Kolecki, 2015). Due to this serious health risk, the FDA removed it from the market in 2004.

People need to be reminded that such OTC remedies are drugs and can have significant side effects and interactions with the other medications they are taking. A very good example of this is St. John's Wort. It is a widely used herbal medicine that has been shown to be effective in mild to moderate depression. Research has shown that it works to increase serotonin (i.e., the neurotransmitter which leads to a happy mood), very similar to prescription drugs used to treat depression. Because it increases serotonin in the brain, it may lead to serotonin syndrome, if

TABLE 10-10 Common Herbal Medicines and Dietary Supplements Used by Adults Age 65+

Supplement or Herbal Medicine	Proposed Use	Percentage Using Weekly
Lutein	Eye health	15.0 (women), 13.4 (men)
Glucosamine	Joint health	9.8 (women), 4.3 (men)
Chondroitin	Joint health	7.0 (women), 3.9 (men)
Saw palmetto	Prostate health	2.6 (men)
Gingko biloba	Memory	4.0 (women), 2.2 (men)

Data from Kelly et al. (2005).

TABLE 10-11 Side Effects of Herbal Medicines

Herbal Medicine	Side Effects and Drug–Drug Interactions
Gingko Biloba	Bleeding, increases effects of anticoagulants, hypoglycemic agents (diabetes), decreases effects of anticonvulsants
Kava	Sedation, liver damage, increases effects of other sedatives
Ginseng	Increases effect of anticoagulants
Garlic	Bleeding, increases effects of anticoagulants, hypoglycemic agents (diabetes)
Ginger	Increases effects of anticoagulants, hypoglycemic agents; decreases effectiveness of antihypertensive agents

Data from Marko & DerMarderosian (2016).

used with other drugs that increase serotonin. Moreover, it will induce the drug metabolizing enzyme cytochrome P450-3A4, one of the major drug metabolizing enzymes in the liver (Markowitz et al., 2003). This, then, can lead to decreased blood levels of other drugs, such as alprazolam (Xanax), a sedative-hypnotic drug. A number of other herbal remedies that have significant side effects or drug–drug interactions can be found in **TABLE 10-11** (Marko & DerMarderosian, 2016).

Because nutraceuticals are not regulated, manufacturers cannot advertise that they are treatments for any diseases. Because they are not treatments for a specific disease, there is no dosage that can be recommended for taking the supplements. Consumers are expected to find the proper dosage themselves, for any given indication (if proper guidelines even exist). Compared to FDA-regulated drugs, there is little money to be made in nutraceuticals. As a result, large research studies have generally not been done to determine if they are effective as claimed. Today, a few well-controlled studies are underway, yet more research is still needed to determine how nutraceuticals can best be used (Lawvere & Mahoney, 2005).

▶ Polypharmacy

A key issue in the pharmacotherapeutics in the older patient is polypharmacy. Due to the increased incidence of chronic disease and added media pressure from the pharmaceutical industry to consume their products, older patients are taking significantly more medications than younger patients (**FIGURE 10-5**). There is also an iatrogenic (i.e., physician

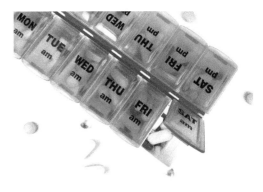

FIGURE 10-5 Older adults are taking significantly more pills than younger patients. Weekly pill boxes, like the one pictured, help patients keep track of when to take which pills.

© JLMcAnally/Shutterstock

TABLE 10-12 Medication Errors Leading to Polypharmacy

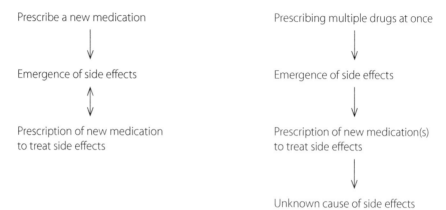

Prescribe a new medication
↓
Emergence of side effects
↑↓
Prescription of new medication
to treat side effects

Prescribing multiple drugs at once
↓
Emergence of side effects
↓
Prescription of new medication(s)
to treat side effects
↓
Unknown cause of side effects

Data from Figure 1, Merel and Paauw, (2017), p. 1579.

induced) component to polypharmacy, with practitioners adding additional medications to treat side effects (**TABLE 10-12**).

A number of basic commonsense steps are generally taken to reduce the number of drugs prescribed for a patient (**TABLE 10-13**). The first step is being aware of all medications being taken (as well as dosages), including herbal and dietary supplements. This is usually best done by asking people to bring everything that they are taking, no matter how seemingly minor, to an office visit (sometimes referred to as a "brown bag review"). Medications and supplements can be identified and the problems they are used to treat can be determined. Care should be taken to ensure that the person is not using two different trade names of the same drug.

Understanding the clinical signs associated with each medicine, its possible side effects, and how the drug is being taken are important principles to consider. Eliminating medications with no therapeutic benefit or where the medication is not indicated is important. In the older adult, a review may lead to changing medications to obtain a more favorable side effect profile. For example, changing from an antidepressant with

TABLE 10-13 A Stepwise Approach to Polypharmacy

Use nonpharmacologic treatments, if at all possible

Disclose all medications being used

Identify medications by generic name and drug class

Identify the clinical indication of each medication

Know the side effect profile of each medication

Identify risk factors for an adverse drug reaction

Eliminate medications with no therapeutic benefit

Eliminate medication with no clinical indication

Substitute a safer medication

In the older adult, avoid a drug with anticholinergic side effects

Avoid treating an adverse drug reaction with a drug

Use a single drug with a less frequent dosing schedule

anticholinergic side effects to one that does not have these side effects may provide the person with a better quality of life. Avoid treating side effects with another drug, if at all possible. Choosing a drug that is taken once a day will improve compliance compared to a drug that must be taken three times a day. Review of medications on a regular basis will also aid in avoiding the problems of polypharmacy.

One key principle in the use of multiple medications is, if possible, is to only start one drug at a time. This will avoid later challenges in determining the source of side effects when multiple medications are started at the same time. This approach requires patience as it may take some time for the drug to reach therapeutic levels in the blood. Hence, determining if a drug is working and if it is producing any side effects will only be uncovered when the full effect of the medication has been reached, which can be a variable time frame. When starting a new therapeutic agent, it is also important to know if the dose should be adjusted downward because of either hepatic or renal metabolism (as noted at the beginning of this chapter). Use the phrases to "Go Low and Go Slow" and "KISS—Keep It Simple Seriously" when evaluating medications in the older patient.

▶ Summary

Pharmacotherapeutics in the older adult is complicated. This may be the most challenging area of geriatric medicine. The physiologic changes that occur with aging lead to significant changes in both pharmacokinetics (i.e., what the body does to a drug) and pharmacodynamics (i.e., what the drug does to the body). The variability of these changes relating to chronologic aging adds to the challenge. The need for multiple medications to treat multiple chronic diseases over long periods of time can lead to even more potential complications. Two things will reduce the toxicity associated with these challenges. First, medical schools must devote significant resources to training future physicians in these issues. And most importantly, the entire healthcare team must be alerted to the issues presented in this chapter so that medication-related concerns can be discussed with the patient and the entire team to resolve any potential issues.

🔍 CASE STUDIES

Case 1: M.R. is a 75-year-old woman who is being treated by a physical therapist post hip replacement. Her medications include desipramine for chronic pain. She takes diphenhydramine to help her sleep. She is then started on hyoscyamine for diarrhea. She now is showing worsening memory problems and disorientation.

1. **What do these drugs have in common that might lead to this presentation?**
2. **How do these drugs act to produce these symptoms?**

Case 2: Confusion due to benzodiazepine
A 75-year-old man is brought to the emergency room by his daughter. She states that over the past few days his cognitive abilities have shown a marked decrease. He now appears disoriented. His medical history includes hypertension, hypercholesterolemia, and atrial fibrillation. His medications include simvastatin, quinapril, and warfarin. He has recently been complaining of difficulty sleeping and has been started on a long-acting benzodiazepine, alprazolam.

1. **How does addition of benzodiazepine cause disorientation?**
2. **What role might the patient's age play in the metabolism of his medications?**
3. **How might the physician change the prescription to avoid these side effects**

TEST YOUR KNOWLEDGE

Review Questions

1. What is the major organ of drug metabolism?
   a. Large intestine
   b. Pancreas
   c. Kidney
   d. Liver

2. Dora, a 78-year-old woman, was not feeling well, so she went to her doctor. After reviewing her medical history and performing a physical examination, the physician diagnosed her with anticholinergic syndrome, which he attributed to one of the four medications she was taking. Which of Dora's medications is likely causing her anticholinergic syndrome symptoms?
   a. Zestoretic (an ACE inhibitor)
   b. Doxepin (an antidepressant)
   c. Lasix (a diuretic)
   d. Naproxen (an NSAID)

3. Which group of people consumes more nutraceuticals than any other age group?
   a. Adolescents
   b. Young adults
   c. Middle-aged adults
   d. Older adults

4. Anticholinergic syndrome refers to a collection of symptoms related to the effects of agents that block which neurotransmitter?
   a. Dopamine
   b. Norepinephrine
   c. Acetylcholine
   d. Serotonin

5. A drug must be tested in older populations in order to receive federal approval.
   a. True
   b. False

Learning Activities

1. Describe how pharmaceutical companies show the FDA that drugs are safe and effective, identify the ideal method of doing so, and explain the problems associated with this method.
2. Explain how pharmacokinetics differs from pharmacodynamics.
3. Imagine that you are working with a patient who has dementia and trying to develop the precise dose for a medication being used to relieve pain. What difficulties might you encounter and what can you do to overcome them?

4. Do you feel that strict limits should be placed on the use of medications with misuse potential? Why or why not? What types of limits would you recommend, if any?
5. Imagine that a friend tells you she is considering taking kava to help reduce her feelings of anxiety and wants your opinion. She is not currently taking any type of medication and has no diagnosed medical conditions. Would you recommend that she take this herbal supplement? Why or why not?

References

Beers, M. H. (1997). Explicit criteria for determining potentially inappropriate medication use by the elderly. *Archives of Internal Medicine, 157*, 1531–1536. doi:10.1001/archinte.1997.00440350031003

Beers, M. H., Ouslander, J. G., Rollingher, I., Reuben, D. B., Brooks, J., & Beck, J. C. (1991). Explicit criteria for determining inappropriate medication use in nursing home residents. UCLA Division of Geriatric Medicine. *Archives of Intern Medicine, 151*, 1825–1832. doi:10.1001/archinte.1991.00400090107019

Bowie, M. W., & Slattum, P. W. (2007). Pharmacodynamics in older adults: A review. *American Journal of Geriatric Pharmacotherapy, 5*, 263–303.

Cusack, B. J. (2004). Pharmacokinetics in older persons. *American Journal of Geriatric Pharmacotherapy, 2*, 274–302. doi:10.1016/j.amjopharm.2004.12.005

Editorial. (2014). Geriatrics—the care of the aged. *Journal of the American Medical Association, 312*(11), 1159–1159. doi:10.1001/jama.2014.10855 (Reprinted from Editorial. (1937). *Journal of the American Medical Association, 109*(26), 2143-2144.

Eslick, G. D., Howe, P. R. C., Smith, C., Priest, R., & Bensoussan, A. (2009). Benefits of fish oil supplementation in hyperlipidemia: A systematic review and meta-analysis. *International Journal of Cardiology, 136*, 4–16. doi:10.1016/j.ijcard.2008.03.092

Fick, D. M., Cooper, J. W., Wade, W. E., Waller, J. L., Maclean, J. R., & Beers, M. H. (2003). Updating the Beers criteria for potentially inappropriate medication use in older adults: Results of a US consensus panel of experts. *Archives of Internal Medicine, 163*, 2716–2724. doi:10.1001/archinte.163.22.2716

Gallagher, P., Ryan, C., Byrne, S., Kennedy, J., & O'Mahony, D. (2008). STOPP (screening tool of older person's prescriptions) and START (screening tool to alert doctors to right treatment). consensus validation. *International Journal of Clinical Pharmacology and Therapeutics, 46*, 72–83. doi:10.1093/ageing/afn197

Kelly, J. P., Kaufman, D. W., Kelley, K., Rosenberg, L., Anderson, T. E., & Mitchell, A. A. (2005). Recent trends in use of herbal and other natural products. *Archives of Internal Medicine, 165*, 281–286. doi:10.1001/archinte.165.3.281

Kolecki, P. (2015). Sympathomimetic toxicity. Retrieved from https://emedicine.medscape.com/article/818583 -overview?pa=1dR2uPMi7lC0TvR4KZaFd6go9772 zhy6hP026pKMn7xYSYXnIiKGgma0tAwQQyS98 SIvl8zjYv73GUyW5rsbWA%3D%3D

Lawvere, S., & Mahoney, M. C. (2005). St. John's Wort. *American Family Physician, 72*, 2249–2254.

Lynch, T., & Price, A. (2007). The effect of cytochrome P450 metabolism on drug response, interactions, and adverse effects. *American Family Physician, 76*, 391–396.

Marko, M. G., & DerMarderosian, A. (2016). Overview of dietary supplements. *Merck Manual: Professional Version*. Retrieved from http://www.merckmanuals.com /professional/special-subjects/dietary-supplements /overview-of-dietary-supplements

Markowitz, J. S., Donovan, J. L., DeVane, C. L., Taylor, R. M., Ruan, Y., Wang, J. S., & Chavin, K. D. (2003). Effect of St John's Wort on drug metabolism by induction of cytochrome P450 3A4 enzyme. *Journal of the American Medical Association, 290*, 1500–1504. doi:10.1001/jama.290.11.1500

Mather, M. (2016). The affective neuroscience of aging. *Annual Review of Psychology, 67*, 213–238. doi:10.1146/ annurev-psych-122414-033540

McLean, A. J., & Le Couteur, D. G. (2004). Aging biology and geriatric clinical pharmacology. *Pharmacological Reviews, 56*, 163–184. doi:10.1124/pr.56.2.4

Medina-Walpole, A., & Pacala, J. T. (2016). *Geriatrics review syllabus* (9th ed.). American Geriatrics Society. New York, NY: Author.

Merel, S. E., & Paauw, D. S. (2017). Common drug side effects and drug-drug interactions in elderly adults in primary care. *Journal of the American Geriatrics Society, 65*(7), 1578–1585.

O'Mahony, D., O'Sullivan, D., Byrne, S., O'Connor, M. N., Ryan, C., & Gallagher, P. (2015). STOPP/START criteria for potentially inappropriate prescribing in older people: Version 2. *Age and Ageing, 44*(2), 213–218.

Patton, R. (2002). Alcohol consumption and mortality: Falls and the elderly. *The British Medical Journal, 325*, 191.

Qato, D. M., Wilder, J., Schumm, L. P., Gillet, V., & Alexander, G. C. (2016). Changes in prescription and over-the-counter medication and dietary supplement use among older adults in the United States, 2005 vs 2011. *Journal of the American Medical Association Internal Medicine, 176*, 473–482. doi:10.1001/ jamainternmed.2015.8581

Ruscin, J. M., & Linnebur, S. A. (2017). Drug therapy in the elderly. *Merck Manual/Professional/ Geriatrics*. Retrieved from http://www.merckmanuals .com/professional/geriatrics/drug-therapy-in-the -elderly/introduction-to-drug-therapy-in-the-elderly

Weinstein, J. R., & Anderson, S. (2010). The aging kidney: Physiological changes. *Advances in Chronic Kidney Disease, 17*, 302–307.

CHAPTER 11

Nutrition and Aging

Kathryn H. Thompson, PhD, RD

CHAPTER OUTLINE

BEHAVIORAL OBJECTIVES

Upon completion of this chapter, the reader will be able to:

1. Demonstrate knowledge of current research on the impact of aging on nutrition status for healthy individuals and individuals with chronic diseases.
2. Describe the importance of early screening and intervention for nutritional risk in older adults.
3. Identify screening tools for the assessment of nutritional risk in the older adult.
4. Recognize the multiple factors that affect nutrition status in older adults (physiologic, social, psychological, economic, and environmental).
5. Describe the physiologic impact of aging on dietary intake and absorption.

(continues)

(*continued*)

6. Use MyPlate to advise the older adult about the implementation of the 2015–2020 Dietary Guidelines for Americans.
7. Describe the basics of the Mediterranean diet and the DASH diet for the treatment of common chronic diseases in the older adult.
8. Recognize the impact of polypharmacy on nutritional status and drug–nutrient interactions in older adults.
9. Describe the appropriate use of nutritional supplements for the older adult.

KEY TERMS

Anorexia	Dehydration	Malnutrition
Cachexia	Diabetes	Mediterranean diet
Calcium	Dietary fiber	Nutritional supplements
Carbohydrate	Dietary Guidelines for Americans	Overnutrition
Cardiovascular disease	Dysphagia	Protein
Celiac disease	Gluten	Vitamin B$_{12}$
Cholesterol	Hypertension	Vitamin D
DASH (Dietary Approach to Stop Hypertension) diet	Lactose intolerance	Weight loss
	Malabsorption	

▶ Introduction

The importance of good nutrition throughout the life span and its contribution to health and quality of life cannot be overestimated. The average life expectancy of individuals in the United States has increased from 68 years in 1950 to 79 years in 2013. By 2060, it is projected that the number of Americans who are 65 or older will more than double to over 98 million and account for nearly 24% of the total U.S. population (Mather, Jacobsen, & Pollard, 2015).

Older adults are a heterogeneous population with health and abilities ranging from healthy and high functioning to frail with complete dependence on others for care. There is a wide range of **malnutrition** prevalence rates reported for this age group ranging from 12–70% in hospitalized patients (Corkins et al., 2014) to 1.5–67% in nursing home residents (Bell, Lee, & Tamura, 2015) and 5.8% in community dwelling adults

(DiMaria-Ghalili, Michael, & Rosso, 2013; Kaiser et al., 2010), which makes it somewhat challenging to address. Moreover, the prevalence of chronic disease in the older adult population is high. Among Medicare beneficiaries, two-thirds are diagnosed with at least two chronic diseases, and 14% have six or more (Centers for Medicare and Medicaid Services, 2012). However, many of these chronic diseases can be managed successfully with nutrition intervention, which can improve both quality and quantity of life.

For many older adults, late life can be a time of great change socially, economically, psychologically, and physically. With the death of a spouse and/or friends, many older adults find themselves increasingly isolated, living alone, and eating meals alone. Living on a fixed income often results in less money available for food purchases. Older adults may become more limited in their mobility due to joint, muscular, and related health problems. Whether experienced separately or in combination, these factors influence the nutritional status of older adults.

The Older Americans Act Reauthorization Act of 2016 (S.192, 2016) places special emphasis on integrated health promotion and disease prevention through nutrition education of older adults to improve their health (Food and Nutrition Board, Institute of Medicine, & Committee on Nutrition Services for Medicare Beneficiaries, 2000). To realize these goals, providers are advised to offer early nutrition screening and intervention for problems of **weight loss**, nutrient deficiencies, and **overnutrition**. States must utilize the expertise of dietitians or other individuals with equivalent education and training to provide these services. All nutritional recommendations and treatment plans should be developed after consideration of individual variations in physiological status, environmental influences, and social support (as discussed further in this chapter).

▶ Screening

The Nutrition Screening Initiative

One of the best ways to achieve high-quality nutrition care for older adults is to promote early screening and intervention. Since 1989, the American Dietetic Association, the National Council on Aging, and the American Academy of Family Physicians have collaborated in an effort called the Nutrition Screening Initiative (NSI) to encourage early and routine screening and intervention for nutrition risk in older adults (White, Ham, Lipschitz, Dwyer, & Wellman, 1991). Guiding the NSI is the underlying premise that nutrition status is a *vital sign*, just as important in evaluating a person's health and well-being as the traditional vital signs of blood pressure and pulse. Moreover, the NSI strives to increase older adults' awareness about nutrition and health and offers healthcare practitioners the

tools to do so. Specifically, the NSI developed the DETERMINE (an acronym described in **FIGURE 11-1**) questionnaire, which can be used to identify whether an individual is at risk for compromised nutritional well-being and assess for change in level of nutritional risk over time (**FIGURE 11-2**).

There are a number of other nutrition screening tools that can be used by non-nutrition trained staff to assess the risk of malnutrition for the older patient. One of the simplest is the Malnutrition Screening Tool (MST), which consists of three simple questions:

- Have you lost weight recently without trying?
- If yes, how much weight have you lost?
- Have you been eating poorly because of decreased appetite?

The first question is scored as 0 (No) or 2 (Unsure), the second question is scored from 1 to 4 based on the amount of weight lost with a score of 2 entered for unsure, and the third question is scored as 0 (No) and 1 (Yes). A total score of 2 or more indicates the older adult is at risk of malnutrition and further assessment is warranted (Anthony, 2008).

The Malnutrition Universal Screening Tool (MUST) is yet another screening tool that has been validated for use in both hospitals and nursing homes. Through the use of this tool, malnutrition risk is determined by assessing body mass index (BMI), unintentional weight loss, and the severity of acute disease (Avelino-Silva & Jaluul, 2017). BMI is used to define normal weight, overweight, and obesity at all ages and is determined by dividing a person's weight in kilograms by his or her height in meters squared. In studies comparing the reliability, validity, and ease of use of the screening tools, both the MST (Skipper, Ferguson, Thompson, Castellanos, & Porcari, 2012) and the MUST (Poulia et al., 2012, 2017) have been shown to perform very well and are recommended for screening older adults in both in-patient and out-patient settings.

The Nutrition Checklist is based on the Warning Signs described below. Use the word <u>DETERMINE</u> to remind you of the Warning Signs.

Disease

Any disease, illness or chronic condition which causes you to change the way you eat, or makes it hard for you to eat, puts your nutritional health at risk. Four out of five adults have chronic diseases that are affected by diet. Confusion or memory loss that keeps getting worse is estimated to affect one out of five or more of older adults. This can make it hard to remember what, when or if you've eaten. Feeling sad or depressed, which happens to about one in eight older adults, can cause big changes in appetite, digestion, energy level, weight and well-being.

Eating Poorly

Eating too little and eating too much both lead to poor health. Eating the same foods day after day or not eating fruit, vegetables, and milk products daily will also cause poor nutritional health. One in five adults skip meals daily. Only 13% of adults eat the minimum amount of fruit and vegetables needed. One in four older adults drink too much alcohol. Many health problems become worse if you drink more than one or two alcoholic beverages per day.

Tooth Loss/Mouth Pain

A healthy mouth, teeth and gums are needed to eat. Missing, loose or rotten teeth or dentures which don't fit well, or cause mouth sores, make it hard to eat.

Economic Hardship

As many as 40% of older Americans have incomes of less than $6,000 per year. Having less -- or choosing to spend less -- than $25-30 per week for food makes it very hard to get the foods you need to stay healthy.

Reduced Social Contact

One-third of all older people live alone. Being with people daily has a positive effect on morale, well-being and eating.

Multiple Medicines

Many older Americans must take medicines for health problems. Almost half of older Americans take multiple medicines daily. Growing old may change the way we respond to drugs. The more medicines you take, the greater the chance for side effects such as increased or decreased appetite, change in taste, constipation, weakness, drowsiness, diarrhea, nausea, and others. Vitamins or minerals, when taken in large doses, act like drugs and can cause harm. Alert your doctor to everything you take.

Involuntary Weight Loss/Gain

Losing or gaining a lot of weight when you are not trying to do so is an important warning sign that must not be ignored. Being overweight or underweight also increases your chance of poor health.

Needs Assistance In Self Care

Although most older people are able to eat, one of every five have trouble walking, shopping, buying and cooking food, especially as they get older.

Elder Years Above Age 80

Most older people lead full and productive lives. But as age increases, risk of frailty and health problems increase. Checking your nutritional health regularly makes good sense.

The Nutrition Screening Initiative • 1010 Wisconsin Avenue, NW • Suite 800 • Washington, DC 20007
The Nutrition Screening Initiative is funded in part by a grant from Ross Products Division of Abbott Laboratories, Inc.

FIGURE 11-1 Factors that influence nutrition risk: the DETERMINE tool.

The National Resource Center on Nutrition & Aging

The Warning Signs of poor nutritional health are often overlooked. Use this Checklist to find out if you or someone you know is at nutritional risk.

Read the statements below. Circle the number in the "yes" column for those that apply to you or someone you know. For each "yes" answer, score the number in the box. Total your nutritional score.

DETERMINE YOUR NUTRITIONAL HEALTH

	YES
I have an illness or condition that made me change the kind and/or amount of food I eat.	2
I eat fewer than 2 meals per day.	3
I eat few fruits or vegetables or milk products.	2
I have 3 or more drinks of beer, liquor or wine almost every day.	2
I have tooth or mouth problems that make it hard for me to eat.	2
I don't always have enough money to buy the food I need.	4
I eat alone most of the time.	1
I take 3 or more different prescribed or over-the-counter drugs a day.	1
Without wanting to, I have lost or gained 10 pounds in the last 6 months.	2
I am not always physically able to shop, cook and/or feed myself.	2
	TOTAL

Total Your Nutritional Score. If it's –

0-2   **Good!** Recheck your nutritional score in 6 months.

3-5   **You are at moderate nutritional risk.** See what can be done to improve your eating habits and lifestyle. Your office on aging, senior nutrition program, senior citizens center or health department can help. Recheck your nutritional score in 3 months.

6 or more   **You are at high nutritional risk.** Bring this Checklist the next time you see your doctor, dietitian or other qualified health or social service professional. Talk with them about any problems you may have. Ask for help to improve your nutritional health.

Remember that Warning Signs suggest risk, but do not represent a diagnosis of any condition. Turn the page to learn more about the Warnings Signs of poor nutritional health.

These materials are developed and distributed by the Nutrition Screening Initiative, a project of:

 AMERICAN ACADEMY OF FAMILY PHYSICIANS

 THE AMERICAN DIETETIC ASSOCIATION

THE NATIONAL COUNCIL ON THE AGING, INC.

 The Nutrition Screening Initiative • 1010 Wisconsin Avenue, NW • Suite 800 • Washington, DC 20007
The Nutrition Screening Initiative is funded in part by a grant from Ross Products Division of Abbott Laboratories, Inc.

FIGURE 11-2 The DETERMINE screening tool.

The National Resource Center on Nutrition & Aging

Patients who have been identified as "at risk" for malnutrition should be evaluated further using a nutrition assessment tool. Nutrition assessment tools are useful in quantifying risk and determining severity and duration of the malnutrition, as well as identifying possible causes for the deficits. These assessment tools are used and relied upon by clinicians, dietitians, and other healthcare professionals with nutritional training because of their ease in use and reliability and validity in identifying nutrition risk. For example, the Subjective Global Assessment (SGA) is a widely used tool to classify patients from well-nourished to severely malnourished. When using the SGA, the clinician records patient weight history, diet history, primary diagnosis, stress level, and changes in functional status. However, clinical judgment is needed in analyzing the information provided. The Mini Nutritional Assessment (MNA) includes anthropometric measurements, diet history, appetite, feeding mode, and laboratory measures of nutritional status. The MNA was developed especially for use with older adults in hospitals, nursing homes, and the community (Avelino-Silva & Jaluul, 2017).

Both the SGA and the MNA include an assessment of weight, muscle mass (mid-arm or calf circumference), and mobility or functional capacity. The inclusion of these criteria is recommended in a consensus statement from the Academy of Nutrition and Dietetics and the American Society for Parenteral and Enteral Nutrition (White et al., 2012) on the diagnosis of malnutrition, which needs to include two or more of the following six characteristics:

- Insufficient energy intake
- Weight loss
- Loss of muscle mass
- Loss of subcutaneous fat
- Localized generalized fluid accumulation that may mask weight loss
- Diminished functional status as measured by handgrip strength

Undernutrition: Weight and Malnutrition

Because the older population is heterogeneous, the prevalence of malnutrition will vary depending on multiple factors, including age distribution and living situation. Results of the MNA survey conducted in Europe, the United States, and South Africa showed that the prevalence of malnutrition in older adults was 22.8%. The highest rates of malnutrition were found among individuals living in institutional settings (50.5%) and the lowest rates among people living in the community (5.8%; Kaiser et al., 2010).

Decreases in body weight are common in adults ages 65–90, and should be considered a warning sign for nutritional risk. There is a strong association between undernutrition and increased morbidity and mortality (Sullivan, 1995). Involuntary weight loss may be caused by inadequate dietary intake, loss of appetite, muscle atrophy, and/or the inflammatory effects of disease. Many older adults may experience a combination of these factors, resulting in nutritional deficiencies in addition to weight loss.

Inadequate Dietary Intake

Many older adults live and eat alone, and their social isolation is associated with decreased food intake. However, studies have shown that food intake can be improved when older adults are able to eat with others (de Castro & Brewer, 1992; Locher, Robinson, Roth, Ritchie, & Burgio, 2005). Older adults are often on fixed incomes, which may limit their ability to purchase food. Chronic disease and the medications needed to manage these conditions may also create a financial burden, forcing individuals to choose between buying food or medications.

Inadequate nutritional intake and unexplained weight loss in older adults is often associated with malignancy or depression. In several small studies of patients with unexplained weight loss, malignancy was a factor in 6%–36% of the patients evaluated (Rabino-vitz, Pitlik, Leifer, Garty, & Rosenfeld, 1986; Thompson & Morris, 1991; Wilson, Vaswani, Liu, Morley, & Miller, 1998). Depression is also associated with decreased food intake in both institutional and community settings. Wilson and colleagues (1998) reviewed the charts of over 1,000 patients and found that depression was a cause of weight loss in 30% of the older patients. In comparison, only 15% of the younger patients were found to have weight loss associated with depression.

Dysphagia, the decreased ability or inability to swallow, is a condition that commonly occurs after a stroke, with Parkinson's disease, or with other motility or structural disorders of the esophagus. Approximately 7%–10% of older adults experience dysphagia and thus are at risk for poor nutritional intake (Achem & Devault, 2005; Keller, 1993). Dementia also is associated with poor nutritional intake. Inadequate energy and **protein** intake are commonly seen in persons with Alzheimer's disease. The lack of proper caloric intake is a predictive factor of morbidity and mortality (White, 1998).

Chewing difficulty related to poor dental health also increases the risk for malnutrition and weight loss for the older adult. Individuals with missing teeth or poorly fitting dentures or for whom chewing is painful often limit their food choices to soft foods and liquids. A limited variety of foods in the diet increases the risk for nutrient deficiencies in addition to lowered caloric intake. Because poor nutrition can contribute to poor dental health, it is important to encourage appropriate dental care with an older individual (Gil-Montoya, Ferreira de Mello, Barrios, Gonzalez-Moles, & Bravo, 2015) (see Chapter 12).

The physiological changes associated with aging can result in **anorexia** or decreased appetite, caused by a general reduction in gastrointestinal motility. Prolonged satiety from a decrease in the rate of gastric emptying can inhibit food intake (Horowitz et al., 1984).

Decreased gastrointestinal motility may also be a factor in the development of constipation, a frequent complaint of older adults.

A decrease in appetite can also be the result of declines in the senses of taste and smell (Rolls, 1999). Age decreases the ability to detect odors and to recognize the taste of salt and other specific tastes.

Reduced taste and smell acuity also can be caused by certain drugs and medications. **TABLE 11-1** presents a summary of the effects of different categories of drugs on appetite.

Food intake typically decreases with age (Morley, 2001; Roberts, 2000) because the basal metabolic rate decreases, resulting in a decrease in energy needs. Moreover, the regulation of food intake through hormones involved in satiety can be impaired, resulting in further reduced food intake (Parker & Chapman, 2004) and inappropriate weight loss in the older adult. An extreme example of this would be **cachexia**, which is a complex metabolic syndrome associated with underlying illness and distinguished by loss of muscle with or without loss of fat mass (Evans et al., 2008). Cachexia is associated with the production of inflammatory cytokines that stimulate fat and muscle breakdown as well as anorexia. This condition is often resistant to nutritional intervention and must be treated by addressing the illness leading to the production of the cytokines (Martinez, Arnalich, & Hernanz, 1993; Oldenburg et al., 1993).

Decreased Absorption of Nutrients

Other gastrointestinal changes that can affect food intake and absorption include **lactose intolerance**. Individuals with lactose intolerance experience intestinal gas, diarrhea, and cramping when they consume dairy products or other foods containing lactose. Lactose intolerance is caused by decreased intestinal lactase production. Lactase is an enzyme that converts lactose into the absorbable sugars

TABLE 11-1 Drugs That Affect Appetite

Examples of Drugs That Increase Appetite	Examples of Drugs That Decrease Appetite
Alcohol	Antibiotics
Antihistamines	Bulk agents
Corticosteroids	Indomethacin
Insulin	Digoxin
Thyroid hormone	Glucagon
Psychoactive drugs	Morphine
	Fluoxetine

Data from Beers, Porter, Jones, Kaplan, & Berkwits (2006).

glucose and galactose. Without the enzyme, lactose cannot be absorbed and subsequently becomes food for intestinal bacteria resulting in intestinal disturbances such as gas, bloating, diarrhea, and cramping. Lactose intolerance is more common in Native American people as well as ethnic groups originating from Asia, Africa, and the Mediterranean. When the condition is severe, it can decrease the absorptive capacity of the intestinal cells and can cause **malabsorption** of many nutrients, but the most common nutritional risk is inadequate calcium intake due to avoidance of dairy products (Heaney, 2013).

Celiac disease is more common in older adults than was originally thought. About 25% of newly diagnosed patients are over the age of 60. Individuals with celiac disease have a sensitivity to the protein gliadin, which is a component of **gluten** found in wheat and some other grains. For persons with celiac disease, consumption of gliadin or gluten

causes damage to intestinal villi and malabsorption of fats, fat-soluble vitamins such as **vitamin D**, and minerals such as **calcium** and iron (Holt, 2007).

Vitamin B$_{12}$ deficiency is characterized by a reversible anemia and irreversible loss of neurological function (Clarke, 2008). Vitamin B$_{12}$ absorption is a complex process requiring the gastric secretion of acid and intrinsic factor. The secretion of both these components, especially acid, decreases with age making older adults more likely to develop a deficiency of vitamin B$_{12}$. Absorption of this vitamin can be further compromised by medications for heartburn, gastroesophageal reflux, or **diabetes**, which are commonly taken by older adults. Vitamin B$_{12}$ deficiency may also contribute to age-related cognitive decline (Stover, 2010).

The ability to synthesize vitamin D in the skin by sunlight decreases with aging. Older adults often have limited exposure to sunlight if they spend most of their time indoors or use sun screens to try to avoid sunlight exposure to prevent sun-related skin aging or skin cancer. Low vitamin D levels decrease muscle strength and increase the risk of falls and contribute to the development of osteoporosis, a disease in which the bones become porous and fragile and the risk of fracture increases substantially (Boucher, 2012).

Dehydration is a common and potentially serious condition in older adults and can have a mortality rate of up to 50% if not adequately treated. Aging is associated with a decrease in total body water, a decline in thirst perception, and a decrease in renal water conservation capacity, all of which contribute to the prevalence of dehydration among older adults. Cognitive impairment is a significant risk factor for dehydration, since even if thirst is recognized, the individual may forget to drink. Issues with incontinence or mobility make it difficult to use the bathroom, and this too may cause older adults to limit their fluid intake. Because the symptoms of dehydration in an older adult can be difficult to recognize or even may be absent, prevention is paramount (Faes, Spigt, & Olde Rikkert, 2007).

▶ Treatment of Weight Loss and Other Nutritional Problems Related to Aging

Weight Loss

Conducting regular body measurements in older adults is one of the simplest ways to assess nutritional adequacy. When an older adult loses 5% or more of his or her body weight in 1 month or 10% or more in 6 months, healthcare providers need to identify the cause for the weight loss. Once the cause has been identified, it is important to treat the condition and provide appropriate nutritional support to return the person to their ideal weight. Treatable causes of weight loss include anorexia and dysphagia. The general causes of weight loss in the elderly can be identified using the mnemonic MEALS ON WHEELS, developed by Morley (1997).

M: medications
E: emotional (depression)
A: alcoholism, anorexia nervosa, or abuse of elders
L: late-life paranoia
S: swallowing disorders
O: oral factors (e.g., poorly fitting dentures, caries)
N: no money
W: wandering and other dementia-related behaviors
H: hyperthyroidism, hypothyroidism, hyperparathyroidism, hypoadrenalism
E: enteric problems, malabsorption
E: eating problems (e.g., inability to feed self)
L: low-salt, low-cholesterol diet
S: shopping and meal preparation problems

A referral to a registered dietitian for intervention is appropriate when weight loss is due to inadequate food intake. When dietary restrictions such as sodium restriction for **hypertension** or **carbohydrate** restriction for diabetes, both of which can decrease the palatability of the diet, are associated with weight loss, modification of the dietary restrictions can be considered. The need for assistance with shopping, food preparation, and feeding also should be assessed. Meal planning and food purchases need to align with the individual's food preferences. Nutrient supplements can also be considered. The nutrient density of foods can be increased by adding egg whites, tofu or milk powder, or healthy oils to foods such as puddings, sauces, vegetables, grains, and pasta. Including healthy snacks, such as nuts and high-calorie **nutritional supplements**, can also be helpful to prevent weight loss and promote the return to a healthy weight.

Treatment of Gastrointestinal Problems

Constipation

Constipation is often treated by increasing fluid and dietary fiber intake. Older adults often limit their intake of fluids. This may be unintentional and related to decreases in their ability to sense thirst, or it may be intentional, especially when they have concerns about incontinence. Limiting fluid intake is a major concern when fiber intake is increased. **Dietary fiber** absorbs fluid and the combination of fiber and fluid aids in moving waste material through the large intestine. The hydrated fiber softens the stools and makes them much easier to pass (Marlett, McBurney, & Slavin, 2002). Thus, any recommendation to increase dietary fiber intake must be accompanied by a recommendation to increase fluid intake. Failure to do so increases the risk for fecal impaction. Ensuring adequate fiber intake may also reduce the incidence of diverticulosis, small sacs in the wall of the colon, and may also lessen the risk of certain types of colon cancer (Giovannucci, Stampfer, Colditz, Rimm, & Willett, 1992; Marlett et al., 2002).

Malabsorption

The two most common causes of malabsorption in older adults are lactose intolerance and celiac disease. Lactose intolerance or lactose malabsorption is treated by eliminating lactose from the diet. Lactose is a sugar found in all dairy products. There are a growing number of commercially available dairy options available for individuals who can no longer consume lactose. These dairy products are treated with the enzyme lactase, which converts the lactose to glucose and galactose, sugars that can be readily absorbed. The bacteria in yogurt with active cultures and acidophilus milk can provide a source of the enzyme lactase, so that these products are well tolerated by some individuals. Although these products are widely available,

individuals with lactose intolerance may not consume enough to meet their calcium needs, so calcium supplements might need to be considered.

Individuals with celiac disease, also known as gluten-induced enteropathy, must avoid all products containing gluten in order to avoid intestinal damage caused by the immune response to the gluten and the accompanying malabsorption. Gluten is found in the cereal grains wheat, barley, and rye. Any products containing these grains or their derivatives contain gluten and must be avoided to prevent intestinal damage and malabsorption. Gluten is found in most breads, cereals, and many other processed foods. It is important to carefully read labels to prevent the accidental consumption of gluten. Fortunately, there are many gluten-free products available commercially, so that food choices need not be as restricted as much as they were before these products became readily obtainable.

Inadequate Intake or Absorption of Vitamins and Minerals

Routine multivitamin and mineral supplementation in the absence of compromised nutritional status is controversial. There is little clinical evidence to support this practice. In 2007, the National Institutes of Health reported insufficient evidence to recommend for or against the use of multivitamins or minerals for the prevention of chronic disease in the general population (Panel, 2007). Since then, several meta-analyses and authoritative reviews have been published and each supports this conclusion (Kamangar & Emadi, 2012). A multivitamin supplement should be used to ensure adequate intake of nutrients whenever there is the suspicion of poor or inadequate food intake, laboratory results reveal a deficiency, or there is some other reason why individuals may not be getting enough nutrients through their diet.

Because older adults have decreased ability to absorb vitamin B_{12}, they can benefit from supplemental B_{12} in the form of a multivitamin and mineral supplement or in fortified foods such as fortified breakfast cereals. Supplemental vitamin B_{12}, including what is added to fortified foods, is more easily absorbed than B_{12} found naturally in food (Baik & Russell, 1999). Daily recommended intake is 10–15 micrograms (Institute of Medicine (U.S.) Standing Committee on the Scientific Evaluation of Dietary Reference Intakes and Its Panel on Folate, Other B Vitamins, and Choline, 1998).

There is also an age-related decrease in the ability to synthesize vitamin D. Older adults at highest risk for vitamin D deficiency include persons who are institutionalized, restricted to living in their homes, or have limited sun exposure (MacLaughlin & Holick, 1985). Inadequate vitamin D status has been associated with muscle weakness, functional impairments, depression, and an increased risk of falls (Gerdhem, Ringsberg, Obrant, & Akesson, 2005). The daily recommended intake of vitamin D for adults up to age 70 years is 600 international units; after age 70, the dosage increases to 800 international units (Institute of Medicine (U.S.) Committee to Review Dietary Reference Intakes for Vitamin D and Calcium, 2011). Many older adults will not meet their vitamin D requirements, especially if dairy intake is limited, so vitamin D supplements should be considered.

Calcium absorption also decreases with age. Because dairy products are a major source of calcium, individuals with lactose intolerance or persons who avoid dairy products should be evaluated for the need for calcium supplements. The recommendation for calcium intake in adults over age 51 is 1,200 mg per day (Institute of Medicine (U.S.) Committee to Review Dietary Reference Intakes for Vitamin D and Calcium, 2011). Generally speaking, a multivitamin and mineral supplement does not include enough calcium to meet the requirement, so additional supplements will be needed.

Dehydration

Dehydration is a common problem in older adults. Signs and symptoms can range from dry mouth, dark urine, and fatigue and lethargy to confusion and weakness (Keller, 2010). Symptoms are often difficult to recognize in the older adult or they may be absent, so it is important to develop strategies for prevention. Older adults should try to consume the equivalent of at least six cups of fluid a day. Making older adults aware of this requirement is often effective in meeting this need (Faes et al., 2007). In addition, older adults should be encouraged to consume fluids with their meals as well as between meals. Juice and sugary drinks should be limited, with water as the best alternative. Many fruits and vegetables also have significant water content. These as well as soups can be included in the diet to increase fluid consumption (Keller, 2010).

Overnutrition

Overnutrition is a condition of excess nutrient and energy intake over time. It can be considered a form of malnutrition when it leads to morbid obesity. In the general population, overnutrition (i.e., BMI of 25.1–29.9, defined as overweight, or a BMI of 30 or greater, defined as obese) is associated with an increase in all causes of mortality, as well as morbidity related to hypertension, dyslipidemia, type 2 diabetes, osteoarthritis, and other chronic diseases. However, some evidence suggests that the mortality risk of overweight may decrease with age. Results from a meta-analysis of individuals over age 65 showed that the lowest risk of mortality by all causes among the 197,940 individuals included in the studies occurred at a BMI of 27.5. Mortality risk began to increase at a BMI less than 23, suggesting that the best weight for height in older adults may be higher than that for younger adults (Winter, MacInnis, Wattanapenpaiboon, & Nowson, 2014), and care should be taken when making recommendations for weight loss in the older adult population.

Recommendations for older adults regarding weight loss must be made on an individual basis. Persons with a high-risk profile for **cardiovascular disease** or diabetes, or individuals who are experiencing a decrease in the quality of life due to excess weight, may benefit from losing weight. Any weight loss should be pursued cautiously, with care taken to provide adequate calcium and vitamin D supplementation as well as exercise in order to prevent loss of muscle mass and a decrease in bone density.

Cardiovascular Disease

Although weight loss in late life may be controversial, there is mounting evidence to support the positive effect of making dietary changes for the primary prevention of cardiovascular disease in older adults. Most recently, data from the PREDIMED trial showed a relative risk reduction for cardiovascular disease of 30% in both men and women who were consuming a **Mediterranean diet** supplemented with either nuts or olive oil as compared to a low-fat control diet. The study participants ranged in age from 55 to 80 years, and 92% were diagnosed as overweight or obese. The participants had either type 2 diabetes or at least three major risk factors for cardiovascular disease such as smoking, hypertension, dyslipidemia, being overweight, or a family history of premature coronary heart disease. Their diet was energy (calorie) unrestricted, and participants did not lose significant amounts of weight, suggesting the relative risk reduction was the result of the composition of the diet (Estruch et al., 2013).

Diabetes

Care for the older adult with diabetes should include a medical nutritional evaluation by a dietitian. The dietitian can tailor a nutrition prescription based on the medical, lifestyle, and personal needs of the individual. Older people who have diabetes may need regular help in adhering to a diet to manage blood glucose levels, whether or not they are insulin dependent. Working with a physician and dietitian to formulate a diet plan and to develop workable menus that provide good glucose control, and take into consideration food preferences and lifestyle habits is recommended. The emphasis for the plan should be on foods that are low on the glycemic index such as whole grains, beans, and vegetables. These foods cause only minimal increases in blood glucose levels when eaten. The planned diet should be rich in fruits, vegetables, and minimally processed carbohydrates. Sugary beverages which will rapidly increase blood glucose levels should be avoided. The obese older adult with diabetes may benefit from modest weight loss; however, because weight loss in older adults is associated with increased risk of morbidity and mortality, this should be addressed in the medical nutrition evaluation (Wedick, Barrett-Connor, Knoke, & Wingard, 2002). Two good dietary patterns that support persons with diabetes are the Mediterranean diet and the **DASH (Dietary Approach to Stop Hypertension) diet**, as recommended in the 2015–2020 **Dietary Guidelines for Americans** (U.S. Department of Health and Human Services and U.S. Department of Agriculture, 2015).

▶ General Nutrition Recommendations

Because the older adult population is heterogeneous, all dietary recommendations must be mindful of individual needs. A good resource is the Dietary Guidelines for Americans 2015–2020 (**FIGURE 11-3**; U.S. Department of Health and Human Services and U.S. Department of Agriculture, 2015). The guidelines provide food-based guidance that can help individuals improve and maintain overall health and reduce their risk of chronic disease. An overarching focus is on making food choices to support healthy eating patterns. There are five general guidelines for older adults:

1. Follow a healthy eating pattern across the life span.
2. Focus on variety, nutrient density, and amount.

Guidelines That Encourage Healthy Eating Patterns

1. **Follow a healthy eating pattern across the lifespan.** All food and beverage choices matter. Choose a healthy eating pattern at an appropriate calorie level to help achieve and maintain a healthy body weight, support nutrient adequacy, and reduce the risk of chronic disease.

Follow a healthy eating pattern over time to help support a healthy body weight and reduce the risk of chronic disease.

- A healthy eating pattern includes: fruits, vegetables, protein, dairy, grains, and oils.
- A healthy eating pattern limits: saturated fats and *trans* fats, added sugars, and sodium.

2. **Focus on variety, nutrient density, and amount.** To meet nutrient needs within calorie limits, choose a variety of nutrient-dense foods across and within all food groups in recommended amounts.

Choose a variety of nutrient-dense foods from each food group in recommended amounts. Examples include

- Fruits: apples, grapes
- Vegetables: lettuce, celery
- Protein: chicken breast, unsalted walnuts
- Dairy: fat-free milk
- Grains: whole-grain bread
- Oils: mayonnaise

3. **Limit calories from added sugars and saturated fats and reduce sodium intake.** Consume an eating pattern low in added sugars, saturated fats, and sodium. Cut back on foods and beverages higher in these components to amounts that fit within healthy eating patterns.

Consume an eating pattern low in added sugars, saturated fats, and sodium. Examples include

- Saturated fats: ice cream, burger
- Added sugars: aerated drinks, muffin
- Sodium: pizza, sandwich

4. **Shift to healthier food and beverage choices.** Choose nutrient-dense foods and beverages across and within all food groups in place of less healthy choices. Consider cultural and personal preferences to make these shifts easier to accomplish and maintain.

Replace typical food and beverages choices with more nutrient-dense options. Be sure to consider personal preferences to maintain shifts over time. For example, replacing macaroni and cheese with vegetable salads.

5. **Support healthy eating patterns for all.** Everyone has a role in helping to create and support healthy eating patterns in multiple settings nationwide, from home to school to work to communities.

Everyone has a role in helping to create and support healthy eating patterns in places where we learn, work, live, and play.

FIGURE 11-3 Dietary Guidelines for Americans 2015–2020.

Reproduced from U.S. Department of Health and Human Services, Office of Disease Prevention and Health Promotion. 2015-2020 Dietary Guidelines. www.health.gov/dietaryguidelines/2015/

3. Limit calories from added sugars and saturated fats and reduce sodium intake.
4. Shift to healthier food and beverage choices.
5. Support healthy eating patterns for all.

The guidelines focus on healthy eating, yet recognize the critical and complementary role of physical activity in promoting good health and preventing disease.

Diet plans consistent with the recommendations in the Dietary Guidelines include "Healthy U.S.-Style Eating Pattern," "Dietary Approaches to Stop Hypertension (DASH)" dietary pattern, "Healthy Mediterranean-Style Eating Pattern," and "Healthy Vegetarian Eating Pattern." All of these dietary patterns are rich in fruits and vegetables, low-fat or nonfat dairy, and whole grains. They tend to be higher in fiber, low to moderate in fat, and rich in potassium, calcium, and magnesium. The meal plans are consistent with dietary recommendations for the treatment of hypertension, heart disease, and diabetes (U.S. Department of Health and Human Services and U.S. Department of Agriculture, 2015). Sample 2,000 kcal meal patterns with recommended servings from each group are shown in **TABLE 11-2**.

The appropriate caloric level will vary for each individual based on specific caloric needs to maintain a healthy weight. The Recommended Dietary Allowance (RDA) for energy for individuals over the age of 50 years is 1,900 kcal for females and 2,300 kcal for males. These average estimates should be adjusted for body size and physical activity to maintain normal weight (National Research Council (U.S.) Subcommittee on the Tenth Edition of the Recommended Dietary Allowances, 1989).

There are many resources available on the Internet to assist healthcare professionals as they help their clients or patients implement these recommendations. For example, MyPlate is part of a communications initiative from the U.S. Department of Agriculture to help Americans adopt healthier eating habits based on the 2015–2020 Dietary Guidelines for Americans. MyPlate uses a graphic of a dinner plate to illustrate serving size in the five food groups—dairy, protein, fruits, vegetables, and grains. The food groups are arranged on the plate to emphasize the importance of choosing a diet rich in fruits and vegetables, which are illustrated as covering half the plate. **FIGURE 11-4** is a graphic which illustrates the five food groups included on MyPlate with some guidance on selections within each group.

MyPlate is part of a larger communications initiative that includes the website ChooseMyPlate.gov, which is a good resource for healthcare professionals as well as consumers. There is a special section on this website that focuses on older adults (www .choosemyplate.gov/older-adult) and includes multiple resources for individuals on healthy eating. Tips for adapting the MyPlate eating plan for a vegetarian diet can be found on the ChooseMyPlate.gov website (www .choosemyplate.gov/protein-foods-vegetarian).

Nutrition scientists at Tufts University Jean Mayer USDA Human Nutrition Research Center on Aging collaborated with AARP to produce an adaptation of MyPlate for older adults (hnrca.tufts.edu/myplate/). This modified resource provides graphic examples of foods that fit into a healthy eating pattern with special focus on the nutritional needs of adults age 50+ (**FIGURE 11-5**). The value added to this resource is that it also emphasizes important habits that contribute to good health, including the need for regular exercise, plenty of fluid intake, and the use of fortified foods or supplements to meet daily requirements for vitamins B_{12} and D.

Additional nutrition information for older adults can be found at these websites:

■ Nutrition.gov
■ Older Individuals: www.nutrition.gov /subject/life-stages/seniors
■ National Institute on Aging, Healthy Eating: www.nia.nih.gov/health/healthy-eating

TABLE 11-2 Healthy Eating Patterns for 2,000 kcal Diets

Food Group	Healthy U.S.-Style Eating Pattern	Healthy Mediterranean-Style Eating Pattern	Healthy Vegetarian-Style Eating Pattern
Vegetables	2½ c-eq/day	2½ c-eq/day	2½ c-eq/day
Dark green	1½ c-eq/week	1½ c-eq/week	1½ c-eq/week
Red and orange	5½ c-eq/week	5½ c-eq/week	5½ c-eq/week
Legumes (beans and peas)	1½ c-eq/week	1½ c-eq/week	3 c-eq/week
Starchy	5 c-eq/week	5 c-eq/week	5 c-eq/week
Other	4 c-eq/week	4 c-eq/week	4 c-eq/week
Fruits	2 c-eq/day	2½ c-eq/day	2 c-eq/day
Grains	6 oz-eq/day	6 oz-eq/day	6½ oz-eq/day
Whole grains	≥ 3 oz-eq/day	≥ 3 oz-eq/day	≥ 3½ oz-eq/day
Refined grains	≤ 3 oz-eq/day	≤ 3 oz-eq/day	≤ 3 oz-eq/day
Dairy	3 c-eq/day	2 c-eq/day	3 c-eq/day
Protein foods	5½ oz-eq/day	6½ oz-eq/day	3½ oz-eq/day
Seafood	8 oz-eq/week	15 oz-eq/week	-
Meats, poultry, eggs	26 oz-eq/week	26 oz-eq/week	3 oz-eq/week (eggs)
Nuts, seeds, soy products	5 oz-eq/week	5 oz-eq/week	14 oz-eq/week
Oils	27 g/day	27 g/day	27 g/day
Limit on calories for other uses (% of calories)	270 kcal/day (14%)	260 kcal/day (13%)	290 kcal/day (15%)

Note: c = cup; eq = equivalent; g = gram; oz = ounce
Data from U.S. Department of Health and Human Services, Office of Disease Prevention and Health Promotion. 2015-2020 Dietary Guidelines. www.health.gov/dietaryguidelines/2015

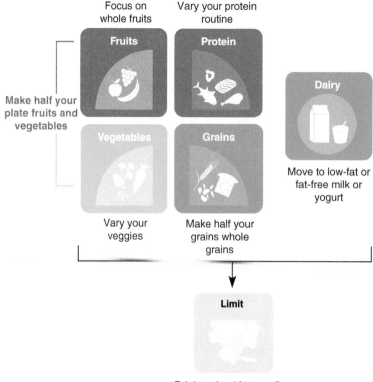

Focus on
whole fruits

Vary your protein
routine

Fruits

Protein

Dairy

Make half your
plate fruits and
vegetables

Vegetables

Grains

Move to low-fat or
fat-free milk or
yogurt

Vary your
veggies

Make half your
grains whole
grains

Limit

Drink and eat less sodium,
saturated fat, and added sugars

FIGURE 11-4 MyPlate.

Data from Choose My Plate. U.S. Department of Agriculture. www.choosemyplate.gov/myplate-mywins

▶ Drug and Nutrient Interactions

More than 90% of older adults aged 57–85 take at least one medication daily. These medications include prescription medications, over-the-counter (OTC) medications, or dietary supplements. Dietary supplements are products that supplement the diet and contain dietary ingredients such as vitamins, minerals, herbs, amino acids, and other substances taken orally. More than one-third of older adults use five or more prescription medications concurrently, and two-thirds use prescription medications with OTC medications and dietary supplements. The use of multiple drugs concurrently, known as polypharmacy, places one in six older

adults at risk for major drug–drug interactions. The majority of these interactions are estimated to involve interactions between medications and dietary supplements (Qato, Wilder, Schumm, Gillet, & Alexander, 2016).

Antihyperlipidemic drugs such as statins, taken to lower **cholesterol** levels, can interact with niacin, a nutritional supplement (vitamin B$_2$), increasing the risk of muscle damage. Grapefruit juice in particular affects the metabolism of a large number of drugs, including statins. It increases the conversion of statins to an active form that can lead to higher serum levels of the drug. Warfarin is an anticoagulant drug (sold under the name Coumadin) used to decrease blood clotting to prevent strokes, heart attacks, deep vein thrombosis, and pulmonary emboli. Garlic interacts with

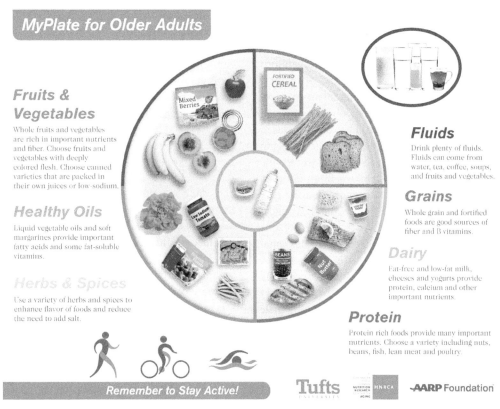

FIGURE 11-5 My Food Plate.
© 2016 Tufts University.

warfarin, increasing anticoagulation of blood, which increases the risk of bleeding. Vegetables, especially green leafy vegetables that are high in vitamin K, may decrease the effectiveness of warfarin and thus increase the risk of clotting (Leibovitch, Deamer, & Sanderson, 2004). These are only a few examples, but they illustrate the necessity for older adults to consult a physician, dietitian, and/or pharmacist to avoid complications related to polypharmacy and drug-nutrient interactions.

Alcohol

Alcohol use in late life does not necessarily decrease with age, as its use is deeply embedded in daily routines (e.g., wine with dinner or a nightcap) and social functions

(e.g., weddings, holidays, and special events). Typically, unless drinking alcohol directly inhibits or exacerbates the effectiveness of medications, contributes to loss of balance and mobility, or interferes with health and nutrition due to abuse, alcohol use is not patently discouraged. Researchers continue to explore if and how alcohol might actually benefit the aging body (e.g., antioxidants, relaxation), but consensus has not been achieved.

The focus on alcohol use by healthcare practitioners should be on whether drinking has increased and why. Increased use of alcohol in later life is generally brought on by a social change, such as the death of a spouse, loss of a close friendship, feelings of loneliness, or the stress of being a caregiver. About one-third of older drinkers begin to misuse alcohol (i.e., they are exceeding recommended drinking limits) later in life as a coping strategy. This type of drinker is often classified as "late onset" and is generally viewed as receptive to interventions that help reduce consumption and offer alternative coping strategies. The other two-thirds of older drinkers who misuse alcohol are referred to as early onset drinkers. They have misused alcohol in the past and are either bringing their drinking habits with them into late life or have resumed their drinking in an effort to cope with life changes. Depending on the person and circumstances, early onset drinkers can be receptive to interventions. For persons who are dependent on alcohol, professional substance abuse intervention is warranted. A growing concern among prevention specialists and healthcare practitioners is that members of the baby boom generation are bringing their drinking (and drugging) habits with them into late life, and services are not currently available to support them. Healthcare professionals need to be aware of the potential for alcohol-use disorders in the older adult and should be ready to make referrals to other appropriate healthcare professionals and community support groups.

Nutritionally speaking, alcohol abuse compromises health and can lead to malnutrition for several reasons. First, alcohol is energy dense and can add calories to the diet when consumed immoderately. This can lead to weight gain. If the alcohol replaces nutrient-rich food in the diet, then the risk for nutrient deficien-cies increases. Alcohol also interferes with the normal absorption of vitamin B_{12}, folic acid, and vitamin C, and the metabolism of vitamins D and B_6, and increases the need for B vitamins and magnesium. All these may result in multiple nutritional deficiencies that can impair health (Ferreira & Weems, 2008).

▶ Summary

The value of appropriate nutrition screening and intervention cannot be overemphasized in the care of older adults. Good nutrition not only optimizes health and well-being, but also helps prevent or deter the onset of many chronic health conditions. Healthcare providers need to be aware of the many changes related to nutrition that occur with age and remain alert to the ways in which nutrition can affect quality of life. Gaining knowledge about the basic principles of nutrition and how they can be applied to encourage healthy eating is essential in caring for older adults. Moreover, healthcare professionals need to be aware of how the aging process can alter nutritional status (as well as how nutritional status can impact the aging process). With careful screening, counseling, and referral if necessary, healthcare professionals can ensure optimal nutritional well-being for their older clients. Promoting quality nutrition is a crucial component of providing the best health care possible for the older population.

🔍 CASE STUDIES

Case 1: Joan is an 82-year-old woman whose husband died last year. Now, she lives alone on a fixed income in a small apartment and has no family members or friends who live in her community. She was referred to you by a social worker, who is concerned because Joan told him that she has lost 20 pounds in the past year. Joan is 5'5" tall and her current weight is 110 pounds.

1. **What factors likely contributed to Joan's weight loss?**
2. **What are some other possible causes of Joan's weight loss that you should inquire about?**
3. **What can you recommend to help Joan return to a healthier weight?**

Case 2: Carli is a nurse who works in a hospital. One of her patients is Stanley, a 65-year-old man who passed out in his kitchen this morning, fell, and cut his head open. When his daughter brought him to the emergency room, she said that he had been acting lethargic and confused before he fell. To be on the safe side, after cleaning and stitching Stanley's wound, his doctor decided to keep him in the hospital for observation overnight. When Carli came in to check on Stanley, he quietly asked if she could help him with his urinal, as he did not feel strong enough to get to the bathroom on his own. He apologized for his raspy voice, telling her that his mouth was a bit dry. Carli assisted him and then went to empty his urinal. As she did, she noticed that it was nearly orange in color.

1. **What condition does Stanley likely have and how can you tell?**
2. **Describe three things that Stanley can do to help alleviate his condition and explain the reasoning for each.**

TEST YOUR KNOWLEDGE

Review Questions

1. An important factor to consider when working with the older adult population is that
   a. It is a heterogeneous population.
   b. All suffer from chronic diseases.
   c. It is an economically disadvantaged population.
   d. All are underweight.

2. According to the Academy of Nutrition and Dietetics and the American Society for Parenteral and Enteral Nutrition, nutrition screening tools should include an assessment of
   a. Weight
   b. Muscle mass
   c. Functional capacity
   d. All of the above

3. In which of the following groups is the prevalence of malnutrition highest?
   a. Residents of long-term care facilities
   b. Residents of retirement communities for active older adults
   c. Older adults ages 60–80 living in a small town
   d. Attendees of a college program for seniors

4. Poor dietary intake is associated with
   a. Depression, dysphagia, and dementia
   b. Poverty, living with a spouse, and hypertension
   c. Constipation, diabetes, and Alzheimer's disease
   d. Dyslipidemia, lack of exercise, and alcohol

5. The focus on alcohol use in older adults should be on:
   a. The type of alcohol the older adult drinks
   b. Whether the older adult drinks alone or with others
   c. Whether the older adult's drinking has increased and why
   d. How much of the older adult's budget is spent on alcohol

Learning Activities

1. Using the MST, assess three random people for malnutrition and explain your findings.
2. Determine the BMI of an individual (with their permission). Explain how you determined his or her BMI, and determine which BMI classification he or she falls into.
3. The Academy of Nutrition and Dietetics and the American Society for Parenteral and Enteral Nutrition developed a set of criteria for diagnosing malnutrition. Identify these criteria and explain how they are used to determine whether an individual has malnutrition.
4. Explain what the mnemonic MEALS ON WHEELS is used for and what each letter stands for.
5. Describe your current diet and discuss whether it will be appropriate as you age and why, or how it might need to change to improve your chances for optimal aging.

References

Achem, S. R., & Devault, K. R. (2005). Dysphagia in aging. *Journal of Clinical Gastroenterology, 39*(5), 357–371.

Anthony, P. S. (2008). Nutrition screening tools for hospitalized patients. *Nutrition in Clinical Practice, 23*(4), 373–382. doi:10.1177/0884533608321130

Avelino-Silva, T. J., & Jaluul, O. (2017). Malnutrition in hospitalized older patients: Management strategies to improve patient care and clinical outcomes. *International Journal of Gerontology, 11*(2), 56–61. doi:10.1016/j.ijge.2016.11.002

Baik, H. W., & Russell, R. M. (1999). Vitamin B$_{12}$ deficiency in the elderly. *Annual Review of Nutrition, 19*, 357–377.

Bell, C. L., Lee, A. S. W., & Tamura, B. K. (2015). Malnutrition in the nursing home: *Current Opinion in Clinical Nutrition and Metabolic Care, 18*(1), 17–23. doi:10.1097/MCO.0000000000000130

Beers, M. H., Porter, R. S., Jones, T. V., Kaplan, J. L., & Berkwits, M. (2006). *Nutrition: General considerations. The Merck Manual* (18th ed.). Whitehouse Station, NJ: Merck & Co.

Boucher, B. J. (2012). The problems of vitamin D insufficiency in older people. *Aging and Disease, 3*(4), 313–329.

Centers for Medicare and Medicaid Services. (2012). *Chronic conditions among Medicare beneficiaries, Chartbook, 2012 Edition.* Baltimore, MD.

Clarke, R. (2008). B-vitamins and prevention of dementia. *Proceedings of the Nutrition Society, 67*(01), 75–81. doi:10.1017/S0029665108006046

Corkins, M. R., Guenter, P., DiMaria-Ghalili, R. A., Jensen, G. L., Malone, A., Miller, S., ... Resnick, H. E. (2014). Malnutrition diagnoses in hospitalized patients: United States, 2010. *Journal of Parenteral and Enteral Nutrition, 38*(2), 186–195.

de Castro, J. M., & Brewer, E. M. (1992). The amount eaten in meals by humans is a power function of the number of people present. *Physiology and Behavior, 51*, 121–125.

DiMaria-Ghalili, R. A., Michael, Y. L., & Rosso, A. L. (2013). Malnutrition in a sample of community dwelling older Pennsylvanians. *Journal of Aging Research and Clinical Practice, 2.*

Estruch, R., Ros, E., Salas-Salvadó, J., Covas, M.-I., Corella, D., Arós, F., ... Martínez-González, M. A. (2013). Primary prevention of cardiovascular disease with a Mediterranean diet. *New England Journal of Medicine, 368*(14), 1279–1290. doi:10.1056/NEJMoa1200303

Evans, W. J., Morley, J. E., Argilés, J., Bales, C., Baracos, V., Guttridge, D., ... Anker, S. D. (2008). Cachexia: A new definition. *Clinical Nutrition, 27*(6), 793–799. doi:10.1016/j.clnu.2008.06.013

Faes, M. C., Spigt, M. G., & Olde Rikkert, M. G. M. (2007). Dehydration in geriatrics. *Geriatrics and Aging, 10*(9), 590–596.

Ferreira, M. P., & Weems, M. K. S. (2008). Alcohol consumption by aging adults in the United States: Health benefits and detriments. *Journal of the American Dietetic Association, 108*(10), 1668–1676. doi:10.1016/j.jada.2008.07.011

Food and Nutrition Board, Institute of Medicine, & Committee on Nutrition Services for Medicare Beneficiaries. (2000). *Role of nutrition in maintaining health in the nation's elderly: Evaluating coverage of nutrition services for the Medicare population.* National Academies Press. Retrieved from http://www.nap.edu/9741

Gerdhem, P., Ringsberg, K. A. M., Obrant, K. J., & Akesson, K. (2005). Association between 25-hydroxy vitamin D levels, physical activity, muscle strength and fractures in the prospective population-based OPRA Study of Elderly Women. *Osteoporosis International, 16*(11), 1425–1431. doi:10.1007/s00198-005-1860-1

Gil-Montoya, J., Ferreira de Mello, A. L., Barrios, R., Gonzalez-Moles, M. A., & Bravo, M. (2015). Oral health in the elderly patient and its impact on general well-being: A nonsystematic review. *Clinical Interventions in Aging*, 461. doi:10.2147/CIA.S54630

Giovannucci, E., Stampfer, M. J., Colditz, G., Rimm, E. B., & Willett, W. C. (1992). Relationship of diet to risk of colorectal adenoma in men. *Journal of the National Cancer Institute, 84*(2), 91–98.

Heaney, R. P. (2013). Dairy intake, dietary adequacy, and lactose intolerance. *Advances in Nutrition: An International Review Journal, 4*(2), 151–156. doi:10.3945/an.112.003368

Holt, P. R. (2007). Intestinal malabsorption in the elderly. *Digestive Diseases, 25*(2), 144–150. doi:10.1159/000099479

Horowitz, M., Maddern, G. J., Chatterton, B. E., Collins, P. J., Harding, P. E., & Shearman, D. J. C. (1984). Changes in gastric emptying rates with age. *Clinical Science, 67*(2), 213–218.

Institute of Medicine (U.S.) Committee to Review Dietary Reference Intakes for Vitamin D and Calcium. (2011). *Dietary reference intakes for calcium and vitamin D.* Washington, DC: National Academies Press (U.S.). Retrieved from https://www.ncbi.nlm.nih.gov/books/NBK56070/ doi: 10.17226/13050

Institute of Medicine (U.S.) Standing Committee on the Scientific Evaluation of Dietary Reference Intakes and its Panel on Folate, Other B Vitamins, and Choline. (1998). *Dietary reference intakes for thiamin, riboflavin, niacin, vitamin B$_6$, folate, vitamin B$_{12}$, pantothenic acid, biotin, and choline.* Washington, DC: National Academies Press (U.S.). doi:10.17226/6015

Kaiser, M. J., Bauer, J. M., Rämsch, C., Uter, W., Guigoz, Y., Cederholm, T., ... Sieber, C. C. (2010). Frequency of malnutrition in older adults: A multinational perspective using the mini nutritional assessment. *Journal of the American Geriatrics Society, 58*(9), 1734–1738. doi:10.1111/j.1532-5415.2010.03016.x

Kamangar, F., & Emadi, A. (2012). Vitamin and mineral supplements: Do we really need them? *International Journal of Preventive Medicine, 3*(3), 221.

Keller, H. H. (1993). Malnutrition in institutionalized elderly: How and why? *Journal of the American Geriatrics Society, 41*(11), 1212–1218.

Keller, M. (2010). Defeating dehydration-patient monitoring is key. *Aging Well, 3*(4), 24.

Leibovitch, E. R., Deamer, R. L., & Sanderson, L. A. (2004). Food-drug interactions: Careful drug selection and patient counseling can reduce the risk in older patients. *Geriatrics, 59*(March), 19–33.

Locher, J. L., Robinson, C. O., Roth, D. L., Ritchie, C. S., & Burgio, K. L. (2005). The effect of the presence of others on caloric intake in homebound older adults. *The Journals of Gerontology Series A: Biological Sciences and Medical Sciences, 60*(11), 1475–1478.

MacLaughlin, J., & Holick, M. F. (1985). Aging decreases the capacity of human skin to produce vitamin D$_3$. *Journal of Clinical Investigation, 76*(4), 1536.

Marlett, J. A., McBurney, M. I., & Slavin, J. L. (2002). Position of American Dietetic Association: Health implications of dietary fiber. *Jornal of the American Dietetic Association, 102*(7), 993–1000.

Martinez, M., Arnalich, F., & Hernanz, A. (1993). Alterations of anorectic cytokine levels from plasma and cerebrospinal fluid in idiopathic senile anorexia. *Mechanisms of Ageing and Development, 72*, 145–153.

Mather, M., Jacobsen, L. A., & Pollard, K. M. (2015). *Aging in the United States* (Population Bulletin 70 No. 2).

Morley, J. E. (2001). Decreased food intake with aging. *The Journals of Gerontology Series A: Biological Sciences and Medical Sciences, 56*(Suppl 2), 81–88.

National Research Council (U.S.) Subcommittee on the Tenth Edition of the Recommended Dietary Allowances. (1989). *Recommended dietary allowances: 3, energy.* (10th edition). Washington, DC: National Academies Press (U.S.). Retrieved from https://www.ncbi.nlm.nih.gov/books/NBK234938/

Oldenburg, H. S. A., Rogy, M. A., Lazarus, D. D., van Zee, K. J., Keeler, B. P., Chizzonite, R. A., ... Moldawer, L. L. (1993). Cachexia and the acute-phase protein response in inflammation are regulated by interleukin-6. *European Journal of Immunology, 23*(8), 1889–1894.

Panel, N. S. S. (2007). National Institutes of Health State-of-the-Science Conference Statement: Multivitamin/Mineral supplements and chronic disease prevention. *The American Journal of Clinical Nutrition, 85*(1), 257S–264S.

Parker, B. A., & Chapman, I. M. (2004). Food intake and ageing—the role of the gut. *Mechanisms of Ageing and Development, 125*(12), 859–866. doi:10.1016/j.mad.2004.05.006

Poulia, K.-A., Klek, S., Doundoulakis, I., Bouras, E., Karayiannis, D., Baschali, A., ... Chourdakis, M. (2017). The two most popular malnutrition screening tools in the light of the new ESPEN consensus definition of the diagnostic criteria for malnutrition. *Clinical Nutrition, 36*(4), 1130–1135. doi:10.1016/j.clnu.2016.07.014

Poulia, K.-A., Yannakoulia, M., Karageorgou, D., Gamaletsou, M., Panagiotakos, D. B., Sipsas, N. V., & Zampelas, A. (2012). Evaluation of the efficacy of six nutritional screening tools to predict malnutrition in the elderly. *Clinical Nutrition, 31*(3), 378–385. doi:10.1016/j.clnu.2011.11.017

Qato, D. M., Wilder, J., Schumm, L. P., Gillet, V., & Alexander, G. C. (2016). Changes in prescription and over-the-counter medication and dietary supplement use among older adults in the United States, 2005 vs 2011. *JAMA Internal Medicine, 176*(4), 473. doi:10.1001/jamainternmed.2015.8581

Rabinovitz, M., Pitlik, S. D., Leifer, M., Garty, M., & Rosenfeld, J. B. (1986). Unintentional weight loss: A retrospective analysis of 154 cases. *Archives of Internal Medicine, 146*(1), 186–187.

Roberts, S. B. (2000). A review of age-related changes in energy regulation and suggested mechanisms. *Mechanisms of Ageing and Development, 116*, 157–167.

Rolls, B. J. (1999). Do chemosensory changes influence food intake in the elderly? *Physiology & Behavior, 66*(2), 193–197.

S.192-Older Americans Act Reauthorization Act of 2016, Pub. L. No. 114–144 (2016). Retrieved from https://www.congress.gov/bill/114th-congress/senate-bill/192

Skipper, A., Ferguson, M., Thompson, K., Castellanos, V. H., & Porcari, J. (2012). Nutrition screening tools: An analysis of the evidence. *Journal of Parenteral and Enteral Nutrition, 36*(3), 292–298. doi:10.1177/0148607111414023

Stover, P. J. (2010). Vitamin B$_{12}$ and older adults: *Current Opinion in Clinical Nutrition and Metabolic Care, 13*(1), 24–27. doi:10.1097/MCO.0b013e328333d157

Sullivan, D. H. (1995). Impact of nutritional status on health outcomes of nursing home residents. *Journal of the American Geriatrics Society, 43*(2), 195–96.

Thompson, M. P., & Morris, L. K. (1991). Unexplained weight loss in the ambulatory elderly. *Journal of the American Geriatrics Society, 39*(5), 497–500.

U.S. Department of Health and Human Services and U.S. Department of Agriculture. (2015). *2015–2020 Dietary guidelines for Americans* (8th Edition). Retrieved from http://health.gov/dietaryguidelines/2015/guidelines/

Wedick, N. M., Barrett-Connor, E., Knoke, J. D., & Wingard, D. L. (2002). The relationship between weight loss and all-cause mortality in older men and women with and without diabetes mellitus: The Rancho Bernardo Study. *Journal of the American Geriatrics Society, 50*(11), 1810–1815.

White, H. (1998). Weight change in Alzheimer's disease. *Journal of Nutrition, Health, and Aging, 2*(2), 110–112.

White, J. V., Guenter, P., Jensen, G., Malone, A., Schofield, M., Group, A. M. W., … of Directors, A. B. (2012). Consensus statement of the Academy of Nutrition and Dietetics/American Society for Parenteral and Enteral Nutrition: characteristics recommended for the identification and documentation of adult malnutrition (undernutrition). *Journal of the Academy of Nutrition and Dietetics, 112*(5), 730–738.

White, J. V., Ham, R. J., Lipschitz, D. A., Dwyer, J. T., & Wellman, N. S. (1991). Consensus of the nutrition screening initiative: Risk factors and indicators of poor nutritional status in older Americans. *Journal of the American Dietetic Association, 91*(7), 783–787.

Wilson, M.-M. G., Vaswani, S., Liu, D., Morley, J. E., & Miller, D. K. (1998). Prevalence and causes of undernutrition in medical outpatients. *The American Journal of Medicine, 104*(1), 56–63.

Winter, J. E., MacInnis, R. J., Wattanapenpaiboon, N., & Nowson, C. A. (2014). BMI and all-cause mortality in older adults: A meta-analysis. *American Journal of Clinical Nutrition, 99*(4), 875–890. doi:10.3945/ajcn.113.068122

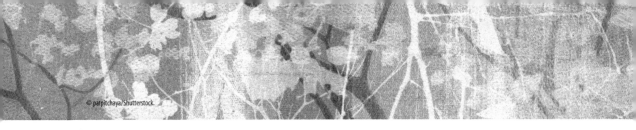

© patpitchaya/Shutterstock.

CHAPTER 12

Perspectives on Oral Care in Healthy Aging and Prevention for the Older Adult

Marji Harmer-Beem, RDH, MS

CHAPTER OUTLINE

BEHAVIORAL OBJECTIVES

Upon completion of this chapter, the reader will be able to:

1. Explain and discuss *Oral Health in America: A Report of the Surgeon General*, highlighting themes that relate to the oral health and well-being of older adults.
2. Identify the percentages of periodontal disease, edentulism, and oral and pharyngeal cancers in the elderly.
3. Recognize dry mouth (xerostomia) and describe the risk factors it poses for the well-being of the older adult.

(continues)

(*continued*)

4. List dental changes of aging versus signs of a disease state.
5. Review oral health of the older adult and its correlates to well-being.
6. List societal and personal barriers for the older adult seeking dental care.
7. Describe common oral conditions the healthcare professional may encounter.
8. Describe a simple oral screening procedure that the healthcare professional can do.
9. Name the basic role of the interprofessional healthcare provider in assisting the older person with oral health concerns.
10. List new models for oral health care to help alleviate oral health disparities.

KEY TERMS

Attrition	Fluoride varnish	Root caries
Dental caries	Oral and pharyngeal (throat)	Stereognosis
Dental plaque (biofilm)	cancers	Streptococcus mutans
Edentulism	Oral screening	Xerostomia
Fluoride gel	Periodontal disease	

▶ Introduction

In 1605, Migel de Cevantes Saavedra wrote *Don Quixote*. In that novel, he wrote, and dental professionals agree, "every tooth in a man's head is more valuable than a diamond" (Saavedra, 1822), because oral pain, missing teeth, and the inability to chew can adversely affect overall health. Health promotion is the focus of all health professionals serving individuals of all ages. In this chapter, the emphasis on oral health is presented as important to the overall health and well-being in older adults. The well-educated health provider understands that oral health is a determinant of overall health (Shay, 2004). Factors that influence dental well-being and its determinates are appropriate for all providers to know (Shay, 2004; U.S. Department of Health and Human Services, 2000).

As the relative proportion of older adults in the U.S. population steadily increases, so does the need for healthcare providers to have knowledge of the biological systems that affect the health and well-being of this diverse population. The oral cavity is no exception.

Older adults can present with a variety of medical and dental histories. They tend to have a disproportionate number of chronic conditions and diseases that are managed rather than cured (e.g., cardiovascular disease, arthritis, visual impairment). These conditions can impair the older adults' functioning throughout the day and limit their daily choices (Shay, 2004).

Rarely does the average person reflect on how important the mouth is to daily life, functioning, and health. General health and oral health are concepts that should be interpreted as a single entity and should not be separated. Oral health means more than healthy teeth to the older adult. Damage to the face and skull complex, whether from illness, injury, or disorder, can result in the loss of health, self-esteem, and well-being (U.S. Department of Health and Human Services, 2000).

Healthy aging is as individualized as personal lifestyle, culture, social connections, and family history. The goal of healthy aging from the oral perspective is to differentiate aging processes and disease, retain as many natural teeth as possible, preserve good health and function, and provide older persons seeking oral care with effective disease preventive measures. Preventive measures are easily managed by a knowledgeable interprofessional team. Using simple provider-based and self-initiated daily measures such as effective toothbrushing, flossing, and a fluoride regime can prevent dental-related disease (U.S. Department of Health and Human Services, 2000).

▶ Oral Health in America: A Report of the Surgeon General

The oral structures, much like the rest of the body, show signs of aging. An understanding of the significance of the oral cavity to a person's general well-being is vital for the healthcare professional. In the 2000 report, *Oral Health in America*, then-Surgeon General David Satcher was the first person ever to alert Americans to the full implication of oral health and its link to general health (U.S. Department of Health and Human Services, 2000). The increasing evidence that oral disease impacts endocrine (e.g., diabetes), cardiovascular, and pulmonary health, particularly but not exclusively in frail elders, may provide many older people the needed incentive to seek care (Shay, 2004; Lalla, 2017). The oral cavity, with its bacterial plaque, is a portal for infection and may lead to aspiration pneumonia, a serious infection in the lungs (Shay, Scannapieco, Terpenning, Smith, & Taylor, 2005). Bacteria traveling via the blood to remote sites from the oral cavity can infect artificial joints or the heart with endocarditis; these are other serious and life threatening infections of oral origin (Rai, Kaur, Goel, & Bhatnagar, 2011). The report stresses two important overarching themes: the "silent epidemic" of oral diseases affecting older people, and maintaining a clean and healthy oral cavity. Maintaining clean and healthy oral cavity plays a primary role in reducing needless pain and

suffering, and therefore preventing associated physical, financial, and social costs, which can be especially devastating for the country's most vulnerable older population (U.S. Department of Health and Human Services, 2000).

Oral health is fundamental to general health. In the early 1900s, most Americans could expect to lose their teeth by middle age amid pain and suffering. Older people today have lived through some of the most technologically advanced discoveries of all time and unprecedented biomedical progress. This is reflected in the oral restorative materials used, from acrylic dentures designed to last 50 years to porcelain, composite (resin) white fillings, amalgam (silver) fillings, and titanium implants. The first wave of the baby boomer generation was the first group to grow up in the age of dental prevention. Public health measures, such as fluoride in municipal water supplies, have decreased **dental caries** (dental decay) rates over the past 50 years. Toothpastes, mouth rinses, and sonic toothbrushes also have contributed to positive results (Shay, 2004).

▶ Oral Structures and Chronic Oral Diseases

Oral structures of the craniofacial complex include the vermillion border (lips); oral mucosa, which is the lining of the cheeks; gums; tongue; and oral pharynx (**FIGURE 12-1**; Shay et al., 2005). Structures that are not readily seen include the salivary glands, the muscles of chewing, and the upper and lower jaws. The health of these structures is integral to psychosocial well-being. For example, emotions are expressed using the oral structures, food is enjoyed, and communication is enhanced (U.S. Department of Health and Human Services, 2000). It may come as no surprise that experiencing tooth loss has been highly correlated with low self-perception of quality

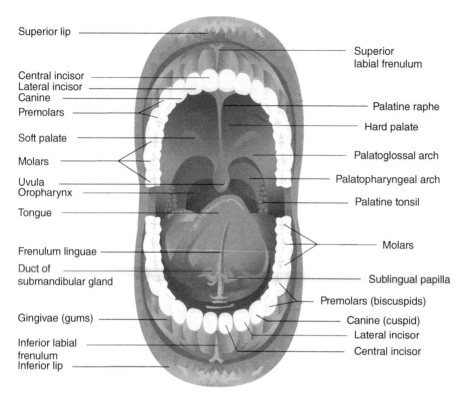

Superior lip

Superior labial frenulum

Central incisor
Lateral incisor
Canine
Premolars

Palatine raphe

Hard palate

Soft palate

Palatoglossal arch

Molars

Palatopharyngeal arch

Uvula
Oropharynx

Palatine tonsil

Tongue

Frenulum linguae

Molars

Duct of
submandibular gland

Sublingual papilla

Premolars (biscuspids)

Gingivae (gums)

Canine (cuspid)

Lateral incisor

Inferior labial
frenulum
Inferior lip

Central incisor

FIGURE 12-1 Normal structures of the mouth.
© stockshoppe/ShutterStock

of life (Haikal, Paula, Martins, Moreira, & Ferreira, 2011).

The healthcare professional has a responsibility to support oral health in the older adult. Chronic oral disease in older adults includes **periodontal disease, edentulism, oral and pharyngeal cancers**, decreased saliva flow, and caries. **FIGURE 12-2** shows occurrences that may be encountered in the oral cavity of the older adult, such as wear on the teeth and restoration of the teeth.

Periodontal disease is the inflammatory reaction and dissolution of the bone structures that hold the teeth within the jaws. Bad breath, food pocketing in the gums, gum recession, pus, and loose teeth are all problems that can accompany this disease. **Dental plaque (biofilm)**, which is an accumulation

of pathogenic bacteria combined with the individual's immune response, can cause periodontal disease. **FIGURE 12-3** illustrates the physical outcomes associated with periodontal disease and have a significant impact on general health.

- Pain
- The inability to chew food
- Decreased caloric intake and subsequent loss of weight
- Root caries due to recession of the gum tissue
- Loose teeth
- Tooth loss
- Speech difficulties
- Decreased self-esteem
- Chronic systemic inflammation

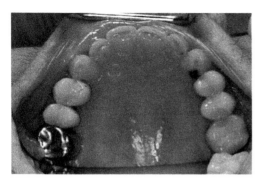

FIGURE 12-2 Many restorations, including posterior porcelain and metal full coverage crowns, and wear (incisal attrition) of anterior teeth of an 83-year-old woman.

Courtesy of Natalie Morin, University of New England

Twenty-three percent of older adults ages 65–74 have severe periodontal disease (U.S. Department of Health and Human Services, 2000). Inflammatory periodontal disease has been associated with poor cardiovascular health, ischemic stroke (U.S. Department of Health and Human Services, 2000) and dementia (Stein, Derosiers, Donegan, Yepes, & Kryscio, 2007; Delwel et al., 2018). Inflammatory mediators, such as cytokines,

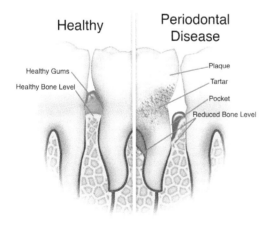

FIGURE 12-3 A comparison of healthy and diseased gums.

© Highforge Solutions/ShutterStock

may facilitate these diseases (Rai et al., 2011). In a longitudinal study investigating dementia among nuns, a review of dental records revealed that individuals with the fewest teeth had the highest risk of both prevalence and incidence of dementia (Stein et al., 2007). Periodontal bone loss is also recognized as a risk factor for osteoporosis (Koduganti, Gorthi, Reddy, & Sandeep, 2009).

The causes of edentulism or toothlessness are diverse. Currently, about 30% of adults age 65 and older are edentulous (those having lost all their teeth) compared to 46% in the 1980s (U.S. Department of Health and Human Services, 2000). Clearly, there is a trend that people are keeping their teeth longer. Yet, statistics show that U.S. states with the greatest prevalence of toothlessness are also the states with the greatest poverty rate (Christie, 2010; Centers for Disease Control and Prevention, 2004). Edentulism greatly affects food choices, which subsequently impacts nutritional state. Diet plays a pivotal role in oral health, and balanced nutrition with high fiber foods can slow the degenerative progression of oral tissue disease (Schwartz, Kaye, Nunn, Spiro, & Garcia, 2012).

Dental caries, also known as cavities or tooth decay, is a bacterial infection attributed to **Streptococcus mutans**. The process of decay starts with the dental biofilm metabolizing food particles through fermentation and by producing an acid substrate, which in turn demineralizes the hard (mineral) structure of the tooth, turning the surface to which the dental biofilm adheres into dark cavitation, also known as cavities (**FIGURE 12-4**). Untreated caries is a major cause of tooth loss. **Root caries** in older individuals pose a unique problem because root surfaces that are left exposed as a result of recessed gums from periodontal disease are at greater risk for decay (Shay, 2002). Caries often go untreated due to lack of sensitivity in the vulnerable teeth; without symptoms, the older adult may not perceive a need to visit the dentist.

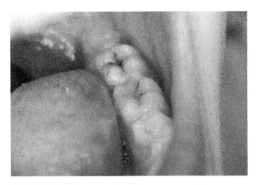

FIGURE 12-4 Untreated cavities may result in tooth loss.

© Avramenko Kostiantyn/Shutterstock

Oral and pharyngeal (throat) cancers are diseases found primarily in older adults, many of whom have a poor prognosis for recovery. Approximately, 31,000 cases are diagnosed each year, mostly in older people (National Cancer Institute, n.d.). Survival rates at the 5-year mark are 62.9% for Whites and 37.2% for African Americans (National Cancer Institute, n.d.). The survival rate for all races increases to 82.4% when localized lesions are included (**TABLE 12-1**). Early diagnosis and treatment can do much to allay suffering and to preserve the form and function of the oral cavity. Healthcare providers should be attuned to these diseases and recommend regular examinations of the oral cavity. Smoking is often the cause of these cancers. Smoking is well known as a detriment to health at any age, and therefore smoking cessation should be encouraged.

Separating Oral Aging from Disease

Xerostomia or dry mouth is associated with decreased saliva flow. Saliva is important in many ways. It protects against excess wear on tooth surfaces, aids in cleansing the oral cavity of debris, flushes acids, maintains oral pH, and makes minerals like calcium and phosphorus available to remineralize early carious lesions on enamel and root surfaces of teeth (Llena-Puy, 2006; Shay & Ship, 1995). Dry mouth can lead to uncomfortable swallowing, speech difficulties, mouth sores, and the cavitation of the hard tooth structure, resulting in tooth decay. With xerostomia, the clearance of food particles is also difficult.

The most common cause of dry mouth in older adults is the use of prescription and over-the-counter medicines. Over 400 commonly used medications cause dry mouth (Centers for Disease Control and Prevention, Division

TABLE 12-1 Oral Cancer Survival Rate at 5 Years Based on Stage of Disease

Stage at Diagnosis	Stage Distribution (%)	5-Year Relative Survival (%)
Localized (confined to primary site)	30	83.7
Regional (spread to regional lymph nodes)	47	64.2
Distant (cancer has metastasized)	19	38.5
Unknown (unstaged)	4	47.9

Reproduced from SEER Stat Fact Sheets: Oral Cavity and Pharynx, www.seer.cancer.gov/statfacts/html/oralcav.html; Young JL Jr, Roffers SD, Ries LAG, Fritz AG, Hurlbut AA (eds). SEER Summary Staging Manual - 2000: Codes and Coding Instructions, National Cancer Institute, NIH Pub. No. 01-4969, Bethesda, MD, 2001.

of Oral Health, 2006). Five out of six persons age 65+ are taking at least one medication and almost half of older adults take three or more medications (Haikal et al., 2011). Individuals living in long-term care facilities are prescribed an average of eight drugs (Shay, 2004). The more medications taken, the higher the risk that at least one medication will cause pharmaceutical inhibition of salivary flow, making it difficult to swallow, speak, and wear dentures.

Severe xerostomia is life altering. For older adults with medication-related xerostomia and whose drug therapy cannot be changed, drug schedules should be modified if possible to achieve maximum drug effect during the day, because nighttime xerostomia is more likely to cause caries (Merck Manual Professional Version, 2016). As a treatment for xerostomia causing caries, custom-fitted acrylic night guards carrying **fluoride gel** may also help limit caries in older adults (Merck Manual Professional Version, 2016). For all drugs, easy to take formulations, such as liquids should be considered and sublingual doses should be avoided, because with a dry mouth, swallowing is difficult. Key recommendations for reducing xerostomia include lubricating the mouth and throat with water before swallowing capsules and tablets or before using sublingual nitroglycerin (Merck Manual Professional Version, 2016). The older adult with xerostomia should also avoid decongestants and antihistamines to prevent drying the mouth (Merck Manual Professional Version, 2016). Dry mouth without an obvious cause needs to be investigated.

Dry mouth is not a sign of aging; most frequently, it is related to pharmacological inhibition or other disease states such as uncontrolled diabetes, Sjögren's syndrome (an immune disorder characterized by dry eyes and dry mouth; Mayo Clinic, 2017), or autoimmune diseases (Merck Manual Professional Version, 2016). Tooth wear and breakdown over time can be related to dry mouth, because lubrication prevents wear.

Tooth loss is not a sign of aging, and currently there is an increasing trend for tooth preservation (Qualtrough & Mannocci, 2011). As older people keep their teeth into old age, tooth decay (caries) and gum disease (periodontal disease) become lifelong concerns (Haikal et al., 2011). **TABLE 12-2** lists common oral conditions and treatments for older adults that the healthcare professional may encounter during their work.

Other facial structures undergo atrophy, wasting away, or shrinking, (Penna, Stark, Esienhardt, Bannasch & Iblner, 2009; Hihara et al., 2017) and the temporomandibular joint (TMJ), or the jaw joint may be susceptible to arthritic changes, making chewing and opening the mouth more difficult (Rai et al., 2011). Changes in oral motor functions in older adults tend to be mild. Tongue **stereognosis**, or the ability to sense and distinguish objects by the touch of the tongue, allows an individual to perceive problems or alterations in the mouth (Rai et al., 2011). This particular sensory system declines with age. Having healthy, natural teeth is associated with good oral stereognostic ability, whereas people experiencing edentulousness usually show a decreased oral stereognostic ability (Jacobs, Bou Serhal, & van Steenberghe, 1998).

Taste disorders are common among older people and often go unrecognized and underestimated. The culprit for most complaints about altered taste are medication related (21.7%), zinc deficiency (14.5%), and oral and systemic diseases (7.4% and 6.4%, respectively; Imposcopi, Inelmen, Sergi, Miotto, & Manzato, 2012). Assessment of taste and gustatory functioning or pertaining to eating should be part of any comprehensive geriatric assessment (Imposcopi et al., 2012).

Color changes in the teeth may arise from long-term intake of food with coloring agents (e.g., coffee) or from prolonged tobacco use (**FIGURE 12-5**). Occlusal or incisal **attrition** (Figure 12-2) may be derived from long-term dietary habits, occupational factors, bruxism

TABLE 12-2 Summary of the Most Common Oral Conditions and Treatment Considerations

Condition	Treatment Consideration
Oral lesions	Oral lesions that do not heal should be biopsied by an oral surgeon.
Dental caries	Tooth restoration, fillings, and crowns; extraction for severe unrestorable teeth with caries.
Edentulism	Prevention of tooth loss, fabrication of prostheses (dentures), dental implants, regular check-ups to reduce the risk of mouth sores, ulcers, and tissue overgrowths.
Periodontal disease	Daily toothbrushing and flossing after every meal, water irrigation, antimicrobial rinses, systemic antimicrobial therapy, tooth scaling and root debridement, surgical periodontal therapy.
Xerostomia	Preventive therapy, fluoride therapy, frequent oral hygiene visits, salivary substitutes, medications that stimulate saliva.
Candidiasis/thrush infection	Topical antifungal agents; patients using inhaled steroids should rinse mouth after use of inhaler.

Data from Rai, Kaur, Goel, & Bhatnagar (2011).

(grinding the teeth), or xerostomia. Teeth displaying attrition may be more brittle and more prone to chipping and loss of surface detail. Loss of tooth imbrications (the ridges or seams of tissue on the tooth) is a sign of the aging tooth (Rai et al., 2011).

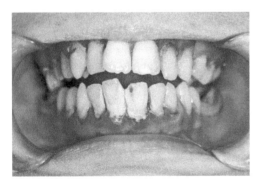

FIGURE 12-5 Drinking coffee and smoking cigarettes are two common causes of discoloration in teeth.
© Lighthunter/Shutterstock

The aging of the dental pulp results in a shrinking nerve, which can contribute to undetected disease because the older person may not perceive pain until the dental disease is far advanced. The pulp becomes smaller with the physiologic laying down of secondary dentin, probably in response to trauma and the wear and tear of continued use over time (Morse, 1991).

The mouth is a mirror to overall health, so when the oral cavity is pink, moist, and clean and lacks signs of inflammation, this can be a predictor of general good health. Healthy teeth lack bacterial film, the progenitor of dental disease. The tongue is velvety in appearance and breath is not unpleasant. Unpleasant breath (halitosis) may be a sign of disease. Diseases other than dental disease that can cause halitosis include alcohol abuse, uncontrolled diabetes, kidney failure, bowel obstruction, and sinusitis. Many systemic diseases also have primary signs and symptoms in the oral cavity, for example, blood diseases such as leukemia and anemia.

Oral health is directly related to quality of life of the older adult (Rai et al., 2011). Poorer scores on quality of life ratings by men and women who are unable to leave home are found in those who have the presence of oral problems such as dry mouth and tooth decay. Well-being correlates linked to oral health include the number of missing teeth and years of education (Strömberg, Holmèn, Hagman-Gustafsson, Gabre, & Wårdh, 2012). Unfortunately, most older people viewed limitations (including dental disease) as a consequence of aging and not as problems that can be solved (Haikal et al., 2011). The healthcare professional is positioned to make a difference in the lives of older adults by recognizing oral problems and referring individuals to the proper professional for treatment, as dental problems are often solvable.

▶ Recognizing Barriers to Care

There are a number of reasons why older adults do not access dental and preventive care. Not having the money to pay for services seems like an apparent cause, but this may be more related to the value placed on dental care than a true lack of funds. Values are instilled early in life and are carried throughout life. Not perceiving the need for dental care is a major barrier to obtaining proper dental care. Lifestyle behaviors can also inform an elder's choice. For example, if an older adult is informed of a diagnosis that is not covered by insurance and costs more than he or she can comfortably spend, or accessing care would require accepting charity, the person may choose not to receive the prescribed dental treatment. Older adults who recognize their health needs and seek care do so because they not only value their well-being, but also perceive that they can afford care.

Accessibility of dental care is another barrier. Millions of older adults live in rural and inner city areas where dentists choose not to practice. Even when individuals have the ability to pay, a dental office or dental care may not be available. The problem becomes exacerbated when transportation to receive care is also not readily available or timely (American Dental Hygienists' Association, 2001).

Physical access is particularly problematic for older people who have disabilities or are restricted to their homes (Stromberg et al., 2012). Disability was identified as second only to financial challenges as a barrier to receiving dental care (Stromberg et al., 2012). Older adults requiring moderate to heavy supportive care, including assistance with oral care routines, reported a lower general quality of life (Stromberg et al., 2012). As more older adults "age in place" and are cared for in the home rather than in long-term care facilities, oral care services should include delivery of in-home prevention and care by dentists and dental hygienist professionals affiliated with home health organizations.

Financial and economic barriers also explain lack of dental care among older adults. Loss of dental insurance at retirement or not having access to dental insurance has affected older adults' dental health outcomes (U.S. Department of Health and Human Services, 2000). Access to affordable health care, including dental care, has yet to be a reality in the United States for persons age 65 or older. Reimbursements for dental and medical services are typically low and do not cover all expenses incurred (U.S. Department of Health and Human Services, 2000). Socioeconomic status, the number of oral symptoms, and location of the home are all associated with general health status (Brennan & Singh, 2012; Toner, Ferguson, & Sokal, 2009). However, independent of socioeconomic status, poor oral health was associated with worse general health and the need for dental prostheses or dentures (de Andrade, Lebrao, Santos, Teixeira, & de Oliveira Duarte, 2012; Rouleau et al., 2011).

▶ The Interprofessional Role in Oral Care and Prevention

The 21st century offers the healthcare professional an opportunity to reassess current curricular structures and practice models to begin dissolving traditional disciplinary barriers and to begin including an interprofessional healthcare team approach for health education, health promotion, and disease prevention (Dounis, Ditmyer, McClain, Cappelli, & Mobley, 2010). Oral health professionals are vital members of the healthcare team. Proper education and training should encourage students in dental sciences to act as team members who can use their expertise in the realm of oral care and education to improve the overall quality of life for the older adults of the future (Dounis et al., 2010).

Prevention

Caregivers and oral health professionals can promote straightforward and safe measures to reverse, arrest, and prevent oral disease in older adults (Joshi, Souminen, Knuuttila, & Bernabé, 2018; U.S. Department of Health and Human Services, 2000). Preventive regimes for the older adult include antimicrobial mouth rinses (e.g., chlorhexidine gluconate 0.12%), fluoride rinses, gels, or toothpastes, and removal of biofilm and hard deposits that are retentive to biofilm. Five percent sodium **fluoride varnish** is used in extended and/or long-term care facilities and the private homes of people who are medically compromised to arrest or decrease the development of dental caries (Hong, Watkins, Ettinger, & Wefel, 2005). Educating older adults about the manual removal of disease-causing biofilm by toothbrushing two or three times a day with a soft bristle toothbrush is important and can reduce gum pocketing (Joshi et al., 2018), equally important is the consistent and effective use of dental floss. Older adults with arthritis may appreciate an electric toothbrush or built-up handles and grips to better manipulate the tools to promote oral cleanliness.

Approximately, 5% of Americans aged 65 and over live in nursing facilities where oral care can be problematic (U.S. Department of Health and Human Services, 2000). Because of the lack of training and perceived time, nursing home and other long-term care facility workers have limited capacity to deliver needed oral healthcare services, even though most residents are at risk for oral diseases (U.S. Department of Health and Human Services, 2000). Conducting risk assessments and implementing anticipatory guidance management (i.e., teaching ahead of need) can make inroads toward realizing true oral prevention outcomes.

Caregivers of older adults must consider the functional capacity of the care recipient when planning for oral hygiene. Higher level functioning capacity is a factor for successful independent living and is an indicator for effectively completing crucial oral hygiene behaviors (Moriya et al., 2013). Otherwise, it is the caregiver's duty to provide basic oral hygiene to the older adult whose functioning will not allow for self-initiated dental hygiene practices. Education and motivation of the family, other caregivers, and long-term care facility staff are essential if oral diseases are to be avoided (Niessen & Fedele, 2002).

Oral prostheses (or removable dentures) require removing and rinsing the dentures after eating. The older adult, caregiver, or healthcare professional needs to clean the mouth with gauze or a soft bristle brush to remove film from the gum tissues. The person should also scrub the dentures at least once per day (**FIGURE 12-6**). Dentures need to be handled carefully. Most types of dentures need to remain moist to keep their shape. The dentures should be placed in water or a mild denture-soaking solution overnight (Carr, n.d.), and then rinsed thoroughly. Denture adhesives may increase bite strength but are not a substitute for a well-fitting denture (Kalra, Nadiger, & Shah, 2012).

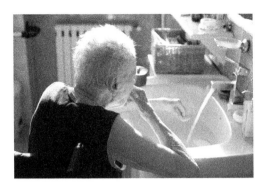

The older adult needs to consistently wear the dentures to ensure continued proper fit and to deter bone loss that accompanies endentulism. Most elders stop wearing dentures because they do not fit or are uncomfortable when loose.

However, changes can be offset if dentures are worn regularly. Many users cope with changes in fit by using adhesives specifically developed to keep dentures snug in the mouth. However, dentures may need to be refined and replaced with some frequency over time.

Simple Oral Screening

Recognizing oral conditions through a simple **oral screening** procedure may save an elder's life and provide early detection of oral or pharyngeal cancers and other oral conditions needing attention. Risk factors for oral and pharyngeal cancer include alcohol and tobacco use, older age, excessive sun exposure, human papilloma virus (HPV), and a diet low in fruits and vegetables. Oral candidiasis or oral yeast infection can appear as a red or white lesion and as cracks at the corners of the mouth. **TABLE 12-3** outlines simple procedures and what to look for

TABLE 12-3 Six Steps to Examining the Oral Cavity

Steps	What to Look For
Examine head, neck, face, and lips	Look for asymmetry, crusts, fissuring, growths, or color change. Palpate lymph nodes.
Labial and buccal mucosa	Pull upper lip up toward nose and observe gums, teeth, and inner lips. Repeat for the lower lip, pulling toward chin. Observe for color, texture, and swelling abnormalities.
Gums	Stretch the mouth, looking at the gums for bleeding, pus, or growths; perform from back to front in all sections.
Tongue	Observe the back, sides, and undersurface of the tongue, looking for swelling, coating, or variation in size, coloration, or texture. Gauze squares may assist full protrusion of the tongue, pulling laterally.
Floor of the mouth	With the tongue elevated and tip to the roof of the mouth, observe the floor of the mouth for color changes, swellings, and surface abnormalities.
Oral pharynx	Have patients tilt their head back and say "ah" while you observe the palate, tonsil area, uvula, and back of the throat for swellings and red or white lesions.

Data from Detecting Oral Cancer: A Guide for Health Care Professionals. National Institutes of Health, National Institute of Dental and Craniofacial Research. http://www.nidcr.nih.gov/oralhealth/topics/oralcancer/detectingoralcancer.htm

during a straightforward screening. It should take no longer than a few minutes, with a flashlight and a tongue depressor to aid visualization. To promote the well-being of the older adult, the healthcare team can examine the oral cavity, take a history, inform the person of the results, and recommend follow-up for a diagnosis as needed.

▶ New Models of Care

New models of oral health care include healthcare teams that are interprofessional in nature. Interprofessional teams can deliver more flexible and individualized care with shared learning from other professions. Different health professionals can come together to learn about gerontology, share experiences, and expertise, and gain knowledge and insights into providing better care for the older adult. There are many interprofessional programs currently operational, such as the Program for Outreach to Interprofessional Services and Education (POISE) and Area Health Education Centers (AHEC). These programs aim to develop, implement, evaluate, and sustain interprofessional education and training for healthcare learners, while emphasizing improved access to health services for the geriatric population in medically and dentally underserved areas (Toner et al., 2009).

There is also room for developing home and community-based programs in oral health (Shahidi, Casado, & Friedman, 2008). Suggested public health priorities for programming include:

- Integrating oral health into medical care.
- Implementing community programs to promote healthy behaviors and improve access to preventive services.
- Developing a comprehensive strategy to address the oral health needs of long-term care residents.
- Assessing the feasibility of preventive and basic restorative services to eliminate pain and infection (Griffin, Jones, Brunson, Griffin, & Bailey, 2012).

Because many physicians and dentists resist accepting low or no reimbursement rates from insurance companies, the financial burden of oral health care is placed on clients. If they cannot afford care, it is not sought. Therefore, prevention activities make sense as a means of keeping older people functioning at optimal levels. Relying on well-trained mid-level providers (e.g., physician assistant, nurse practitioner, and advanced dental hygiene practitioner or dental therapist) to provide care can help keep costs affordable and accessible, and provide a viable alternative to the present system (American Dental Hygienists' Association, 2001; American Dental Hygienists' Association, Division of Communication, 2012). Other models of care include training the workforce to specifically work with older adults and other underserved populations. Allowing mid-level practitioners or independently practicing allied health and dental hygiene professionals to treat people in their homes would fill a serious gap in services (American Dental Hygienists' Association, 2001; American Dental Hygienists' Association, Division of Communication, 2012).

▶ Summary

It is imperative for healthcare professionals in every discipline to realize that oral health cannot be separated from general health and well-being. Each professional should be able to differentiate between typical age-related or disease-related physiologies. Social issues such as poverty affect oral health and general health. Level of oral health is highly correlated to the older adult's nutritional status and their general quality of life. The importance of dental health to well-being cannot be overstated. Preventive oral health measures, such as effective brushing, mechanical control of pathogenic biofilm, and the use of safe fluorides, are effective measures for older people. Being aware of the directions of change, such as trends toward less edentulism in older adults and the link between oral health and general health, will better inform priorities and planning for the health and comfort of our diverse older population.

🔍 CASE STUDIES

Case 1: Ms. May, an 80-year-old woman, grew up in a small rural community that did not have fluorinated water until she was in her late teens. She had dental issues throughout her childhood, and by the time she entered college, she had a full upper denture. Ms. May did not have dental insurance, so she only went to the dentist when something hurt. By the time Ms. May retired, her lower teeth were restored with many fillings and crowns. During a recent visit to her dentist, he diagnosed her with inflammatory periodontal disease and recommended that she have routine cleanings every three months to control the biofilm causing her red swollen gums. Tragically, Ms. May had a stroke (right cerebrovascular accident [CVA]) with left hemiplegia soon after, and was sent to a rehabilitation hospital.

1. **What preventive methods could have helped Ms. May avoid tooth loss?**
2. **Is it possible that Ms. May's periodontal disease had anything to do with her stroke? Why or why not?**
3. **How should she care for her denture?**

Case 2: Mrs. Jones had not been to a dentist in a number of years and did not really want to go to her dental appointment this morning. However, she was starting to get concerned about the pain in her jaws and she recently noticed that two of her teeth were starting to become loose. The notion of losing a tooth was finally enough to spur her to visit the dentist, Dr. Carson. While examining her teeth, Dr. Carson noticed that Mrs. Jones had bits of food stuck in little pockets around her teeth in her gums along with a bad case of halitosis. "So what's the verdict, doctor?" Mrs. Jones asked. "Do I just need to start brushing more often?" "You're going to need to do a bit more than just brush more often," Dr. Carson replied. "You have a condition we need to discuss."

1. **What condition does Mrs. Jones have and how do you know?**
2. **What will likely happen to Mrs. Jones if she does not address this condition?**
3. **Besides daily toothbrushing, what else might Mrs. Jones need to do and/or have done to her in order to treat her condition?**

TEST YOUR KNOWLEDGE

Review Questions

1. Examining the oral cavity entails six steps. Which of the following is not a part of those six steps?
   a. Palpating the lymph nodes
   b. Stretching the mouth to look for bleeding
   c. Having the person say "ah" to observe the palate
   d. Having the person touch tongue to nose

2. What percentage of persons over 65 have severe periodontal disease?
   a. 10%
   b. 23%
   c. 45%
   d. 73%

3. Recession of gum tissue causes all of the following except:
   a. Weight gain
   b. Pain
   c. Root caries
   d. Decreased self-esteem

4. The ability to sense objects by the touch of the tongue in the mouth is essential for the perception of oral self-cleanliness. The lack of touch sense in the mouth is called
   a. Periodontal disease
   b. Sjögren's syndrome
   c. Stereognosis
   d. Taste disorder

5. Taste disorders are common among the elderly, and often go unrecognized and underestimated. Which of the following is *not* a widespread reason for taste complaint?
   a. Medication use
   b. Mineral deficiency
   c. Systemic diseases
   d. Lack of interest in food

Learning Activities

1. Examine classmates' mouths with a flashlight and tongue depressor for signs of oral health. Compare and contrast color, texture, moisture, and lack of inflammation (redness), being mindful of infection control. The goal is to have an interprofessional perspective of oral well-being.

2. Interview older family members and friends about attitudes regarding oral health, access to preventive oral health, disparities that affect the older adult, and policies that the elder thinks could help oral health outcomes and disparities, if they are identified. Class members will report the findings to the larger group, categorizing similar answers.

3. Search online for the keywords *periodontal disease* and *general health*. Create a bibliography in class that shows the link between oral health and general health.

4. Search the web for professionals who treat the older population and create an interprofessional referral base for potential senior dental patients in your area.

5. Imagine that you work in a nursing facility and one of your patients has xerostomia, but does not think it is a big deal. Describe what you would say to this patient to explain the importance of treating this condition.

References

American Dental Hygienists' Association. (2001). Access to Care Position Paper. Retrieved July 28, 2013, from http://www.adha.org/resourcesdocs/7112_Access_to_Care_Position_Paper.pdf

American Dental Hygienists' Association, Division of Communications. (2012). Mid-level Oral Health Providers: An Update. Accessed November, 12–15.

Brennan, D. S., & Singh, K. A. (2012). Dietary, self-reported oral health and socio-demographic predictors of general health status among older adults. *Journal of Nutrition Health and Aging, 16*(5), 437–441.

Carr, A. (n.d.) Denture Care: How do I clean dentures? *Mayo Clinic.* Retrieved June 28, 2013, from http://www.mayoclinic.com/health/denturecare/AN02028

Centers for Disease Control and Prevention. (2004). *Behavioral risk factor surveillance system survey data.* Atlanta, GA: Department of Health and Human Services, Centers for Disease Control and Prevention.

Centers for Disease Control and Prevention, Division of Oral Health. (2006). *Oral health for older Americans.* Retrieved June 28, 2013, from http://www.cdc.gov/OralHealth/publications/factsheets/adult_older.htm

Christie, L. (2010). America's wealthiest (and poorest) states. *CNN Money, Sept.* Retrieved June 28, 2013, from http://money.cnn.com/2010/09/16/news/economy/Americas_wealthiest_states/indexhtm

de Andrade, F. B., Lebrao, M. L., Santos, J. L., Teixeira, D. S., & de Oliveira Duarte, Y. A. (2012). Relationship between oral health-related quality of life, oral health, socioeconomic, and general heath factors in elderly Brazilians. *Journal of the American Geriatrics Society, 60*(9), 1755–1760.

Delwel, S., Binnekade T. T., Perez, R. S. G. M., Hertogh, C. M. P. M., Scherder, E. J. A., & Lobbezoo, F. (2018). Oral hygiene and oral health in older people with dementia: A comprehensive review with focus on oral soft tissues. *Clinical Oral Investigations, 22*(1), 93–108.

Dounis, G., Ditmyer, N. M., McClain, M. A., Cappelli, D. P., & Mobley, C. C. (2010). Preparing the dental workforce for oral disease prevention in an aging population. *Journal of Dental Education, 74*(10), 1086–1094.

Griffin, S. O., Jones J. A., Brunson, D., Griffin P. M., & Bailey, W. D. (2012). Burden of oral disease among older adults and implication for public health priorities. *American Journal of Public Health, 120*(3), 411–418.

Haikal, D. S., Paula, A. M., Martins, A. M., Moreira, A. N., & Ferreira E. F. (2011). Self-perception of oral health and impact on quality of life among the elderly: A quantitive-qualitative approach [Abstract]. *Ciência & Saúde Coletiva, 16*, 3317–3329.

Hihara, H., Kanetaka, H., Kanno, A., Koeda, S., Nakasato, N., Kawashima, R., & Sasaki, K. (2017). Evaluating age-related change in lip somatosensation using somatosensory evoked magnetic fields. *PLoS ONE, 12*(6), e0179323. doi:10.1371/journal.pone.0179323

Hong, L., Watkins, C. A., Ettinger, R. L., & Wefel, J. S. (2005). Effect of topical fluoride and fluoride varnish on in vitro root surface lesions. *American Journal of Dentistry, 18*(3), 182–187.

Imposcopi, A., Inelman, E. M., Sergi, G., Miotto, F., & Manzato, E. (2012). Taste loss in the elderly: Epidemiology, causes, and consequences. *Aging Clinical and Experimental Research, 24*(6), 570–579. doi:10.3275/8520

Jacobs, R., Bou Serhal, C., & van Steenberghe, D. (1998). Oral stereognosis: A review of the literature. *Clinical Oral Investigations, 2*(1), 3–10.

Joshi, S., Suominen, A. L., Knuuttila, M., Bernabé, E. (2018). Toothbrushing behaviour and periodontal pocketing: An 11-year longitudinal study. *Journal of Clinical Periodontology, 45*(2), 196–203. doi:10.1111/jcpe.12844

Kalra, P., Nadiger, R., & Shah, F. K. (2012). An investigation into the effect of denture adhesives on incisal bite force of complete denture wearers using pressure transducers—a clinical study. *Journal of Advanced Prosthodontics, 4*(2), 97–102.

Koduganti, R. R., Gorthi, C., Reddy, V., & Sandeep, N. (2009). Osteoporosis: A risk factor for periodontitis. *Journal of the Indian Society of Periodontology, 13*(2), 90–96.

Lalla, E. (2017). Clinical management of patients with diabetes and periodontal disease: Ideas whose time has come. *Compendium of Continuing Education in Dentistry, 38*(8 Suppl), 14–19, 20 quiz.

Llena-Puy, C. (2006). The rôle of saliva in maintaining oral health and as an aid to diagnosis. *Medicina Oral, Patologia, Cirugia Bucal, 11*(5), 449–455.

Mayo Clinic. (2017). Sjogren's syndrome. Retrieved from https://www.mayoclinic.org/diseases-conditions/sjogrens-syndrome/symptoms-causes/syc-20353216

Moriya, S., Tei, K., Yamazaki, Y., Hata, H., Kitagawa, Y., Inoue, N., & Miura, H. (2013). Relationships between higher-level functional capacity and dental health behaviors in community-dwelling older adults. *Gerodontology, 30*, 133–140. doi:10.1111/j.1741-2358.2012.00654.x

Morse, D. R. (1991). Age related changes of the dental pulp complex and their relationship to systemic aging. *Oral Surgery, Oral Medicine, Oral Pathology, 72*(6), 721–745.

Murchisen, D. F. (2016). Xerostomia. In *Merck Manual Professional Version* on-line. Retrieved from https://www.merckmanuals.com/professional/dental-disorders/symptoms-of-dental-and-oral-disorders/xerostomia

National Cancer Institute. (n.d.) Surveillance epidemiology and end results (SEER). SEER stat fact sheets: Oral cavity and pharynx, stage distribution and 5-year relative survival by stage at diagnosis for 2007–2013, all races, both sexes. *National Cancer Institute* online. Retrieved from http://www.seer.cancer.gov/statfacts/html/oralcav.html

National Institute of Dental and Craniofacial Research. (2013). Detecting Oral Cancer: A Guide for Health Care Professionals. Bethesda, MD: National Institutes of Health. Retrieved from http://www.nidcr.nih.gov/oralhealth/topics/oralcancer/detectingoralcancer.htm

Niessen, L. C., & Fedele, D. J. (2002). Aging successfully: Oral health for the prime of life. *Compendium of Continuing Education in Dentistry, 23*(Suppl 10), 4–11.

Penna, V., Stark, G. B., Esienhardt, S. U., Bannasch, H., & Iblner, N. (2009). The aging lip: A comparative histological analysis of age-related changes of the upper lip complex. *Plastic and Reconstructive Surgery, 124,* 624–628.

Qualtrough, A. J., & Mannocci, F. (2011). Endodontics and the older patient. *Dental Update, 38,* 559–562, 564–566.

Rai, S., Kaur, M., Goel, S., & Bhatnagar, P. (2011). Moral and professional responsibility of oral physician toward geriatric patient with interdisciplinary management—the time to act is now! *Journal of Midlife Health, 2,* 18–24. doi:10.4103/0976-7800.83261

Rouleau, T., Harrington, A., Brennan, M., Hammond, F., Hirsh, M., Nussbaum, M., & Bockenek, W. (2011). Receipt of dental care and barriers encountered by persons with disabilities. *Special Care Dentistry, 31*(2), 63–67.

Saavedra, M. D. C. (1822). *The history of the ingenious gentleman, Don Quixote of La Mancha* (P. A. Motteux, Trans.). Edinburgh: Hurst, Robinson & Co.

Schwartz, N., Kaye, E. K., Nunn, M. E., Spiro, A. 3rd, & Garcia, R. I. (2012). High fiber foods reduce periodontal disease progression in men aged 65 and older: The Veterans Affairs normative aging study/dental longitudinal study. *Journal of the American Geriatrics Society, 60*(4), 676–683.

Shahidi, A., Casado, Y., & Friedman, P. K. (2008). Taking dentistry to the geriatric patient: A home visit model. *Journal of the Massachusetts Dental Society, 57*(3), 46–48.

Shay, K. (2002). Infectious complications of dental and periodontal diseases in the elderly. *Clinical Infectious Diseases, 34*(9), 1215–1223.

Shay, K. (2004). The evolving impact of aging America on dental practice. *Journal of Contemporary Dental Practice, 5*(4), 101–110.

Shay, K., Scannapieco, F. A., Terpenning, M. S., Smith, B. J., & Taylor, G. W. (2005). Nosocomial pneumonia and oral health. *Special Care in Dentistry, 25*(4), 179–187.

Shay, K., & Ship, J. A. (1995). The importance of oral health in the older patient. *Journal of the American Geriatrics Society, 43*(12), 1414–1422.

Stein, P. S., Desrosiers, M., Donegan, S. J., Yepes, J. F., & Kryscio, R. J. (2007). Tooth loss, dementia and neuropathology in the Nun study. *Journal of the American Dental Association, 38*(10), 1314–1322; quiz 1381–1382.

Strömberg, E., Holmèn, A., Hagman-Gustafsson, M. L., Gabre, P., & Wårdh, I. (2012) Oral health-related quality-of-life in homebound elderly dependent on moderate and substantial supportive care for daily living. *Acta Odontologica Scandinavica, 71*(3–4), 771–777. doi:10.3109/00016357.2012.734398

Toner, J. A., Ferguson, K. D., & Sokal, R. D. (2009). Continuing interprofessional education in geriatrics and gerontology in medically underserved areas. *Journal of Continuing Education in the Health Professions, 29,* 157–160.

U.S. Department of Health and Human Services. (2000). *Oral health in America: A report of the surgeon general—Executive summary.* Rockville, MD: U.S. Department of Health and Human Services, National Institute of Dental and Craniofacial Research, National Institutes of Health. Retrieved from https://www.nidcr.nih.gov/DataStatistics/SurgeonGeneral/Documents/hck1ocv.@www.surgeon.fullrpt.pdf

Young, J. L. Jr., Roffers, S. D., Ries L. A. G., Fritz, A. G., & Hurlbut, A. A. (Eds.). SEER Summary Staging Manual—2000: Codes and Coding Instructions, National Cancer Institute, NIH Pub. No. 01-4969.

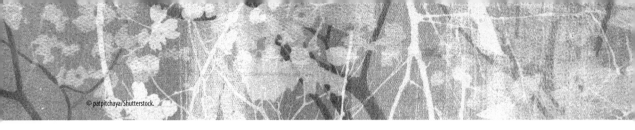

© patpitchaya/Shutterstock.

CHAPTER 13

Sexuality and Aging

Nancy MacRae, MS, OTR/L, FAOTA

BEHAVIORAL OBJECTIVES

Upon completion of this chapter, the reader will be able to:

1. Explain the difference between the terms sex and gender.
2. Describe the different components that influence sexuality.
3. Recognize the importance of intimacy in feelings of sexuality.
4. Describe complications associated with common diseases that can interfere with sexual functioning and the expression of sexuality.
5. Demonstrate a conversation with a client using the PLISSIT model approach.

(continues)

(*continued*)

6. Describe the role prescription drugs can play in sexual expression.
7. Describe gender differences in sexual functioning in late life.
8. Identify causes of inappropriate client sexual behavior and explain potential appropriate responses.
9. Describe some of the challenges institutions face in supporting the sexual activities of older residents.

KEY TERMS

Bisexual	Lesbian	Sexual orientation
Estrogen replacement therapy	Libido	Sexual preference
Gay male	Menopause	Sexuality
Gender	PLISSIT model	Transgender
Intimacy	Sex	

▶ Introduction

In generations past, discussions about sexuality were only conducted behind closed doors. Then, U.S. society demanded that people were discreet regardless of their **sexual orientation** (i.e., who they are sexually attracted to) and sexual activities. After all, proper ladies and gentlemen did not publicly divulge their intimate secrets. Fast forward to the sexual revolution of the 1960s when the pendulum started to swing in the opposite direction. Today, in our Internet-based society, we are more concerned about people sharing too much information about their sex lives than sharing too little. However, it is important to recognize that many older adults remain reluctant to open up about their sexuality. For this reason, healthcare professionals must remain client centered and recognize that **sex** and **sexuality** continue to be important and subsequently impact health in late life. Moreover, interactions with older clients need to be culturally sensitive to promote open and frank discussions about sexual functioning.

Research on sexual functioning and sexuality would be nearly nonexistent if not for the emergence of birth control options and the major shift in social norms and expectations that occurred in the mid-20th century. In 1960, when the first birth control pill became available for purchase, women were given the opportunity to personally control their own fertility and reproduction for the first time in history. At the same time, social expectations of women began to shift and they were no longer viewed as just wives, mothers, and daughters. Women were granted access into the workplace and they began to raise their voices on issues important to them. The sexual revolution and the women's liberation movement during the 1960s–1980s were intricately intertwined and provided social and political platforms for adults to advocate for change, including the ability to express their sexuality and sexual orientation.

Even though society has taken a giant step toward accepting new roles for women and different expressions of sexuality by both men and women, there is more to learn about sexual functioning and sexuality, especially during the second half of life. In this chapter, the text covers influences on sexual functioning in late life, practitioner responses to inappropriate sexual behaviors (ISBs), and sexual functioning of older adults with special needs.

▶ Sex and Sexuality

Sex refers to the anatomy of an individual's reproductive system (and related secondary characteristics) as well as the act of copulation or intercourse. **Gender** refers to the social roles, behaviors, and norms that a society deems appropriate for a given sex. Madison Avenue has used sex and gender as marketing tools for years because it helps sell products. Sexual innuendo pervades our society. We see sexual images and stereotypes portrayed daily in advertisements, print media, songs, movies, television, and social media. Jokes with sexual connotations are frequently interjected into daily life. Yet, as prevalent as sex is within our society, little time or attention is devoted to understanding the quality and capacity of our sexual being, that is, our sexuality. Sexuality is a core characteristic of who we are. It is how we think about and express our sexual interests and sexual identity. Even though sexuality includes sexual activities, it is also a state of mind. We can be sexual without engaging in sex.

Exploring our sexuality is a lifelong process, a lifelong adventure. What we learn about sexuality, whether explicit or not, frames how we perceive ourselves and can greatly influence how we act. Taking stock of what sexuality encompasses can help us realize how very basic it is to our sense of self. Dailey (1981) conceptualized sexuality through the use of the "Circles of Sexuality" model. The model consists of a ring of overlapping circles that represent the five core components of sexuality. The components include sensuality, **intimacy**, sexual identity, sexual health and reproduction, and sexualization. Dailey also suggested that not only can personal values and expectations influence how each component intersects, but these also influence how

individuals see themselves as sexual beings. FORGE, a national transgender antiviolence organization (FORGE, n.d. [a]), modified the five circles by adding power to the sexualization circle to address issues of power and control often experienced by members of the **lesbian**, **gay male**, **bisexual**, and **transgender** (LGBT) community (**FIGURE 13-1**; FORGE, n.d. [b]).

Similar models and frameworks also suggest that sexuality is influenced by personal values and ability to be intimate with another person in a mutually satisfying manner. Specifically:

- Feelings and beliefs about what it means to be male or female
- Relationship(s) with people of similar or other genders
- How relationships are established, especially close and intimate ones
- How feelings are expressed

Family, cultural, and religious environments influence the development of sexuality. If we have been loved and nurtured and our sense of competence has been fostered and strengthened by the people we love, we will be more likely to have healthy self-images and a fair amount of success in both initiating and sustaining personal relationships. Conversely, if we encountered abuse in our past, it is likely that we will not develop a positive sense of self-worth and may have difficulty developing and maintaining trusting relationships.

Sexuality is also influenced by our self-perception as sexual beings and how our first expressions of overt sexual feelings were received by others. Reactions of embarrassment, ridicule, shame, or censure can leave lasting scars. Conversely, shared feelings of acceptance, encouragement, and enjoyment lead to a more positive conclusion. Fostering the ability to say "no" and accepting the responsibility that accompanies the expression of sexuality will also strengthen one's feeling of self-efficacy in this realm.

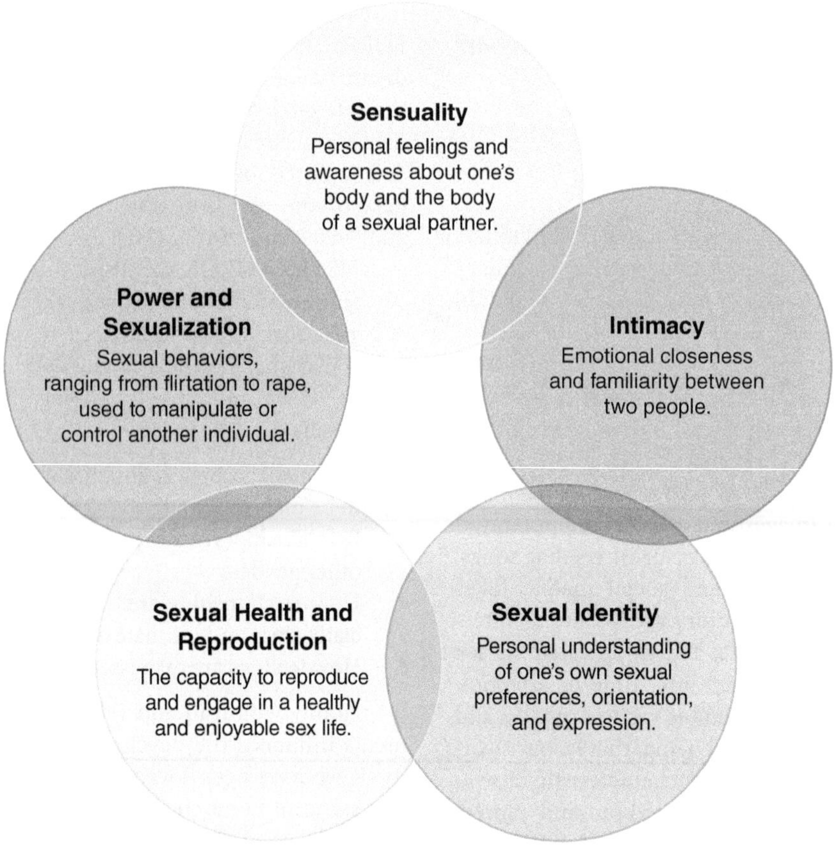

FIGURE 13-1 Dailey's original "Circles of Sexuality" model was modified by FORGE to include a "Power and Sexualization" circle representing the complex issues of power and control that members of the LGBT community face.

Developed by Dr. Dennis M. Dailey, Professor Emeritus, University of Kansas, Lawrence, Kansas.

▶ Aging and Sexuality

Deeply embedded in our youth-oriented society is the assumption that sex and sexuality are provinces of only the young. Older men are depicted as "dirty old men" if they show any interest in sex, and older women are assumed to be "sexless." Yet, sexual identity does not disappear as the years pass. Sexual feelings and urges simply change, just as other aspects of our being change and evolve. As age increases, older adults may have fewer sexual encounters, but may find more pleasure and satisfaction by linking sex and intimacy to quality of life.

Satisfaction with one's own sexual behavior has been found to be associated with health, not age (Chao et al., 2011).

Betty Friedan, in her seminal 1993 book *The Fountain of Age*, examined aging and sexuality and challenged the reader to look at how social values victimize both sexes: women by the feminine mystique; men by a lifetime of machismo (Friedan, 1993, p. 14). Images of youthful erection always leading to intercourse and an excessive emphasis on performance are a heavy burden for both older men *and* women to live up to and impose unrealistic expectations and barriers to intimacy. Pleasuring, cuddling, and touching have been found to be more important among older adults (Boston Women's Health Book Collective, 2005; Wilkins & Warnok, 2009), who tend to view their total sexual experience through a qualitative rather than a quantitative lens.

In a study on sexuality using a nationally representative sample of older adults, Lindau and colleagues (2007) defined sexual activity in late life as "any mutually voluntary activity with another person that involves sexual contact, whether or not intercourse or orgasm occurs" (Lindau et al., 2007, p. 762). Study participants revealed that sexual experiences were more than meeting or exceeding a standard of performance. First, the two people involved define the parameters of the sexual relationship. Second, an infinite variety of possibilities may prove satisfying to one or both partners. The main challenge for women remains finding a partner with whom to be intimate (Boston Women's Health Book Collective, 2005; Starr & Weiner, 1981; Wilkins & Warnok, 2009).

A 2009 study supported the Lindau findings and suggested a strong association existed between physical health and sexual activity among older adults (Wilkins & Warnok, 2009). As in the Lindau study (Lindau et al., 2007), each participant reported at least one of the following benefits from engaging in mutually agreeable sex: improved health (both mental and physical), increased life span, more solid relationships, and/or a bona fide escape from reality. These findings were substantiated by Block and colleagues in 2012, thus further supporting the idea that the association between health and sexual activity is stronger than the association between age and sexual activity.

In the original Lindau study (Lindau et al., 2007), a majority of older adults surveyed reported sexuality as an important component of their lives and engaged regularly in an intimate sexual relationship. Among participants reporting some sexual problems, sexual activity only began to substantially decrease after the age of 74. Fifty percent of the sexually active older adults were bothered by at least one problem: erectile dysfunction for males and low **libido** (i.e., sexual drive), vaginal lubrication, and climax difficulties for females. Also notable was that participants reportedly welcomed the opportunity to discuss their sexuality, a topic rarely brought up by their physicians.

In another U.S. study, Laumann, Das, and Waite (2008) analyzed data from the 2005–2006 National Social Life, Health, and Aging Project with a sample of 3,000 women and men ages 57–85. In their interviews, they found that with the exception of men's erectile and orgasmic problems, biological aging did not result in increased sexual issues for either sex. Rather, sexual problems identified by participants occurred in response to the multiple stressors in their lives stemming from their physical health, mental health, and intimate relationships. Stress, anxiety, and depression, along with poor mental health, were strongly associated with women's reports of sexual problems, but less so with men's problems. Furthermore, sexual health was directly affected by the strength and quality of the intimate relationship.

A British study by Gott and Hinchliff (2003) examined the views of older adults on the importance of sex in their lives. The study utilized a combination of quantitative and qualitative data. Similar to Lindau and colleague's findings (2007), participants welcomed the chance to discuss sex. Study outcomes underscored sex as an important part of a close relationship. Health problems and widowhood often led to a reprioritization of the role of sex in older adults' lives and the difficulty of maintaining physical intimacy. Even when intercourse was viewed as no longer possible, it remained centrally important.

In a study of older adults with lower socioeconomic status, researchers (Ginsberg, Pomerantz, & Kramer-Felley, 2005) found that the 179 participants wanted to engage in sexual activities more frequently than they did, but could not due to a lack of available partners. Touching and kissing were reportedly most desired; mutual stroking, masturbation, and intercourse were less desired and also infrequently experienced. The researchers also found that age and health status predicted preferences for sexual activity.

▶ Intimacy

What is evident across the literature on sexuality and older adults is the importance of intimacy (Boston Women's Health Book Collective, 2005; Butler, Lewis, Hoffman, & Whitehead, 1994). Sexual intimacy requires self-acceptance and risk taking. It involves purposely losing control of oneself and acquiescing to what is happening. When the result of sexual intimacy is satisfying, feelings of positive self-esteem and trust are reinforced.

Intimacy needs to be included as a component of meaningful sexuality. Women, as kin keepers, have traditionally nurtured a capacity for connection and engagement with others in all forms of intimacy. Men may have many friends, but deep and honest disclosure that is so vital to intimacy may not be a part of male friendships. Carl Gustav Jung, the father of analytic psychology, described the midlife years after age 40 as the "afternoon" and "evening" of life (Jung, 1933, p. 108), and suggested that each sex learns to know its polarities, the sexually opposite side of their nature: for the male, his feminine qualities; for the female, her male traits (Lachman, 2004). Coming to terms with these unused and unfamiliar characteristics can involve stress and anxiety, but reconciling the differences can lead to a freedom of expression previously unknown (Butler et al., 1994). This "crossover" may be a key to vital aging. "Disengagement from the roles and goals of youth and from activities and ties that no longer have any personal meaning may, in fact, be necessary to make the shift to a new kind of engagement in age" (Friedan, 1993, p. 181). Embracing changes

in gender roles can enhance sexual activity, particularly with women not only showing more initiative, but also expecting more closeness and disclosure from their partners. Couples who persevere through these growth trials can find a new depth and richness in their relationships (Miracle & Miracle, 2009). They will then be ready to reinvest in different ways of communicating with each other. They continue to want to genuinely touch, know, and love each other (**FIGURE 13-2**). Such renewed ties of intimacy can lead to a sense of control of life and an acceptance rather than a fear of aging (Comacho & Reyes-Ortiz, 2005).

Eastman-McArthur and colleagues (2011) conducted a qualitative research study involving older adults attending a course about sex and intimacy. The learners' beliefs

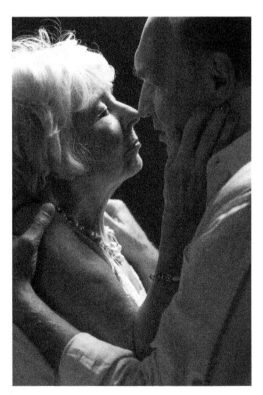

FIGURE 13-2 Older couples need to embrace the changes that come with age and continue to touch, know, and love each other.
© photographee.edu/Shutterstock

about their own sexuality and their challenges in expressing sexuality were categorized into themes: needing to be empowered with knowledge gained about sexuality, not feeling alone due to validation about sexual experience, decreasing inhibitions, help accepting body changes and sexual responding, increasing comfort about own sexuality, communicating more openly, nurturing relationships, and enhancing sexual responses. Such findings reinforce that older adults not only want and need to discuss sexuality, but also have a desire for more education. These results underscore the importance of participatory education, in which learners are equal participants in discussions with instructors so that the type and depth of information sought is obtained.

▶ Physiologic Changes in Sexual Functioning

Women

Undeniable changes occur in both men and women in the physiologic aspects of their sexual functioning as they age. Signs of physical aging begin to be seen in both men and women as bodies begin to show the effects of gravity and waistlines begin to widen. The changes each person encounters, regardless of sex, do not need to preclude sexual activity because reduced sexual hormones affect only response time and perhaps the intensity of the physical response. Knowing about and understanding the effect of these changes, combined with appropriate adaptations, can actually enhance rather than deter sexual satisfaction in late life (Eastman-McArthur, Koch, & Brick, 2011).

Menopause, a natural and often anticipated life transition, is the cessation of menstruation. It is part of the climacteric, a period of time lasting from 6 to 15 years that leads up to and follows the occurrence of the last menstrual period. Menopause is usually accepted as the beginning of a woman's second

half of life and is a physiologic marker for changes in her sexual functioning. The average age of the last period of American women is approximately 52 years, with an average range from ages 45 to 55 (Northrup, 2010).

Much has been written in feminist texts (Friedan, 1993; Northrup, 1994; Siegal et al., 1987; Cacchioni & Tiefer, 2012) about the "medicalization" of sex and menopause, with large portions of the medical field viewing menopause as a "deficiency" disease. This medicalization has intruded into the lives of young women with the creation of a new category of disease: female sexual dysfunction, which was often cited by researchers who were associated with drug companies and encouraged women to seek out their medical cures (Taylor & Gosney, 2011; Moynihan, 2003). How menopause is approached and managed by women is overwhelmingly influenced by the combination of their cultural, religious, and family experiences as well as their level of acceptance of the aging process.

Ironically, during the first half of the 20th century in the United States, medical intervention was seldom used for menopause because it was viewed as a natural event. Now that 50 million women are nearing menopausal age, an incredible market for manufactured hormones exists (Starr & Weiner, 1981). **Estrogen replacement therapy** (ERT) or hormone replacement therapy was recommended by physicians to treat this "deficiency disease," with its accompanying hot flashes, sweating, and vaginal dryness, and to reduce the likelihood of developing osteoporosis or heart disease. Debates regarding the necessity for ERT abound because of an increased likelihood of developing uterine or breast cancer, heart disease, stroke, and cognitive decline with this treatment (Lobo, 2017; Mayo Clinic, 2015). In the Women's Health Initiative Memory Study (National Institutes of Health, 2005), women over age 65 using ERT were found to be at higher risk of mild cognitive impairment and women undergoing estrogen plus progestin therapies had twice the rate of dementia as women not undergoing those two treatments. Yet, these findings led to an abrupt cessation of the use of ERT. Now the pendulum has swung back, and recent data shows that healthy woman under age 60 have a favorable risk–benefit profile for using ERT for a limited timeframe (Lobo, 2017; Mayo Clinic, 2015). In using ERT, the final decision must be made by the individual based on her own health status and unique family medical history. Natural treatment approaches (e.g., use of homeopathic and herbal remedies, diet, and mind and body practices such as yoga, tai chi, and acupuncture) are now more available to help women manage any physical changes occurring during the menopausal years (Brett & Keenan, 2007; National Center for Complementary and Alternative Medicine, 2013; Northrup, 2010; Weed, 1992).

Even though the likelihood of women's sexual dysfunction increases with age, older women continue to regularly engage in and enjoy sex (Wilkins & Warnok, 2009). However, decreased hormone levels (e.g., estrogen) along with coexisting medical and psychiatric illnesses can impact sexual functioning. In a study on sexual activity and satisfaction of more than 3,000 healthy community-dwelling older women, Trompeter and colleagues (2012) focused on understanding sexual satisfaction rather than sexual dysfunction, which led to some unexpected findings. Despite general concerns surrounding menopause, the majority of sexually active participants reported frequent arousal, lubrication, and orgasm into old age, even while experiencing lower sexual desire. Study findings also suggested that sexual activity was not necessary to attain sexual satisfaction, supporting a nonlinear model of sexuality in older women. That is, women engage in sexual activity for reasons other than sexual desire, like sustenance of a relationship, validation, and nurturance; touching, caressing, and the like (Bancroft, 2007; Bradford & Meston, 2007), reaffirming that good physical and emotional health are positively related to engagement in sexual activity. Decreasing

amounts of estrogen account for many of the signs exhibited at menopause (**TABLE 13-1**).

An obvious omission from this list of changes is a decrease in libido or sexual drive. Sexual desire and activity are not necessarily related. Not all aging women are concerned about decreased libido (Trompeter, Bettencourt, & Barrett-Connor, 2012; Wilkins & Warnock, 2009). Basson (2006) suggested that women participate in sexual activity for a number of reasons, primarily a desire for intimacy and not necessarily for biological urges. Libido can actually increase during postmenopause because of the elimination of pregnancy fears, decreased child care responsibilities, an increase in energy and a zest for life, and improved self-awareness and confidence.

In a study of 964 participants, Nusbaum and colleagues (2004) found that if desire decreases, it is likely the result of health problems, side effects of medications, or a lack of available partners. Women age 65 and older reported one or more sexual concerns, a similar number to younger women. They also reported that their partner's sexual difficulties were a significant barrier to their sexual activities. Yet, despite similar reports throughout adulthood, physicians tend not to initiate discussions about sexuality and concerns about sexual activity with their female patients. When they do, they isolate the identified problems and seldom address partners' difficulties, which can directly affect women's sexual satisfaction (Nusbaum, Singh, & Pyles, 2004).

Men

Sexual functioning also changes for men as they age, but these changes are less dramatic than those experienced by perimenopausal women. A gradual decrease in circulating testosterone after age 60 accounts for physical changes affecting arousal, orgasm, postorgasm, and extragenital structure, although this decrease in testosterone does not by itself signal a decrease in potency as other factors need to be considered (**TABLE 13-2**; Miracle & Miracle, 2009).

TABLE 13-1 Signs Exhibited at Menopause

Vaginal changes	Thinning of walls Decreased lubrication Foreshortening of vagina Delayed and reduced expansion of the vagina[a]
Vasomotor changes leading to hot flashes or flushes	Blood flows to skin, causing a 4–8° F skin temperature increase Sweating Increased heart rate Chills Tingling of skin
Less rapid and extreme vascular responses to sexual arousal	Waning of flush Reduced increase in breast volume during arousal[b]
Orgasm with fewer contractions	
Bladder and urethral changes	Increased need to urinate, particularly immediately after intercourse Irritability—a variant of "honeymoon cystitis"[b]
Diminished fatty tissue of mons	Labia majora become susceptible to mechanical trauma from repetitive bumping or rubbing during intercourse
Clitoral area is more susceptible to irritation by forceful manipulation[c]	

[a]Miracle and Miracle (2009)
[b]Weed (1992)
[c]Farage & Maibach (2006)

TABLE 13-2 Changes in Sexual Functioning for Older Men

Arousal	Delayed and less firm erection with longer intervals to ejaculation Less clear sense of impending orgasm
Orgasm	Abbreviated ejaculation Decreased expulsive urethral contractions Decreased force of seminal fluid expulsion Reduced amount of semen ejaculation; ejaculation may not occur with every intercourse
Postorgasm	Rapid loss of erection Longer time needed between erections
Extragenital	Decreased swelling and erection of nipples Absence of flush Reduced elevation of testicles[a]

[a]Weed (1992; Northrup (2010)

Knowing about and accepting these changes can diminish a man's fears of performance and contribute to increased sexual pleasure. Recognizing the need for more prolonged and direct stimulation can also lead to lengthened and more engaging lovemaking sessions, possibly offering a more profound sense of pleasure than earlier in life. The technique of "stuffing," when a partially erect penis is stuffed into the vagina and the woman tightens her vaginal muscles rhythmically to stimulate both partners, can be an effective technique to facilitating a positive sexual experience.

▶ Gender Differences

The meaning of sexuality can change as one ages. Even though men and women have adopted distinctive sexual styles and roles during their lifetimes, some older women may find themselves experiencing new cultural expectations for sexual behavior. These cultural changes may include different sexual scripts, whereby the woman can assume the lead, asking for dates, or paying her share of expenses on dates. Increased opportunities and subsequent accomplishments in the workplace have also been shown to support engagement in role transitions (e.g., after the loss or change of partner), an increase in self-esteem, and the promotion of one's own sexual agency (Leiblum, 1990; McCormick, 2010; Wiederman, 2015)

Masturbation or sexual self-stimulation is a normal part of sexual expression. It is a safe way to relieve sexual tension and avoid both pregnancy and sexually transmitted diseases. Masturbation often continues throughout life. In one study with nearly 2,000 older adults with an average age of 60, Schick and colleagues (2010) found that 63% of male and 46% of female participants reported masturbating in the last year. In addition to preserving sexual functioning when a partner is not available, masturbation may enhance feelings of autonomy. However, masturbation was not the favored sexual activity of the majority of

those participants (men and women) who engaged in it. Rather, masturbation was viewed as a substitute sexual activity, and if given a choice 85% of women and 89% of men preferred interpersonal rather than solo sexual activity. Among all participants, 66% of men and 67% of women reported engaging in sexual intercourse a few times a month.

In a longitudinal study by Duke University, begun in 1954, interviews with 254 older men and women revealed a lasting difference in how they viewed sexual activity and that it remains more stable over time than previously thought (Pfeiffer, Verwoerdt, & Davis, 1972; Steinke, 1997). Study findings indicated that 75% of men in their 70s engaged in intercourse at least once a month, whereas more than a third of men in their early 60s and nearly 30% of men in their late 60s reported engaging in weekly intercourse. The majority of women were not sexually active, primarily due to a lack of partners or a decreased libido in their current male partner, which is termed "voluntary celibacy" (Bradford & Meston, 2007). However, findings from the same study indicated nearly one-half of married women ages 66–71 were sexually active and approximately 30% of women close to age 80 were sexually active (Pfeiffer et al., 1972; Steinke, 1997). Other more recent studies (Lindau et al., 2007) confirmed those findings. Even in the oldest age group, participants closer to age 80 who were sexually active stated that they engaged in a sexual activity 2–3 times a month and 23% reported sexual activity once a week or more (Lindau et al., 2007; Sharpe, 2004). Yet another longitudinal study spanning from 1989 to 2014 (Twenge, Sherman, & Wells, 2017) found American adults are engaging in less sex since the late 1990s. The authors hypothesize that the reduction may be due to the increasing number of people without steady partners and a decline in sexual activities among those with partners. Similarly, an AARP (2009) survey of 1,670 adults age 45 and older also detected a decrease in the frequency of sexual activity and in the overall sexual satisfaction among participants.

In interviews with 10 healthy, active, divorced or single women age 60 and older, Crose and Drake (1993) found that although the women reported a decrease in sexual encounters, they maintained a consistent or increased level of sexual satisfaction compared to when they were young. These women also felt that they displayed more positive sexual attitudes over time, sexual encounters had become less pressured, pregnancy was no longer a fear, and seeking pleasure for themselves was an acceptable goal. Masturbation was increasingly used by the women to relieve sexual tension. They also noted that a stimulating relationship was a prerequisite to sex. As women maintain and renew ties of intimacy in late life with both men and women, they are provided a sense of control in their lives (Friedan, 1993).

▶ Raising the Subject of Sexual Functioning

Because sexual functioning and sexuality are primal aspects of our lives, they need to be included as part of functional evaluations across the life span, even into end-of-life care (Stausmire, 2004). Sexual activities are part of daily life and fall within the scope of practice for many healthcare practitioners (American Occupational Therapy Association, 2014, p. 18; Friedman, 1997), and as such, need to be regularly included in healthcare assessments. Reminding the clients being evaluated that the subject of sex is just another aspect of daily life that needs to be considered in an assessment helps normalize the conversation so that effective interventions can be pursued. This invitation for discussion also provides an opportunity for them to talk about their functioning.

Time and practice are needed for practitioners to normalize the conversation about sexual functioning with their older patients. The first step is to recognize one's own level of comfort with the subject, including the acceptance of one's own sexuality. This self-evaluation is not easy and requires a level of maturity and a period of introspection. The second step is to start engaging patients. A simple and straightforward way to begin questioning is with a phrase such as, "I do not want to make you feel uncomfortable, but I am now asking all my clients about any issues they may be having with their sexual functioning…." The more frequently the subject is broached, the easier it becomes to ask. When questions are included routinely in the interview process clients will expect those questions, which can lead to better rates of disclosure about sexual problems. The same approach has been embraced by practitioners engaged in conversations concerning other sensitive issues such as family violence or abuse and substance misuse.

After establishing that an older adult has concerns or complaints about their sexual functioning, a practitioner might consider asking open-ended questions to obtain more details. For example:

- How do you express your sexuality?
- How have your sexual relationships changed as you have aged?
- What (information or interventions) can I provide to help you?

It is invaluable for practitioners to possess knowledge, skills, and abilities when helping individuals work through their concerns about sexual functioning (**FIGURE 13-3**). Practitioners should be able to demonstrate:

- Sensitivity while discussing a sensitive issue
- Empathy and understanding of the effect of the loss of sexual functioning on the mind, spirit, and body
- Knowledge of the physiological changes related to the medical diagnosis
- Cultural competency and respect for gender and cultural differences in sexual expression
- Familiarity with potential strategies for intervention
- Knowledge of available referral resources

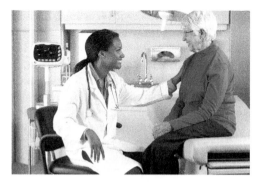

FIGURE 13-3 Practitioners must be able to demonstrate several qualities, including empathy, cultural competency, and knowledge of changes as well as available referral resources.
© Monkey Business Images/Shutterstock

In the course of working with an individual, practitioners should be aware of their own and their client's faulty assumptions. Common misperceptions include:

- The client will initiate discussion about sexual functioning, if it is important.
- The client's sexual preference aligns with the practitioner's views of sexuality.
- The client is monogamous.
- The client shares the practitioner's views on morality.
- The client's age explicitly correlates with increased or decreased libido.

Practitioners also need to be sensitive to indirect and sometimes awkward attempts by the client (e.g., jokes, hints) to bring up the topic, suggesting a desire to initiate a conversation.

Working with older adults when discussing sexual functioning can provide them with many benefits. Eastmen-McArthur, Koch, and Brick (2011) conducted a qualitative study with older adult students taking a course on sexuality. In the feedback collected, the students cited feeling empowered with their newly gained knowledge and having their experiences with sexuality and aging validated. The information they received reportedly helped them feel less alone, decreased their inhibitions, helped them accept the physical changes occurring in their aging bodies, increased their comfort with their sexuality and enhanced their sexual responses, helped them communicate more openly about sex, and supported them in nurturing relationships.

▶ Assessing and Addressing Sexual Functioning

Like other healthcare issues, sexual functioning can also be assessed and addressed effectively. One helpful tool to addressing problems in sexual functioning is the four-level **PLISSIT model** (Annon, 1976). The model not only helps the practitioner identify the level of intervention needed by a client or patient, but also assists the practitioner in understanding the level at which he or she can comfortably provide the needed intervention. Annon's model also provides a way for differentiating sexual problems and concerns and how to treat them. Specifically, the schema can help distinguish persons who are likely to respond to sex education and brief sex therapy from persons who require intensive psychotherapy.

In the model, each ascending level requires more expertise from practitioners than the previous level, so the interventions provided need to remain within the practitioner's own level of expertise and competence. Knowledge of resources available within a treatment site or community is a necessary prerequisite of using this approach so that referrals can be handled smoothly and without causing patient embarrassment or anxiety.

The four levels of treatment within the PLISSIT model are:

- *Permission*: The client is given permission to discuss any concerns and is reassured as a sexual being. This level affords an opportunity for practitioners to provide a nonjudgmental and relaxed environment in which to share their knowledge. For example, since sexual activity is considered an activity of daily living (ADL; American Occupational Therapy Association, 2014), occupational therapy practitioners will bring up sexuality in their initial assessment of the client. This inquiry opens the door to the topic and invites the client to bring up any concerns at a later time. By raising the subject of sexual functioning with an individual who has suffered a stroke, for example, they will be aware that the issue will be addressed later in the rehabilitation process.

- *Limited information*: Specific factual information directly relevant to the particular sexual concern is provided on a one-on-one basis; myths and misconceptions, particularly about disabilities, can be dispelled. The practitioner can assure the client that sexual functioning can be resumed.
- *Specific suggestions*: Strategies or alternatives are provided to change or influence the specific problem behavior. Positioning, adaptive equipment, and timing are examples of what might be discussed. With the client's permission, the partner can be included to provide individualized strategies to facilitate sexual activity.
- *Intensive therapy*: Long-term treatment for chronic sexual problems is provided by a licensed qualified professional. This client's need is an important determination as most practitioners are not trained to offer this kind of treatment.

In using the PLISSIT model, healthcare practitioners need to proceed only to the level at which they feel comfortable and for which they feel prepared. Experienced providers will likely feel comfortable working with people within the first three levels (i.e., obtaining permission, offering limited information, and making specific suggestions). They likely possess the experience, insights, and cultural competence to support a client with appropriate

referral sources and to dispel misinformation and myths about sexual dysfunction. Information about coping with disability and its potential impact on sexual expression, cultural norms, and expectations for treatment can be presented and discussed. Calmly communicating information in an accepting nonjudgmental manner and making referrals to other practitioners, such as occupational therapists and psychologists, when needed is crucial.

A second model on sexual health is the Recognition Model (Cauldrick, Sadlo, & Cross, 2010). The model has five stages and is recommended for a team-based approach, because working to resolve issues as a team will help normalize the conversation about sex and sexuality, provide consistency in dealing with clients, and value the individual as a sexual being. The team takes steps that:

1. Recognize the individual as a sexual being
2. Permit and facilitate opportunities to communicate and engage
3. Explore the sexual concerns and problems of the individual
4. Address issues of sexual problems within the team's realm of expertise
5. Refer individual to an appropriate level of treatment

Practitioners using the Recognition Model will need to be experienced so they can be confident and competent for their interventions to be successful.

A third approach to addressing issues with sexual functioning is to explore areas of concern with regard to sexual performance. Concerns frequently arise after illness, injury, long-term disability, or chronic health problem. General concerns fall into four categories: self-esteem, body image, relationships, and family (Fox, 1990).

Soon after disability occurs or as a chronic condition worsens, questions about self-worth as a sexual being can arise. Concerns about whether the body can be trusted to function and doubts about how accepting a partner will be of physical changes and needs intersect with questions about self-esteem. Anxiety may surface regarding the ability to maintain or initiate new social and intimate relationships. Questions about how to engage in sexual relations and fulfill the role of a partner may also need to be addressed.

Practitioners who are comfortable with their own sexuality and have an interest in treating older adults are better positioned to treat problems with sexual functioning. Approaching sexuality from a positive, open viewpoint using a strengths-based perspective of what a person can achieve rather than a deficit model of what they cannot do can make a crucial difference in treatment success (Joe, 1996). In light of the ever-increasing numbers of older adults in the population, health-care practitioners need to be knowledgeable about the sexual functioning of older adults and proactive in promoting their good health (Langer-Most & Langer, 2010).

Sexual Functioning and Health Problems

Knowledge about specific health diagnostic categories commonly associated with old age and coexisting with chronic health conditions is necessary in order to deal effectively and sensitively with issues in sexual functioning. Combining a psychosocial approach with a health diagnostic approach (refer to PLISSIT model) helps assess and address areas of concern related to sexuality by persons who are in less than optimal physical health or who are physically challenged.

Arthritis

Limitations imposed by arthritis and rheumatism affect more than 50% of people age 65 and older (Lawrence et al, 2008). Forms of arthritis, including osteoarthritis, rheumatoid arthritis, gout syndrome, and fibromyalgia, occur most frequently in women, obese people, and persons who do not exercise regularly

(Hattjar, 2012). Sore joints, limitations in range of motion, loss of mobility, and pain or discomfort with movement can impede sexual performance and affect quality of life. Yet, regular sexual activity can lead to adrenal gland production of cortisone and production of endorphins that can decrease stress and lead to less pain and discomfort, as well as lessen the symptoms of depression (Doheny, 2012; Joe, 1996;). The following suggestions for older adults can help them cope with the challenges arthritis may cause:

- Rest prior to sexual activity to prevent fatigue or engage at times when energy is greatest (energy conservation).
- Place a pillow under painful limbs.
- Use aspirin prophylactically, if medically allowed, for pain before sexual activity.
- Use a hot shower or other thermal heat source before sexual activity or use a heated blanket or mattress pad.
- Experiment with alternative positions that do not put prolonged pressure on involved joints (joint protection).
- Use alternatives to intercourse such as mutual masturbation or oral sex.
- Empty bladder before sexual activity to increase comfort.
- Exercise regularly to increase or maintain joint mobility.
- Communicate and discuss fears and discomfort with partner.

Heart Disease

Heart disease can lead to anxiety about and avoidance of sexual activity. However, the energy expended during the average sexual act approximates walking rapidly or climbing one or two flights of stairs. Four to five weeks after a coronary attack, an individual is usually ready to resume sexual activities (albeit with medical permission). Nonetheless, it is not uncommon for men to report sexual difficulties for up to a year after recovery. Fear of sudden death during sex, low physical endurance, and medication-induced erectile problems often feed a man's anxiety. In fact, death during coitus accounts for less than 1% of sudden coronary deaths, and of these, 90% typically occur in men involved in extramarital relations, which may be attributed to relationship stress and being in an unfamiliar location (Chen, Zhang, & Tan, 2009; Lewis, 1985; Parzeller, Raschka, & Bratzke, 2001). Women with heart disease are less likely to develop subsequent sexual problems. Coitus in general continues to be regarded as a positive physical activity that can contribute to good physical health, much like walking or other daily activities, even for persons with heart disease (Chen, Zhang, & Tan, 2009). Following are suggestions for coping with the effects of heart disease during sexual activity:

- Take a less active role in the sexual act.
- Learn and use relaxation or de-stressing techniques.
- Use masturbation as an alternative to intercourse.
- Use foreplay to enable the heart to warm up slowly.
- Avoid sexual activity when anxious or fatigued or when the weather is extremely hot, cold, or humid.
- Use positions that both conserve energy and are non-weight-bearing (i.e., sitting or side-lying; Laflin, 2002).
- Use an activity configuration (i.e., an analysis of how a person spends his/her time during the day) to determine energy and desire to participate in sexual activity (Hattjar, 2012).

Cerebrovascular Accidents

Cerebrovascular accidents (CVAs or strokes) can lead to sensory losses, perceptual problems, loss of strength and mobility, visual problems, and/or communication problems. Suggestions for improving sexual functioning of older adults with a CVA diagnosis may include engaging the intact senses of touch, smell, and vision rather than speech in addition to the following:

- Experiment with comfortable positions.
- Keep partner within the visual field.

- Use heated blankets or mattress pads to facilitate relaxation.
- Use a manual vibrator for stimulation to compensate for weakness or incoordination.
- Stimulate areas that remain responsive to touch (Laflin, 2002).

Cancer

In 2016, over one and a half million people in the United States were diagnosed with cancer and over one half million died from the disease (National Cancer Institute, 2018). The prevalence of cancer in women include breast, lung, and colorectal cancers, while men are more apt to be diagnosed with lung, prostate, and colorectal cancers. Coping with the aftermath of cancer and its treatments (e.g., chemotherapy, radiation, and excision) includes acceptance of emotional and physical changes that can alter body image and self-esteem (Ganz & Greendale, 2007). Suggestions for older adults adjusting to life with cancer are as follows:

- Use vaginal lubricants.
- Engage in fantasy and massage, and use sex toys or vibrators to increase arousal.
- Request medication changes to facilitate sexual functioning.
- Schedule sex during times with the most energy.
- Be creative and open to trying new things.
- Assess how the body has changed and responds to sexual stimulation.
- Incorporate relaxation techniques to increase interest in sexual activity.
- Engage in pelvic floor (i.e., Kegel) exercises to build muscles between the legs.
- Use pillows, bolsters, wedges (Hattjar, 2012, p. 50–54).

An approach to improve sexual functioning is one that does not rely on diagnostic categories, but symptomatology or the presenting problem. **TABLE 13-3** provides a list of common presenting problems with possible diagnosis, precautions, and potential solutions to resolve each issue.

TABLE 13-3 Presenting Problems in Sexual Functioning and Potential Solutions

Presenting Problem	Possible Diagnoses	Precautions	Potential Solutions
Decreased endurance	Arthritis Cardiac disease Post-CVA Parkinson's disease Multiple sclerosis	Avoid extreme temperatures, heat, cold, and humidity. Avoid anxiety and fatigue. Avoid sexual activity until 1 hour after a large meal. Avoid alcohol.	Rest prior to sexual activity. Schedule sexual activity for the best energy time during the day. Utilize sexual positions and techniques that require less energy:<ul><li>Affected partner lying on back (no energy expended to support weight on arms)</li><li>Both partners in spoon side-lying position with back of one to front of another (no overworking of muscles to support weight)</li><li>Ample direct genital foreplay</li><li>Masturbation as an alternative</li></ul>
Pain, stiff joints, or decreased range of motion	Arthritis	Respect pain. Support painful area. Do not continue painful motion. Avoid staying in one position for too long. Be well rested.	Place pillow under affected limbs. Precede sexual activity with a warm bath, hot shower, or other heat source. Take aspirin prophylactically for pain prior to sexual activity. Exercise regularly to increase or maintain joint mobility. Use a heated blanket or mattress pad. Use relaxation techniques. Experiment with alternative positions that do not put prolonged pressure on involved joints:<ul><li>Rear entry supported by woman</li><li>Non-affected partner on top</li></ul>Use prescribed muscle relaxants to manage high tone (stiff muscles) prior to sexual activity.
Contractures	Arthritis Post-CVA	Avoid stress to contractures.	Use comfortable positions. Work within pain-free range of movement.
Tremors	Parkinson's disease Medication-related side effect		Use positions that incorporate weight bearing on affected limbs. Either decrease or increase movement, depending on which produces fewer tremors.

Presenting Problem	Possible Diagnoses	Precautions	Potential Solutions
Bladder/bowel dysfunction	Post-CVA Spinal cord injury	Have towels nearby in advance.	Discuss fears and concerns with partner before sexual activity. Determine safest time during urinary schedule for sexual activity. Use protective covering on mattress. Man can wear condom for small amounts of urinary incontinence during sexual activity. Empty bladder before sexual activity. If on a catheterization program, catheterize and empty bladder before sexual activity. Secure indwelling catheter prior to sexual activity (woman, to abdomen; man, to penis) Use extension on tubing for bedside drainage bag for more maneuverability.

Data from Ellis & Dennison (2014); Hattjar (2012); Kaufman, Silverberg, & Odette (2003); Laflin (2002).

▶ Medication Effects

Medications can also affect sexual functioning. Therefore, it is important for prescribers, practitioners, and users to communicate about the potential side effects of medications on sexual functioning. Honest and open reporting of concerns to providers needs to be encouraged. Different formularies of a required medication may be available and eliminate or reduce the identified sexual problem. A list of commonly used prescription medications and their possible side effects is included in **TABLE 13-4**, along with some of the drugs prescribed to treat sexual dysfunction.

▶ Inappropriate Sexual Behaviors Toward Practitioners

A client's inappropriate sexual behavior (ISB) toward a practitioner can interfere with care and intervention services. ISB is a form of sexual

harassment. Because of its unwelcome nature, ISB can interfere with an individual's work performance and create a hostile, offensive work environment. Sexual harassment is a form of sexual discrimination and it violates Title VII of the Civil Rights Act of 1964 (Civil Rights Act Title VII, 1964). Key challenges in reporting ISB are that definitions of ISB vary and practitioner's interpretation of an ISB event can vary depending on personal sensitivity to the appropriateness of the behavior.

A client's ISB can range from attempts of flattery and offensive jokes, to asking for a date and/or deliberate touching, to exposure and attempts at sexual fondling (Friedman, 2007). This range of behaviors is common in the healthcare field and occurs along a continuum of mild to severe behaviors (McComas, Hebert, Geacomin, Kaplan, & Dulberg, 1993; Schulte & Kay, 1994; Zook, 2000). Possible causes for ISB include disinhibition arising from neurological conditions such as dementia, long-term sexual dysfunctioning, fear of losing sexual functioning, and an attempt to gain power or control over the practitioner and the intervention process.

TABLE 13-4 Drug-Induced Sexual Dysfunction

Drug	Potential Effects
Alcohol (ethanol)	Libido enhanced at low doses; dose-related progressive decline due to central nervous system depressant effects; can result in failure of erection in men and reduced vaginal vasodilation and delayed orgasm in women; can also cause disinhibition, impaired judgment, and decreased ability to enjoy sexual encounter
Amphetamines	Libido enhanced at low doses; possible erectile dysfunction in men with higher doses; may cause hyperexcitability, tremulousness, and anxiety
Anticonvulsants	Reduced libido; can cause drowsiness, irritability, dizziness, confusion, ataxia, and slurred speech, as well as nausea, constipation, and/or diarrhea, which may interfere with sexual activity
Antidepressants	
Tricyclics; monoamine oxidase inhibitors (MAOIs)	Decreased libido, erectile dysfunction, impotence, delayed and/or painful ejaculation, and anorgasmia in men; decreased libido, delayed orgasm, and anorgasmia in women
Selective serotonin reuptake inhibitors	Drugs that cause delayed orgasm or no orgasm at all
Trazodone	Priapism, increased libido in women
Antihypertensives	
Diuretics	Decreased libido, erectile dysfunction, impotence, gynecomastia
Beta-blockers	Erectile dysfunction, decreased libido, impotence
Alpha-blockers	Erectile dysfunction, priapism (i.e., prolonged erection)
Calcium-channel blockers and methyldopa, clonidine, hydralazine	Erectile dysfunction
Barbiturates and benzodiazepines	Libido enhanced at low doses; progressive decline with higher doses due to central nervous system depressant effects
Cocaine	Erectile dysfunction, ejaculatory dysfunction, anorgasmia

Data from Lee & Sharfi (1982); Nolin & Aldridge (1982); Smith & Talbert (1986); Thompson (1995); Troutman (1997).

Ignoring ISB is one response option, but may result in only weakening the therapeutic relationship (Schneider, Wierakoon, & Heard, 1999). Friedman (2007) recommended that practitioners not ignore ISB. Indeed, practitioners should not accept any behavior from a client that they would not accept from anyone else (Miracle & Miracle, 2009). Immediate reporting of repeated behavior must occur, and an interprofessional behavioral plan, which is appropriate for clients with decreased inhibition, may need to be developed.

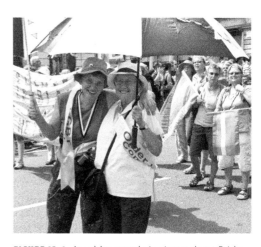

FIGURE 13-4 An older couple is pictured at a Pride Parade in London.
© Padmayogini/Shutterstock

▶ Special Populations

Even though society has become more inclusive in accepting people with lifestyles and living situations unlike their own, research and practice has yet to catch up with identifying the nuances in providing quality health care to marginalized or high-risk populations. Current information and best practices for working with LGBT and other special populations are provided.

Older Lesbians and Gay Males

Older lesbians and gay males are a diverse group—a group whose popular image is often portrayed negatively. Although their **sexual preferences** may differ from heterosexuals, they share some of the same issues with their sexuality in late life. However, when ageism is added to homophobia, the challenges lesbians and gay males face in addressing sexuality becomes compounded. Social stereotypes of lonely, depressed, oversexed, unattractive, and unemotional older lesbians and gay men are myths (**FIGURE 13-4**). Friend's (1991, p. 99) account of older lesbians and gay males suggested they are "psychologically well-adjusted, self-accepting, and adapting well to the aging process." Moreover, a majority of the older lesbians studied were described as happy and well adjusted (Friend, 1991). Still, lesbians and gay males have legitimate reasons to remain fearful about accessing adequate health care as they age and their health deteriorates (Fenge & Hicks, 2011).

Just as healthcare practitioners often overlook issues with sexuality when interacting with older clients, they also ignore issues of sexuality with older lesbians and gay males. As a result, clients can become (or remain) marginalized and harbor concerns about confidentiality, especially concerning their sexual orientation. Older lesbians, in particular, and gay males fear discrimination and lack of sensitivity by healthcare professionals because they do not perceive they are treated respectfully and with dignity (MetLife Mature Market Institute, 2006).

Researchers with the Gay and Grey Project (Fenge, Fannin, Armstrong, Hicks, & Taylor, 2009) conducted at Bournemouth University in England worked with individuals age 50 and older, and found that only 14% of participants had informed their healthcare practitioners about their sexual orientation. Such secrecy has previously been shown to lead to an increased risk of developing heart disease, engaging in self-harm and suicide, and fearing the quality of care provided in late life. Secrecy can also lead to internalization of loss and grief when a partner leaves the relationship or dies, because such loss and grief are not openly acknowledged by society. Social support is often provided not by blood relative and families, but with a chosen family or fictive kin, which highlights the importance of building and maintaining social capital in their personal lives (Gray, 2009). Healthcare practitioners need to be sensitive to and connect with their client's personal narratives through the use of sensitive, inclusive language. By doing so, it will empower clients' agency and provide them with culturally safe services (Crameri, Barrett, Latham, & Whyte, 2015).

Using social construction theory, Friend (1991) proposed that the social framework of heterosexuality has led to the social construction of same-sex identity as one of sickness. Indeed, up until 1973, homosexuality was listed as a mental illness in the Diagnostic Statistical Manual (DSM) of the American Psychiatric Association (APA; Drescher, 2015). Today's older lesbian and gay males have had to reconstruct the meaning of their sexual identity while living in a heterosexually dominated society. They have also had to declare their sexuality many times over, something heterosexuals do not need to even consider. Cass (1979) identified the seven stages of self-identity that lesbians and gay males progress through as identity, confusion, comparison, tolerance, acceptance, pride, and synthesis. She suggested that if stages were mastered at appropriate ages of development, maturity would be facilitated. The inability to master certain stages could ultimately lead to immaturity and feelings of incompetence (Coleman, Butcher, & Carson, 1984). Reconstructing or developing sexual identities outside of the social norm often result in conflicts with family and friends as well as advocacy to initiate social change. Members of the LGBT community may be the only people who need to inform their family of origin about their changed group membership status—a event commonly referred to as "coming out" (Elliot, 1993).

Efforts to find a niche in society can lead to the need to make many adjustments throughout life. These on-going adjustments can actually facilitate older lesbians and gay males ability to manage the aging process, as these experiences help develop a "crisis competence." Flexibility in gender roles and a redefinition of family may provide a unique lens or perspective on other crises faced during their lives (Friend, 1991; Ginsberg et al., 2005). The fact that they may not be able to count on family in old age has encouraged this group to plan differently for that time in their life.

Pope (1979) made a number of recommendations for practitioners working with older lesbians and gay males, which should be applied to all older adults:

- Take a nonjudgmental approach.
- Assess for their stage of development with their sexual identity.
- Develop an awareness of a client's culture.
- Develop an awareness of societal discrimination against the client.
- Recognize the importance of sex in the lives of older adults.
- Accept that clients may need a variety of sexual behaviors to satisfy need.
- Nurture an open mind and remain nonjudgmental of sexual activity in late life.

If healthcare providers are unable to appropriately address sexual issues with clients regardless of sexual orientation, they have the responsibility to refer them to more appropriate providers for their sexual care (Hinchliff, Gott, & Galena, 2005).

Like many older men and women, lesbians and gay males may experience sexual difficulties in late life. However, the changes they experience can create a different challenge when both partners are undergoing changes at the same time (Leiblum, 1990). Thus, expectations can be difficult during shared times of change if each partner assumes that the other will intuitively know how the other feels and what the other wants or needs just because they are the same sex. The assumption is highly unrealistic and, as with any type of relationship, requires good communication between partners.

Transgender Adults

Transgender is an umbrella term for persons whose gender identity, gender expression, or behavior does not conform to that typically associated with the sex to which they were assigned at birth. The opposite term is cisgender—a person who identifies with the gender they were assigned at birth. Persons who identify as transgender often possess an internal awareness of being male, female, or something different, and are further labeled as gender nonconforming. Transgender people or "trans" communicate their identity through their outward appearance. Yet, it is important to note that not every person who presents as gender nonconforming will identify as a transgender person. In fact, gender is increasingly being viewed as existing on a spectrum. In addition to being male, female, or transgender, individuals may be nonbinary (i.e., a person who does not identify strictly as male or female) or agender (i.e., a person who does not identify as male or female; American Psychiatric Association, 2017).

Not surprisingly, gender nonconforming persons have faced and continue to face challenges blending into society and obtaining the quality of life they seek. They are not protected under gender equality laws in the United States, and thus face discrimination at work, school, in obtaining housing, and in receiving health care, to name a few. As a result, gender nonconforming people often live outside of mainstream society, and accurate statistics about them are limited. Recent estimates based on a 2015 survey of 28,000 people suggest that older transgender adults comprise approximately 0.5% percent of the population age 65 and older (James et al., 2016.)

Older transgender adults are marginalized in society and are hesitant to seek medical assistance. In a 2013 study (Fredriksen-Goldsen et al., 2013), researchers found that older transgender adults had significantly poorer health (i.e., physical health, disability, depressive symptomatology, and perceived stress) than lesbians and gay males, who are known to have some of the same problems. Concealment of their gender identity (as transgendered) related to higher levels of stress, and they reported lower levels of social support (Fredriksen-Goldsen et al., 2013).

Healthcare practitioners need to be straightforward in asking people how they wish to be addressed, use sensitive questioning and language, and provide a supportive environment (Alegria, 2011; Barrett et al., 2015). Practitioners also need to provide culturally safe services, during which institutionalized discrimination is understood and providers genuinely attempt to understand the unique experiences, histories, and power imbalance of transgender or other gender nonconforming persons. Families of choice also need to be included in treatment and care.

Adults with Physical Disabilities

Nosek and colleagues (1996; Nosek, Foley, Hughes, & Howland, 2001; Nosek, Howland, Rinala, Young, & Chanpong, 2001; Nosek, Hughes, Swedlund, Taylor, & Swank, 2003) conducted a national study of women experiencing physical disabilities and evaluated them using both quantitative and qualitative analyses. The study sample included 881 women: 475 with disabilities and 406 able-bodied women, who served as the comparative group. The researchers discovered that women shared concerns about issues surrounding their sense of self, relationships, sexuality, and health care. Their findings underscore the importance of addressing psychosocial factors when addressing sexual functioning. For example:

■ Women with disabilities were less satisfied with their frequency of dating and the constraints placed on them in attracting partners.

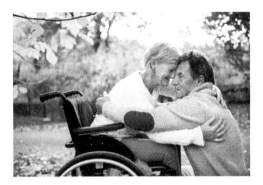

FIGURE 13-5 While women with disabilities may have different issues with sexual functioning than able-bodied women, many engage in intimate sexual relationships.

© Halfpoint/Shutterstock

- Women with disabilities were less likely to have friendships evolve into romantic relationships.
- Over 80% of all participants (with or without disabilities) had experienced at least one serious relationship or marriage (**FIGURE 13-5**).
- Women with disabilities had experienced emotional, physical, or sexual abuse as frequently as nondisabled women, but for longer periods of time.
- Women with disabilities reported as much sexual desire as women without disabilities, but not as much opportunity for sexual activity.
- Women with disabilities had significantly lower levels of sexual satisfaction with their sexual lives than women without disabilities.
- Forty-one percent of the women with disabilities did not feel they had adequate information about how their disability affected their sexual functioning.

In a study of men and women, Taleporos and McCabe (2005) found differences in the relationship between the severity and duration of a physical disability and body esteem. Men with physical disabilities devalued the lower parts of their bodies more than women, threatening their body image because it contradicted the masculine ideal of strength and machismo. Age uniquely predicted self-esteem and body esteem in women, with women more likely to possess poorer body image than men as they age. An earlier study by the same research team found that body esteem in women was most closely related to self-esteem, whereas for men it was related to sexual esteem (Taleporos & McCabe, 2002).

For couples with one of the partners experiencing a disability, there is often a decline in the frequency of sexual activity, a change in the approaches used to engage in sex, and a decline in both sexual satisfaction and interest. Still, the desire for more sexual satisfaction was expressed (Sadoughi, Leshner, & Fine, 1971). Fear, feelings of discomfort, and increased stress affecting their roles and personal boundaries contribute to the physical limitations. Partners who formed relationships after the disability manifested reported greater satisfaction (both with frequency and variety of sexual activity; Kreuter, Sullivan, & Siosteen, 1994). The longer a partner acted as a caretaker in a relationship established prior to the disability, the more difficult achieving intimacy became after the onset of the disability (Miller, 1994). Furthermore, when one partner sustained a disability in old age (permanent or transient), the ability to adjust and form a new identity as a sexual being was challenged, which often led to dissatisfaction with sexual activity or a latency period before reengaging in sexual activity (Parker & Yau, 2012). Associating with other people and social activities appeared to be the strongest predictor of positive marital adjustment (Urey, Viar, & Henggeler, 1987).

By recognizing the importance of sexuality and sexual activity as vital aspects in the lives of older adults, healthcare professionals can help clients maintain or enhance their self-esteem and increase their options for intimacy. Armed with more realistic expectations about aging and disability-related changes, the information that couples need, plus appropriate educational strategies, the professional can better assist in the development of adaptive coping strategies.

▶ Adults Living in Institutions

When adults become dependent on medical care and are institutionalized, their need for intimacy and sexual expression does not disappear. In actuality, their requirement for intimacy and personal validation may increase, as they are forced to cope within their new restrictive environment. Kaplan wrote that "sex is among the last pleasure-giving biological processes to deteriorate, it is potentially an enduring source of gratification at a time when these are becoming fewer and fewer, and a link to the joys of youth" (Kaplan, 1990, p. 204). Indeed, people who are institutionalized may suffer from what Ghusen (1995) terms "emotional malnutrition." Long-term care residents report they support the sexual rights of their peers, whether or not they personally are sexually active (Steinke, 1997). Healthcare providers must acknowledge these needs and rights in order to provide truly person-centered care. The need to address sexual relations in nursing homes has been an increasingly relevant issue as the older population grows. While sexual activity among competent consenting adults cannot be regulated by law, there is discussion about including sexual activity in advanced directives in the future (Tenenbaum, 2012).

Some institutions have set aside a room where couples may spend time alone to pursue intimate relations or simply help coordinate private couple time for residents who have a roommate, who is not their partner (Galindo & Kaiser, 1995; Roach, 2004). Staff need to receive training on accepting resident expressions of intimacy and sexuality (e.g., masturbation, hand holding, kissing, touching, petting; Ghusen, 1995; Steinke, 1997), how to respond when discovering acts of sexual expression, as well as how to discreetly redirect residents into private areas if needed. Most importantly, staff need to be reminded that residents' rights, regardless of sexual preference, orientation, and identity must be respected (Tenenbaum, 2012).

Ghusen (1995) offered specific training goals for healthcare practitioners. Specifically:

- Be aware of myths and realities surrounding sex and sexuality in late life
- Be educated about older adults' sexual needs
- Be responsible for shielding residents from abuse
- Be aware of their own prejudices and biases

Ghusen also recommended that practitioners provide older adults with alternate outlets for sexual expression that maintain and restore ego strength. Additionally, the needs of the partners of adults who are institutionalized need to be recognized and addressed. Providing time and space for intimacy when it is desired is important, as is offering counseling and understanding from staff (Lichtenberg, 2014; McCartney, Izeman, Rogers, & Cohen, 1987).

In discussions about the sexual activities of persons who are institutionalized, their competency or ability to give informed consent to engage in sex is a point of contention. Determining whether an older adult is capable of making a choice to engage in sexual activities and not being taken advantage of by a partner (whether this is another resident, spouse/partner, acquaintance, or staff member) is crucial. Guidelines proposed by Lichtenberg (1994 and 2014) for use in long-term care settings (Miracle & Miracle, 2009; McCartney et al., 1987) suggest the capacity for decision-making regarding sexual activity should be assumed until proven otherwise. Staff must prove a person does not have such capacity by adhering to established institutional guidelines and conducting an assessment, including an interview with the resident. Each individual case needs to include a cognitive capacity analysis of the older adult (see Chapter 8). The ability to communicate choice, an understanding of the choice, an appreciation of consequences and reasoning, and rationale of choice also needs to be assessed. This can occur with the use of a semi-structured interview, one that centers on the relationship in question, whether the involved person can avoid exploitation and his/her awareness of any potential risks. Lichtenberg (2014) further believes staff policies around sexuality and capacity assessment need to be created, annual training needs to occur, and case discussions need to be encouraged.

Despite what staff may think, individuals are allowed to make choices even when their actions lead to failure or place them at risk for poor outcomes. The dignity of risk must be afforded residents as it is a fundamental human right (Tarzia, Fetherstonhaugh, & Bauer, 2012). Protecting the residents' right to consent and dignity of risk is not an easy task for practitioners. Sexual decision-making poses many ethical and legal dimensions for healthcare providers and requires thoughtful discussions on a case-by-case basis. Conversations must include the interprofessional treatment team so that better and more humane decisions can be reached (Miracle & Miracle, 2009). Moreover, such discussions must occur within the parameters of a person-centered philosophy and the decisions made must include the resident involved (or their healthcare proxy).

Borrell (2012) advocated that institutions adopt a specific process to prepare for addressing concerns about resident sexual activity before it occurs. Recommendations included assembling key stakeholders, learning about the issues, conducting focus groups for values clarification, reviewing sample policies, creating working definitions of key concepts, identifying interventions, drafting a working policy document that defines consent and risk, and implementing and then evaluating the policy. Lichtenberg (2014) further believes staff policies about sexuality and capacity assessment need to be created, annual training needs to occur, and case discussions need to be encouraged.

▶ Adults Infected with HIV

In 2015, people over age 50 accounted for 17% (6,735) of the 39,513 HIV diagnoses in the United States. Nearly half (49%) of these new diagnoses were among gay and bisexual (i.e., a person attracted to both males and females) men, 15% were among heterosexual men, 23% were among heterosexual women, and 12% among persons who inject drugs (Centers for Disease Control and Prevention, 2015). From 2010 to 2014, there was an 18% increase in HIV diagnosis among gay males and bisexual women. The incidence of HIV is rising faster among adults age 50 and older than in younger age groups, with an infection ratio between males to females of approximately 9:1 (National Institute on Aging, 2017; Feldman, Fillit, & McCormick, 1994).

The largest risk factor for contracting HIV infection continues to be unprotected sex. Older adults know less about HIV/AIDS and other sexually transmitted diseases than younger adults. In the 2010 study by Schick and colleagues, two-thirds of the participants age 50 and older reported not using a condom. Moreover, atrophic vaginal tissue changes and decreased lubrication in older women make them particularly susceptible to lesions that may readily admit HIV (Whipple & Scura, 1996; Illa et al., 2008). HIV infection among older adults is associated with faster disease progression, leading to higher rates of morbidity and mortality than those infected at a younger age (Smith, Delpech, Brown, & Rice, 2010).

Barriers to diagnosing HIV in older people abound, including physicians not asking older patients about their sexual activity or their drug (e.g., heroin) use, limited testing of older adults for HIV, and the reluctance of older adults to share information about their sexual activity (Stall & Catania, 1994). Healthcare practitioners also tend to hold ageist beliefs about sex in late life (Miracle & Miracle, 2009) and are unlikely to seek out information about sexual activity. Similarly, older adults may be more likely to conceal their sexual status due to fear of discrimination or prejudice. Nonspecific symptoms related to HIV infection may also be overlooked because of the high level of chronic illnesses in the older population (Miracle & Miracle, 2009). Unfortunately, a delay in diagnosis can shorten survival time, as can the addition of the comorbidities prevalent in older adults (Goodroad, 2003).

AIDS Dementia Complex (ADC) is one of the most common and clinically important central nervous system complications of late HIV-1 infection. ADC is a source of great morbidity, and when severe, is associated with limited survival. Neurocognitive deficits are a pronounced consequence of HIV-AIDS. Evidence now suggests that older adults with HIV are at higher risk for developing cognitive impairments (Gorman, Foley, Ettenhofer, Hinkin, & van Gorp, 2009). Watkins and Treisman (2015) describe these cognitive impairments as including emotional changes and impairments in attention, executive function, and memory. They also found that with the use of HAART medications (a customized set of prescribed medications based on how much virus is in the blood), there are less frequent cognitive issues. In this post-HAART era, mild motor neurocognitive disorders and depression are more predictive of the severity of HIV-dementia (Watkins & Treisman, 2015).

Client education about safe sexual practices have been almost exclusively directed at younger cohorts. This is due in part to social stereotypes that depict older adults as no longer interested or engaging in sexual activities. Consequently, safe sex practices often are not discussed with them. A few HIV interventions have targeted HIV-positive older adults. One such program is Project ROADMAP (Re-educating Older Adults in Maintaining AIDS Prevention), which focuses on reducing high-risk sexual behavior among HIV-positive older adults served in primary care clinics (Illa et al., 2010).

Recommendations to improve safe sex practices in late life include fostering an increased awareness on the part of healthcare practitioners, particularly physicians, of the need to routinely include sexual functioning and histories as part of the medical examinations (Wallace, Paauw, & Spach, 1993; Whipple & Scura, 1996). A 2007 study supported the willingness of older adults to talk about sexuality in their lives (Landau et al., 2007). This open conversation process also involves dispelling the stereotype that older adults are sexually inactive. Healthcare practitioners need to be aware of the different ways sexually transmitted diseases (STDs) may be transmitted among older adults and appropriate modes of treatment. They also need to remain sensitive as to how safe sex information is acknowledged by clients/patients and shared with their partners (Stall & Catania, 1994). Offering nonjudgmental, plain language information and responses to queries may begin to improve the situation for adults of all ages.

▶ Summary

Acknowledging the sexuality of older adults and the role of sexual functioning in maintaining quality of life helps healthcare practitioners support their older clients. Being respectful of a client's sexual identity by providing empathy, offering appropriate information, adaptations, and strategies to resolve challenges in their sexual functioning provide an invaluable service. Advocating for person-centered care and respectful policies in institutions for older residents can facilitate maintaining their roles as vital sexual beings. Tact, discretion, and judicious use of humor also can be useful tools upon which healthcare practitioners can rely. When healthcare practitioners routinely incorporate questions and discussions about sexual functioning in their practices, it helps normalize the conversation about sex and sexuality, and enables clients the opportunity to discuss their concerns in a safe and supportive environment. Collaborative problem solving can also help empower clients to address problems with sexual functioning. Helping clients achieve intimacy with another person is a valuable and important objective in the missions of healthcare practitioners in supporting their clients' well-being and quality of life.

🔍 CASE STUDIES

Case 1: Sally is a 58-year-old postmenopausal female. She was diagnosed with rheumatoid arthritis eight years ago. Sally is married to Jack, a 59-year-old male. They have one 3-year-old grandson, with whom they spend every weekend. Sally works 40–50 hours each week as the cake decorator for a local bakery, and her job can be stressful, especially during wedding season. Jack works full time as well and appears to share household responsibilities with Sally. Sally reports no complaints with her health and relationship, except that she is simply too tired at the end of the day to even think about engaging in sex with Jack.

1. **What factors are likely contributing to Sally's disinterest in sex and why?**
2. **Describe five changes you would recommend to Sally to improve her sexual relationship with Jack.**

Case 2: Harry is a 70-year-old gay male, who recently moved into an assisted living facility that is part of a continuing care retirement community, because he has been experiencing increasing forgetfulness, depression, and diabetes, which he can no longer manage himself. Prior to relocating, he lived with his partner, Jim, for decades. Jim plans to move into the independent living portion of the community and visits Harry almost daily. Harry and Jim have not had sex since Harry moved, but they are planning to resume their sexual relationship when Jim moves in. Harry also recently switched to a new primary care physician because his previous doctor's office is located over an hour from his new home. He likes his new physician, but has not yet revealed to him that he is gay, although the doctor quietly suspects it.

1. **If Harry and Jim want to have sex, should the staff at the facility prevent them from doing so? Why or why not?**
2. **Why do you think Harry has not told his doctor that he is gay? Is he justified in doing so?**
3. **What should Harry's doctor do to ensure that he is providing appropriate care to Harry (and any other gay or lesbian patients)?**

TEST YOUR KNOWLEDGE

Review Questions

1. Daily's "Circles of Sexuality" model includes which of the following five components?
   a. Sensuality, intimacy, sexual identity, sexual health and reproduction, and sexualization
   b. Sex, gender, sexual identity, sexual health and reproduction, and intimacy
   c. Intimacy, sensuality, gender identity, sexual activity, and sexual health
   d. Sexual health, gender identity, sex, sexual activity, and intimacy

2. One helpful tool to addressing problems in sexual functioning is the four-level PLISSIT model. Which of the following statements best described the model?
   a. It helps the practitioner identify the level of intervention needed by a client.
   b. It provides a way to address all sexual problems in the same manner.
   c. It guides the practitioner in providing basic sex education and brief sex therapy to each client.
   d. It is an assessment tool that does not require an intervention by the practitioner.

3. A client's ISB toward a practitioner can interfere with care and intervention services. Which of the following is a false statement about ISB?
   a. ISB is a form of sexual harassment.
   b. ISB can interfere with an individual's work performance and create a hostile, offensive work environment.
   c. Sexual harassment is not a form of sexual discrimination.
   d. A practitioner's interpretation of an ISB event can vary depending on personal sensitivity to the appropriateness of the behavior.

4. Gender is another term for sex.
   a. True
   b. False

5. Embracing changes in gender roles can enhance sexual activity in late life.
   a. True
   b. False

Learning Activities

1. What effects has peer pressure had on your sexuality?

2. How can one's cohort effects influence one's sexuality?

3. Bring in advertisements and/or jokes that depict older adults and sexuality in both positive and negative ways. Discuss their veracity and the stereotypes they defy or confirm.

4. Describe what considerations a practitioner needs to make when working with an individual who is transgender.

5. Using a model (PLISSIT or Recognition), and considering the four areas of sexual concern, develop a plan that addresses the specific diagnosis, age, and concerns of the following clients. Also discuss who might be involved in their care using a team approach:
   a. A woman, age 72, with a total hip replacement and arthritis who is interested in continuing sex with her partner.
   b. A 65-year-old man with congestive heart failure who is very concerned about continuing his sexual relationship with his 55-year-old wife.
   c. A 70-year-old man post right cerebrovascular accident who is experiencing both sensory changes (decreased sensation on the left side, decreased left visual field) and decreased endurance. Despite these, he wishes to maintain an intimate relationship with his wife of more than 50 years.

6. Describe your first discoveries of sexual feelings.

7. How have your family, culture, and religion affected:
   a. Your own sexuality
   b. Your views on the sexuality of others?

References

AARP. (2009). *Sex, romance, and relationship: AARP survey of midlife and other adults.* Retrieved from https://assets.aarp.org/rgcenter/general/srr_09

Alegria, C. A. (2011). Transgender identity and health care: Implications for psychosocial and physical evaluation. *Journal of the American Academy of Nurse Practitioners, 23,* 175–182.

American Occupational Therapy Association. (2014). Occupational therapy practice framework: Domain & process. *American Journal of Occupational Therapy, 68,* S1–S48.

American Psychiatric Association. (2013). *Diagnostic and statistical manual of mental disorders* (5th ed.). Arlington, VA: American Psychiatric Publishing

Annon, J. S. (1976). The PLISSIT model: A proposed conceptual scheme for the behavioral treatment of sexual problems. *Journal of Sex Education and Therapy, 2*(2), 1–15.

Bancroft, J. H. J. (2007). Sex and aging. *New England Journal of Medicine, 357,* 820–822.

Barrett, C., Whyte, C., Comfort, J., Lyons, A., & Crameri, P. (2015). Social connection, relationships and older lesbian and gay people. *Sexual and Relationship Therapy, 30,* 131–142.

Basson, R. (2006). Sexual desire and arousal disorders in women. *New England Journal of Medicine, 354,* 1497–1506.

Borrell, L. J. (2012). Too much or too little care, closeness and love: How to establish boundaries and guidelines for intimacy, sexuality and sexual behavior in assisted living and nursing home environments. *Senior Psychiatric Connection Continuing Education Series #5.* Retrieved from http://www.seniorpsychiatry.com/articles/toomuchtoolittle.pdf

Boston Women's Health Book Collective (2005). *Our bodies, our selves.* New York, NY: Touchstone.

Bradford, A., & Meston, C. M. (2007). Senior sexual health: The effects of aging on sexuality. In L. VandeCreek, F. L. Peterson, & J. W. Bley (Eds.), *Innovations in clinical practice: Focus on sexual health* (pp. 35–45). Sarasota, FL: Professional Resources Press.

Brett, K., & Keenan, N. L. (2007). Complementary and alternative medicine use among midlife women for reasons including menopause in the United States: 2002. *Menopause, 14,* 300–307.

Butler, R. N., Lewis, M. I., Hoffman, E., & Whitehead, E. D. (1994). Love and sex after 60: How physical changes affect intimate expression. A roundtable discussion: Part 1. *Geriatrics, 49*(9), 21–27.

Cacchioni, T., & Tiefer, L. (2012). Why medicalization? Introduction to the special issue of medicalization of sex. *Journal of Sex Research, 49,* 307–310.

Cass, V. (1979). Homosexual identity formation: A theoretical model. *Journal of Homosexuality, 4,* 219–235.

Cauldrick, L., Sadlo, G., & Cross, V. (2010). Proposing a new sexual health model of practice for disability teams: The Recognition Model. *International Journal of Theory and Rehabilitation, 17*(6), 290–299.

Centers for Disease Control and Prevention. (2013). HIV testing and risk behaviors among gay, bisexual, and other men who have sex with men- United States. *MMWR: Morbidity & Mortality Weekly Report, 62*(47), 958.

Chao, J. K., Lin, Y. C., Ma, M. C., Lai, C. J., Ku, Y. C., Kuo, W. H., & Chao, I. C. (2011). Relationship among sexual desire, sexual satisfaction, and quality of life in middle-aged and older adults. *Journal of Sex & Marital Therapy, 37*(5), 386–403.

Chen, X., Zhang, Q., & Tan, Q. (2009). Cardiovascular effects of sexual activity. *Indian Journal of Medical Research, 130,* 681–688.

Civil Rights Act Title VII (1964). Retrieved from https://www.eeoc.gov/laws/statutes/titlevii.cfm

Coleman, J. C., Butcher, J. N., & Carson, R. C. (1984). *Abnormal psychology and modern life* (7th ed.). Glenview, IL: Scott, Foresman and Company.

Comacho, M. E., & Reyes-Ortiz, C. A. (2005). Sexual dysfunction in the elderly: Age or disease? *International Journal of Impotence Research, 17,* S52–S56.

Crameri, P., Barrett, C., Latham, J. R., & Whyte, C. (2015). Innovation and translation: It is more than sex and clothes: Culturally safe services for older lesbian, gay, bisexual, transgender and intersex people. *Australian Journal on Aging, 34,* 21–25.

Crose, R., & Drake, L. K. (1993). Older women's sexuality. *Clinical Gerontologist, 12*(4), 51.

Dailey, D. (1981). *Sexual expression and aging.* In F. Berghorn & D. Schafer (Eds.), *The dynamics of aging* (pp. 311–333). Boulder, CO: Westview Press.

Doheny, K. (2012). 10 Surprising health benefits of sex. Retrieved from http://www.webmd.com/sex-relationships/guide/10-surprising-health-benefits-of-sex

Drescher, J. (2015). Out of DSM; Depathologizing homosexuality. *Behavioral Sciences, 5,* 565–575. doi: 10.3390/bs5040565

Eastman-McArthur, H., Koch, P., & Brick, P. (2011). Can people become older, wiser, & sexually smarter?: Qualitative evaluation of a sexual education course for older adults. Presentation at Eastern Region Meeting for Scientific Study of Sexuality. Philadelphia, PA.

Elliot, J. E. (1993). Career development with lesbian and gay clients. *Career Development Quarterly, 41*(3), 210–226.

Ellis, K., & Dennison, C. (2014). *Sex and intimacy for wounded veterans.* The Sager Group.

Farage, M., & Maibach, H. (2006). Lifetime changes in the vulva and vagina. *Archives of Gynecology and Obstetrics, 273*(4), 195–202.

Feldman, M., Fillit, H., & McCormick, W. C. (1994). The growing risk of AIDS in older patients. *Patient Care, 10,* 61–71.

Fenge, L., & Hicks, C. (2011). Hidden lives: The importance of recognizing the needs and experiences of older lesbians and gay men within healthcare practice. *Diversity in Health and Care, 8,* 147–154.

Fenge, L. A., Fannin, A. Armstrong, A., Hicks, C., & Taylor, V. (2009). Lifting the lid on sexuality and ageing: The experiences of volunteer researchers. *Qualitative, Social Work, 8,* 509–524. doi: 10.1177/1473325009345783

FORGE. (n.d.[a]). *Home page.* Retrieved from: http://forge-forward.org/about/

FORGE. (n.d.[b]). *The 5 circles of sexuality: Overview and implications for transgender people.* Retrieved from http://forge-forward.org/wp-content/docs/HANDOUT-circles-of-sexuality-eli-r-green.pdf

Fox, S. (1990). Dismissing taboos: OTs integrate sexuality into "whole reason" treatment approach. *Advance for Occupational Therapists,* 13–17.

Fredriksen-Goldsen, K. J., Cook-Daniels, L., Kim, H. J., Erosheva, E. A., Emlet, C. A., Hoy-Ellis, C. P., . . . Muraco, A. (2013). Physical and mental health of transgender older adults: An at-risk and underserved population. *The Gerontologist, 54,* 488–500.

Friedan, B. (1993). *The fountain of age.* New York, NY: Simon and Schuster.

Friedman, J. D. (1997). Sexual expression: The forgotten component of ADL. *OT Practice, 2*(1), 20–25.

Friedman, J. D. (2007). Inappropriate patient sexual behavior: Part I: Understanding this prevalent situation. *Advance for Occupational Therapy Practitioners, 23*(19), 46–47.

Friend, R. A. (1991). Older lesbian and gay people: A theory of successful aging. *Journal of Homosexuality, 20*(3–4), 99–118.

Galindo, D., & Kaiser, F. E. (1995). Sexual health after 60. *Patient Care, 29,* 25–38.

Ganz, P. A., & Greendale, G. A. (2007). Female sexual desire – beyond testosterone. *Journal of the National Cancer Institute, 99,* 659–661.

Ghusen, H. (1995). Sexuality in institutionalized patients. *Physical Medicine and Rehabilitation, 9*(2), 475–486.

Ginsberg, T. B., Pomerantz, S. C., & Kramer-Felley, V. (2005). Sexuality in older adults: Behaviours and preferences. *Age and Ageing, 34,* 475–480.

Goodroad, B. K. (2003). HIV and AIDS in people older than 50. A continuing concern. *Journal of Gerontological Nursing, 29*(40), 18–24.

Gorman, A. A., Foley, J. M., Ettenhofer, M .L., Hinkin, C. H., & van Gorp, W. G. (2009). Functional consequences of HIV-associated neuropsychological impairment. *Neuropsychology Review, 19*(2), 186–203. doi: 10.1007/s11065-009-9095-0

Gott, M., & Hinchliff, S. (2003). How important is sex in later life? The views of older people. *Social Science and Medicine, 56,* 1617–1628.

Gray, A. (2009). The social capital of older people. *Ageing & Society, 29,* 5–31.

Hattjar, B. (2012). *Sexuality and occupational therapy: Strategies for persons with disabilities.* Bethesda, MD: AOTA Press.

Hinchliff, S., Gott, M., & Galena, E. (2005). "I daresay I might find it embarrassing": General practitioners' perspectives on discussing sexual issues with lesbian and gay patients. *Health and Social Care in the Community, 13*(4), 345–353.

Illa, L., Brickman, A., Saint-Jean, G., Echenique, M., Metsch, L. Eisdorfer, C. . . . Sanchez-Martinez, M. (2008). Sexual risk behaviors in late middle age & older HIV seropositive adults. *AIDS and Behavior, 12*(6), 935–942.

Illa, L., Echenique, M., Jean, G. S., Bustamante-Avallaneda, V., Metsch, L. Mendez-Mulet, L., & Eisdorfer, C. (2010). Project ROADMAP: Reeducating older adults in maintaining AIDS prevention: A secondary intervention for older HIV-positive adults. *AIDS Education and Prevention, 22*(2), 138–147.

James, S. E., Herman, J. L., Rankin, S., Keisling, M., Mottet, L., & Anafi, M. (2016). *The report of the 2015 U.S. transgender survey.* Washington, DC: National Center for Transgender Equality. Retrieved from https://www.transequality.org/sites/default/files/docs/USTS-Full-Report-FINAL.PDF

Joe, B. E. (1996, September 19). Coming to terms with sexuality. *OT Week,* 214–216.

Jung, C. G. (1933). *Modern man in search of a soul.* New York, NY: Harcourt, Brace, & World.

Kaplan, H. S. (1990). Sex, intimacy, and the aging process. *Journal of the American Academy of Psychoanalysis, 18*(2), 185–205.

Kaufman, M., Silverberg, C., & Odette, F. (2003). *The ultimate guide to sex and disability.* San Francisco, CA: Cleis Press.

Kreuter, M., Sullivan, M., & Siosteen, A. (1994). Sexual adjustment after spinal cord injury (SCI) focusing on partner experiences. *Paraplegia, 32,* 225–235.

Lachman, M. E. (2004). Development in midlife. *Annual Review of Psychology, 55,* 305–331.

Laflin, M. (2002). Sexuality and elderly individuals. In C.B. Lewis (Ed.), *Aging: The health care challenge* (4th ed.) (pp. 278–200). Philadelphia, PA: F. A. Davis.

Langer-Most, O., & Langer, N. (2010). Aging and sexuality: How much do gynecologists know and care? *Journal of Women and Aging, 22*(4), 283–289.

Laumann, E. O, Das, A., & Waite, L. J. (2008). Sexual dysfunction among older adults: Prevalence and risk factors from a nationally representative US probability sample of men and women, aged 57–85 years of age. *Journal of Sexual Medicine, 5,* 2300–2311.

Lawrence, R. C., Felson, D. T., Helmick, C. G., Arnold, L. M., Choi, H., Deyo, R. A., . . . Jordan, J. M. (2008). Estimates of the prevalence of arthritis and other rheumatic conditions in the US: Part 2. *Arthritis & Rheumatism, 58*(1), 26–35.

Lee, M., & Sharfi, R. (1982). More on drug-induced sexual dysfunction. *Clinical Pharmacy, 1,* 397.

Leiblum, S. R. (1990). Sexuality and the midlife woman. *Psychology of Women Quarterly, 14,* 495.

Lewis, C. B. (1985). *Aging: The health care challenge.* Philadelphia, PA: F. A. Davis.

Lichtenberg, P. A. (1994). *A guide to psychological practice in geriatric long-term care.* New York, NY: Haworth Press.

Lichtenberg, P. A. (2014). Sexuality and physical intimacy in long term care. *Occupational Therapy in Health Care, 28,* 42–50.

Lindau, S. T., Schumm, P., Laumann, E., Levinson, W., O'Muircheartaigh, C. H., & Waite, L. J. (2007). A study of sexuality and health among older adults in the United States. *New England Journal of Medicine, 357*(8), 762–766.

Lobo, R. A. (2017). Hormone-replacement therapy: Current thinking. *Nature Reviews Endocrinology, 13,* 220–231.

Mayo Clinic (2015). *Hormone therapy: Is it right for you?* Retrieved from https://www.mayoclinic.org/diseases-conditions/menopause/in-depth/hormone-therapy/ART-20046372?pg=1

McCartney, J. R., Izeman, H., Rogers, D., & Cohen, N. (1987). Sexuality and the institutionalized elderly. *Journal of the American Geriatrics Society, 35, 331–333.* doi:10.1111/j.1532-5415.1987.tb04640.x

McComas, J., Hebert, C., Geacomin, C., Kaplan, D., & Dulberg, C. (1993). Experiences of students and practicing physical therapists with inappropriate patient sexual behavior. *Journal of Physical Therapy, 73,* 762–769.

McCormick, N. B. (2010). Sexual scripts: Social and therapeutic implications. *Sexual and Relationship Therapy, 25,* 96–120.

MetLife Mature Market Institute. (2006). *Out and aging: The MetLife study of lesbian and gay baby boomers.* Retrieved from https://www.metlife.com/assets/cao/mmi/publications/studies/mmi-out-aging-lesbian-gay-retirement.pdf

Miller, L. (1994). Sex and the brain-injured patient: Regaining love, pleasure and intimacy. *Journal of Cognitive Rehabilitation, 12*(3), 12–20.

Miracle, A. W., & Miracle, T. S. (2009). Sexuality in late adulthood. In B.R. Bonder & V. Dal Bello-Haas (Eds.), *Functional performance in older adults* (pp. 409–426). Philadelphia, PA: F. A. Davis.

Moynihan, R. (2003). The making of a disease: Female sexual dysfunction. *British Medical Journal, 326,* 45–47.

National Cancer Institute. (2018, April). *Cancer statistics.* Retrieved from https://www.cancer.gov/about-cancer/understanding/statistics

National Center for Complementary and Alternative Medicine. (2013). *Menopausal symptoms and complementary health practices.* Retrieved from http://nccam.nih.gov/health/menopause/menopausesymptoms

National Institute on Aging. (2007). News releases: Study sheds new light on intimate lives of older Americans. Retrieved from http://www.nih.gov/news/pr/aug2007/nia-22.htm

National Institutes of Health. (2005). *Facts about menopausal hormone therapy.* Retrieved from http://www.nhlbi.nih.gov/health/women/pht_facts.pdf

Nolin, T. D., Aldridge, S. D. (1982). Drug-induced sexual dysfunction. *Clinical Pharmacy, 1,* 141–147.

Northrup, C. (1994). *Women's bodies, women's wisdom.* New York, NY: Bantam.

Northrup, C. (2010). *Women's bodies, women's wisdom: Creating physical and emotional health and healing* (Rev. ed.). New York, NY: Bantam.

Nosek, M. A., Foley, C. C., Hughes, R. B., & Howland, C. A. (2001). Vulnerabilities for abuse among women with physical disabilities. *Sexuality and Disability, 19*(3), 177–189.

Nosek, M. A., Howland, C., Rinala, D. H., Young, M. E., & Chanpong, G. F. (2001). National study of women with physical disabilities: Final report. *Sexuality and Disability, 19*(1), 5–39.

Nosek, M. A., Hughes, R. B., Swedlund, N., Taylor, H. B., & Swank, P. (2003). Self-esteem and women with disabilities. *Social Science and Medicine, 56,* 1737–1747.

Nosek, M. A., Rintala, D. H., Young, M. E., Howland, C. A., Foley, C. C., Rossi, D., & Chanpong, G. (1996). Sexual functioning among women with physical disabilities. *Archives of Physical Medicine and Rehabilitation, 77*(2), 107–115.

Nusbaum, M. R. H., Singh, A. R., & Pyles, A. A. (2004). Sexual healthcare needs of women aged 65 and older. *Journal of the American Geriatrics Society, 52,* 117–122.

Parker, M. G., & Yau, M. K. (2012). Sexuality, identity and women with spinal cord injury. *Sexuality and Disability, 30,* 15–27. doi: 10.1007/s11195-011-9222-8

Parzeller, M., Raschka, C., & Bratzke, H. (2001). Sudden cardiovascular death in correlation with sexual activity—results of a medicolegal postmortem study from 1972–1998. *European Heart Journal, 22*(7), 610–611.

Pfeiffer, E., Verwoerdt, A., & Davis, G. C. (1972). Sexual behavior in middle life. *American Journal of Psychiatry, 128*(10), 1262–1267.

Pope, M. (1979). Sexual issues for older lesbians and gays. *Topics in Geriatric Rehabilitation, 12*(4), 53–60.

Roach, S. M. (2004). Sexual behavior of nursing home residents: Staff perceptions and responses. *Journal of Advanced Nursing, 48*(4), 372–379.

Sadoughi, W., Leshner, M., & Fine, H. L. (1971). Sexual adjustment in a chronically ill and physically disabled population: A pilot study. *Archives of Physical Medicine and Rehabilitation, 52*(7), 311–317.

Schick, V., Herbenick, D., Riece, M., Sanders, S. A., Dodge, B., Middlestadt, S. E., Fortenberry, J. D. (2010). Sexual behaviors, condom use, and sexual health of Americans over 50: Implications for sexual health promotion for older adults. *Journal of Sexual Medicine, 7*(Suppl 5), 315–329.

Schneider, J., Wierakoon, P., & Heard, R. (1999). Inappropriate client sexual behaviour in occupational therapy. *Occupational Therapy International, 6*(3), 176–194.

Schulte, H. M., & Kay, J. (1994). Medical students' perceptions of patient-initiated sexual behavior. *Academic Medicine, 69*, 842–846.

Sharpe, T. H. (2004). Introduction to sexuality in late life. *The Family Journal, 12*, 199–205.

Siegal, D. L., Costlaw, J., Lopez, M. C., Taub, M., & Kronenberg, F. (1987). Menopause: Entering our third age. In P. B. Doress & D. L. Siegal (Eds.), *Ourselves, growing older: Women aging with knowledge and power* (pp. 116–126). New York, NY: Touchstone Books.

Smith, R. D., Delpech, V. C., Brown, A. E., & Rice, B. D. (2010). HIV transmission and high rates of late diagnoses among adults aged 50 years and over. *AIDS, 24*, 2109–2115. doi:10.1097/QAD.0b013e32833c7b9c

Smith, R. J., Talbert, R. L. (1986). Sexual dysfunction with antihypertensive and antipsychotic agents. *Clinical Pharmacy, 5*, 373–384.

Stall, R., & Catania, J. (1994). AIDS risk behaviors among late middle-aged and elderly Americans: The National AIDS Behavioral Surveys. *Archives of Internal Medicine, 154*, 57–63.

Starr, B. D., & Weiner, M. B. (1981). *The Starr–Weiner report on sex and sexuality in the mature years.* New York, NY: Stein and Day.

Stausmire, J. M. (2004). Sexuality at the end of life. *American Journal of Hospice and Palliative Care, 21*, 33–39.

Steinke, E. E. (1997). Sexuality in aging: Implications for nursing facility staff. *Journal of Continuing Education in Nursing, 28*(2), 59–63.

Taleporos, G., & McCabe, M. P. (2002). The impact of sexual esteem, body esteem, and sexual satisfaction on psychological well-being in people with physical disability. *Sexuality and Disability, 20*(3), 177–183.

Taleporos, G., & McCabe, M. P. (2005). The relationship between the severity and duration of physical disability and body esteem. *Psychology and Health, 20*(5), 637–650.

Tarzia, L., Fetherstonhaugh, D., & Bauer, M. (2012). Dementia, sexuality and consent in residential aged care facilities. *Journal of Medical Ethics, 3*, 609–613.

Taylor, A., & Gosney, M. A. (2011). Sexuality in older age: Essential considerations for healthcare professions. *Age and Ageing, 40*(5), 538–543.

Tenenbaum, E. (2012). Sexual expression and intimacy between nursing home residents with dementia: Balancing the current interests and prior values of heterosexual and LGBT Residents. *Temple Political and Civil Rights Law Review, 459.* Retrieved from http://papers.ssrn.com/sol3/papers.cfm?abstract_id=2149841

Thompson, J. F. (1995). Geriatric urologic disorders. In L. Y. Young & M. A. Koda-Kimble (Eds.), *Applied Therapeutics: The Clinical Use of Drugs* (pp. 103–111). Vancouver, WA: Clinical Therapeutics.

Trompeter, S. E., Bettencourt, R., & Barrett-Connor, E. (2012). Sexual activity and satisfaction in healthy community-dwelling older women. *American Journal of Medicine, 125*, 37–43.

Troutman, W. G. (1997). Drug-induced sexual dysfunction. In P. O. Anderson & J. E. Knoben (Eds.), *Handbook of Clinical Drug Data* (p. 686). Stamford, CT: Appleton & Lange.

Twenge, J. M., Sherman, N. A., & Wells, B. E. (2017). Declines in sexual frequency among American adults, 1989–2014. *Archives of Sexual Behavior, 46*, 2389–2401.

Urey, J. R., Viar, V., & Henggeler, S. W. (1987). Prediction of marital adjustment among spinal injured persons. *Rehabilitation Nursing, 12*, 26–27.

Wallace, J. I., Paauw, D. S., & Spach, D. H. (1993). HIV infection in older patients: When to suspect the unexpected. *Geriatrics, 48*(6), 61–70.

Watkins, C. C., & Treisman, G. J. (2015). Cognitive impairment in patients with AIDS–prevalence and severity. *HIV/AIDS (Auckland, NZ), 7*, 35. doi: 10.2147/HIV.S39665

Weed, S. S. (1992). *Menopausal years: The wise woman way.* Woodstock, NY: Ash Tree.

Whipple, B., & Scura, K .W. (1996). The overlooked epidemic: HIV in older adults. *American Journal of Nursing, 96*(2), 23–28.

Wiederman, M. W. (2015). Sexual script theory: Past, present and future. In J. D. DeLamater & R. F. Plante (eds.), *Handbook of the sociology of sexualities* (pp. 7–22). Cham, Switzerland: Springer.

Wilkins, K. M., & Warnock, J. K. (2009). Sexual dysfunction in older women. *Primary Psychiatry, 16*(3), 59–65.

Zook, R. (2000). Sexual harassment in the workplace. *American Journal of Nursing, 100*(12), 24.

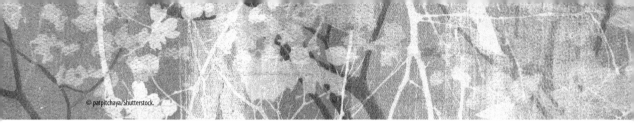
© patpitchaya/Shutterstock.

CHAPTER 14

Reframing Aging Issues to Ensure a Better Future

Raven H. Weaver, PhD

BEHAVIORAL OBJECTIVES

Upon completion of this chapter, the reader will be able to:

1. Understand that countries throughout the world are experiencing aging at different rates because of different social, political, economic, and environmental opportunities and able to explain some of the reasons for this and consequences of it.
2. Describe ways in which structural inequalities create unequal opportunities for healthy aging and explain the challenges for policies to be relevant to current societal needs.

(continues)

(continued)

3. Understand and describe the respective and collaborative roles of the family and healthcare professionals in caring for frail older adults.
4. Explain how individual beliefs influence health in late life.
5. Identify the critical role of healthcare professionals in the field of aging in shaping a more positive social environment for the future.

KEY TERMS

Age composition	Cumulative advantage/	Healthy life expectancy
Aging network	disadvantage framework	Structural lag
Caregiver support ratio	Direct care workforce	Telehealth
Compassionate ageism	Elderspeak	
Cultural competencies	Filial expectations of care	

▶ Aging: A Global Perspective

It is hard to believe that nearly two-thirds of all humans who have ever lived beyond age 65 are alive today! According to a report from the U.S. Census Bureau, in 2015 the global population over age 65 was 562 million people, or 8% of the entire world population. In some countries such as Japan, Germany, Italy, Greece, and Sweden more than 20% of their population is made up of people age 65 and older (He, Goodkind, & Kowal, 2016). By 2050, the older population is expected to nearly triple to 1.6 billion people, or nearly 17% of the world's projected population (He et al., 2016).

Not surprisingly, developed nations currently are sustaining larger older populations than undeveloped nations due to better access to healthcare and technology, and greater economic prosperity that affords a healthy quality of life. The shifting **age composition** or distribution by age within populations is occurring at very uneven rates with the most significant changes in the developing world. Developing countries have relatively young populations.

For example, 27 countries in Africa have a life expectancy at birth below age 60. As a result, the vast majority of African countries have a younger age structure, with less than 5% of the total population being age 65 and older (He et al., 2016). The younger population is a product of recent improvements in nutrition, vaccinations, and sanitation that contributed to higher fertility levels (Holden, 1996). The collective focus of government, communities, and individuals to address economic, social, and political problems can directly influence opportunities to grow old.

Over the next 50 years, the rate of aging is expected to outpace previous growth. That is, the projected length of time (in years) for a country to double its older adult population from 7% to 14% will be shorter than in the past. For example, according to the U.S. Census Bureau report by He and colleagues (2016), Chile will take 26 years to double its aging population (1999 and 2025). Remarkably, it took South Korea only 18 years to experience the same proportional doubling (2000–2018; World Population Review, 2018). In comparison, it took 69 years for the United States (1944–2013) and 115 years for France

(1865–1980) to double its population of persons age 65 and older (He et al., 2016).

Population aging is a global issue. In both developed and developing nations, nearly every aspect of life is affected by the unprecedented rate of population growth, including the family, the workplace, and the healthcare system. Nations worldwide are examining how they can best adapt to the needs of their growing aging populations. They are looking for innovative solutions to address challenges related to living and working longer, managing chronic diseases, maintaining independence, receiving care from family members, training the workforce on age-specific issues, accessing long-term services and supports (LTSS), utilizing health care, and ensuring economic security, among many other challenges and opportunities. Actions taken in the United States or other countries are not readily transferable to or implementable in other nations due to fundamental differences in culture and infrastructure, such as healthcare and social service systems. However, learning what other countries are doing can be informative and guide the development of policy. Not only can an examination of current policies and practices provide potential solutions, but also can learning about the aging experience through the lens of gender, socioeconomic status, race, ethnicity, culture, marital status, sexual orientation, and religion.

Failure to think deeply about population aging is a weakness in gerontology as a discipline. That is, nations, including the United States, cannot rely solely on known trends within their populations to accurately project them into the future. Although projections may provide a loose guide for preparing for the future, unknown realities remain. Much of our interest in and concern over our aging society stems from the fact that older adults are already the most heterogeneous and complex demographic. Moreover, people are living longer than ever before. The population referred to as the "oldest-old" (persons age 85+) will

be increasing in size. By 2050, more than one of three older adults (37.1%) will be age 85+, compared to only one in four older adults (25.4%) in 2015 (He et al., 2016). The oldest-old will also be more racially and ethnically diverse. In 2012, only about 16% of persons age 85+ were non-White, yet by 2050, about 30% of the oldest-old population is expected to be non-White (Ortman, Velkoff, & Hogan, 2014).

Other structural changes among the older adult population are anticipated, including the narrowing of the gap between women and men's life expectancy, which will reduce the sex ratio (number of females to males). Racial and ethnic composition will also become increasingly diverse. Non-Hispanic Whites are expected to remain the largest group, although by 2044 will no longer constitute more than 50% of the total population (Colby & Ortman, 2015). Thus, the profile of older adults of future generations in the United States is expected to be characteristically different from older adults of today, notably including more males, a diversity of race and ethnic backgrounds, increased longevity, more years of high physical functioning, and individuals with more formal education.

In the following sections of this chapter, the discussion will focus on how aging in the United States needs to be viewed as (1) a social enterprise, (2) a family endeavor, and (3) an individual experience. At each level, concerns about how perspectives and circumstances may evolve and result in the need for change are described. Issues that have caught the attention of researchers, government and community planners, and the public are presented to provide context for understanding and thinking about how these issues may affect older adults' experiences in the future and to help reframe how society, family, and individuals view "aging" and older adults as an opportunity for economic and cultural growth. In conclusion, some of the roles and responsibilities for future healthcare professionals in the aging field are highlighted.

▶ Aging as a Social Enterprise

Starting in the 1930s, there was considerable support from the U.S. government to provide assistance to a "deserving" older adult population. Social Security was established in 1935 followed by Medicare, Medicaid, and the Older Americans Act (OAA) in 1965. These and subsequent programs based on need (income based) and entitlement (benefits received after paying into a program) assistance were designed to address basic needs in late life. Collectively, the programs have contributed to enhanced economic security, social engagement, health, and well-being among older adults. Social Security alone effectively reduced the overall rate of poverty among older Americans from 35.2% in 1959 to 9.3% in 2016 (U.S. Census Bureau, 2017). Medicare is a federal program that provides a reliable system of health coverage for persons after exiting the work force after age 65 or after becoming disabled (**FIGURE 14-1**). In 2015, 17% of the overall U.S. population was covered by Medicare, of which 84% were eligible based on age (Kaiser Family Foundation, 2015). Medicaid is the primary need-based insurance program that provides health coverage for low-income individuals. Medicaid has become the primary source of insurance for LTSS for older adults. Low-income older adults with complex and often costly healthcare needs may become

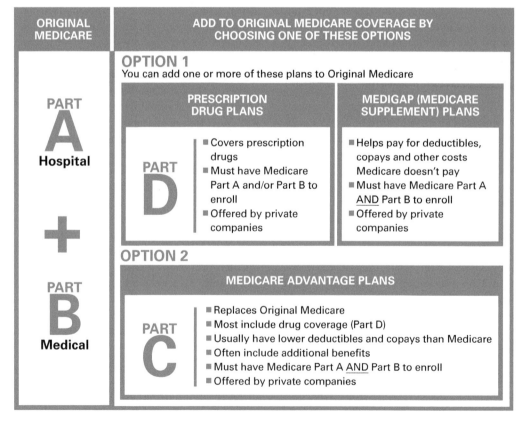

FIGURE 14-1 The four main components of Medicare coverage.

dual-eligible beneficiaries of Medicare and Medicaid. Additional opportunities to enrich the lives of older adults and help keep them independent are provided by a coordinated system of services and supports, effectively known as the **aging network** (O'Shaughnessy, 2008). The aging network refers to all agencies, programs, and activities supported by the OAA. The OAA typically receives bipartisan support, but reauthorization of funds to support OAA programming can be challenging. Most recently, the long-overdue OAA Reauthorization Act of 2016 occurred 5 years after the previous legislation expired.

As each generation reaches age 65, it distinguishes itself from the previous generation by bringing new challenges and demands. Governments are challenged to enact policies that keep pace with changing needs of each successive cohort. Members of the baby boom generation (born 1946–1964) started turning age 65 in 2011. Due to the continued large number of people turning age 65 each day (estimated at 10,000/day), policymakers have been forced to look to the future and the viability of supporting them (via Social Security, Medicare, and Medicaid) as they age. When policies do not keep pace with changing demographics and social circumstances, they often fall short of meeting the needs of the current aging population, resulting in **structural lag** (Wilmoth, 2014), that is, a lag between policy (providing structure) and reality. Ensuring public policy is responsive to the lived experience of individuals can be daunting. Increases in life expectancy, delayed retirement, labor force participation, evolving marriage and family structures, and changes in racial and ethnic compositions contribute to structural lag, both separately and combined. A long-term consequence of structural lag is increased social, economic, and health inequalities among older adults. Thus, there is a need to look beyond "average" improvements and recognize the more nuanced reality that sheds critical awareness about disparities rooted in structural (policy based) inequalities.

Structural Inequalities

Using a life course perspective grounds our understanding of how biopsychosocial factors influence health and well-being throughout life (Baltes, Reese, & Lipsitt, 1980). These factors contribute to the considerable heterogeneity among older individuals. Put another way, "lurking just beneath the surface of overall improved wellbeing… are great disparities in need, notably by race, gender, age, and living arrangement" (Hudson, 2014, p. 16). Other social factors such as socioeconomic status, sexual orientation, sexual identity, and marital status also contribute to experiences of aging and late-life outcomes. According to the **cumulative advantage/disadvantage (CAD) framework**, a lifetime of exposures and experiences accumulate and provide a partial explanation for health disparities found in late life (Dannefer, 2003). Older people who are simultaneously members of two (or more) disadvantaged groups may experience double or multiple jeopardies (e.g., experiences of devaluation of multiple group memberships such as race, age, and gender). Thus, aging is not uniform across the population. Instead, increasingly diverse trajectories are observed. These trajectories are not only based solely on personal choices or health behaviors, but also influenced by environmental exposures, systemic inequalities, access to health services, and other factors.

The CAD framework encourages us to think about the complicated patterns that contribute to health inequalities in late life. Individuals experiencing cumulative disadvantage may be particularly vulnerable to adverse health outcomes that could be preventable. Exposure to adverse childhood experiences typically increase risk for negative events and outcomes in the future. For instance, children in families with fewer economic resources may be less likely to use health services, which may result in poorer health outcomes. Yet, we need to better understand the specific mechanisms related to social, economic, and psychological resources and how they interact and contribute to individuals' development, specifically in relation to late-life outcomes. With a better understanding, there is potential to identify modifiable factors and disrupt the inequalities that disproportionately affect older adults who are members of the disadvantaged social groups.

Socioeconomic Security

Educational Attainment

Education is considered a key factor in gaining access to employment opportunities, achieving economic prosperity, and enabling retirement security, all of which contribute to well-being in late life. As new generations approach retirement age, the education attainment gap between older adults and the overall population continues to shrink. Older adults reported significantly lower college degree completion rates (27%) compared to the overall U.S. adult population (33%; Ryan & Bauman, 2016). However, newer cohorts of older adults report more years of schooling than previous cohorts. In 1965, 24% of older adults completed high school and only 5% had a college degree (U.S. Census Bureau, 2013). Fifty years later, in 2015, 84% of older adults had completed high school and 27% had completed a 4-year college degree (Ryan & Bauman, 2016). Sex-based differences in educational attainment have dissipated, with near-equal bachelor degree completion rates for women (33%) and men (32%) in 2015 (Ryan & Bauman, 2016), compared to the unequal rate between women (15%) and men (25%) in 2007 (Munnell, Soto, & Golub-Sass, 2008). Racial differences in educational attainment remain pronounced, but increased rates of degrees conferred have been observed. In 2007, completion rates for bachelor degrees were 21% for Whites, 10% for Blacks, and 9% for Hispanics (Federal Interagency Forum on Aging-related Statistics, 2008). By 2015, the completion rates increased to 33% for Whites, 23% for Blacks, and16% for Hispanics; nearly 54% of Asians have at least a Bachelor's degree (Ryan & Bauman, 2016).

Regarding high school completion rates, in 2015, Hispanic populations were less likely to have completed high school (67%) compared to non-Hispanic White (93%), Black (87%), and Asian populations (89%). These data provide a profile of older adults that demonstrates increased educational attainment over the last six decades. Because higher educational attainment is associated with reduced poverty, improved health, and lower mortality, the changing educational landscape bodes well for improved health and well-being among the aging population in the future.

Employment Opportunities

Older adults are physically and mentally able to work longer today than in the past. In 1967, the Age Discrimination in Employment Act eliminated mandatory retirement in most professions, encouraging participation in the labor force beyond age 65 to enhance economic security in late life. This policy, in addition to improvements in health and increased life expectancy, have opened possibilities for older adults to work longer or begin new careers. According to the U.S. Bureau of Labor Statistics (2017), labor force participation among older adults continues to rise (**FIGURE 14-2**).

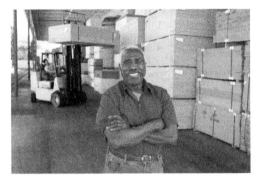

FIGURE 14-2 While the standard retirement age is 65, many older adults choose to continue working either full or part time; continued engagement may reflect financial necessity or a desire to remain social and productive.
© sirtravelalot/Shutterstock

Nearly one in five adults age 65+ reported being employed full or part time (U.S. Bureau of Labor Statistics, 2017). Women's labor force participation has increased substantially over the last seven decades. Less than one-third of women were in the workforce in the 1940s, but participation rates topped 56.7% in 2015. Even so, labor force participation still remains lowest for women across all races and ethnicities.

Despite the economic recessions in the 2000s, overall labor force participation rates have persisted among older workers. Typically, individuals with higher educational attainment remain in the workforce longer than their less-educated counterparts. For example, older workers are more likely to be employed in management, legal, and community and social service occupations compared to accommodations, food preparation and serving, and construction-related professions (Desilver, 2016). Individuals with less education often have more physically demanding jobs that offer lower wages than cognitively demanding jobs. Ironically, these older workers may be least able (physically) but most in need (for financial reasons) to continue working. Thus, older adults face different motives for employment in late life. For some older workers, financial need is the primary impetus for remaining in the workforce. For others, working helps them feel useful, provides socialization through the workplace, or provides something to do, or the opportunity to feel productive. Remaining engaged in the workplace may contribute to individuals' sense of life purpose, which can decrease risk of physical decline among older adults (Kim, Kawachi, Chen, & Kubzansky, 2017).

Financial Security in Retirement

Historically, individual retirement income was conceptualized as a three-legged stool, with each source contributing to its balance. Contributions were to come from Social Security, workplace pension, and personal savings. Although never intended to be a primary resource, Social Security currently provides the largest source of retirement income for older adults and has substantially improved older adults' economic security (see Chapter 6). But it alone is not enough to completely avert the risk of poverty. Pensions and personal savings also contribute to financial security, but these components of the three-legged stool are largely influenced by individuals' occupation and income across the life course. Individuals with higher paying jobs are more likely to accrue a retirement pension and have enough money to save for retirement (personal savings), which reduces their reliance on Social Security and risk of poverty in late life.

Some older workers are financially able to retire at earlier ages because of general economic growth, the availability of private retirement plans, and enhanced Social Security benefits that can give a boost to planned retirement income. Conversely, other individuals are prematurely forced out of the workforce due to their inability to perform a physically demanding job, poor health, or lack of employment options. Although Social Security is considered a successful supplemental income policy, there is considerable variability of success in keeping individuals out of poverty when examined by race/ethnicity, age, sex, marital status, and level of education attainment. Across all racial and ethnic groups, the risk of poverty increases with advancing age, with high disparities between White, Black, and Hispanic older adults living in poverty—7.5%, 18.3%, and 19.5% respectively (Gonyea, 2014). Women are at greater risk of poverty than men. Older married couples have lower rates of poverty compared to their unmarried counterparts. Moreover, individuals living alone are more likely to confront poverty than individuals living with others. To best illustrate the disparities among older adults living in poverty, the rate of White men (age 65–74) living in poverty is 6.9%, while the rate of Black women (age 85+) living in poverty is 24.9% (Gonyea, 2014). The disadvantages experienced early in life lead to inequalities later in life. Older individuals with the greatest need to continue working into late life are most likely not able to continue working because of cumulative disadvantages that negatively affect their health; a situation not likely to change in the near future.

Health Inequalities

Overall improvements in health have been observed among older adults. People are living longer and experiencing more years of high physical functioning. Rates of disability (e.g., limitations with personal care and other daily activities) have declined significantly. However, the chance to grow old and have relatively good health is unequal (Abramson, 2016). That is, individuals age with unequal opportunities, with disparities in material resources, neighborhood contexts, and healthcare access that amplify socioeconomic and racial inequalities. Disability is not inevitable in late life, but the risk of disability associated with chronic conditions increases with age. Older adults are at increased risk for increased chronic health conditions, limitations in mobility, cognitive impairments, poverty, social isolation, hospitalization, and long-term care facility placement.

People who have the greatest need often have the fewest resources available upon which to rely. That is, individuals with lower socioeconomic status (SES) have poorer health throughout their lifetimes and tend to die earlier than individuals enjoying a higher SES. Thus, aging is a stratified process that reflects the accumulation of exposure to risks and structural inequalities from birth onward. Specifically, minority populations in the United States have higher rates of mortality and morbidity and poorer physical and mental health when compared to non-Hispanic White populations. Health disparities experienced by older groups of racial/ethnic minorities can be partially explained by the accumulative effects of factors such as differential access to medical care, inadequate health insurance, exposure to environmental pollutants, and employment in low-paying and often physically demanding occupations.

Geographic disparities continue to prevail, as well. Rural areas are expected to harbor a disproportionate share of the aging population growth in the coming years. Individuals living in rural areas have higher rates of poverty and chronic disease compared to their urban counterparts. The rural-urban mortality gap continues to widen, with higher rates of premature deaths in rural areas. In rural areas, availability of and access to services tend to be more limited. In addition, hospital closures and risk of closure is high in rural areas. Some critical access hospitals are more than 35 miles away from another hospital, significantly raising emergency response times in times of critical need.

Telehealth is a new approach to healthcare that supports and promotes long distance clinical health care and health-related education through telecommunications technologies to connect patients and healthcare providers (**FIGURE 14-3**). In rural areas, telehealth has potential to reduce the burden of travel, improve monitoring of health conditions, and enhance timely communication between patients and providers. In addition, patient-centered health care is

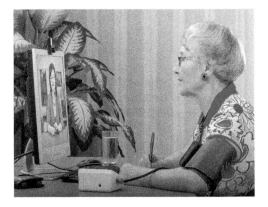

FIGURE 14-3 Technology has made it possible for healthcare providers to work with patients long distance.
© verbaska/Shutterstock

critical, specifically promoting communication, health literacy, medication management, and health and lifestyle behavior changes. With telehealth services receiving Medicaid reimbursement in 48 states and the District of Columbia (National Conference of State Legislatures, 2016), it is likely that telehealth will become more common. More than half of hospitals and just 30% of patients were utilizing telehealth in 2013. However, recent studies reveal that more than 70% of individuals are comfortable communicating with healthcare providers via technology, and thus are open to using telehealth services (American Hospital Association, 2015). Telehealth practices tend to improve patient outcomes (e.g., decreased hospital readmission, increased adherence to medication) and encourage patient empowerment and communication with providers (Kruse et al., 2017). The potential of increasing access to low-cost, high-quality services through telehealth may be a fruitful approach to reduce the rising costs of health care.

Healthcare

Rising healthcare costs are a major social concern. In 2016, older adults represented 15% of the overall population, but more than one-third of total healthcare costs were spent on the individuals age 65+ (Sawyer & Sroczynski, 2017). As might be expected, the need for health care increases with age, resulting in the highest costs of health care among the oldest-old (age 85+). A large portion of healthcare expenditures specifically cover prescription drugs, nursing home care, and home health services. The rising costs of prescription drugs continues to outpace inflation (Hackett, 2017). Another driving force behind increasing healthcare expenditures is related to the cost of advanced medical technology and expensive treatments for life-threatening diseases like heart disease and cancer (Murthy & Ketenci, 2017). Yet, the health benefits of technological innovations (e.g., new procedures, new equipment) may outweigh the concerns about

rising healthcare cost. Still, other social factors, like low socioeconomic status and multiple chronic health conditions, are also directly linked to high healthcare costs. Black and Hispanic populations have higher rates of disease and disability and lower frequency of accessing health care compared to their White counterparts. Low utilization rates coupled with financial barriers and/or not having needed health insurance coverage results in higher overall healthcare costs.

Healthcare for older adults is available through a variety of insurance programs, often combining individual resources (out-of-pocket expensive or private insurance) with public health insurance (Medicare) and need-based insurance (Medicaid). Since 1965, when Medicare and Medicaid were created, these government programs have played a significant role in health care for older adults and will likely continue to do so. In 2016, Medicare covered 47.8 million adults age 65+, regardless of income, medical history, or health status (Centers for Medicare and Medicaid Services, 2017). Medicare helps cover the costs of health and medical care services among older Americans. On average, older adults' annual out-of-pocket expenses were $6,150 in 2013, with 53% spent on medical and long-term services. The remaining portion was spent on monthly premiums (Kaiser Family Foundation, 2017a). Medicare covers services like hospitalization, physician visits, and prescription drugs, but only provided limited post-acute care in a skilled nursing facility or home health care and covers some preventive services and hospice care (see Chapter 6). LTSS, dental services, eyeglasses, and hearing aids are essential for many older adults, but are not covered under Medicare.

Gaps in healthcare coverage for older adults often lead to reliance on supplemental insurance programs, including Medicaid, to help cover their basic health needs. Medicaid is available to low-income individuals, regardless of age. Typically, older adults exhaust their personal financial resources before becoming eligible for Medicaid insurance to cover their medical and long-term care expenses. In fact, Medicaid has unintentionally become the major source of coverage for LTSS, including home-based care, community-based care, and nursing home care (Reaves & Musumeci, 2015). Currently, more than half of older adults' long-term care expenses are funded through Medicaid. Medicaid equally provides services to older individuals in the community as well as institutional settings (e.g., nursing facilities). Yet, Medicaid spending is disproportionately spent on older adults in institutional settings (Kaiser Family Foundation, 2017b). State and federal governments jointly fund Medicaid, which gives states considerable control over eligibility criteria and service options available for beneficiaries. Medicaid is not only the largest source on federal revenue for states, but it is also a big expenditure for states. Not surprisingly, efforts to balance state and federal budgets often incite debate about how to restructure Medicaid (see Chapter 6). As pressure to reduce costs of social insurance programs, whether it be by cutting Medicare benefits or tightening eligibility criteria for Medicaid, the older population continues to expand. Thus, fiscal challenges surrounding Medicare and Medicaid are likely to continue, keeping old-age politics front and center.

In an effort to reduce coverage disparities, the Affordable Care Act (ACA) expanded healthcare coverage for more than 16 million U.S. residents (Health and Human Services, 2015). It also has provided protection to individuals with preexisting health conditions, which disproportionately describes older people. Prior to the ACA, individuals with preexisting conditions could be denied coverage based on their conditions. At this writing, ACA law ensures access to adequate and affordable health insurance to them. If the law remains intact, there are immediate benefits to older adults, including free preventive health services, prescription drug discounts, and expansion of employer health insurance coverage for early retirees between the ages of

55 and 65. In addition, there are probable long-term benefits among the younger population, such as the potential to reduce health risks as a result of earlier detection and prevention of health issues that adversely affect late life. When implemented, the ACA policymakers encouraged states to expand Medicaid coverage to insure more low-income individuals and families (Clemans-Cope, Long, Coughlin, Yemane, & Resnick, 2013). Currently, 31 states and the District of Columbia have increased health coverage through Medicaid expansion (Kaiser Family Foundation, 2016). However, with ongoing discussions and efforts to repeat the ACA, it is difficult to project whether this initiative for expanding healthcare coverage will have the opportunity to impact health in late life.

▶ Aging as a Family Affair

Family Caregiving

Strong **filial expectations of care** (i.e., it is the family's responsibility to care for their own members) hold across the life course, starting with care for young children and extending to care for elderly parents. Family members provide more than 90% of long-term care to frail and disabled older adults (James, Hughes, & Rocco, 2016). In the United States, there are 34.2 million family caregivers currently providing help to someone over age 50 (Family Caregiver Alliance, 2015). Currently, there are seven potential caregivers between the age of 45 and 64 to every one high-risk person age 80+. Yet, changing demographic trends in the family are creating a new reality for family caregiving. For example, although the number of living generations has increased, there are fewer members in each generation. As family size decreases, fewer potential family members will be available to provide care. As a result, the 7:1 **caregiver support ratio** is projected to decline to 4:1 by 2030 and to 3:1 by 2050 when all the "baby boomers" have reached the high-risk years of late old age (Redfoot, Feinberg, & Houser, 2013). As the caregiver support ratio decreases, older adults will be less able to rely on family caregivers compared to the past, thus increasing tension between filial caregiving expectations and the reality of potential caregivers' ability and aspirations to provide care.

Families often provide the front line of direct care and support. Informal caregivers (i.e., family, friends, and community members) typically contribute their time and energy to help address older adults' care needs free of cost. They play an integral role in keeping older adults in their homes and in the community. Often, informal caregivers spend an average of 20 hours a week providing unpaid help, often in addition to full-time employment and other responsibilities. Caregiving within the conventional family structure (i.e., husband, wife, and children) can be explained by the hierarchical compensatory model of care (Cantor, 1991), which suggests spouses are the preferred caregiver, followed by adult children, extended kin, and then formal service providers. However, this conventional heteronormative family formation is becoming more uncommon. Families are more diverse, as demonstrated by demographic and social trend that reflect variations of family by age, generation, marital status, sexual orientation, parental status, and geography (Roberto & Blieszner, 2015). These changes come with new expectations of providing care to older adults, which may not align with the hierarchical compensatory model of care. Caregiving in stepfamilies may be insufficient due to fragile filial commitment between stepchildren and aging stepparents. Caregiving arrangements may vary by sexual orientation, too. LGBT persons tend to rely more on friends to provide care, but may experience caregiving challenges because their chosen family (i.e., friends) often lack the social and legal sanctions for involvement in healthcare

decision-making. With a broader conceptualization of family, it is critical for researchers to explore how family members interact and cooperate to address caregiving issues.

Family care is thought to be one possible solution to personal and economic challenges, but the concept of family care needs to be strengthened (e.g., improving caregiver support policy; Poo, 2015) and should be diversified to include new family structures. A healthy caregiver can better address the care needs of older adults to deter premature decline in health and well-being and subsequent institutionalization. Thus, it will be important to attend to the needs of caregivers to reduce risk of burnout (i.e., physical, emotional, and mental exhaustion) and adverse health outcomes. Policymakers who address this caregiving need may be able to nurture the strong role that caregivers currently play in the health of older adults.

Emotional and Health Impacts

Caregiving can be both stressful and rewarding. The caregiving experience is shaped by factors such as the care recipient's level of need, the caregiver's own problems, the caregiver's strengths, and the availability of support. In addition to providing care, caregivers may be dealing with challenges in their work and personal lives. The majority of caregivers would like more information about caregiving-related topics (e.g., safety and home modifications, managing caregiver stress levels, dealing with care recipients' challenging behaviors) to help them navigate complex medical, cognitive, and behavior care needs (AARP, 2015). Having more information and support would likely reduce risk of adverse health outcomes for the caregiver. Caregivers are more likely than non-caregivers to report fair or poor health (AARP, 2015). They are at increased risk of health problems, including high levels of stress, depression and anxiety, and chronic physical health concerns. As the number of hours providing care and the intensity of care increases, caregivers report higher levels of physical and emotional stress. Despite the accumulation of health risks associated with caregiving, caregivers are more likely than non-caregivers to miss or delay seeking preventive healthcare visits (James et al., 2016). In an effort to prioritize the needs of care recipients, caregivers may neglect their own health and subsequently increase their risk of preventable adverse health outcomes.

For a balanced perspective on family care, it is important to consider the positive psychosocial health benefits associated with caregiving. Maintaining caregivers' social engagement (Pinto, 2016) and obtaining access to information and resources (Hong, Hasche, & Lee, 2011) can protect caregivers from negative outcomes associated with caregiving. Caregivers have different motives for helping, including their personal bond with the care recipient, a lack of alternative care arrangements, or a desire to avoid moving the care recipients to residential care (for both personal and monetary reasons). Spouses who tend to have a strong commitment to caregiving and keeping their spouse from being institutionalized, report more positive feelings about caregiving than adult children (Broese van Groenou, De Boer, & Iedema, 2013). Other caregivers feel useful and helpful, ultimately viewing the act of caregiving as a rewarding experience (Brown & Brown, 2014).

Not surprisingly, older adults also benefit from receiving informal care. Through informal care, older adults may be able to retain a sense of autonomy or independence even as their need for care increases. Care recipients who participated in the Cash and Counseling Demonstration program were allowed to hire (and pay) family members and friends to provide care (**FIGURE 14-4**; Castora-Binkley, Noelker, Ejaz, & Rose, 2010). When compared to participants who also lived at home but relied on traditional agency-based services and reported similar benefits to the program, participants who relied on informal caregivers and were in control of their care arrangements

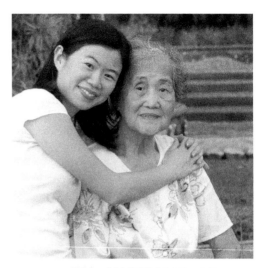

FIGURE 14-4 Informal caregiving is when a family member, friend, or community provides care usually for free.
© wong sze yuen/Shutterstock

expressed less concern about inadequate care. Thus, when older adults are afforded flexibility and control over getting their care needs met, they typically experience greater satisfaction and report higher quality of life (Crist, 2005).

Economic Costs

Informal caregivers are rarely compensated for the time spent providing assistance. The caregiving services they provide translate to an estimated value of $470 billion per year in the United States. (Reinhard, Feinberg, Choula, & Houser, 2015). Caregiving responsibilities may interfere with employment (e.g., having to reduce work hours, take unpaid time off, and forfeit wages and benefits) and can create a financial burden for the caregiver. Yet, financial obligations to provide care still fall on older adults and their families. According to AARP (2015), about one in five caregivers reported financial stress.

Informal caregiving is a critical yet an overlooked component of the long-term care system that is rarely included in estimates of long-term care expenditures. Social and political arguments have been made for increasing pressure on families to provide care of older family members as a remedy for fixing public sector financing challenges. Historically, government support is available to complement family caregiving efforts only after family resources have been exhausted. Attempts to shift more care on families would (once again) have unequal ramifications for disadvantaged groups who have experienced inequalities throughout the life course. For example, the demand for caregiving for persons with dementia such as Alzheimer's disease is already high and expected to increase. In 2016, more than 15 million individuals provided unpaid care for more than 5.4 million persons with Alzheimer's disease or other forms of dementia. By 2050, more than 16 million U.S. adults are expected to have Alzheimer's disease (Alzheimer's Association, 2017). Yet, the caregiver burden on Black families will be greatest, given that Black individuals are about twice as likely than White individuals to be affected by the disease (Alzheimer's Association, 2017). Greater prevalence of Alzheimer's disease will undoubtedly increase the demands on families to take care of their own, while reinforcing the need for better services and supports for caregivers.

Currently, caregiver policies are a patchwork of uncoordinated services that do not meet the current, much less the future needs of caregivers. Caregivers remain vulnerable to experiencing negative emotional and physical health outcomes, financial losses, job instability and retirement insecurity, and declining social networks. Family caregiving is considered "a public issue that can no longer be ignored and calls for national policies to acknowledge and support [caregivers]" (Feinberg, 2014, p. 65). Suggesting that families take on more responsibility sounds like an easy answer, but it would be problematic and unfeasible given the declining ratio of potential caregivers to those needing care. Creative solutions need to be developed and examined for efficacy. Policies and programs are needed to promote financial support, flexible employment, and social support for the informal caregiving workforce. Appropriate training to enhance caregivers' skills for dealing with complex care needs should be developed and made readily available. Solutions like these may help to alleviate caregiver burden and stress, and thus contribute to enhanced caregiver well-being.

The Family and Medical Leave Act (FMLA) of 1993 allows eligible employees up to 12 weeks of unpaid, job-protected leave. To be eligible, employees must have worked for the employer for at least 12 months and for the equivalent of full-time services (U.S. Department of Labor, n.d.). Individuals in greatest need (e.g., low-wage earners, part-time workers) are not typically eligible. Qualifying reasons for taking protected leave vary, but include caregiving for spouse, children, or parent with a serious health condition (U.S. Department of Labor, n.d.). Thus, nonconventional caregiving expectations, like greater reliance of friends in the LGBT+ community, are not recognized under FMLA. With increasingly diverse family structures, modifying policies like FMLA can extend protections for new caregiving arrangements and compensate for cumulative disadvantage across the life course (Angel & Settersten, 2015). A future goal is to provide LTSS that not only benefit individual caregivers but are culturally competent, innovative, and effective for providing care to older adults across diverse settings and circumstances. The evidence-based A Matter of Balance (AMOB) program, for instance, originally was a professional-led health promotion program to reduce rate of falling among older adults. To reach older adults in diverse settings while keeping costs down, researchers modified the program to become a trained volunteer lay leader model (Healy et al., 2008), which continues to be an effective approach for fall prevention among older adults (Walters & Troutman-Jordan, 2017). More innovative programs such as AMOB that will enhance the health and safety of older adults will be needed in the future.

Formal Caregiving

Despite their best efforts, family caregivers cannot address all the needs of their loved ones. Financial resources and family caregiving options are often exhausted before turning to formal caregiving. An estimated 70% of older adults can expect to use some form of formal long-term care at some point after age 65 (Administration of Community Living, n.d.). Professional caregivers are called upon, often as a last resort, to provide services and supports to help care recipients remain in their homes and communities for as long as possible. Affordable services and supports are available through Medicaid or the OAA for vulnerable families (e.g., income at or below the poverty level; physical and mental disabilities; frailty; social or geographical isolation). Typically, support services complement rather than replace ongoing family care or provide assistance when family care is unavailable.

For more than 25 years, there has been a shift in state policy and healthcare delivery systems to increase community-based, noninstitutional care and services to accommodate individual preferences to remain in their homes as they age (Farber, Shinkle, Lynott, Fox-Grage, & Harrell, 2011). Since 2013, a slight majority (53%) of Medicaid long-term care spending has been on HCBS, reflecting the long-standing preference for individuals to remain in their homes (Eiken, Sredl, Burwell, & Saucier, 2016). The resultant home and community-based services (HCBS) are part of a coordinated system of care that is person centered, effective, and efficient in addressing diverse needs of older adults. HCBS help with medical and nonmedical needs of people with chronic conditions that often limit mobility, functioning, and self-care. The availability and type of noninstitutional services vary considerably within each community. Typical service options include in-home assistance with meals, homemaker services, personal care, transportation, telephone monitoring, respite for family members, daycare, and legal services (Medicaid.gov,

n.d.). As personal limitations increase and level of care and support intensifies, individuals may require around-the-clock care and supervision as well as more intensive or skilled nursing care, which is available in nursing facilities.

The shift toward using HCBS is considered a change that contributes positively to the quality of life of recipients. A hallmark of most HCBS is that it promotes person-centered care, independence, and autonomy (Alkema, 2013). Despite its virtues, longstanding criticisms of HCBS systems center on its bureaucratic nature and fragmented funding. Eligibility for services is often based on income and varies from state to state. In addition, near-risk populations who perceive a need for assistance but do not meet the criteria for receiving services are overlooked. A variety of resources pay for services, which contributes to service fragmentation. Financing can come from Medicare, Medicaid, Social Services (Title XX of the Social Security Act), Supplemental Security Income (Title XVI of the Social Security Act), Administration on Aging, Veterans Administration, and Housing and Urban Development (Kart & Kinney, 2000). The cost-effectiveness of fragmented funding is less clear. The cost of health services and care continues to outpace nearly all other segments of the economy. In 2017, the median annual cost for a semi-private room in a nursing home was $85,775. In comparison, the cost of a home health aide was $49,192 and attendance at an adult day health center was $18,200 (Genworth Financial, 2017). Researchers have calculated that the expenditure per community resident compared to nursing home resident is approximately one-third less costly (Houser, Fox-Grage, & Ujvari, 2012; Kaye, Harrington, & LaPlante, 2010; Lehning & Austin, 2010). Long-term evaluations of demonstration projects (e.g., Money Follows the Person, which promotes living in the least restrictive environment) comparing the costs of community care to institutional care have been favorable (Irvin et al., 2015), but cost-effectiveness analyses have not yet provided clear evidence that home-based care is more cost effective (Konetzka, 2016). Thus, more research is needed to assess the overall cost-effectiveness of institutional alternatives.

A major part of the formal caregiving workforce is the direct care workforce (DCW), which is comprised of nursing assistants, home health aides, and personal care or home care aides who provide supportive, nonmedical services (**FIGURE 14-5**). Collectively, the workforce is one of the fastest growing occupations with high demand for new jobs. According to the Paraprofessional Healthcare Institute (Paraprofessional Healthcare Institute, 2017a), about 9 in 10 direct care workers are women and their median age is 41 years. Non-White individuals comprise more than half of the workforce, about 20% of workers were born outside the United States, and 23% of workers live below the federal poverty line. With low educational attainment requirements, only 19% of the workforce has an Associate's or higher degree. Not surprisingly, becoming part of the DCW is an employment option for individuals who encounter educational or language barriers when seeking employment.

The number of DCWs needs to grow with our rapidly aging population. Unfortunately, this paraprofessional group is plagued with challenges. Workers continue to be perceived as unskilled, untrained, underpaid, and over-worked (Cantor, 1991), and perceptions have

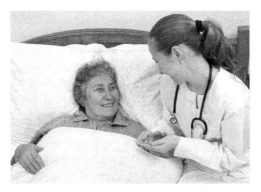

FIGURE 14-5 Direct care aides are able to provide care for older adults within their homes.
© Ocskay/Shutterstock

not evolved much over time. Training requirements for the workforce have been viewed as inadequate and vary by occupation and state. Minimal federal standards require just 75 hours of training for home health aides, with less than one-third of all states requiring more training. For personal care aides (who only provide help with activities of daily living), there are no federal training standards in place (Paraprofessional Healthcare Institute, 2017b).

The industry reports an acute shortage of direct care workers (Stone, 2017). Despite minimal barriers to becoming a DCW, agencies find it increasingly difficult to recruit and retain competent and committed workers. These jobs are complex and require significant skill and knowledge with limited supervision and support (Stone, 2017). Yet, low wages, limited hours, and insignificant healthcare benefits are unattractive to workers, thus weakening the worker pool. As Stone described, "The direct care workforce is undervalued by society, policymakers, providers, and, even more problematic, consumers and their families" (2017, p. 97).

In 2017, the median hourly wage for home care workers was just over $10, hardly a living wage, especially when most workers report being unable to obtain full-time hours (Paraprofessional Healthcare Institute, 2017c). The inability to obtain full-time position status also affects their ability to qualify or pay for health coverage. Not surprisingly, many workers support themselves and their families by heavy reliance on public benefits. If the industry offered living wages and extended labor protections, workers would be better able to support their families. Then, it would be easier to recruit and retain workers, which is especially important as the demand for workers continues to rise.

Developing innovative training for this highly diverse workforce has the potential to reduce workforce instability (Raynor, 2014). Through training, the role of workers could be potentially elevated with increased focus on issues important to service funders such as quality of care and reduction of costs for care recipients. For example, the Coaching Supervision program trains supervisors through a coaching and leadership program as a means to enhance workplace relationships, reduce workforce turnover, and improve care outcomes (Paraprofessional Healthcare Institute, 2017d). By creating a better work environment (e.g., one that provides a living wage and offers career advancement opportunities), workers and their families as well as clients and their families will benefit from improved economic well-being.

▶ Aging as an Individual Experience

Self-Perceptions and Attitudes

Ageism is prejudice or discrimination against a person based on their age. Stereotypes about and ageism directed toward older adults is a societal problem that will likely affect all of us. Thus, it is one form of inequality we will all experience, should we live long enough. Two forms of ageism are prevalent, one at the societal level and the other at the individual level. At the societal level, the concept of **compassionate ageism** contributed to the development of old-age policies (e.g., Social Security) designed to alleviate the burden of growing old. Thus, compassionate ageism is based on an underlying belief that all older adults are poor, frail, and thus deserving of help. Ageism is embedded in nearly all social institutions (e.g., work, law, and medicine), evident when people assume all older adults are alike and refer to them using false stereotypes (e.g., older adults are less productive in the workplace; aging inevitably leads to dementia and incompetence that impeded decision-making; depression is a normal part of aging). Institutionalized ageism restricts the lives and livelihood of older adults by limiting their work opportunities and restricting access to health care.

The United States is a youth-oriented society, so we all tend to hold some level of ageist beliefs, whether we are aware of it or not. Regardless of age, our self-perceptions about age affect our own behaviors and health. Langer and Rodin (1976) conducted groundbreaking research that focused on the illusion of control, aging, and decision-making. In a classic study, older nursing home residents who were given control over their daily schedule performed better on memory tests and had lower mortality rates compared to their counterparts who were not given the same control. Langer found that actively challenging ingrained behaviors about old age can lead to enhanced functional performance and well-being (Langer, 2009). The role of enhanced personal responsibility and choice on older adults' general sense of well-being has continued to be reported (Mooney, Elliot, Douthit, Marquis, & Seplaki, 2016).

Ageist ideas and stereotypes that are perpetuated throughout society can affect individuals' health at any age. Levy and colleagues' portfolio of research demonstrates how self-perceptions can influence health outcomes in late life. For example, having negative attitudes about aging is associated with adverse health outcomes (e.g., lower quality of life, earlier mortality). Recent studies have shown that older adults with negative attitudes had worse memory performance (Levy, Zonderman, Slade, & Ferrucci, 2012) and displayed greater prevalence of Alzheimer's disease biomarkers after death (Levy et al., 2016).

Conversely, Levy's work also reveals advantages of having positive attitudes toward aging. Older adults with positive attitudes have greater longevity and likelihood of engaging in positive health practices than their peers with negative attitudes—they are less lonely, have a greater will to live, and are more likely to fully recover from a disability (Levy & Myers, 2004; Levy, Pilver, Chung, & Slade, 2014; Levy, Slade, Kunkel, & Kasl, 2002). Further research suggests that perceptions of aging and everyday functioning are shaped by culture and contextual setting, including family, leisure, finances, and workplace (O'Brien et al., 2017).

The effects of negative and outdated stereotypes (e.g., mental and physical deterioration are inevitable; older adults are not interested in sex and intimacy; older adults are financially well-off; aging leads to loneliness; older adults cannot adapt to new situations) extend beyond not just individuals, but also to the family, community, and society as a whole. The good news is, the narrative around aging is malleable and beliefs and stereotypes have and will continue to shift over time. Raising awareness about how our age-based perceptions and biases influence health and well-being is a critical first step in changing the negative narratives surrounding aging and later life. Still, the process of unlearning ageism is complex. Today, the prevalence of ageism is magnified by social media, television, and film that promotes a youth-oriented culture that perpetuates ageism and age stereotypes. News outlets refer to the "graying of America" or the "silver tsunami" to capture an increasingly older population with labels that evoke negative feelings. With ageist references all too prevalent, embracing old age as a valued status in our society is difficult. Now, ageism goes beyond conflict between young and old, but is prevalent even within groups of older adults (e.g., young-old versus oldest-old). Indeed, according to Levy (2009), due to unflattering ageist stereotypes being ingrained into peoples' psyches since childhood, older adults are often the worst perpetrators of these negative stereotypes. What you hear often enough, you start to believe. All of us need to work on busting these ageist stereotypes. Rather than viewing older adults as unproductive in late life, we can adjust our views to redefine productivity, forging new pathways for older adults in society. For example, many older adults hold the important role of grandparent, caregiver, volunteer, or may be involved in civic and social activities. In addition, ageist stereotyping intersects with other 'isms' like sexism, classism, and racism. For

instance, older women face greater scrutiny than older men regarding beauty standards. The reality of an aging population has been portrayed as a catastrophic event, devastating to overcoming. Instead, we need to learn to view (in a genuine way) the aging population in a more positive light, filled with opportunity and growth.

Awareness is the first step. Opportunities that strengthen generational interaction and interdependence can disrupt the negative narratives surrounding aging. One strategy is to increase intergenerational contact between youth and older adults, which has potential to reduce anxiety about aging, increase knowledge about aging, and increase empathy among younger generations (Jarrott & Savla, 2015). Coming together and working to create a society that better serves *all* members of our society is a lofty but achievable goal. Changing the narratives encourages a new and more accurate foundational belief about aging: "old" is different than "young," but "old" is acceptable and valued in our society (Calasanti, 2015).

Health Behaviors

Most of us are living longer and life will continue to offer opportunities for growth and personal enhancement. Cumulative inequality theory suggests that early disadvantage in childhood increases risk of exposure to additional risks later in life. Thus, late life is a reflection of the unique combination of influences throughout life (e.g., different social and environmental contexts) that contribute to unequal opportunities. Increased life expectancy, therefore, does not equate to increased **healthy life expectancy** (He et al., 2016). Instead, many individuals are at risk of living more years with functional limitations and poorer health. Older adults may face physical, cognitive, and emotional vulnerabilities and experience environmental barriers (e.g., unsafe neighborhood) that shape their opportunities to expand their healthy life expectancy.

Various factors contribute to health outcomes across the life course. Early childhood disadvantage is associated with health problems in adulthood and the development of new health problems later on (Ferraro, Schafer, & Wilkinson, 2016). Individual and familial beliefs about aging affect health, too. Individuals with negative self-perceptions about aging perceive more barriers to care and delay healthcare utilization (Sun & Smith, 2017). Recent studies question whether this link between self-perceptions of aging and health is applicable across diverse populations. Racial and ethnic minority groups tend to have lower socioeconomic positions, which partially explains racial disparities in health in late life. Yet, Menkin and colleagues (2017) found that age expectations related to functional ability and health expectations were not the same across racial/ethnic minority populations. For example, Black older adults anticipated the least functional decline, while Chinese Americans expected the most decline.

Prevention has the potential to improve the likelihood of healthier years throughout life. Health promotion and prevention were intended to be key components of the ACA of 2010, but preventive services among older adults have been slow to implement (Jensen, Salloum, Hu, Ferdows, & Tarraf, 2015). Primary care offices are in a position to support prevention programs and efforts with the appropriate supports and incentives to conduct preventive screenings. Normalizing the provider-patient conversation about the benefits of prevention has the potential to enhance quality of life and healthy life expectancy. Interventions can target modifiable factors to reduce risk of further decline and prevent unnecessary health disparities. For example, adult day programs have been found to reduce caregiver stress and contribute to participants' physical, emotional, and cognitive health. However, more research is needed to understand programmatic features that attract and retain at-risk participants and caregivers (e.g., low income, rural dwelling, minority race/

ethnicity). In sum, individuals have different experiences and opportunities throughout life that affect their views and thus their help-seeking and help-accepting behaviors. Some individuals are naturally more resilient in coping with challenges than others. Regardless, preventative interventions can promote health and well-being across the life course, having long-term impacts on all members of our society. We have a personal responsibility to create the change we want to see, specifically surrounding what it means to grow old. Actions that directly affect one individual or a group of individuals indirectly affect all individuals; thus, confirming the interconnectedness of our society in redefining our future, for elders now and for elders in the years to come.

▶ Aging and the Healthcare Workforce

Older adults are destined to become even more racially and ethnically diverse in the coming years. Yet, a few broad conclusions can still be made about how to reframe aging issues in the hopes of ensuring a better future. Exposure to risk and adverse experiences in early life leave certain groups (e.g., low income, racial/ethnic minorities) more vulnerable in late life. Thus, the concerns facing our current aging population will persist and potentially intensify in the future. First, structural inequalities (e.g., barriers to education, economic security) contribute to unequal opportunities throughout life that adversely affect health in late life. Unless specifically addressed, these inequalities are likely to proliferate. Second, strong family commitments to provide care for one another are likely to continue, but filial expectations can contribute to the development of adverse outcomes for caregivers (e.g., health, social, emotional, financial, and physical). Support for informal caregivers is a growing need, and person-centered collaborations with the **direct care workforce** could potentially alleviate some of the unique challenges associated with each group (e.g., burnout among informal caregivers; turnover for formal caregivers). Third, attitudes and stereotypes about aging are malleable. Efforts to modify individuals' perceptions about aging have the potential to contribute to the health and well-being of citizens in our aging society and around the world. If aging issues go unaddressed, there are potential negative long-term ramifications for our aging society: individuals will continue to have internalized negative beliefs about aging that adversely affect health; providing care to older adults will continue to take its toll (e.g., financially, socially, physically) on informal and formal caregivers; and systemic inequalities will continue to provide unequal opportunities for health and well-being in late life. Each of us, as family members and healthcare professionals, has a role in raising awareness and making a difference to better meet the needs of current and future older adults.

Responsibilities of Healthcare Professionals

Future healthcare professionals have many opportunities to enhance the quality of life among older adults. The first step is awareness of how ageism can be communicated followed by reflection on one's own personal biases toward age. The healthcare community is not safe from the harmful effects of ageism; it is alive and well in many healthcare settings, even in subtle ways. Ageism "permeates the attitudes of medical providers, the mindset of older patients, and the structure of the healthcare system, having a potentially profound influence on the type and amount of care offered, requested, and received" (Ouchida & Lachs, 2015). For example, healthcare providers may engage in overtreatment by providing aggressive treatment that does not align with older adults' wishes. Conversely, they may engage in undertreatment by ignoring symptoms of conditions infrequently associated with older adults (e.g., alcohol/drug use, intimate partner

violence, sexual activity). Communication can also be problematic. Some health professionals speak indirectly to older adults by talking to their caregiver instead. Others may use **elderspeak** (i.e., a slower, exaggerated, and louder intonation of simpler vocabulary and sentence structure) when communicating with older adults. This inappropriate communication style is demeaning, assumes a lack of awareness and understanding by the older person, and can be harmful to their self-esteem. Further, individuals may be exposed to persistent discrimination through other unconscious biases of healthcare professionals (e.g., biased treatment recommendations; poorer quality of patient-provider communication), which contribute to health disparities (Williams & Wyatt, 2015). The effects of discrimination, whether based on age, race, gender, sexuality, mental health, and/or social standing, can easily lead to an undesirable quality or level of care.

Next, healthcare professionals have a unique opportunity to empower and encourage decision-making among older adult clients. Empowering the older individual in health communication and decision-making can lead to improved quality of services. Lifespan theory of control explains that at any age, perceived personal control about a situation influences health (Barlow, Wrosch, Heckhausen, & Schulz, 2016; Schulz & Heckhausen, 1999). Individuals can adjust to difficult situations by using different strategies to maintain control. For example, an individual experiencing mobility issues may choose to use a cane and modify their living environment to maintain control over their physical functioning. Another approach is to disengage from or downgrade an expectation about a specific goal. For example, an older adult with arthritis in her hands and finger joints may choose to continue typing letters to stay connected with friends and family, but give up playing piano to reduce the amount of pain she experiences. This strategy is used to manage losses and sustain basic functioning, which creates a sense of control over changing circumstances. These types of modifications have potential to enhance personal responsibility and choice, which may contribute to older adults' general sense of well-being and good health. Conversely, low sense of personal control negatively influences late life health outcomes. Sense of control may decline with age, but having higher educational attainment is associated with higher control beliefs across the life span (Lachman, Neupert, & Agrigoroaei, 2011). Healthcare professionals using a person-centered approach that encourages older adult and family involvement in decision-making processes typically develop a strong partnership that is beneficial for older adults' health.

Last, healthcare professionals must develop skills to enhance their **cultural competencies** to meet the diverse needs of an aging population. When older adults' experience losses (e.g., physical limitations, normative cognitive decline, declining health), coping strategies may be shaped by context, culture, and psychosocial factors. Because the older population is culturally diverse and is expected to become even more diverse, services and supports need to be culturally responsive (Jongen, McCalman, Bainbridge, & Clifford, 2017). Future studies will need to examine the unique experiences of racial and ethnic minorities (Chiu, Feuz, McMahan, Miao, & Sudore, 2016). Other service areas that need to be improved include, but are not limited to, eHealth technologies (Barakat, Woolrych, Sixsmith, Kearns, & Kort, 2013), health and human service practices for LGBT populations (Erdley, Anklam, & Reardon, 2014; Fredriksen-Goldsen, Hoy-Ellis, Goldsen, Emlet, & Hooyman, 2014), and differences based on geographic residence such as rural versus urban (Brossoie & Roberto, 2015).

One way to enhance cultural competency is through greater collaboration between healthcare professionals and informal caregivers. Collaboration can help clarify the communication of cultural needs and preferences as well as ensure a seamless, uninterrupted network of services for persons with increasingly complex care needs.

Some health issues tend to be overlooked in late life because they are considered more salient for younger individuals. For example, intellectual and developmental disabilities (Heller, Fisher, Marks, & Hsieh, 2014) and intimate partner violence (Brossoie & Roberto, 2015) are not commonly considered issues older adults' experience; yet, these can greatly influence their health and well-being. Professionals may lack awareness about how these issues may continue to affect individuals in late life. As a result, minimal collaboration tends to occur between providers and these professionals. Some evidence suggests that interprofessional collaboration enhances healthcare processes and outcomes, including reduced risk of hospitalization and institutionalization (Trivedi et al., 2013). If healthcare professionals within the aging network collaborate with public health and medical care professionals, it is likely that older adults' health and functioning will improve. More research is still needed to understand whether and how collaboration is effective across different settings and among increasingly diverse older adults.

Caregiving is a public health concern, as it affects nearly everyone in some capacity (e.g., emotional, psychological, social, physical, financial health, and well-being). As Former First Lady Rosalyn Carter once said: "There are only four kinds of people in the world: those who have been caregivers, those who are currently caregivers, those who will be caregivers, and those who will need caregivers" (Alzheimer's Association, n.d.). Unequal distribution of resources throughout life contribute to health inequities that compound in late life. Older adults and their families may not have the available resources to provide adequate care to ensure a quality of life. It would be difficult for younger generations to handle substantially more of the care responsibilities for older family members. Future healthcare professionals in the field of aging will provide care for older adults who can no longer care for themselves. As such, caregiving should be viewed as a lifelong, interdependent, intergenerational sharing of long-term care responsibilities.

▶ Summary

In conclusion, the basic facts about aging are indisputable: nations around the world are aging at different rates and these nations are responding differently to the associated challenges of an aging society. Aging is now a more visible national phenomenon. Demographers have relentlessly drawn the attention of researchers, healthcare providers, and policymakers to the realities of a graying population. These challenges will likely persist and intensify as the older population continues to grow. To address these problems effectively, aging issues need to be reframed as a shared national concern, not as the sole responsibility for older adults and their families to resolve. Solutions will require innovation and creativity that break from previous patterns and strategies that worked in the past. Instead, older adults need to be seen as a more central part of the national fabric of our society. Limited resources are available to conduct good science to inform the future of aging programs through rigorous studies. Thus, stronger partnerships should be created between aging service professionals to improve coordination within the healthcare system. Practitioners, researchers, and policymakers must find a common language to communication progress made in their respective fields (Lindberg, 2017). Professionals in the field of aging can improve the health and well-being of the increasingly diverse aging population in the United States and globally.

Collectively, we (as individuals and as a nation) have much to lose if we do not address the growing costs and burden of caring for an aging world. It is perplexing that aging is not highly valued in our society, even as we all hope to reach old age. So, we need to ask ourselves what do we want for our future older selves? How can we change the pervasive negative attitudes about aging that infiltrate interactions at the individual, family, and societal level? All members of society have a responsibility to "disrupt ageism" and "change the conversation about what it means to grow older" (Jenkins, 2017, p. S115). Social change is slow, but addressing major concerns with structural inequalities in society, caregiving challenges, and internalized beliefs will propel the status of older adults into new territory that is better for all members of society.

🔍 CASE STUDIES

Case 1: Patty is a 74-year-old Black woman, living alone in suburban America. Although she describes her quality of life as good, she needs help with basic activities of daily living. Patty has no nearby family, as her children have lived across the country for nearly 20 years. Although she still talks with them on a weekly basis, she sometimes lacks companionship. This isolation from family may be linked to recent symptoms of depression.

After church one Sunday, Patty talked with a friend about her ongoing challenges with her daily care needs. This friend recommended that Patty apply for assistance through the local Area Agency on Aging to receive some help. She did, and found out that she was eligible to receive personal care and home health services.

1. **Describe the typical worker that will help Patty with her daily needs.**
2. **What types of services will Patty's formal caregivers likely provide?**
3. **What are some of the challenges that her direct care worker may experience?**

Case 2: Jack, a 67-year-old White man, and Tim, a 68-year old Black man, have been friends for over 60 years. They attended school together for many years in Detroit until Jack transferred to a different school when his father got promoted and they moved to a more affluent community. The same year,

Tim's father was seriously injured in a car accident and could no longer work. Tim dropped out of school and got a job on an assembly line at an automobile manufacturing company to help support his family. Jack went to college, earned a degree, and had a career in finance. Tim was laid off in his 40s when his company moved the manufacturing facility overseas. After that, he had difficulty finding work, and held down a number of jobs before a series of medical conditions forced him to retire. Today, Jack is relatively healthy, lives in an upper middle class neighborhood, and is planning to retire next year, at which point his full pension and postretirement medical benefits will kick in. Tim lives in a small house in a rural community about 30 miles away from the closest city. He is on a fixed income and his health is failing.

1. **What are some examples of situations and conditions that Jack and Tim are both at an increased risk for now that they are older adults?**
2. **From a statistical standpoint, which friend, Jack or Tim, is likely to live longer, and why?**
3. **Is Tim a good candidate for telehealth services? Why or why not?**

TEST YOUR KNOWLEDGE

Review Questions

1. Future growth in older populations will occur
   a. at the same rate across the world.
   b. faster in developed nations.
   c. faster in developing nations.
   d. faster in urban areas.

2. Recent trends suggest that older adults _____ than previous cohorts.
   a. have lower educational attainment
   b. are retiring earlier
   c. are more racially and ethnically diverse
   d. have greater risk of poverty

3. For future older Americans, family caregivers will
   a. be more available to assist with care than they are today.
   b. be less available than they are today because of decreasing family size.
   c. be less available than they are today because of a declining willingness to help.
   d. be more inclined to provide financial support but not actual care.

4. Which of the following is true regarding how attitudes and stereotypes about aging influence health in late life?
   a. Attitudes/stereotypes do not affect health and wellbeing in late life.
   b. Negative attitudes/stereotypes are associated with worse memory and early mortality.
   c. Positive attitudes/stereotypes are associated with individuals working longer.
   d. Attitudes/stereotypes do not affect wealthy older adults' health and well-being.

5. How will the older population of Baby Boomers be different from their older predecessors of today?
   a. More educated
   b. More healthy
   c. Less impoverished
   d. Higher likelihood of not living alone
   e. All of the above

Learning Activities

1. Choose a developing nation and research information about its aging population. What major issues do older adults face in this country? What are the age-specific social issues? What are some similarities and differences between this country and the U.S.?

2. Take a look at the Family and Medical Leave Act policy (www.opm.gov /policy-data-oversight/pay-leave /leave-administration/fact-sheets /family-and-medical-leave/). With changing and diverse family arrangements, identify several specific examples that demonstrate how this policy is experiencing structural lag.

3. Develop a 6-week curriculum for a Family Caregiver Training course. What topic should be the focus of each week? How would you decide what topics to cover? How would you recruit participants to join?

4. Take the AGE Implicit Association Test from Project Implicit (implicit .harvard.edu/implicit/takeatest .html). Are you surprised by your results? Why or why not? What do you think the results reflect about our society?

5. Interview three middle-aged individuals about what future concerns they have as they become older adults in an ever-aging society.

References

AARP. (2015). Caregiving in the U.S. *Research Report.*

Abramson, C. M. (2016). Unequal aging: Lessons from inequality's end game. *Public Policy & Aging Report, 26,* 68–72. doi:10.1093/ppar/prw006

Administration of Community Living. (n.d.) *Who needs care?* Retrieved from https://longtermcare.acl.gov/the -basics/who-needs-care.html

Alkema, G. E. (2013). *Current issues and potential solutions for addressing America's long-term care financing crisis.* Retrieved from http://www.thescanfoundation .org/shaping-affordable-pathways-aging-dignity -current-issues-and-potential-solutions-addressing -america

Alzheimer's Association. (n.d.). Caregiver Resources. Retrieved from https://www.alz.org/cacentral/in_my _community_21690.asp

Alzheimer's Association. (2017). 2017 Alzheimer's Disease facts and figures. Retrieved from https://www.alz.org /facts/overview.asp

American Hospital Association. (2015). The promise of telehealth for hospitals, health systems, and their communities. *TrendWatch.* Retrieved from http://www .aha.org/research/reports/tw/15jan-tw-telehealth.pdf

Angel, J. L., & Settersten, R. A. (2015). What changing American families mean for aging policies. *Public Policy & Aging Report, 25,* 78–82. doi:10.1093/ppar/prv011

Baltes, P., Reese, H., & Lipsitt, L. (1980). Life-span developmental psychology. *Annual Review of Psychology, 31,* 65–110.

Barakat, A., Woolrych, R. D., Sixsmith, A., Kearns, W. D., & Kort, H. S. (2013). eHealth technology competencies for health professionals working in home care to support older adults to age in place: Outcomes of a two-day collaborative workshop. *Medicine 2.0, 2*(2), 1–10. doi:10.2196/med20.2711

Barlow, M. A., Wrosch, C., Heckhausen, J., & Schulz, R. (2016). Control strategies for managing physical health problems in old age: Evidence for the motivational theory of life-span development. In J. W. Reich & F. J. Infurna (Eds.), *Perceived control: Theory, research, and practice in the first 50 years* (pp. 281–309). New York, NY: Oxford University Press.

Broese van Groenou, M., De Boer, A., & Iedema, J. (2013). Positive and negative evaluation of caregiving among three different types of informal care relationships. *European Journal of Ageing, 10,* 301–311. doi:10.1007 /s10433-013-0276-6

Brossoie, N., & Roberto, K. A. (2015). Community professionals' response to intimate partner violence against rural older women. *Journal of Elder Abuse & Neglect, 27,* 470–488. doi:10.1080/08946566.2015. 1095664

Brown, R. M., & Brown, S. L. (2014). Informal caregiving: A reappraisal of effects on caregivers. *Social Issues and Policy Review, 8,* 74–102. doi:10.1111/sipr.12002

Calasanti, T. (2015). Combating ageism: How successful is successful aging? *The Gerontologist, 56,* 1093–1101. doi:10.1093/geront/gnv076

Cantor, M. H. (1991). Family and community: Changing roles in an aging society. *Gerontologist, 31,* 337–346. doi:10.1093/geront/31.3.337

Castora-Binkley, M., Noelker, L. S., Ejaz, F. K., & Rose, M. (2010). Inclusion of caregiver supports and services in home- and community-based service programs: Recent reports from state units on aging. *Journal of Aging & Social Policy, 23,* 19–33. doi:10.1080/08959420.2011.532001

Centers for Medicare and Medicaid Services. (2017). Annual report of the boards of trustees of the federal hospital insurance and federal supplementary medical insurance trust funds. Retrieved from https://www.cms.gov/Research-Statistics-Data-and-Systems/Statistics-Trends-and-Reports/ReportsTrustFunds/Downloads/TR2017.pdf

Chiu, C., Feuz, M. A., McMahan, R. D., Miao, Y., & Sudore, R. L. (2016). "Doctor, make my decisions": Decision control preferences, advance care planning, and satisfaction with communication among diverse older adults. *Journal of Pain and Symptom Management, 51,* 33–40. doi:10.1016/j.jpainsymman.2015.07.018

Clemans-Cope, L., Long, S. K., Coughlin, T. A., Yemane, A., & Resnick, D. (2013). The expansion of Medicaid coverage under the ACA: Implications for health care access, use, and spending for vulnerable low-income adults. *The Journal of Health Care Organization, Provision, and Financing, 50,* 135–149. doi:10.1177/0046958013513675

Colby, S. L., & Ortman, J. M. (2015). Projections of the size and composition of the U.S. population: 2014 to 2060. *United States Census Bureau.* Retrieved from https://www.census.gov/content/dam/Census/library/publications/2015/demo/p25-1143.pdf

Crist, J. D. (2005). The meaning for elders of receiving family care. *Journal of Advanced Nursing, 49,* 485–493. doi:10.1111/j.1365-2648.2004.03321.x

Dannefer, D. (2003). Cumulative advantage/disadvantage and the life course: Cross-fertilizing age and social science theory. *The Journals of Gerontology Series B: Psychological Sciences and Social Sciences, 58,* S327–S337. doi:10.1093/geronb/58.6.S327

Desilver, D. (2016). More older Americans are working, and working more, than they used to. Pew Research Center. Retrieved from: http://www.pewresearch.org/fact-tank/2016/06/20/more-older-americans-are-working-and-working-more-than-they-used-to/

Eiken, S., Sredl, K., Burwell, B., & Saucier, P. (2016). Medicaid expenditures for long-term services and supports (LTSS) in FY 2014. *Medicaid.gov*

Erdley, S. D., Anklam, D. D., & Reardon, C. C. (2014). Breaking barriers and building bridges: Understanding the pervasive needs of older LGBT adults and the value of social work in health care. *Journal of Gerontological Social Work, 57,* 362–385. doi:10.1080/01634372.2013.871381

Family Caregiver Alliance. (2015). Caregiver statistics: Demographics. Retrieved from https://www.caregiver.org/caregiver-statistics-demographics

Farber, N., Shinkle, D., Lynott, J., Fox-Grage, W., & Harrell, R. (2011). *Aging in place: A state survey of livability policies and practices.* Retrieved from http://assets.aarp.org/rgcenter/ppi/liv-com/aging-in-place-2011-full.pdf

Federal Interagency Forum on Aging–related Statistics. (2008). *Older Americans 2008: Key indicators of well-being. Federal Interagency Forum on aging-related statistics.* Washington, DC: U.S. Government Printing Office.

Feinberg, L. F. (2014). Moving toward person- and family-centered care. *Public Policy & Aging Report, 24,* 97–101. doi:10.1093/ppar/pru027

Ferraro, K. F., Schafer, M. H., & Wilkinson, L. R. (2016). Childhood disadvantage and health problems in middle and later life: Early imprints on physical health? *American Sociological Review, 81,* 107–133. doi:10.1177/0003122415619617

Fredriksen-Goldsen, K. I., Hoy-Ellis, C. P., Goldsen, J., Emlet, C. A., & Hooyman, N. R. (2014). Creating a vision for the future: Key competencies and strategies for culturally competent practice with lesbian, gay, bisexual, and transgender (LGBT) older adults in the health and human services. *Journal of Gerontological Social Work, 57,* 80–107. doi:10.1080/01634372.2014.890690

Genworth Financial (2017). Compare long-term care costs across the United States. Retrieved from: https://www.genworth.com/about-us/industry-expertise/cost-of-care.html

Gonyea, J. G. (2014). The policy challenges of a larger and more diverse oldest-old population. In R. B. Hudson (Ed.), *The new politics of old age policy* (pp. 155–180). Baltimore, MD: Johns Hopkins University Press.

Hackett, B. (2017). Prescription drug costs continue to skyrocket. *AARP Report.*

He, W., Goodkind, D., & Kowal, P. (2016). An Aging World: 2015. *U.S. Census Bureau, International Population Reports (P95/16-1).* Washington, DC: U.S. Government Publishing Office.

Health and Human Services. (2015). Health insurance coverage and the Affordable Care Act. Retrieved from https://aspe.hhs.gov/system/files/pdf/139211/ib_uninsured_change.pdf

Healy, T. C., Peng, C., Haynes, M. S., McMahon, E. M., Botler, J. L., & Gross, L. (2008). The feasibility and effectiveness of translating a matter of balance into a volunteer lay leader model. *Journal of Applied Gerontology, 27,* 34–51. doi:10.1177/0733464807308620

Heller, T., Fisher, D., Marks, B., & Hsieh, K. (2014). Interventions to promote health: Crossing networks of intellectual and developmental disabilities and aging. *Disability and Health Journal, 7*, S24–S32. doi:10.1016/j.dhjo.2013.06.001

Holden, C. (1996). The developing world: New populations of old add to poor nations' burden. *Science, 273*(5271), 46–47. doi:10.1126/science.273.5271.46

Hong, S., Hasche, L., & Lee, M. J. (2011). Service use barriers differentiating care-givers' service use patterns. *Ageing & Society, 31*, 1307–1329. doi:10.1017/S0144686X10001418

Houser, A., Fox-Grage, W., & Ujvari, K. (2012). Across the states 2012: Profiles of long-term services and supports. *AARP Public Policy Institute.*

Hudson, R. B. (2014). Contemporary challenges to aging policy. In R. B. Hudson (Ed.), *The new politics of old age policy* (pp. 3–19). Baltimore, MD: Johns Hopkins University Press.

Irvin, C. V., Denny-Brown, N., Bohl, A., Schurrer, J., Wysocki, A., Couglin, R., & Williams, S. R. (2015). Money Follows the Person 2014: Annual evaluation report. *Report to the U.S. Department of Health and Human Services, Centers for Medicare and Medicaid Services.* Contract #HHSM-500-2010-00026I/HHSM-500-T0010.

James, E., Hughes, M., & Rocco, P. (2016). Addressing the needs of caregivers at risk: A new policy strategy. *University of Pittsburgh Health Policy Institute.*

Jarrott, S. E., & Savla, J. (2015). Mediators of the impact of intergenerational exchange on young adults' images of future older selves. *International Journal of Behavioral Development, 40*, 282–288. doi:10.1177/0165025415581913

Jenkins, J. A. C. (2017). Disrupt aging: A call to action for gerontologists. *The Gerontologist, 57*, S115–S117. doi:10.1093/geront/gnx079

Jensen, G. A., Salloum, R. G., Hu, J., Ferdows, N. B., & Tarraf, W. (2015). A slow start: Use of preventive services among seniors following the Affordable Care Act's enhancement of Medicare benefits in the US. *Preventive Medicine, 76*, 37–42. doi:10.1016/j.ypmed.2015.03.023

Jongen, C., McCalman, J., Bainbridge, R., & Clifford, A. (2017). Services and programs to improve culture competency (pp. 75–97). In C. Jongen, J. McCalman, R. Bainbridge, & A. Clifford (Eds.), *Cultural competence in health: A review of evidence.* Springer Briefs in Public Health. Springer: Singapore. Retrieved from https://link.springer.com/chapter/10.1007/978-981-10-5293-4_6

Kaiser Family Foundation. (2015). Medicare. Retrieved from https://www.kff.org/state-category/medicare/medicare-enrollment/

Kaiser Family Foundation. (2016). Medicaid Expansion Enrollment. Retrieved from https://www.kff.org/health-reform/state-indicator/medicaid-expansion-enrollment/?currentTimeframe=0&sortModel=%7B%22colId%22:%22Location%22,%22sort%22:%22asc%22%7D

Kaiser Family Foundation. (2017a.) An overview of Medicare. Retrieved from https://www.kff.org/medicare/issue-brief/an-overview-of-medicare/

Kaiser Family Foundation. (2017b). Medicaid's role for seniors. Retrieved from http://www.kff.org/infographic/medicaids-role-for-seniors/

Kart, C. S., & Kinney, J. M. (2000). *The realities of aging: An introduction to gerontology* (6th ed.). Boston, MA: Allyn & Bacon.

Kaye, H. S., Harrington, C., & LaPlante, M. P. (2010). Long-term care: Who gets it, who provides it, who pays, and how much? *Health Affairs, 29*, 11–21. doi:10.1377/hlthaff.2009.0535

Kim, E. S., Kawachi, I., Chen, Y., & Kubzansky, L. D. (2017). Association between purpose in life and objective measures of physical function in older adults. *JAMA Psychiatry, 74*, 1039–1045. doi:10.1001/jamapsychiatry.2017.2145

Konetzka, R. T. (2016). Are home- and community-based services cost-effective? *Medical Care, 54*, 219–220. doi:10.1097/MLR.0000000000000514

Kruse, C. S., Krowski, N., Rodriguez, B., Tran, L., Vela, J., & Brooks, M. (2017). Telehealth and patient satisfaction: A systematic review and narrative analysis. *BMJ open, 7*(8), e016242. doi:10.1136/bmjopen-2017-01624

Lachman, M. E., Neupert, S. D., & Agrigoroaei, S. (2011). The relevance of control beliefs for health and aging. In K. W. Schaie & S. L. Willis (Eds.), *Handbook of the psychology of aging* (7th ed.) (pp. 175–190). London: Academic Press.

Langer, E. J. (2009). *Counterclockwise: Mindful health and the power of possibility.* New York, NY: Ballantine Books

Langer, E. J., & Rodin, J. (1976). The effects of choice and enhanced personal responsibility for the aged: A field experiment in an institutional setting. *Journal of Personality and Social Psychology, 34*, 191–198.

Lehning, A. J., & Austin, M. J. (2010). Long-term care in the United States: Policy themes and promising practices. *Journal of Gerontological Social Work, 53*, 43–63. doi:10.1080/01634370903361979

Levy, B. (2009). Stereotype embodiment: A psychosocial approach to aging. *Current Directions in Psychological Science, 18*, 332–336.

Levy, B. R., Ferrucci, L., Zonderman, A. B. Slade, M. D., Troncoso, J., & Resnick, S. M. (2016). A culture–brain link: Negative age stereotypes predict Alzheimer's disease biomarkers. *Psychology and Aging, 31*, 82–88. doi:10.1037/pag0000062

Levy, B. R., & Myers, L.M. (2004). Preventive health behaviors influenced by self-perceptions of aging. *Preventive Medicine, 39*, 625–629. doi:10.1016/j.ypmed.2004.02.029

Levy, B. R., Pilver, C., Chung, P., & Slade, M. D. (2014). Subliminal strengthening: Improving older individuals' physical function over time with an implicit-age-Stereotype intervention. *Psychological Science, 25*, 2127–2135. doi:10.1177/0956797614551970

Levy, B. R., Slade, M.D., Kunkel, S.R., & Kasl, S.V. (2002). Longevity increased by positive self-perceptions of aging. *Journal of Personality and Social Psychology, 83*, 261–270.

Levy, B. R., Zonderman, A. B., Slade, M. D., & Ferrucci, L. (2012). Memory shaped by age stereotypes over time. *Journal of Gerontology: Psychological Sciences, 67*, 432–436. doi:10.1093/geronb/gbr120

Lindberg, B. W. (2017). Stone shares insights on applied research, 2017 Pollack Lecture (Part 2). *Gerontology News*. Washington, DC.

Medicaid.gov (n.d.). Self-directed services. Retrieved from https://www.medicaid.gov/medicaid/ltss/self-directed/index.html

Menkin, J. A., Guan, S. S. A., Araiza, D., Reyes, C. E., Trejo, L., Choi, S. E., ... McCreath, H. E. (2017). Racial/ethnic differences in expectations regarding aging among older adults. *The Gerontologist, 57*, S138–S148. doi:10.1093/geront/gnx078

Mooney, C. J., Elliot, A. J., Douthit, K. Z., Marquis, A., & Seplaki, C. L. (2016). Perceived control mediates effects of socioeconomic status and chronic stress on physical frailty: Findings from the Health and Retirement Study. *The Journals of Gerontology: Series B*. Advance online publication. doi:10.1093/geronb/gbw096

Munnell, A. H., Soto, M., & Golub-Sass, A. (2008). *Are older men healthy enough to work?* Chestnut Hill, MA: Center for Retirement Research at Boston College.

Murthy, V., & Ketenci, N. (2017). Is technology still a major driver of health expenditure in the United States? Evidence from cointegration analysis with multiple structural breaks. *International Journal of Health Economics and Management, 17*, 29–50.

National Conference of State Legislatures. (2016). State coverage for telehealth services. Retrieved from: http://www.ncsl.org/research/health/state-coverage-for-telehealth-services.aspx

O'Brien, E. L., Hess, T. M., Kornadt, A. E., Rothermund, K., Fung, H., & Voss, P. (2017). Context influences on the subjective experience of aging: The impact of culture and domains of functioning. *The Gerontologist, 57*, S127–S137. doi:10.1093/geront/gnx015

Ortman, J. M., Velkoff, V. A., & Hogan, H. (2014). An aging nation: The older population in the United States. *U.S. Census Bureau* #P25–1140.

O'Shaughnessy, C. V. (2008). The aging services network: Accomplishments and challenges in serving a growing elderly population. *National Health Policy Forum*. Retrieved from http://www.nhpf.org/library/details.cfm/2625

Ouchida, K. M., & Lachs, M. S. (2015). Not for doctors only: Ageism in healthcare. *Generations: Journal of the American Society on Aging*. Retrieved from http://www.asaging.org/blog/not-doctors-only-ageism-healthcare

Paraprofessional Healthcare Institute. (2017a). Workforce data center. Retrieved from https://phinational.org/policy-research/workforce-data-center/

Paraprofessional Healthcare Institute. (2017b). Inadequate training and few opportunities to advance. *Issues*. Retrieved from https://phinational.org/issue/training-advanced-roles/

Paraprofessional Healthcare Institute. (2017c). Low wages, insufficient hours, and high rates of poverty. *Issues*. Retrieved from https://phinational.org/issue/wages-benefits/

Paraprofessional Healthcare Institute. (2017d). A leadership training center that achieved widespread impact across care settings. Retrieved from https://phinational.org/impact_story/leadership-training-center-achieved-widespread-impact-across-care-settings/

Pinto, J. M. (2016). Barriers to social participation in caregivers of older people: A systematic review. *Research in Health Science, 1*, 78. doi:10.22158/rhs.v1n2p78

Poo, A. J. (2015). *The age of dignity: Preparing for the elder boom in a changing America*. New York, NY: The New Press.

Raynor, C. (2014). Innovations in training and promoting the direct care workforce. *Public Policy & Aging Report, 24*, 70–72. doi:10.1093/ppar/pru005

Reaves, E. L., & Musumeci, M. (2015). Medicaid and long-term services and supports: A primer. Retrieved from https://www.kff.org/medicaid/report/medicaid-and-long-term-services-and-supports-a-primer/

Redfoot, D., Feinberg, L., & Houser, A. (2013). The aging of the baby boom and the growing care gap: A look at future declines in the availability of family caregivers. *Insight on the Issues, 85*, 1–12.

Reinhard, S. C., Feinberg, L., Choula, R., & Houser, A. (2015). Valuing the invaluable: 2015 update: Undeniable progress, but big gaps remain. *AARP Public Policy Institute*.

Roberto, K. A., & Blieszner, R. (2015). Diverse family structures and the care of older persons. *Canadian Journal on Aging/La Revue canadienne du vieillissement, 34*, 305–320. doi:10.1017/S0714980815000288

Ryan, C. L., & Bauman, K. (2016). Educational attainment in the United States: 2015. *Current Population Reports, P20-578*. United States Census Bureau.

Sawyer, B., & Sroczynski, N. (2017). How do health expenditures vary across the population? *Kasier Family Foundation*. Retrieved from https://www.healthsystemtracker.org/chart-collection/health-expenditures-vary-across-population/#item-people-age-55-account-half-total-health-spending_2015

Schulz, R., & Heckhausen, J. (1999). Aging, culture and control: Setting a new research agenda. *The Journals of Gerontology Series B: Psychological Sciences and Social Sciences, 54*, P139–P145. doi:10.1093/geronb/54B.3.P139

Stone, R. I. (2017). Developing a quality direct care workforce: Searching for solutions. *Public Policy & Aging Report, 27*, 96–100. doi:10.1093/ppar/prx015

Sun, J. K., & Smith, J. (2017). Self-perceptions of aging and perceived barriers to care: Reasons for health care delay. *The Gerontologist, 57*, S216–S226. doi:10.1093/geront/gnx014

Trivedi, D., Goodman, C., Gage, H., Baron, N., Scheibl, F., Iliffe, S., . . . Drennan, V. (2013). The effectiveness of inter-professional working for older people living in the community: A systematic review. *Health & Social Care in the Community, 21*, 113–128. doi:10.1111/j.1365-2524.2012.01067.x

U.S. Bureau of Labor Statistics. (2017). Demographics. Retrieved from https://www.bls.gov/cps/demographics.htm#older

U.S. Census Bureau. (2013). Older Americans month: May 2011. Retrieved from https://www.census.gov/newsroom/releases/archives/facts_for_features_special_editions/cb11-ff08.html

U.S. Census Bureau. (2017). Historical poverty tables: People and families—1959–2016. Retrieved from https://www.census.gov/data/tables/time-series/demo/income-poverty/historical-poverty-people.html

U.S. Department of Labor. (n.d.). FMLA: Fact sheets. Retrieved from https://www.dol.gov/whd/fmla/fact_sheets.htm

Walters, C., & Troutman-Jordan, M. (2017). An investigation of the effectiveness of A Matter of Balance/Volunteer Lay Leader Model (AMOB/VLL): Findings from a community senior center. *Activities, Adaptation & Aging, 42*(1), 69–80. doi:10.1080/01924788.2017.1376174

Williams, D., & Wyatt, R. (2015). Racial bias in health care and health challenges and opportunities. *Journal of the American Medical Association, 314*, 555–556. doi:10.1001/jama.2015.9260

Wilmoth, J. M. (2014). The implications of structural lag for old age policy. In R. B. Hudson (Ed.), *The new politics of old age policy* (pp. 20–38). Baltimore, MD: Johns Hopkins University Press.

World Population Review. (2018). South Korean population 2018. Retrieved from http://worldpopulationreview.com/countries/south-korea-population/

EPILOGUE

Patient[1] Advocacy for Older Adults

Ellen Menard, MBA, BSN, RN

Regula Robnett, PhD, OTR/L, FAOTA

Providing culturally competent care and possessing a high degree of knowledge in aging issues are central to the high performance expectations for today's healthcare professional. Innovations in care can be mind-boggling, especially to your aging patients. They will be counting on you to help them understand and navigate the healthcare maze. They will need you to advocate for them and, if possible, help them to advocate for themselves as they cope with rapid and complex changes in both systemic and personal realms. As an excellent care provider, you want to rise to this challenge. Most patients and/or their families or caregivers will struggle mightily to navigate today's convoluted healthcare network. It is a space where already highly stressed people, who are often very sick as well, are bombarded with foreign-sounding medical and technological words, sterile equipment, distressing smells, odd sounds and sights, and even scarily masked healthcare professionals. The poking, prodding, and questioning that take place can be intimidating, humiliating, and even dehumanizing. These patients need help. Here are some of the key ingredients for successful patient advocacy.

▶ Teamwork

Teamwork is an essential key ingredient to enhance patient advocacy. Complexities in care requirements have increased the need for information sharing and collaboration. For patients to thrive in today's milieu, they require a coherent and cohesive (and when possible, consistent) care team approach. Interprofessional practice puts the patient's goals at the center of concern, and all work together in partnership to make the healthcare experience the best it can be. We owe it to

---

[1]The term patient is used here because of its prevalence in the healthcare literature, but those healthcare professionals who work with clients can use the term client interchangeably with patient throughout.

our patients to be knowledgeable about other care professionals, to confer and join forces with each other, and to refer to one another, as needed. Care team members must be on the "side" of their patients. In practice, they must give their patients a voice, or sometimes be their patients' voices. When they voice the patient's concerns, they will have become their patient's advocate.

An emerging field of professionally trained patient advocates is helping to fill what at times can be a health literacy, communication, and healthcare vacuum. Enlightened hospitals, physician practice groups, insurance companies, and even patients/families themselves may employ these professionals to participate in and guide an individual's care or treatment plan. The role of patient advocate has been listed by U.S. News and World Report (Nemco, 2007) as a rewarding and necessary new healthcare career for "persuasive, persistent," and caring individuals. With or without a professional patient advocate on board, however, the entire healthcare team is still "on point" and each member is fully responsible for their patient's care and safety.

▶ Plain Language

The use of plain language and being aware of appropriate health literacy is another key ingredient to ensure patients get the services and information they need. One might think that any health literacy deficits are a thing of the past, but the reverse actually is true. Consider the degree to which information has become available on the Internet and through social media, along with radio, television, libraries, and other nearly instantaneous ways to retrieve data. The amount of information out there is excessive (and growing exponentially). Envision already stressed patients and their families/caregivers accessing information that is often confusing

and perhaps contradictory to other sources, including their own doctors. Information quests often can lead to more questions, uncertainty, anxiety, and frustration.

The Joint Commission estimates that medical miscommunication accounts for approximately 80% of serious medical errors (FierceHealthCare, 2010). Extension Healthcare (n.d.) estimates that $12 billion are wasted every year due to communication inefficiencies. Think of how easily miscommunications or misunderstandings occur. One has only to imagine the children's game of "telephone" to understand the importance of clear and direct written and spoken language. In addition to speaking concisely in lay terms, paying close attention to the patient's responses and noting the nuances of tone and body language are also crucial. For example, the healthcare professional might say: "Your case is terminal and we need to bring in the hospice people." The patient wonders what terminal means (or where the terminal is) and why hostile people need to be brought in. This may be an extreme example, but we should not assume that patients understand medical jargon and that they are hearing exactly what we are trying to say.

An interesting note is that patients may not even be aware of their lack of comprehension. In a study of emergency room patients and their level of understanding of the care they received and discharge instructions, the majority of patients (78%) demonstrated a deficiency in understanding, especially in the domain of discharge instructions, yet only 20% of the 140 English-speaking patients studied reported being aware of their lack of understanding (Engle et al., 2009). This is just more evidence to support the need for clear communication. We must refrain from assuming that just because patients are told what to do, they actually comprehend the information and are willing and able to follow through. (See Chapter 5 for a more in-depth look at health literacy.)

▶ Listening

Perhaps, it is self-evident (although it is not as widespread as we might expect or hope) that another key to effective patient advocacy is listening. Too often, we listen with biased ears, thus tuning out crucial information that does not fit with our assumptions of what we expect to hear. We cannot be successful as patient advocates unless we open our minds to truly hear what the person has to say. A technique that is helpful for ensuring understanding is to paraphrase what we have just heard and to ask patients if we are on the right track and thus understanding them correctly. Connect with patients, sit down at their level, get to know them, and listen to what they have to say (as well as what they [purposefully] do not say). All of us could listen harder.

Collaborating with and being on the patient's side does not necessarily mean always agreeing with or doing what patients want. Doing so would not serve either the patient or the healthcare team member well. The concept of patient advocacy means that patients (or others who care for and about them) act as their own advocates and are informed and comfortable enough to have a voice and interact productively with the healthcare team, thereby optimizing patient quality and safety outcomes. When the interprofessional team operates within this contemporary frame of reference, optimal health care with improved patient outcomes occur routinely. Patients have better healthcare experiences. Dedicated collaboration helps to prevent errors; it can also save lives.

Although misunderstandings occur among patients of all ages, older patients with potentially decreased sensory or cognitive functioning have unique care needs and are likely to be the most vulnerable population with whom you will work. You owe it to yourself and your profession to be fluent in the language of health care and to partner and collaborate with your fellow team members and patients—actively, proactively, and constructively.

▶ Summary

Patient advocacy is not about having all the answers. It is about establishing partnerships with colleagues and with care recipients. It is about staying current in your field, asking the right questions, listening, and engaging in clear two-way communications. Moreover, as a team member, an "insider," you will know the right resources to access and make the best referrals for best practice. Your involvement will go a long way to help your patients and families with the "when" and "how" to effectively engage their appropriate care provider, whether that provider is a nurse, surgeon, therapist, or any other healthcare professional.

Any person or organization with a stake in a patient's health and wellness is by definition a patient advocate. Innovations and advances in healthcare delivery will add to the intricate nature of the healthcare system. Not only will the layers of complexity continue to increase, but also medical specialization will likely be the norm, and care delivery may become more complicated and less seamless before the situation begins to turn around. Despite the best of intentions, training, and preparation, opportunities for mistakes, errors, or accidents will happen. In fact, in a study of premier hospitals in the United States, after a 10-year period, adverse events had increased and occurred in approximately one-third of all hospital admissions (Classen et al., 2011). These adverse medical events have contributed to as many as 180,000 deaths per year (*Lancet*, 2011). As a professional care provider, this should shock and dismay you. Patients and their families or caregivers need your help and constant vigilance. You can do something. You can begin by embracing your patient advocacy role in collaborating with the healthcare team to help your patients stay far away from the precipice—the danger zone—where they are most vulnerable. Quality and safety must be daily mantras. Being a dedicated and competent patient advocate is a laudable and necessary goal.

References

Classen, D. C., Resar, R., Griffin, F., Federico, F., Frankel, T., Kimmel, N., ... James, B. C. (2011). "Global trigger tool" shows that adverse events in hospitals may be ten times greater than previously measured. *Health Affairs, 30*(4), 581–589.

Engle, K. G., Heisler, M., Smith, D. M., Robinson, D. H., Forman, S. H., & Ubel, P. A. (2009). Patient comprehension of emergency department care and instructions: Are patients aware of when they do not understand? *Annals of Emergency Medicine, 53*(4), 454–461.

Extension Healthcare. (n.d.). Care Team Collaboration Solutions: Impact on Discharge Planning, Readmission Rates, and HCAHPS Scores. Retrieved from http://docplayer.net/34866004-Impact-on-discharge -planning-readmission-rates-and-hcahps-scores.html

FierceHealthcare. (2010, October 21). Joint Commission Center for Transforming Healthcare Tackles Miscommunication Among Caregivers. Retrieved from http://www.fiercehealthcare.com/press-releases/joint -commission-center-transforming-healthcare-tackles -miscommunication-amongcaregi#ixzz2SHiKnYPv

Lancet. (2011). Medical errors in the USA: Human or systemic? [Editorial]. *377*(9774), 1289.

Nemco, M. (2007, December 17). Patient advocate: Ahead of the curve. *U.S. News and World Report.* Retrieved from http://money.usnews.com/money /careers/articles/2007/12/19/ahead-of-the-curve -careers

▶ An Older Patient's True Story

Paulette, a single, trim 79-year-old with thick eyeglasses and hearing aids is alone and sitting at the edge of her hospital bed, with a look a bit like a restrained animal on her very pale face. She came into the hospital for simple colitis surgery 12 days ago and wound up with a serious and debilitating upper respiratory infection (URI). A deep rattling cough is evident, but at her insistence, the doctor has just signed the discharge order for her to go home, where she lives alone with her 60-pound dog. Even though she wore her doctor down and got her way about leaving, she appears to be in a foul mood. A beautiful suit, upscale shoes, and a handbag are on a nearby chair. She wants out! You walk into her room and assess your about to be discharged patient.

Whatever role you play as part of the healthcare team, there are certain patient advocacy actions that should jump out at you as you contemplate the needs of this older woman. In collaboration with your patient and fellow team members, some questions must be asked and resolved before she leaves, or she will present a high risk for readmission. What are the clues or cues? What questions need to be raised? How will you proceed?

Clues and Cues

Older woman
Lives alone
Mood and affect
Pale (scared?)
Trim with nice clothing
Upper respiratory infection/productive cough
Discharge instructions
Large dog at home needs care

Questions to Ask

1. Are any family/support persons expected? When? What other supports does she have (or could she access) in the community?
2. Will she have someone stay at her house or will she be alone? Will home care be required?
3. Does she need a referral for rehabilitation? What rehab services might she need? Who can offer these services?
4. How her eyesight impact her ability to live in her home?
5. Is she safe ambulating without assistance? Does she need a device?

How are her transfers to sitting, standing, getting into and out of the shower, and so on?

6. Considering her visual and hearing impairments and distracted by her own mood, would she likely comprehend the detailed discharge instructions? Will she need enlarged font on the discharge instructions?

7. What is going on with her mood? Is this a change? If so, what is at the bottom of it?

8. Is she in pain or discomfort? Is she fearful? (of what?) Is she too proud (or private) a person to offer up this information?

9. What is her medical status due to her upper respiratory infection? Her surgery? Her cough?

10. What about her dog? Will she be able to handle the 60-pound dog and walk it daily?

11. What about her psychosocial needs? Loneliness/isolation?

12. If her affect today is not the norm for her, what is going on here? Is she depressed?

13. Has her care been compromised during this hospitalization? Has anyone explored and communicated the positives and negatives of her patient experience directly with her? Would she recommend this hospital to others? Why or why not? How does she feel about her doctor? The care team?

Considering the patient's entire story, including medical indications, is Paulette ready to be discharged or is she at a safety risk and vulnerable to readmission? What do you think? If you think she is not ready, yet she has already been discharged by her doctor, what can you do about it now?

Create your own best-case scenario solution for "Paulette."

Case Analysis

Unfortunately, this case presents an all-too-common situation, fraught with peril for the patient. Ideally, these typically busy care team members would have been consulted before the patient was discharged. In this case, the team conferred and ultimately decided Paulette was not ready to go home. They based their determination on the following evidence: The patient was demonstrating a completely different affect than in previous days. Because she had become very ill with her URI in the past week, Paulette had likely become dehydrated and was confused. The look on the patient's face expressed fear and confusion. The patient finally admitted she did not feel well enough to go home. Her independent streak was a deeply embedded personal trait. She was terribly worried about her dog. When priorities, including getting patients home into their own familiar environments or decreasing hospital days and costs, appear to compete, staying on the side of the patient will always serve. For example, readmission of the patient or a preventable fall at home serves neither the patient nor the hospital.

Conclusion

The decision the care team (including the patient's doctor) made, in this case without the patient's immediate concurrence, was to seek a skilled nursing facility (SNF) short-term stay for Paulette. There, she would be helped to get back on her feet, follow her special colon diet safely, get rehabilitation services, and rehydrate. In short, she would be cared for, especially because she was still very ill from her URI and was still so early in recovering from her colon surgery. Taken all together, as a full picture, the patient presented ongoing care needs. Still protesting until she was settled into a local SNF, she did very well and was transferred home within 10 days.

Case Summary

As this case illustrates, the care team's good work serves not just the patient, but ultimately also the hospital. But, think of how proactive collaboration (as well as more effective listening skills) may have reduced this patient's stress level or saved work that had already been started. What if everyone on the team was just too "busy," as is the norm? How would that have served the patient? What if she suffered a fall at home, breaking a hip or worse? Patient safety practices mandate vigilance. Besides, being on the same side as the patient saves the organization money, contributes to an overall positive reputation, and decreases the risks of malpractice, readmission, and excess care charges. What if the team had not revisited the discharge order with Paulette's doctor? "What?," you say, "Challenge a doctor's order?" Wrong frame, entirely. The correct frame is: We are all on the same side—the patient's side. We should not seek to compete with or outdo one another, but to join forces to make each patient care experience the best it can be.

If you were not the patient's nurse in this story, you would have taken the team's concerns to the patient's primary nurse. Any concerns from your own health sciences vector, supported by the context supplied by the answers to the questions, would be fodder for the team's discussion. The patient's nurse would confer with the hospital's discharge coordinator or social worker, or go directly to the attending physician. Were you the patient's respiratory therapist? You would likely have had an excellent grasp of the patient's progress throughout her stay, her developing infection, and current cough. Were you another team member? How would your professional role fit into this scenario? Think of this situation as neither challenging the patient's wishes nor the doctor's discharge order. Many a patient, patient's family, doctor, and healthcare organization have ultimately been grateful for the collaborative work of the care team and their astute patient advocacy roles.

About the Contributing Author Ellen Menard, MBA, BSN, RN, is a nationally recognized patient advocacy expert, speaker, and the author of *The Not So Patient Advocate: How to Get the Care You Want Without Fear or Frustration*. Her *New York Times*–recommended and multi-award-winning book is now in its fourth year of publication, continuing its wide reach to both healthcare practitioners and lay audiences. Besides serving in clinical and managerial roles in hospitals, Menard has 25 years of hospital administrator and corporate senior healthcare executive experience, and most recently was senior vice president for Organizational Effectiveness for Inova Health System.

Answers to Review Questions

Chapter 1

1. b
2. a
3. b
4. b
5. c

Chapter 2

1. d
2. a
3. a
4. c
5. c

Chapter 3

1. a
2. c
3. c
4. b
5. b

Chapter 4

1. c
2. c
3. b
4. c
5. d

Chapter 5

1. d
2. c
3. b
4. c
5. d

Chapter 6

1. 1b, 2f, 3d, 4e, 5c, 6a
2. a
3. a
4. d
5. a

Chapter 7

1. b
2. Cornoary heart disease b, peripheral artery disease d, congenital heart disease c, deep vein thrombosis e, cerebrovascular disease a
3. c
4. c
5. d

Chapter 8

1. c
2. d
3. d
4. a
5. a

Chapter 9

1. c
2. a
3. b
4. c
5. d

Chapter 10

1. d
2. b
3. d
4. c
5. b

Chapter 11

1. a
2. d
3. a
4. a
5. c

Chapter 12

1. d
2. b
3. a
4. c
5. d

Chapter 13

1. a
2. a
3. c
4. b
5. a

Chapter 14

1. c
2. c
3. b
4. b
5. e

Glossary

A

AARP A non-profit non-partisan group that advocates for the needs of older adults and promotes their quality of life.

Accessibility Refers to the ability to navigate through an environment.

Active euthanasia The act to shorten life by taking direct action. For example, a veterinarian engages in active euthanasia when it "puts down" or euthanizes an animal.

Activities of daily living (ADLs) Basic daily activities required to maintain health and wellness. Core ADLs include eating, bathing, dressing, toileting, and transferring/walking.

Activity theory A gerontological theory to examine old age. It posits that older adults are happier and healthier when they remain engaged in daily life and social interactions.

Adult day services Community-based programs and group services with specialized plans of care designed to meet the daytime needs of individuals with functional and/or cognitive impairments.

Adult protective services A local government agency mandated to investigate reports of suspected elder abuse within a community.

Advanced directive A set of legal documents that outline preferred medical treatments and care when an individual can no longer speak for him or herself. Advanced directives typically contain a living will, appointment of a medical power of attorney, and directives for organ and tissue donation.

Age composition The distribution of age groups in a given population. (e.g., 0–18 years or ages 65+).

Age-associated memory impairment (AAMI) The most common age-related cognitive decline that is associated with mild forgetfulness.

Ageism The systematic stereotyping of and discrimination against individuals who are old. Ageism fosters the notion that older adults are not useful and not valued.

Aging in place The ability to live in one's home or community as one ages regardless of age, income, or level of ability.

Aging network Broadly refers to the agencies, programs, and activities that are supported by the Older Americans Act.

Agnosia A loss of a perceptual skill, specifically not understanding the use of common objects.

Alzheimer's disease (AD) An irreversible degenerative brain disease that is the most common form of dementia.

Americans with Disabilities Act A federal civil rights policy for individuals with disabilities. The overarching goal of the Act is to integrate individuals with disabilities into communities and society with the same access and rights as persons without disabilities.

Anorexia A physiological change often associated with aging that can result in decreased appetite; caused by a general reduction in gastrointestinal mobility.

Anosmia The inability to smell.

Apraxia The complete inability to perform coordinated movements without muscular or sensory impairment.

Area agencies on aging Regional agencies that provide information and referrals to community-based services or offer them as part of their mission.

Assisted living facility (ALF) A broad term used to describe several types of congregate living arrangements (e.g., adult group homes, board and care homes, personal care homes, and assisted living facilities). ALFs are designed for individuals who need extra help in their day-to-day lives, but who do not require 24-hour skilled nursing care.

Assistive technology Devices or tools that provide assistive, adaptive, and rehabilitative support to help increase, maintain, or improve the functional capabilities of the user.

Atherosclerosis The development of fatty plaques and the proliferation of connective tissue in the walls of arteries.

Attachment theory The theory suggests that an individual's attachment to nurturing figures (e.g., mother or father) are initially focused on meeting basic needs such as safety and security, with the level and nature of the attachment changing over time.

Attention Being able to focus or concentrate.

Attrition The wearing away of the tooth surface.

Average life expectancy The average length of time a person is expected to live based on location such as country or state.

B

Baby boom generation Americans born after WWII ended—between 1946 and 1964.

Beehive theory The theory suggests that a bereaved individual fluctuates between acceptance and denial, and bewilderment and pain during the grieving process.

Behavior change Seeking to alter daily habits, often to improve health.

Bereavement A feeling of anguish over the death of a loved one.

Biopsychosocial Biological, psychological, and sociological factors that influence aging processes, quality of life, and well-being.

Bisexual A person sexually attracted to both males and females or the state of being sexually attracted to both males and females.

Brain death When a brain ceases to function and is unresponsive to stimuli following a devastating brain injury.

Burnout Excessive and prolonged stress experienced by healthcare professionals caused by the work environment.

C

Cachexia A complex metabolic syndrome associated with underlying illness and distinguished by loss of muscle with or without loss of fat mass.

Calcium A major mineral in the human body needed for movement and to maintain strong bones. Derived from many foods such as dairy products.

Carbohydrate A macronutrient consisting of one or more sugar molecules. Carbohydrates are present in foods such as bread, rice, grains, potatoes, and sugar.

Cardiopulmonary resuscitation (CPR) A life-saving medical technique to revive an individual whose heart has stopped beating by conducting a series of compressions on the chest and breaths into the mouth.

Cardiovascular disease An umbrella term that includes health conditions that restrict or narrow blood vessels, which can lead to a heart attack (e.g., arteriosclerosis, coronary artery disease, and hypertension).

Caregiver A person who provides care for an individual.

Caregiver support ratio The number of potential caregivers for each older person. As the caregiver support ratio decreases, older adults will be less likely to rely on family members for care.

Cataract A condition in which the lens of the eye becomes opaque as the proteins within it become increasingly oxidized, glycosylated, and cross-linked.

Celiac disease A digestive and autoimmune disorder in which the ingestion of gluten may damage the lining of the small intestine.

Centenarian A person at least 100 years old.

Cerebrovascular accident (CVA; stroke) Infarction in the brain that can be hemorrhagic (bleeding in the brain) or ischemic (inadequate blood flow to the brain).

Cholesterol A substance found in every cell in the human body that is necessary for cell functioning. However, the accumulation of cholesterol on the walls of arteries can restrict blood flow and contribute to increased risk for coronary artery disease.

Chore services A home and community-based service for home maintenance activities such as mowing, cleaning gutters, and house cleaning.

Chronic bronchitis Clinically defined as a chronic cough ("smoker's cough") producing sputum, and occurring on most days for at least 3 months' duration over at least 2 consecutive years.

Chronic obstructive pulmonary disease (COPD) An umbrella term for a health condition that includes emphysema and chronic bronchitis.

Chronological age The length of time a person has been alive (e.g., he turned 70 years old on his last birthday).

Circumstantial loss Unexpected experiences, incidents, or events that negatively affect daily life (e.g., divorce, illness, and house fire).

Clinical death When the heart stops circulating blood throughout the body and the lungs are unable to oxygenate the blood—two functions necessary to sustain human life.

Cognition The mental processes that involve thinking, learning, and memory.

Cognitive behavioral therapy (CBT) An evidence-based form of psychological treatment that is used to change personal behaviors and thinking and has shown to be effective in improving personal functioning and quality of life.

Cohousing A type of collaborative housing in which residents actively participate in the design and operation of their own neighborhoods.

Compassion fatigue The burnout or weariness healthcare professionals experience in response to the emotional stress produced in their caregiving positions.

Compassionate ageism The belief that all older adults need help and deserve receiving help through special programs and policies designed specifically for them.

Competency The ability to make personal choices and understand the consequences of those choices, particularly when those choices place the decision-maker or other people at risk.

Complicated grief When individuals are unable to manage their grief and experience symptoms such as intense sorrow, yearning, and emotional pain during the majority of days for more than 12 months.

Compression of morbidity Decreasing the time in which personal and systemic burdens caused by illness are reduced to the shortest time possible before death.

Continuing care retirement community (CCRC) Communities specifically designed to provide a spectrum of lifetime care to residents. Housing arrangements range from independent housing (least restrictive) to skilled nursing home care (most restrictive).

Continuity theory A psychosocial theory in gerontology that theorizes that people remain consistent in how they live their lives, manage their relationships, and exhibit their personalities even though they may experience changes in their physical, mental, and social status.

Contracture A condition generally caused by joint immobilization that result in decreased range of motion, stiffening and subsequent structural changes, and pain upon movement at one or more joints.

Convoy of support A dynamic social network of support that changes (or moves) with an individual through life challenges and transitions.

Crystallized intelligence Intelligence that tends to remain strong in people who are aging typically; it includes skills such as language comprehension, educational qualifications, and life and occupational (job) skills.

Cultural competencies The ability of an individual and/or a healthcare system to engage appropriately and effectively regardless of the different cultures, beliefs, linguistic needs, and healthcare practices of the individuals they treat.

Cumulative advantage/disadvantage framework Using this framework, scholars posit that a lifetime accumulation of exposures and experiences provide a partial explanation for health disparities found in later life. For example, lack of health care in early life leads to health problems in late life.

D

DASH diet Dietary approach to stop hypertension diet (DASH). The program is similar to the Mediterranean diet, which is rich in fruits and vegetables, low in carbohydrates, saturated fats, and sugars.

Death The absence of vital cellular and tissue activity that are necessary to sustain life. The end of a life for a person or other organism.

Death with Dignity Act (DWDA) An Act first passed in Oregon that legally allows residents to end their own lives by utilizing physician-assisted suicide.

Dehydration The loss of water and salts that are essential for normal body function.

Delirium A serious, rapidly developing state of confusion often associated with surgery or hospitalization. The risk for developing delirium is higher for older adults.

Dementia Progressive cognitive impairment that eventually interferes with daily functioning. The prevalence of dementia among 60-year-olds is only 1–2%, but it becomes increasingly more common with advancing age (up to approximately 50%).

Dental caries Also known as cavities or tooth decay; a bacterial infection attributed to streptococcus mutans.

Dental plaque (biofilm) A biofilm (usually yellow) that develops on teeth due to bacterial colonization.

Dependence A physical state that occurs with continued use of a drug and results in symptoms of withdrawal if the drug is discontinued.

Depression A mood disorder characterized by loss of interest in living. Symptoms that accompany depression can include sadness, hopelessness, loss of energy, tearfulness, loss of appetite, insomnia, and/or excessive sleep.

Developmental loss Anticipated events or milestones that occur as a function of personal growth and maturation (e.g., leaving the family home, retirement).

Diabetes A group of metabolic disorders characterized by insufficient insulin production or usage.

Diabetes mellitus A condition in which there is insufficient insulin. This can lead to elevated blood glucose levels or inability to use available insulin.

Diaphragm The dome-shaped skeletal muscle located beneath the lungs; the major muscle of ventilation.

Dietary fiber Non-nutrients that are considered important as a part of a healthy balanced diet because of their crucial role in moving waste material through the large intestine and as a component of medical nutrition therapy.

Dietary Guidelines for Americans A federal nutrition policy issued and updated every 5 years by the U.S. government. It provides guidelines or qualitative statements for making food choices that can people lead a healthy life.

Direct care workforce Members of the caregiving workforce including nursing assistants, home health aides, and personal care or homecare aides who provide supportive, nonmedical services.

Discrimination The act of exhibiting prejudicial behavior towards an individual or group of people.

Disengagement theory The first psychosocial theory on aging that proposed that older adults recognize as their health and abilities decline, their time as industrious citizens is limited before they die. Therefore, they intentionally distance themselves from their social roles and responsibilities to allow younger and healthier adults to take their place as productive members in society.

Diverticulosis The development of small sacs where the large intestinal lining has herniated through the intestinal muscular wall.

Do not resuscitate (DNR) Also called a no code order. A legally binding order directing healthcare practitioners and emergency responders to withhold life-saving treatments such as CPR and advanced cardiac support in the event that the heart stops.

Dual process model of grief In this model, resolving grief is dynamic and oscillates between two orientations. That is, the grief work process shifts between coping with loss (e.g., via therapy, avoidance, denial) and reorienting to daily life (e.g., adjusting to new routines and changes in lifestyle).

Dysphagia The decreased ability or inability to swallow caused by weakness of tongue muscles, poor control of the swallowing reflex, or a lack of coordinated muscular action of the pharynx or esophagus.

Dyspraxia A decreased ability to plan and/or execute purposeful movements.

E

Eden Alternative An innovative nursing home model designed to combat boredom, loneliness, and helplessness. The model is resident centered and encourages residents to be active and engage in communal activities.

Edentulism The condition of being toothless to some degree. Loss of some teeth results in partial edentulism, whereas loss of all teeth is complete edentulism.

Elder abuse Intentional or neglectful acts by a caregiver or trusted individual that lead to or may lead to harm of a vulnerable elder. There are seven main types of elder abuse: physical, psychological, sexual, exploitation, neglect, abandonment, and self-neglect.

Elderspeak A demeaning style of communication with older adults that uses slow, exaggerated, and loud intonation of simpler vocabulary and sentence structure.

Endurance The ability to sustain involvement in a physical activity.

Episodic memory Memory oriented toward the past. This is what most people think of when they think of the global term memory. This type of declarative or conscious memory particularly involves remembering episodes or experiences in our lives (e.g., what we ate for lunch, our last birthday party).

Estrogen replacement therapy (ERT) Also referred to as hormone replacement therapy. ERT is a treatment that includes female hormones to raise estrogen levels in the body. It is usually prescribed to manage discomforts (e.g., hot flashes) associated with menopause.

Euthanasia The act of killing another living being for the purpose of relieving incurable pain and suffering. Euthanasia can take two forms: passive and active.

F

Failure to thrive A deterioration in functioning and subsequent weight loss not related to a specific disease, but often attributed to conditions such as depression, loneliness, social withdrawal, and lack of interest in life.

Fecal incontinence The inability to voluntarily control defecation, because of the weakening of the external anal sphincter muscle or lack of awareness of needing to toilet.

Fictive kin Individuals who take responsibility for engaging in traditional social roles of family members but are not related by birth or marriage to the person they regard as kin.

Filial expectations of care A family's belief that it is their responsibility to care for their own members.

Fluid intelligence Intelligence that involves the speed and accuracy of information processing such as discrimination, making comparisons, and categorization, often deemed to be largely evolutionarily and genetically based.

Fluoride gel Acidic, highly concentrated fluoride product that dentists topically apply to a patient's teeth about twice a year. It can help reduce tooth sensitivity, fight cavities, and strengthen tooth enamel.

Fluoride varnish A highly concentrated form of fluoride that is applied to the tooth's surface by a dentist, dental hygienist, or other healthcare professional.

Food and Drug Administration The federal agency responsible for protecting the public health by regulating public access to over the counter and prescription medications.

Formal caregivers Individuals who are paid to deliver care. Most formal caregivers are employed by agencies that offer caregiving and healthcare services.

Free radicals Molecules that contain at least one unpaired electron in their outer valence shells. Free radicals are unstable and most notably form in the mitochondria of cells, the site of aerobic respiration. The free radical theory on aging is a specific version of the wear and tear theory.

Functional age The age level at which a person can perform. For example, a frail 50 year old man may have a functional age of a 75 year old man.

G

Gastritis Inflammation of the stomach lining.

Gay male A male who is sexually attracted to other males.

Gender Refers to the social roles, behaviors, and norms that a society deems appropriate for a given sex.

Geriatrics A medical term for the study, diagnosis, and treatment of diseases and health problems specific to older adults.

Gerotechnology A professional field that focuses on developing technology to support older adults in their daily lives.

Gerontology The scientific study of aging that examines the biological, psychological, and sociological (biopsychosocial) factors and issues associated with old age and aging.

Gerotranscendence A life stage associated with obtaining maturity and wisdom and moving away from the materialism and self-centeredness of earlier years.

Gluten A component found in cereal grains such as wheat, barley, and rye.

Good death A death that is free from avoidable distress and suffering, in accordance with the dying person's wishes, and reasonably consistent with clinical, cultural, and ethical standards.

Grandfamilies Families in which a grandparent acts as a surrogate parent to a grandchild because the child's parent is unable. Today, most grandfamilies form due to a parent's substance misuse (e.g., opioid addiction and alcohol dependence) and/or incarceration.

Grief Keen mental suffering or distress over affliction or loss, sharp sorrow, or painful regret.

H

Health literacy The degree to which a person has the capacity to obtain, process, and understand basic health information and services needed to make appropriate health decisions.

Healthcare power of attorney (HCPOA) An individual appointed to speak on a person's behalf regarding medical decisions when he or she cannot speak or express their own wishes.

Healthy life expectancy Estimate of one's life-span in a healthy state.

Heterogeneous Mixed or consisting of dissimilar elements or parts. Older adults are a heterogeneous population with varied lifestyles, beliefs, and needs.

Home health Services provided in the home rather than in a hospital or nursing facility. Home health services are ordered as part of a treatment plan, involve skilled nursing care, and are ordered by a physician.

Hospice care Compassionate care provided at the end of life that focuses on pain relief and quality of life rather than curative treatments.

Hydrophilicity A molecule with a strong affinity for water molecules.

Hypertension High blood pressure.

Hyposmia A decreased or diminished sense of smell.

Hypothalamus A small but important structure that controls the activity of the pituitary gland that stimulates or inhibits its hormonal production and release.

I

Incidence The number of new cases (of disease) reported.

Individual or personal autonomy Having the ability to make decisions and choices regarding one's own life including directing one's own care.

Inducibility The ability of enzyme levels to be increased following stimulation either by a drug or other biochemical stimulus.

Infantilizing Treating an adult as if he or she is a child with limited understanding, immature, and weak.

Informal caregivers Individuals who provide direct care without compensation (e.g., family members).

Insomnia The inability to fall asleep and/or stay asleep.

Instrumental activities of daily living (IADLs) Daily activities that enhance the quality of everyday life but require the ability to plan, make decisions, and act. IADLS include tasks such as completing housework, using the telephone, managing money, and shopping.

Intimacy Personal closeness and familiarity between two people. Intimacy is one component of an affectionate and loving relationship. Sexual intimacy is only one form of intimacy.

K

Kyphosis Stiffening of the rib cage over time due to calcification and wedging of cartilage between the ribs and vertebrae resulting in an exaggerated curvature (a "hunchback" posture) of the thoracic spine.

L

Lactose intolerance An inability to break down milk sugar (lactose), the carbohydrate found in many dairy products.

Learned helplessness A condition that develops when living beings learn that their responses are independent of desired outcomes. Consequently, they learn to not respond to stimulation and may become helpless and apathetic.

Least restrictive environment An environment that enables individuals opportunities to function to the highest degree possible and be as independent as possible.

Lesbian A female who is sexually attracted to other females.

Libido Sexual desire or sex drive.

Life expectancy The length of time a person is expected to live.

Lifespan The expanse of time from birth to death.

Limited literacy skills Possessing below basic literacy skills.

Lipophilicity A molecule with an affinity for fat molecules.

Literacy Refers to a constellation of skills such as reading (e.g., word recognition, fluency, drawing inferences from text), writing, speaking, and listening as well as other skills such as thinking analytically and making decisions.

Living will A legal document that instructs health-care providers how an individual wants to be treated if he or she becomes terminally ill or cannot communicate his or her wishes.

Long-distance caregiver A caregiver who lives more than one hour away from the care recipient, but still provides care.

Longevity The length of time lived.

Long-term care insurance (LTCI) Insurance that provides payment or supplementary payment for long-term care.

Long-term care ombudsmen (LTCO) Advocates for the health and welfare of residents in long-term care facilities. LTCOs serve geographic regions within a state.

Long-term memory Permanent or long-term storage (e.g., autobiographic information, early-life experiences, or often-repeated information).

Long-term services and supports Services and supports available to individuals with functional limitations who need assistance with their ADLs and IADls. Long-term services and supports are provided across the continuum of care.

Loss A universal feeling of grief that develops after being deprived of something of value or someone.

M

Malabsorption Difficulty digesting or absorbing nutrients from food. Celiac disease is one of the most common causes of malabsorption.

Malnutrition A physical condition that results from a poorly balanced diet or a deficiency in the digestive processing system.

Mandatory reporters Individuals (e.g., physicians, nurses, rehabilitation specialists, social workers, and direct care workers) who are required by law to report suspected elder abuse.

Maximum life span The oldest age reached by an individual in a population.

Maximum muscle strength Muscle strength at its optimum, which usually occurs in young adulthood.

Meal services A home and community-based service option to ensure recipients have access to a nutritious meal. Home-based meal services include Meals on Wheels, which may provide meals several times a week. Community-based meal sites include congregate meal services, in which participants share a meal and engage in socialization.

Medicaid A means-tested or need-based program jointly sponsored by the states and the federal government to provide health care and other services to people who meet eligibility requirements (e.g., low income).

Medicaid waivers State programs for eligible Medicaid recipients requiring long-term services and supports.

Medicare A federal entitlement program that provides healthcare coverage to persons age 65+ and individuals with long-term disabilities.

Medigap Additional health insurance coverage purchased by Medicare recipients to cover the gaps in healthcare not covered by Medicare Parts A and B.

Mediterranean diet A diet rich in fruits, vegetables, and healthy fats such as olive oil. The diet has been shown to help reduce the risks of heart disease.

Menopause The time in a woman's life when menstruation ceases.

Metastasize The spread of cancer to another part of the body beyond the original cancer site.

Mild cognitive impairment (MCI) Cognitive losses that may portend the diagnosis of Alzheimer's disease (AD); individuals with amnestic or memory-related MCI are at higher risk of developing AD.

Motivational interviewing A psychotherapeutic approach to assist clients in resolving their problems by helping them find the motivation within themselves to affect positive lifestyle changes in their lives.

Motor coordination The combination of body movements that result in an intended action. Fine motor skills utilize small muscle movements (e.g., muscles in the hand for writing) while gross motor skills include major muscle groups (e.g., muscles in the legs, arms, and torso for walking or running).

Myocardial infarction Blockage of the coronary arteries that can cause tissue death to part of the heart. Also referred to as a heart attack.

N

Natural death Dying in old age when the body ceases to function on its own.

Naturally occurring retirement community (NORC) A demographic term used to describe a neighborhood, multi-unit dwelling, or group of buildings in which the residents are older adults. NORCs are not planned retirement communities, they just naturally evolved into communities with older residents.

Nonmedical home care services Home and community-based services that provide assistance in daily care, housekeeping, meal preparation, medication reminders, transportation, and companionship. Individuals providing such services may not need to hold special licenses or accreditation to perform their duties.

Numeracy The possession of numerical and calculating skills such as basic computing, measuring and timing medicines, assessing risk, calculating percentages and statistics, interpreting food labels, and reading medical devices.

Nutritional supplements A product that is added to a diet when it is not consumed in sufficient quantities (e.g., vitamins, minerals, and proteins). Nutritional supplements are typically available for purchase over-the-counter.

O

Obstructive sleep apnea (OSA) A temporary cessation of breathing that, when the trachea is either totally or partially obstructed, causes the body's oxygen level to drop, which then causes the person to wake up repeatedly throughout the night.

Old An age group category used by researchers referring to people ages 65-84. Other age groupings include young-old and old-old.

Old-old An age group category used by researchers referring to people age 85 and older. Other age groupings include young-old and old.

Older adult The preferred term when speaking about individuals age 65 and older.

Older Americans Act (OAA) Federal legislation passed in 1965 to specifically address the needs and rights of older adults. The OAA continues to be reauthorized and is expected to be reauthorized indefinitely. It is one piece of legislation that represents the United States' commitment to promoting the rights and welfare of older adults.

Olfaction Sense of smell.

Oral and pharyngeal (throat) cancers Cancers that form in the tissues of the oropharynx (the part of the throat at the back of the mouth, including the soft palate, the base of the tongue, and the tonsils).

Oral screening A quick review of the oral structures to determine if dental disease or oral problems are present.

Organ and tissue donation An act of donating organs and or tissue to be transplanted in another person's body; generally, but not necessarily after death.

Orientation Awareness of self, surroundings, and time (and sometimes situation).

Osteoarthritis A degenerative joint disease marked by ulceration and destruction of joint cartilage, eventually leading to exposure and destruction of the underlying bone. The normal cushioning effect of cartilage is lost, causing bone to rub on bone.

Osteoporosis A disease in which bone mass and bone density become diminished making them more likely to fracture.

Overnutrition A condition of excess nutrient and energy (caloric) intake over time. It can be considered a form of malnutrition when it leads to morbid obesity.

P

Palliative care Also known as comfort care. Refers to treating symptoms to keep the individual comfortable rather than trying to cure the illness.

Passive euthanasia An act of "standing by" and not taking action to prevent an inevitable death by allowing nature to take its course. For example, allowing a patient to die of an infection rather than treat it.

Peptic ulcer An ulceration of the stomach, esophagus, or duodenum caused by gastric acid.

Perception The brain's ability to make sense of incoming sensory (e.g., auditory, olfactory, gustatory, and visual) information.

Periodontal disease The inflammatory reaction and dissolution of the bony structures that hold the teeth in the jaws.

Persistive vegetative state An irreversible brain state in which activity in the cortex (where complex thinking processes occur) may cease but primal functions regulated in the brain stem (e.g., blinking, swallowing, and breathing) remain strong.

Personality Traits, behaviors, and qualities particular to an individual.

Person-centered care The provision of services in respect to the individual's wishes and needs.

Pharmacodynamics The effects of a drug on a body. Specifically, it is how drug responses change based on the changes in the body's cellular responses to the drug over time.

Pharmacogenomics Study of how a person's genetic background determines both the pharmacokinetic and pharmacodynamic responses to drugs.

Pharmacokinetics Described as what the body does to a drug. Specifically, it is how a drug travels through the body over time and how the body distributes, metabolizes, and excretes it.

Phase process model A type of grief processing model that posits that grieving individuals pass through phases (e.g., acceptance, adjusting to a new life) as they work towards resolving their grief.

Physiatrists Physicians who specialize in rehabilitation.

Physician-assisted suicide Taking one's own life under the guidance of a physician.

Physicochemical properties The relationship between the chemical structure of the drug and its interactions with the body.

Plain language Communication that an individual can understand the first time he or she hears it or reads it.

Plain language guidelines Standards of plain language for designing communication materials for all media formats. Guidelines include areas of content, structure/organization, writing style, and appearance and appeal.

PLISSIT model A four-level model on sexual functioning that helps providers identify the level of intervention needed by a client or patient. It also assists a provider in understanding the level at which he or she can comfortably provide the needed intervention.

Polypharmacy Taking multiple medications at a time.

Polyvictimization When multiple forms of abuse are inflicted on an individual.

Praxis The ability to carry out purposeful motor actions.

Premature death Dying at a young age.

Presbycusis Hearing loss associated with aging.

Presbyopia A condition of the eye in which molecular changes render the lens less elastic and more rigid, which significantly impairs the ability to focus on near objects.

Prevalence Total number of cases (e.g., of disease) reported.

Primary memory This type of memory has limited capacity of just a few items, and involves information that is either used right away or is generally forgotten in a matter of seconds.

Procedural memory Memory that is performance based, for example, remembering how to ride a bicycle or the motoric steps to completing a recipe or self-care task. Because these tasks are often overlearned and have become automatic, this type of memory is often maintained into old age.

Productive aging Making valued contributions to one's own life by engaging in enjoyable, meaningful, and useful activities.

Program of All-Inclusive Care for the Elderly (PACE) A community-based program for people ages 55+ meeting the eligibility requirements for nursing home care. Enrollment in PACE enables participants to live at home and receive comprehensive services, including all medical and supportive services (therapies, day services, meals, counseling, respite, and medication management) at a PACE location.

Prospective memory Relates to remembering to do something in the future (e.g., appointments, medications, meetings, chores).

Protein One of the three macronutrients used as energy sources (calories) by the body. Proteins are essential components of the muscle, skin, and bones.

Q

Quality of Life A standard of well-being for an individual or a population determined by measuring multiple factors such as health status, social connectedness, emotional well-being, and spirituality.

R

Range of motion The ability of a joint to move through its natural pattern of movement.

Reaction time The time it takes to respond to a stimulus (e.g., braking a car when driving).

Reading levels A grading system that accounts for level of fluency in reading. When older adults struggle with limited literacy, numeracy, and English proficiency, they are assessed at low reading levels.

Rehabilitation The process of helping someone regain his or her highest possible level of functioning after an injury or illness.

Restless leg syndrome (RLS) A neurological disorder that causes "creepy crawly feelings" or other unpleasant sensations in the legs such as the irresistible urge to move the legs while in bed or at rest.

Reverse mortgage A financial planning option that can make it possible for some older adults to stay in their homes longer. Borrowers use their homes as collateral, and the bank sets up either an annuity or a line of credit for borrowing money until the home is sold or the loan repaid.

Rituals Meaningful activities that can be undertaken as an individual or as a group. Participating in a ritual can strengthen feelings of social connectedness and belonging, offer psychological support, and provide meaning to a loss.

Root caries Dental caries involving the tooth root in the cementum or cervical area of the tooth.

S

Sandwich generation Adults caught between two caregiving roles: caring for a child and caring for a parent (or even grandparent).

Sarcopenia Loss of muscle mass. This is a common occurrence with aging.

Scotoma A partial loss of vision or decreased vision (blind spots) in an otherwise normal visual field.

Self-neglect A person's inability to understand the consequences of his or her own actions or inaction, which leads to, or may lead to, self-harm or endangerment.

Semantic memory Involves a cumulative knowledge base about the world in general (e.g., language, including the meaning of words and the relationship of words; mathematical facts, symbols, and formulas; vocational information learned during one's career; and the recall of current events and worldly facts).

Senescence The process of physical decline (i.e., cell deterioration) with age.

Senior Service America (SSA) An advocacy group for political and legislative issues that affect older adults. SSA also provides employment and training opportunities nationwide.

Sensory deficits Diminished use or loss of one or more senses (i.e., hearing, taste, vision, touch, and smell).

Sex The anatomy of an individual's reproductive system (and related secondary characteristics) as well as the act of copulation or intercourse.

Sexual orientation A person's sexual identity in relation to the sex to which they are attracted.

Sexual preference Personal choice regarding sexual behavior and activity.

Sexuality How a person thinks about and expresses their sexual interests and sexual identity.

Shame-free environment An environment that provides a feeling of safety and encourages questions without judgement.

Shared housing An informal housing model in which residents may share expenses or exchange services for rent.

Short-term memory Involves remembering information for a short duration. An example of normal short-term memory is being able to recall a seven-digit number (e.g., a telephone number) for a few minutes.

Skip-generation household Similar to grandfamily. Households in which a grandparent (or aunt/uncle) takes on a surrogate parenting role with a child because the parent is unable to do so. Skip-generation households are often formed after a parent's incarceration or when a parent has problems with substance misuse and addiction.

Sleep hygiene Personal activities and habits that precede sleep and are conducive to sleeping soundly.

Sleep restriction Restricting one's time in bed so that most of the time spent in bed is while asleep.

Snowbirds Older adults who move south for the winter to avoid the cold weather at home and all the heating bills and snow removal that accompany living in the cold.

Social roles A set of defined and connected behaviors that define an individual's position in the community and dictate basic behaviors within social groups such as families, workplaces, and communities.

Social Security A federal insurance program also known as the Old-Age, Survivors, and Disability Insurance (OASDI) program, which is funded through payroll taxes. Monthly Social Security benefits remain a large portion of monthly income received by many older adults.

Social Security Act After the Great Depression, there was increased social awareness for the need for policies and programs to assist individuals as they age. The Social Security program was signed into law in 1935 and through its benefits program has helped keep older adults out of poverty.

Stage process model A type of grieving process in which the bereaved must move through stages of grief to work through their grief. Kübler-Ross'

five stages of grief include denial, anger, bargaining, depression, and acceptance.

State units on aging State agencies that administer, manage, and design programs and services for older adults.

Stereognosis The ability to sense objects by the touch of the tongue, allowing one to perceive problems or alterations in the mouth. Can also refer to sensory perception through touch to identify objects.

Stereotypes Conventional, oversimplified, and often formulaic conceptions, options, or images of a person or group of people.

Stimulus control Refers to the amount of time spent in bed attempting to get to sleep or back to sleep. If a person cannot fall asleep within a half hour, it might be best to get out of bed and engage in a relaxing activity.

Streptococcus mutans Anaerobic bacterium in the oral cavity leading to tooth decay.

Structural lag A lag between public policy (providing structure) and reality. When policies do not keep pace with changing demographics and social circumstances, they often fall short of meeting the needs of the current aging population and result in structural lag.

Successful aging The ability to age well in the areas of health, social connections, and well-being. The concept is strongly connected to quality of life and satisfaction with life.

Suicide The deliberate taking of one's own life by using self-directed injurious behavior with an intent to die as a result of that behavior.

Super-centenarian An individual at least 110 years old.

Supplemental Security Income (SSI) A means-tested or need-based welfare program that provides cash assistance and health care coverage to people with low-income and limited assets who are blind, disabled, or age 65 and older.

T

Talk therapy A therapeutic relationship in which a provider and client work together to confront issues that the client wants to resolve. Also referred to as counseling or psychotherapy.

Task-based model A type of phase process model that accommodates an individual's need to work through tasks or phases to work through grief.

Teach-back A technique in which the provider asks the client or patient to state what he or she just heard and what he or she is supposed to do.

Telehealth The use of telecommunication technologies to connect patients with providers in an effort to provide health care in remote areas.

Telephone reassurance A routine telephone contact program in which participants are telephoned each day at a specified time. During the call, the caller conducts a brief reality orientation and assesses the older adult's wellbeing through conversation. If the caller suspects a problem (including if the participant does not answer the phone), the information is reported directly to a designated person for follow-up.

Terminally ill A health condition from which there is no reasonable hope of recovery.

The Joint Commission An independent nonprofit organization that certifies healthcare organizations and programs in the United States using high standards and expectations of quality care.

Tolerance As patients continue to use a drug, the therapeutic effect declines, thus requiring an increased dose to maintain the therapeutic effect.

Total fertility rate (TFR) The average number of live births a child-bearing woman would have in her lifetime. TFRs vary by country and by year.

Transgender An umbrella term for persons whose gender identity, gender expression, or behavior does not conform to that typically associated with the sex to which they were assigned at birth.

Transportation Community-based services created specifically to transport individuals. Some transportation services focus specifically on transport to medical appointments while others operate like a public transportation system.

Trusted individual A person on whom one relies with the expectation that he or she will not take advantage of or abuse the relationship.

U

Universal design The design and composition of an environment so that it can be accessed, understood and used to the greatest extent possible by all people regardless of their age, size, ability, or disability.

Urinary incontinence The loss of voluntary control of micturition (the discharge of urine from the bladder).

V

Village model A resident-governed community service and support model in which members work together to coordinate the nonmedical services and care they need.

Vitamin B_{12} A vitamin important for the normal formation of red blood cells and the health of nerve tissues.

Vitamin D A group of fat-soluble vitamins chemically related to steroids, essential for intestinal absorption and the development of bone and tooth structures.

W

Working memory Actively using or manipulating information from a short-term storage base. For example, recalling a telephone number and actually dialing the number to make a call (one must retain the number while dialing).

Weight loss A reduction of body mass. When an older adult loses 5% or more of his or her body weight in 1 month or 10% or more in 6 months, healthcare providers need to identify the cause for the weight loss.

X

Xerostomia The condition of dry mouth caused by decreased saliva production.

Y

Young-old An age group category used by researchers referring to people ages 50–64. Other age groupings include old and old-old.

Index

Note: Page numbers followed by *f* or *t* indicate material in figures or tables, respectively.